CLINICAL BRAIN IMAGING:
Principles and Applications

CONTEMPORARY NEUROLOGY SERIES AVAILABLE:

Fred Plum, M.D., *Editor-in-Chief*
***Series Editors:* Sid Gilman, M.D., Joseph B. Martin, M.D., Ph.D., Robert B. Daroff, M.D., Stephen G. Waxman, M.D., Ph.D., M-Marsel Mesulam, M.D.**

19 THE DIAGNOSIS OF STUPOR AND COMA, EDITION 3
Fred Plum, M.D., and Jerome B. Posner, M.D.

21 DISORDERS OF THE CEREBELLUM
Sid Gilman, M.D., James R. Bloedel, M.D., Ph.D., and Richard Lechtenberg, M.D.

26 PRINCIPLES OF BEHAVIORAL NEUROLOGY
M-Marsel Mesulam, M.D., *Editor*

28 CLINICAL NEUROENDOCRINOLOGY, EDITION 2
Joseph B. Martin, M.D., Ph.D., F.R.C.P.(C), and Seymour Reichlin, M.D., Ph.D.

29 ADVANCES IN CONTEMPORARY NEUROLOGY
Fred Plum, M.D., *Editor*

30 THE WERNICKE-KORSAKOFF SYNDROME, EDITION 2
Maurice Victor, M.D., Raymond D. Adams, M.D., and George H. Collins, M.D.

31 SEIZURES AND EPILEPSY
Jerome Engel, Jr., M.D., Ph.D.

32 CLINICAL NEUROPHYSIOLOGY OF THE VESTIBULAR SYSTEM, EDITION 2
Robert W. Baloh, M.D., and Vicente Honrubia, M.D.

33 SPINAL CORD COMPRESSION: DIAGNOSIS AND PRINCIPLES OF MANAGEMENT
Thomas N. Byrne, M.D., and Stephen G. Waxman, M.D., Ph.D.

34 GUILLAIN-BARRÉ SYNDROME
Allan H. Ropper, M.D., Eelco F. M. Wijdicks, M.D., and Bradley T. Truax, M.D.

35 THE NEUROLOGY OF EYE MOVEMENTS, EDITION 2
R. John Leigh, M.D., M.R.C.P. (U.K.) and David S. Zee, M.D.

36 DISORDERS OF PERIPHERAL NERVES, EDITION 2
Herbert H. Schaumburg, M.D., Alan R. Berger, M.D., and P.K. Thomas, C.B.E., M.D., D.Sc., F.R.C.P., F.R.C. Path.

37 PRINCIPLES OF DRUG THERAPY IN NEUROLOGY
Michael V. Johnston, M.D., Robert L. Macdonald, M.D., Ph.D., and Anne B. Young, M.D., Ph.D.

38 PRINCIPLES OF GERIATRIC NEUROLOGY
Robert Katzman, M.D. and John W. Rowe, M.D.

CLINICAL BRAIN IMAGING: Principles and Applications

JOHN C. MAZZIOTTA, M.D., Ph.D.
Professor of Neurology and Radiological Sciences
UCLA School of Medicine
Los Angeles, California

SID GILMAN, M.D.
Professor and Chairman
Department of Neurology
University of Michigan Medical School
Ann Arbor, Michigan

F. A. DAVIS COMPANY • Philadelphia

Printed in the United States of America

Last digit indicates print number: 10 9 8 7 6 5 4 3 2 1

As new scientific information becomes available through basic and clinical research, recommended treatments and drug therapies undergo changes. The author(s) and publisher have done everything possible to make this book accurate, up to date, and in accord with accepted standards at the time of publication. The authors, editors, and publisher are not responsible for errors or omissions or for consequences from application of the book, and make no warranty, expressed or implied, in regard to the contents of the book. Any practice described in this book should be applied by the reader in accordance with professional standards of care used in regard to the unique circumstances that may apply in each situation. The reader is advised always to check product information (package inserts) for changes and new information regarding dose and contraindications before administering any drug. Caution is especially urged when using new or infrequently ordered drugs.

Clinical brain imaging : principles and applications / [edited by]
John C. Mazziotta, Sid Gilman.
p. cm.
Includes bibliographical references and index.
ISBN 0-8036-5944-X (hardbound : alk. paper) : $110.00 (approx.)
1. Brain—Imaging. I. Mazziotta, John C. II. Gilman, Sid.
[DNLM: 1. Brain Diseases—diagnosis. 2. Magnetic Resonance Imaging. 3. Tomography, Emission-Computed. 4. Tomography, X-Ray Computed. WL 141 C6406]
RC386.6.D52C55 1992
616.8'04754-dc20
DNLM/DLC 91-28189
for Library of Congress CIP

FOREWORD

The impact of modern imaging techniques on the clinical neurosciences generally has been called "revolutionary." But looking back over my four decades of experience in clinical neurology, "metamorphosis" more adequately describes the sweeping effects on neurology and neurosurgery of these new techniques.

Only those who practiced neurology or neurosurgery before the mid-1970s can fully appreciate the overwhelming change from the period when the clinical examination and other available diagnostic tools were carried to obsessive lengths to be sure no scrap of potentially useful information was ignored. Although seldom spoken of in those early days, a simple form of neuroimaging was being carried out during the history-taking and clinical neurologic examination. Throughout the diagnostic process, the clinician was forming in his or her mind a picture of the pathology that might be going on in the patient. Imagination and past experience were the algorithms used to construct this image.

Before 1973, occasional indirect glimpses of brain disease were obtainable during life by pneumoencephalography and cerebral angiography. Both procedures had two undesirable features: (1) They were so traumatic that the clinician could not readily repeat them as often as might be desired; and (2) most importantly, they were unable to show directly the site of greatest clinical interest, the substance of the brain.

1973 was a landmark year in neuroimaging. At the end of 1972, the EMI group directed by Sir Godfrey Hounsfield first publicly displayed x-ray computed tomography (CT). By modern standards these early images were poor, but to perceptive observers they were spectacular. The full impact of computerized reconstruction of a tomographic tissue section struck home in 1973, and it stimulated others to apply the principle brought into medicine by Hounsfield to produce other possible sources of images.

I felt vindicated by Hounsfield's design, construction, and testing of his x-ray CT scanner because I had described back-projection and reconstruction of a point moved through a head phantom in 1961. The technique utilized a rotate-translate scanning pattern by a photon beam, but there were no suitable computers commercially available in 1960 when this work was done. I used a simple analog integrator network to recover my scanned points.

Also in 1973, Paul Lauterbur described the use of controlled nonuniformities (gradients) in the main magnetic field to localize the source of a nuclear magnetic resonance (NMR) signal. NMR imaging was the result, but because it was felt that the word "nuclear" would be perceived negatively by the public, the "N" was removed and the technique became known as MRI, for magnetic resonance imaging.

In the same year, tomographic computerized reconstruction of tissue positron-emitter distribution was begun with positron annihilation gamma rays. In x-ray CT, the absorption of x-rays collimated into small beams is measured as they sweep out paths in many directions through a slice of the head. The absorption of x-rays in a beam in a given path through the head can be integrated. This absorption was called a line integral; by mathematically manipulating these lines and then adding up all of them in a computer, an image of the slice could be constructed. A similarity was recognized between this line integral through the tissues and the two positron annihilation gamma rays emitted simultaneously in opposite directions. The positron emission tomographic (PET) scanner emerged.

Ordinary gamma-emitting isotopes are of limited interest in the study of living humans. There are no medically useful gamma emitters below sodium in the periodic table, so no atomic substitutions of gamma emitters can be made without denaturing the labeled molecules. The ability to substitute positron-emitting nuclides for several of the light atoms common in tissues, and the ability to image their location (PET scanning) created almost unlimited research possibilities.

In the years following 1973, the radiologic instrument manufacturers and the medical community were so heavily occupied absorbing the phenomenon of x-ray CT that little general interest was shown in developing other imaging modalities. The technology of CT finally stabilized by 1982, but the clinician's appetite had been whetted for direct information about the living patient. Images displaying regionality of many tissue characteristics have been actively pursued since then, revealing not only MRI data but also regional metabolic processes and neurotransmitter receptor activity.

Modern scanning provides so much three-dimensional data that they must be displayed tomographically. It is now possible to do a "living autopsy" that, in many ways, tells more about the patient's pathophysiology than could be inferred retrospectively from a traditional postmortem examination. The great reduction in the number of autopsies performed during the past 20 years has in part been due to the widespread availability of x-ray CT, despite its limited tissue characterization.

In the hope of directly benefiting living patients, the development and application of clinical imaging modalities is being actively pursued. PET scanning will become practical for many hospitals. MRI scanning will become much more elaborate and useful, and there will be other imaging modalities not now foreseen.

This book documents the extent to which modern neuroimaging has come to pervade various subdisciplines within neurology. All the contributors to this volume are recognized authorities in the fields upon which they have written. Several are pioneers. This is the first book to deal in depth with all the computed tomographic imaging techniques. It begins with a concise description of the technology of each method and integrates this with clinical application, providing pertinent observations on the pathophysiologic information that has emerged. It requires only a brief examination of the table of contents to appreciate the completeness of subject coverage and the eminence of the editors and authors.

WILLIAM OLDENDORF, M.D.

PREFACE

Advances in medical imaging have produced revolutionary changes in the practice of medicine. As described in the Foreword by Dr. William Oldendorf, the clinical neurosciences have been, and probably will continue to be, at the forefront of these changes. (In 1975 Dr. Oldendorf won the Lasker Award for his early investigations in this field.) X-ray computed tomography (x-ray CT) was the first of the CT techniques to be clinically useful on a large scale. Initially applied only to the brain, it produced startling images that showed the brain parenchyma directly for the first time.

The need for advanced imaging techniques to study the brain and spinal cord has been a leading force driving the subsequent quest for the ultimate development of all the CT-based techniques, including MRI, PET, and SPECT. The first examples of each technique consistently were directed at the brain.

This text has been written for physicians in training and for practicing clinicians who wish to have an up-to-date review of CT-based techniques. We anticipate that not only clinical neurologists and neurosurgeons will be interested, but also radiologists, nuclear medicine physicians, and psychiatrists.

The initial chapters of the book provide information on the principles of imaging, discussed in language that should be understood by all physicians. The later chapters concern the findings in many of the disease processes commonly encountered, and additional chapters cover specific regions of the brain such as the basal ganglia and the cerebellum. The brain is the focus of the text; the application of imaging to the spinal cord, nerve plexuses, or peripheral nerves is not emphasized.

Rather than attempting to produce an encyclopedic listing of disease entities and images about them, we have focused instead on the pathophysiologic mechanisms of disease processes. The text shows how imaging techniques allow the clinician and investigator to observe the structure and function of the brain as it responds to or recovers from disease. Thus, the reader has a basis for evaluating other, similar conditions.

The future of imaging will undoubtedly be exciting, ever-changing, and accelerating in its pace. In the epilogue, we speculate on some possible directions these advances may take. Surely the future will see integration of structure and function in a synthesis of methodologies devoted to measuring each of these two important features of biological integrity. The number of measurements possible with each technique will increase, particularly in emission tomography (that is, PET and SPECT) as new tracers are developed and validated for the measurement of neurotransmitter systems, molecular biological aspects of brain disorders, and disease-specific ligands. The number and type of measurements will also increase in MRI, with the imaging of isotopes other than hydrogen, and the use of spectroscopy to provide biochemical information about the changing brain in health and disease.

We anticipate that, with time, diagnostic brain imaging will become totally noninvasive. As MR angiography replaces conventional angiography, the final vestiges of invasive diagnostic imaging of the brain will disappear. The result will be an unprecedented amount of information about the patient that can be obtained safely and without hospitalization. Concomitantly, the refinement of modern endovascular techniques will allow therapies to be delivered to the central nervous system by way of percutaneous catheters, avoiding surgical procedures. Finally, the cost and complexity of imaging techniques will continue to decrease, an inevitable and desirable result of advancing technology and the economics of free enterprise.

The imaging techniques described in this text have unveiled new vistas of the brain and the disorders that affect it. We have endeavored to present this information in a fashion useful to the clinician. We hope that this volume will serve as a sound basis for a lifelong interest in the study of neuroimaging as a science to understand brain function and dysfunction, and especially as a tool to care for patients.

JOHN C. MAZZIOTTA, M.D., PH.D.
SID GILMAN, M.D.

ACKNOWLEDGMENTS

We would like to acknowledge all the investigators around the world who shared their ideas, scientific work, and illustrations. Special thanks are extended to Maureen Chang for her editorial assistance and to Lee Griswold for preparing much of the artwork. In addition, the authors and editors wish to acknowledge the encouragement, patience, diligence, and thorough editorial support provided by Dr. Sylvia K. Fields, Ms. Bernice Wissler, and Mr. Robert Craven, Sr. of the F. A. Davis Company.

CONTRIBUTORS

David Brooks, M.D.
MRC Cyclotron Unit
Hammersmith Hospital
London, England

Thomas N. Byrne, M.D.
Associate Clinical Professor
Department of Neurology
Yale University School of Medicine
New Haven, Connecticut

Harry Chugani, M.D.
Associate Professor
Departments of Neurology, Pediatrics, and the Brain Research Institute
UCLA School of Medicine
Los Angeles, California

Rosalind B. Dietrich, M.B.Ch.B.
Associate Professor of Radiological Sciences
Director of Magnetic Resonance Imaging
University of California, Irvine
Orange, California

Burton Drayer, M.D.
Director, MRI
Barrow Neurological Institute
Phoenix, Arizona

Ranjan Duara, M.D.
Associate Professor of Radiology and Neurology
University of Miami School of Medicine
Chief, Section on PET
Division of Nuclear Medicine
Department of Radiology
Mount Sinai Medical Center
Miami Beach, Florida

Richard Frackowiak, M.D.
MRC Cyclotron Unit
Hammersmith Hospital
London, England

Stephen S. Gebarski, M.D.
Associate Professor
Department of Radiology
The University of Michigan
Ann Arbor, Michigan

Wendell A. Gibby, M.D.
Director, MRI
Utah Valley Regional Medical Center
Provo, Utah

Sid Gilman, M.D.
Professor and Chairman
Department of Neurology
The University of Michigan
Ann Arbor, Michigan

Søren Holm, Ph.D.
Department of Clinical Physiology and Nuclear Medicine
Bispebjerg Hospital
Copenhagen, Denmark

Niels A. Lassen, M.D.
Department of Clinical Physiology and Nuclear Medicine
Bispebjerg Hospital
Copenhagen, Denmark

Robert B. Lufkin, M.D.
Associate Professor
Department of Radiological Sciences
UCLA School of Medicine
Los Angeles, California

John C. Mazziotta, M.D., Ph.D.
Professor of Neurology and Radiological Sciences
UCLA School of Medicine
Los Angeles, California

Michael E. Phelps, Ph.D.
Jennifer Jones Simon Professor
Chief, Division of Nuclear Medicine and Biophysics
Chief, Laboratory of Nuclear Medicine
Department of Radiological Sciences
UCLA School of Medicine
Los Angeles, California

William Theodore, M.D.
Clinical Epilepsy Section
NINCDS
National Institutes of Health
Bethesda, Maryland

Jane L. Tyler, M.D.
Veterans Administration Medical Center
Charleston, South Carolina

Robert Zimmerman, M.D.
Professor
Department of Radiology
University of Pennsylvania
Philadelphia, Pennsylvania

CONTENTS

PART I. BASIC PRINCIPLES OF NEUROIMAGING MODALITIES 1

1. X-RAY COMPUTED TOMOGRAPHY 2

Wendell A. Gibby, M.D., and Robert A. Zimmerman, M.D.

PHYSICAL PRINCIPLES OF X-RAY CT 2

FORMATION OF THE X-RAY CT IMAGE 4

ARTIFACTS 7
- Intrinsic X-ray CT Artifacts 7
- Machine-Related Artifacts 9
- Patient-Related Artifacts 9

DOSIMETRY 9
- Direct Radiation 9
- Scatter Radiation 10

CONTRAST AGENTS 10
- Intravenous Contrast Agents 10
- Intrathecal Contrast 18
- Stable Xenon CT 21

CLINICAL APPLICATIONS OF X-RAY CT 23
- Brain 23
- Orbit 26
- Otic Capsule 28
- Spine 28
- Skull 31

THE FUTURE 32

2. MAGNETIC RESONANCE IMAGING 39
Robert B. Lufkin, M.D.

PHYSICAL PRINCIPLES OF MR SCANNING 39
The Nucleus of the Atom 39
Magnetic Properties of the Nucleus 40
Resonance of the Nucleus 41
Transverse Magnetization and the MR Signal 43
T_2 Relaxation 45
T_1 Relaxation 46
Pulsing Sequence 46
MR Contrast Mechanisms 47
Proton Density 47
T_1 and T_2 Contrast Mechanisms 47
Effects of T_1 and TR on Image Contrast 47
Effects of TE and T_2 on Image Contrast 49

FORMATION OF THE MR IMAGE 50
Magnetic Field Gradients 50
Slice Select Gradient (G_{ss}) 50
Two-Dimensional Fourier Transformation Imaging. 51
Pulse Sequence Timing Diagram 53
Image Formation Matrix 53
Spatial Resolution 54
Multiecho Pulse Sequence 55
Multislice Pulse Sequence 57
Orthogonal Scan Plane Selection 57
Effects of Varying TE 58
Effects of Varying TR 58

MRI INSTRUMENTATION 58
Main Magnetic Field 58
Gradient Magnetic Field Generators 63
Radiofrequency (RF) Subsystem 63

MRI CONTRAST AGENTS 64

THE UTILITY OF MRI IN NEUROLOGIC STUDIES ... 66
Strengths 66
Weaknesses 68

3. POSITRON EMISSION TOMOGRAPHY (PET) 71
Michael E. Phelps, Ph.D.

POSITRON DECAY 73

PRODUCTION OF LABELED COMPOUNDS 74
Cyclotron 74
Labeled Compounds 76
Dosimetry 78

PET SCANNERS 79
The Principle of Computed Tomography in PET 79
Sampling Requirements 81
Annihilation Coincidence Detection (ACD) 82
Detectors and Geometric Configuration 83
Spatial Resolution 85
Statistical Noise 86
Partial Volume Effect 87
Axial Resolution and Sampling 89
Efficiency and Temporal Resolution 89

TRACER KINETIC MODELING 89
Definition of Terms 91

THE VALUE OF PET IN NEUROLOGIC AND PSYCHIATRIC DISORDERS 101

4. SINGLE PHOTON EMISSION COMPUTED TOMOGRAPHY (SPECT) 108

Niels A. Lassen, M.D., Ph.D. and Søren Holm, Ph.D.

SPECT IMAGING SYSTEMS 109
Sensitivity 110
Resolution 110
Contrast 110
Attenuation and Scatter 111
Camera-based Systems 114
Dedicated SPECT Systems 114

RADIOISOTOPES USED IN SPECT 115

SPECT IMAGING OF CEREBRAL BLOOD FLOW 119
Xenon 133 119
Technetium 99m-HMPAO 123

RECEPTOR LIGANDS LABELED WITH IODINE 123 129

PART II. NEUROIMAGING IN CLINICAL EVALUATION AND MANAGEMENT 135

5. **EPILEPSY** 136
William H. Theodore, M.D.

AN APPROACH TO THE PATIENT 136

PARTIAL SEIZURES ("LOCALIZATION-RELATED EPILEPSY") 138
X-ray CT and MR Imaging 138
False Localization 143
Cerebral Metabolism and Blood Flow in Partial Seizures 144
Positron Emission Tomography: Interictal Studies 145
Positron Emission Tomography: Ictal Studies 148
Single Photon Emission Computerized Tomography 151
Functional Images in the Localization of Epileptic Sites 151
Pathophysiology of Decreased Metabolism and Blood Flow in Epileptic Foci 152
The Role of PET and SPECT in the Evaluation of Patients for Surgery 152

GENERALIZED SEIZURES 153
Imaging Changes in Primary Generalized Seizures 153
Imaging Changes in Secondary Generalized Epilepsy: Infantile Spasms and the Lennox-Gastaut Syndrome 154

MAGNETIC RESONANCE SPECTROSCOPY 155

PET AND THE NEUROPHARMACOLOGY OF EPILEPSY 155

A STRATEGY FOR IMAGING EVALUATION OF PATIENTS WITH EPILEPSY 156

6. **NEOPLASTIC DISORDERS** 166
Jane L. Tyler, M.D. and Thomas N. Byrne, M.D.

NEUROIMAGING MODALITIES IN THE EVALUATION OF INTRACRANIAL NEOPLASMS 168

SPECIFIC NEOPLASTIC DISORDERS 171
Intracerebral Gliomas 171
Meningiomas 192
Pituitary Adenomas 195

Intracerebral Metastases 198
Other CNS Tumors 200

REMOTE EFFECTS OF INTRACEREBRAL TUMORS 200

RESPONSE OF TUMORS TO TREATMENT 201

THE DIFFERENTIATION OF RADIATION NECROSIS FROM RECURRENT TUMOR 203

7. **CEREBROVASCULAR DISEASE** 217

D.J. Brooks, M.D. and R.S.J. Frackowiak, M.D.

THE PATHOPHYSIOLOGY OF ISCHEMIA 217

THE USE OF STRUCTURAL SCANNING IN THE DIAGNOSIS OF CEREBROVASCULAR DISEASE 219
Cerebral Hemorrhages and Hematomas 219
Subarachnoid, Subdural, and Epidural Hemorrhages 222
Nonhemorrhagic Cerebral Infarcts 223
Vascular Malformations and Extracranial Artery Disease 225
Conclusions: Applications of Structural Scanning 226

THE USE OF FUNCTIONAL IMAGING FOR THE INVESTIGATION OF CEREBROVASCULAR DISEASE 227
Methods of Functional Imaging 227
Clinical Applications of Functional Imaging 229

THE ROLE OF NEUROIMAGING IN THE MANAGEMENT OF CEREBROVASCULAR DISEASE 236
Asymptomatic Carotid Artery Occlusions and Stenoses 236
Symptomatic Carotid Artery Occlusions and Stenoses 237
Treatment of Acute Cerebral Infarction 238

8. MOVEMENT DISORDERS 244
John C. Mazziotta, M.D., Ph.D.

HUNTINGTON'S DISEASE 246
Clinical and Pathologic Features 246
Pneumoencephalography and X-ray CT 247
MRI 248
PET 250
Future Prospects 255

PARKINSON'S DISEASE 256
Clinical and Pathologic Features 256
X-ray CT 257
MRI 257
PET and SPECT 260
Future Prospects 267

PROGRESSIVE SUPRANUCLEAR PALSY 267
Clinical and Pathologic Features 267
X-ray CT 270
MRI 270
PET 270

WILSON'S DISEASE 272
Clinical and Pathological Features 272
X-ray CT 273
MRI 274
PET and SPECT 274

DYSTONIA 275
Clinical and Pathologic Features 275
X-ray CT 276
MRI 276
PET 277

TARDIVE DYSKINESIA 277

MISCELLANEOUS DISORDERS 279

9. DEMENTIA 294
Ranjan Duara, M.D.

CHARACTERISTICS OF DEMENTIA 294
Clinical Symptoms and Signs 294
Pathophysiology 295
Etiology 295

DEGENERATIVE DISORDERS AND NORMAL AGING 297
Normal Aging 297
Alzheimer's Disease 300
Parkinson's Disease 318

Pick's Disease 319
Progressive Supranuclear Palsy (PSP) 322
Neurotransmitter and Neuroreceptor Studies in Degenerative Dementia 325

VASCULAR DISORDERS 325
X-ray CT Studies of Multi-infarct Dementia 327
X-ray CT Studies of Binswanger's Disease 328
MRI Studies 329
PET Studies 331
SPECT Studies 332

NORMAL PRESSURE HYDROCEPHALUS 333
X-ray CT Studies 334
MRI Studies 334
PET and SPECT Studies 336

THE USE OF NEUROIMAGING IN THE DIFFERENTIAL DIAGNOSIS OF DEMENTING CONDITIONS 336

10. MAGNETIC RESONANCE IMAGING OF ADULT WHITE MATTER DISEASE 350
Burton P. Drayer, M.D.

PATHOANATOMY 350
Multiple Sclerosis (MS) and Variants 350
Microangiopathic Leukoencephalopathy 351

MRI STUDIES 353
Technique 353
Multiple Sclerosis 354
Ischemic (Microangiopathic) Leukoencephalopathy . 356

DIFFERENTIAL DIAGNOSIS 362

11. CEREBELLAR DISORDERS 370
Sid Gilman, M.D. and
Stephen S. Gebarski, M.D.

DEGENERATIVE DISEASES 371
Olivopontocerebellar Atrophy (OPCA) 371
Friedreich's Ataxia (FA) 374
Paraneoplastic Cerebellar Degeneration 377

DEMYELINATIVE DISEASE 378

CEREBELLAR ANOMALIES 380
Chiari Malformations 380
Dandy-Walker Syndrome 383
von Hippel-Lindau Disease 383

VASCULAR DISEASE 385
Transient Ischemic Attacks 385
Cerebellar Infarction 387
Cerebellar Hemorrhage 387
Aneurysms 389
Arteriovenous Malformations 390

CEREBELLAR ABSCESS 392

ALCOHOLIC CEREBELLAR DEGENERATION 392

NEOPLASMS 394
Signs and Symptoms of Cerebellar Tumors 394
Intra-Axial Cerebellar Tumors 396
Metastatic Disease of the Cerebellum 397
Extraparenchymal Tumors 397
Cerebellopontine-Angle Schwannoma 402

12. PEDIATRIC DISORDERS 411

Harry T. Chugani, M.D. and
Rosalind B. Dietrich, MB, ChB

NORMAL BRAIN DEVELOPMENT 411
Structural Imaging 412
Functional Imaging 416

BRAIN MALFORMATIONS 424
Clinical/Pathophysiologic Background 424
Structural Imaging 424
Functional Imaging 424
Cerebral Malformations 425
Hamartomas and Arachnoid Cysts 432
Phakomatoses 432

HYPOXIC-ISCHEMIC ENCEPHALOPATHY IN THE NEWBORN 438
Clinical/Pathophysiologic Background 438
Structural Imaging 438
Functional Imaging 441
Clinical/Pathophysiologic Correlations 441

CHILDHOOD EPILEPSY 442
Lennox-Gastaut Syndrome 442
Infantile Spasms 444

METABOLIC DISEASES 447
Clinical/Pathophysiologic Background 447
Structural Imaging 447
Clinical/Pathophysiologic Correlations 448

PRACTICAL CONSIDERATIONS 449

13. EPILOGUE: FUTURE VISIONS 458

John C. Mazziotta, M.D., Ph.D. and Sid Gilman, M.D.

MAGNETIC RESONANCE IMAGING 458
MR Angiography 459
Three-Dimensional MRI 460
Nonproton MRI 460
MR Spectroscopy 461

POSITRON EMISSION TOMOGRAPHY 462
New Ligands and Neurotransmitter Probes 462
Applications to Presymptomatic Individuals 463
Functional Reorganization and Rehabilitation after Brain Injury 463
Animal Studies 464
Clinical Considerations 464

SPECT 465
New Choices in Ligands 465
Improved Spatial Resolution 465

IMAGE INTEGRATION: MERGING STRUCTURE AND FUNCTION 465

INDEX 469

Part I

BASIC PRINCIPLES OF NEUROIMAGING MODALITIES

Chapter 1

X-RAY COMPUTED TOMOGRAPHY

Wendell A. Gibby, M.D., and Robert A. Zimmerman, M.D.

PHYSICAL PRINCIPLES OF X-RAY CT
FORMATION OF THE X-RAY CT IMAGE
ARTIFACTS
DOSIMETRY
CONTRAST AGENTS
CLINICAL APPLICATIONS OF X-RAY CT
THE FUTURE

The introduction of x-ray computed tomography (CT) in 1973 initiated a revolution in clinical medicine by providing the first opportunity directly to image human soft tissues noninvasively and three-dimensionally. The utility of x-ray CT scanning was important in many fields, but the impact upon neurology was particularly noteworthy. X-ray CT scanning quickly obviated pneumoencephalography and reduced the use of angiography to limited, specific situations. Although the subsequent development of other imaging modalities, particularly magnetic resonance imaging (MRI), provided superior imaging capability in many respects, x-ray CT scanning has remained an important tool in the neurologic diagnostic armamentarium. CT scanning is used widely and is superior to other imaging techniques in a number of clinical situations. This chapter will review the physical principles of x-ray CT, the equipment used, the problems related to dosimetry, the use of contrast agents, the current applications of CT, and its future potential.

PHYSICAL PRINCIPLES OF X-RAY CT

An x-ray is an electromagnetic wave that can interact with matter in either a wavelike or particlelike fashion.[40] At the energies used in CT, x-ray photons interact with the electron clouds of atoms, either by scattering or by the photoelectric effect (Fig. 1 – 1). The type of scattering that occurs is known as Compton scatter. This can be conceptualized (Fig. 1 – 1*A*) as an incident photon striking the outer electron of an atom, ejecting the electron in a billiard-ball fashion. The ejected electron, called a recoil electron, causes ionization of the atom, so that the atom alters its electric charge. This electron is quickly absorbed by surrounding atoms. Compton scatter causes two major problems in conventional diagnostic imaging. First, the scattered photons do not convey diagnostic information. Second, the scatter is a major safety hazard to personnel because these photons maintain most of their original energy.

The second type of interaction of x-rays in the CT energy range is the photoelectric effect (Fig. 1 – 1*B*). This involves the inner-shell electrons, which are tightly bound to the nucleus. The photoelectric effect occurs when an incoming photon interacts with the inner orbital electron. This effect can occur only when the energy of the incoming photon is equal to or slightly greater

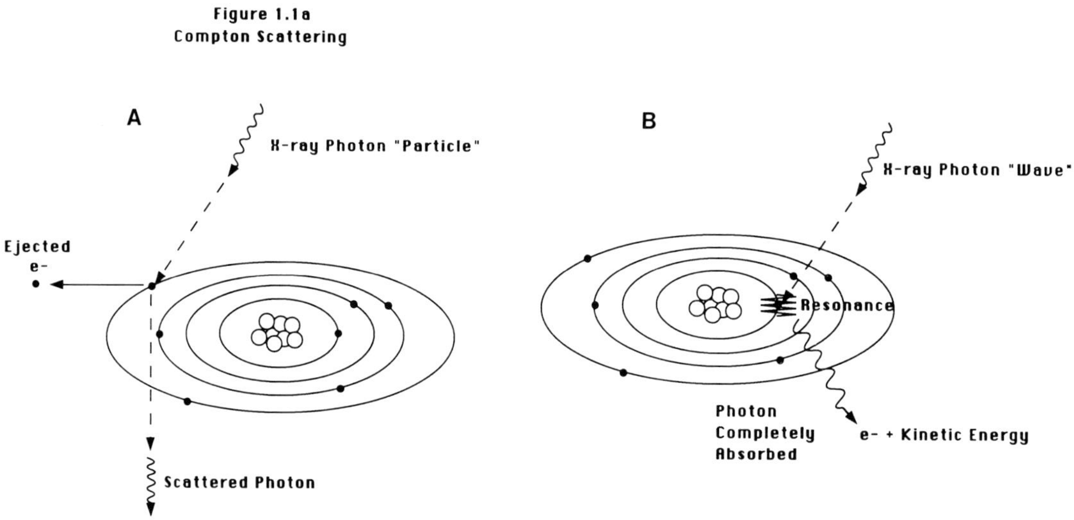

Figure 1–1. Interactions of x-rays (photons) with matter in the diagnostic x-ray energy range. (*A*) Compton scatter. Incoming x-ray photon strikes outer orbital electron, causing ionization of the atom by ejecting the electron. The "scattered" photon is then deflected, retaining the majority of its energy. The electron is quickly absorbed by surrounding atoms. (*B*) Photoelectric effect. An incoming photon interacts with an inner orbital electron. All excess energy (Ke) of the photon above the binding energy is transferred to the electron as kinetic energy, which causes ionization of the atom. The photon is completely absorbed.

than the binding energy of the electron (the *k-edge energy*). The photon disappears completely, the atom is ionized, and any energy of the photon that exceeds the binding energy is transferred to the electron as kinetic energy.

Passage of an x-ray beam through the body causes "beam hardening," which means that the average energy of the photon beam exiting the patient is greater than that entering the patient. The x-ray CT scanner measures linear attenuation of the beam—that is, the reduction in the number of photons as the beam passes through the body. The number of photons attenuated, however, changes with beam energy.[88] If a given area or tissue of the body (such as bone) strongly absorbs the beam, the tissue behind it will not receive the same beam energy as when scanned from a different angle. The attenuation coefficient, which is explained below, will be erroneous. This causes beam-hardening artifacts in the image reconstruction.

Because scanning requires energies in which Compton scatter occurs, marked scattering of photons takes place. If ordinary radiographs were to be produced, this scattering would cause unacceptable image degradation and loss of tissue contrast. With x-ray CT, however, the scatter is significantly reduced by using a collimator (a devicc for producing a beam of parallel x-rays) both for the beam exiting the x-ray tube and for the transmitted x-ray beam exiting the patient at the detectors.

FORMATION OF THE X-RAY CT IMAGE

In x-ray CT, an object is examined by the passage of x-ray beams through the object from several different directions. The result is the formation of a three-dimensional representation of that object. When an x-ray beam passes through the body, its intensity is attenuated logarithmically as a function of distance.[17] A measurement of the intensity of the exiting beam is known as the *linear attenuation coefficient* when the attenuator thickness is 1 cm.

The linear attenuation coefficient is related to the absorption of a given material via both photoelectric interaction and Compton scattering interactions.

For each x-ray beam that is passed through the body, the exiting intensity is measured. The data are then integrated, and a numerical reconstruction of the object made with a digital representation of the image. The intensity of each point (pixel) is displayed on a cathode-ray tube in the form of relative brightness. To normalize the images, water is arbitrarily assigned a CT number of zero. Each of the measured pixel values is subtracted from the relative linear attenuation coefficient of water and then divided by the linear attenuation coefficient of water, which is then multiplied by a magnifying constant, *K*, to give the CT number.[80] In early generation x-ray CT scanners, this magnifying constant was 500 and was called the EMI unit.[82] Later machines utilized a magnifying constant of 1000, called the Hounsfield unit in honor of the inventor of x-ray CT. A 1% change in CT attenuation coefficients with respect to water equals 10 Hounsfield units. Table 1–1 gives the approximate CT Hounsfield units of various body tissues.[8,77,89]

After the x-ray beam exits the patient, it must be transformed into an electronic signal that can be quantified, digitized, reconstructed, and displayed. Three types of detectors are currently used in x-ray CT scanners: a solid-state scintillation detector; a gas-filled ionization chamber; or, less commonly, a scintillation-photomultiplier tube.

Table 1–1 X-RAY CT ATTENUATION VALUES

Substance	*CT Number (in Hounsfield Units)*
Water	0
CSF	4–16
Air	−1000
Fat	−84
Bone	>1000
White matter (adult)	30
Gray matter (adult)	38
Flowing blood (HCT 40)	51
Fresh clotted blood	81
Chronic subdural hematoma	46
Muscle	67
White matter (at age 1 mo)	15
Gray matter (at age 1 mo)	23
Disc material	80–110

The scatter of radiation produced by an x-ray beam is reduced by narrow collimation, which converts the scattered beam into one that has only parallel rays. This is achieved by placing a collimator both on the x-ray tube and at the detector aperture. Collimation is also important in reducing patient dosage, so that all the radiation to which the patient is exposed contributes to image formation and is not simply scattered through the tissues. Collimators also are important in achieving thin slices.

Image reconstruction occurs by one of two methods in current scanners. Most common is the filtered back-projection method. A second method is the Fourier transformation. A detailed explanation of these methods is beyond the scope of this chapter, and discussions of them can be found in a number of review articles.[12,87,115] A simplified analysis of the filtered back-projection method is given in Fig. 1–2. A single point represented in the center has been scanned from six directions (Fig. 1–2*A*). The data sets are then "back-projected" on the matrix and a rough representation of the image is formed (Fig. 1–2*B*). This can be improved by acquiring more views (Fig. 1–2*C*). By filtering the raw data, the abrupt edge transitions can be smoothed and a more pleasing picture obtained (Fig. 1–2*D*, *E*).

The data are then transferred to a hard disk capable of storing multiple images. The disk becomes quickly filled, however, requiring that the images be transferred to a more permanent storage medium such as magnetic tape, floppy disk, or optical disk. Currently, magnetic tapes are commonly used because of their low cost and high data-storage capacity. These are being replaced, however, with optical disks, which cannot be erased and can provide storage capacities of up to 3.6 gigabytes

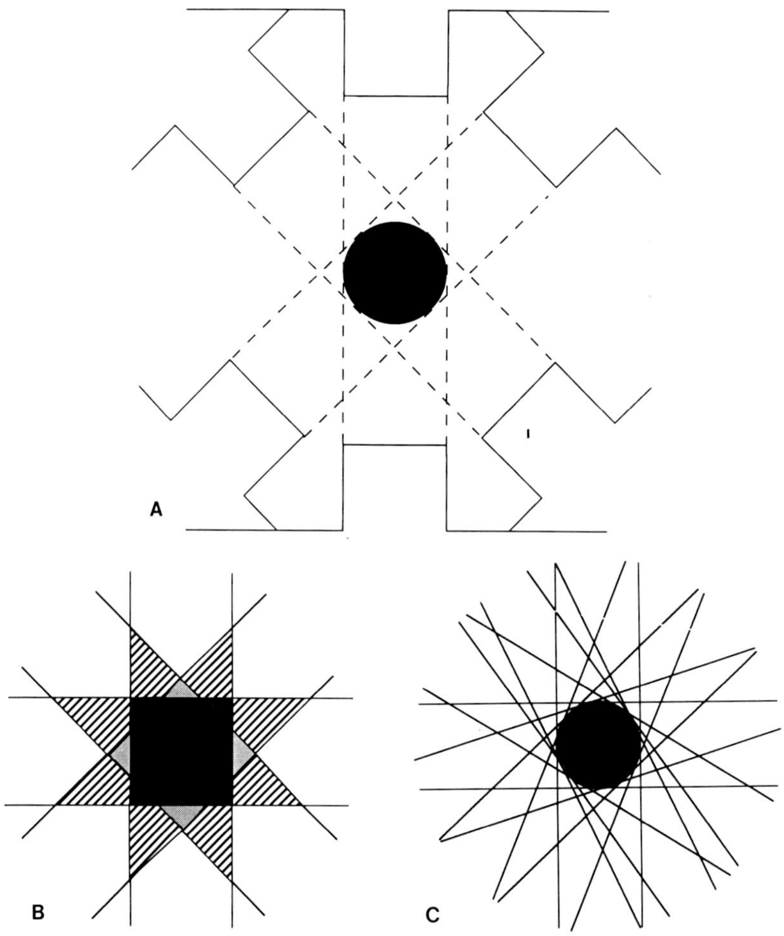

Figure 1–2. (*A*) Filtered back-projection technique of reconstruction. The circular object represented has been scanned from six different directions. The profile of the x-ray output is given as the square wave function seen surrounding the circle. (*B*) The signal output is then back-projected over the matrix, giving a rough image. (*C*) By acquiring many more views, the CT representation of the initial object can be improved. (*D*) Filtered back-projection method. In this instance, the square wave output from the object is first added to a mathematical function or filter, which, when back-projected, improves the edge quality of the picture. (*E*) Back-projection of filtered raw data improves image quality.

—storing 6000 images having a 512 × 512 matrix, the equivalent of 100 magnetic tapes. In addition to the software needed for data acquisition and image reconstruction, specialized software allows region-of-interest measurements of CT numbers, graphics, three-dimensional (3-D) reconstruction, magnification of a given section of the image, and a variety of dynamic functions including image subtraction and region-of-interest intensity measurements over time.

With any imaging system, the ability to detect a pathologic region depends upon the size of the abnormality and the contrast (difference in intensity) between it and adjacent tissue. Lesion detection contrast is defined as the CT number of the lesion minus the CT number of adjacent tissue divided by the CT number of the lesion. Spatial and contrast resolution place limits on the ability of CT to discriminate between normal and pathologic tissue. Another factor is how faithfully the imaging chain (from detector to film output) replicates the information contained in

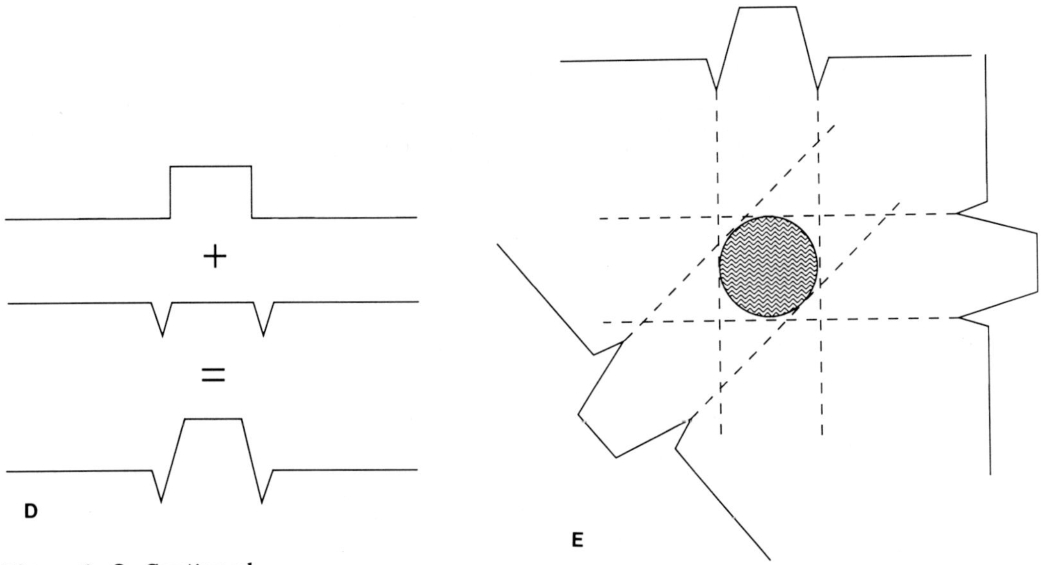

Figure 1–2. *Continued*

these tissues. For instance, if a tumor with density identical to water is suspended in a cylinder of water, then no matter how large the tumor, it will never be seen. Nor can a tumor be seen that is very dense but smaller than the spatial resolution of the scanner.

ARTIFACTS

Artifacts in x-ray CT scanning can be divided into those intrinsic to the scanning process itself, those that result from specific scanner abnormalities, and those that are patient related.

Intrinsic X-ray CT Artifacts

Beam hardening is a common source of artifact, particularly in regions with thick, dense bone such as the petrous bones. As indicated earlier, beam hardening occurs when the average energy of the x-ray beam exiting the patient is greater than that entering the patient because of absorption of the lower-energy x-ray. Lower-energy x-rays are termed "soft" and thus the beam is described as hardened. For areas where the x-ray beam must pass through a great deal of bone, the average effective energy of the x-ray beam is increased and consequently the CT number is erroneously calculated. If, because of beam hardening, a different energy is used to scan one part of the head than another, the effective CT number will be different in each site because attenuation values vary with changes in x-ray beam energy. This is the major cause of the "interpetrous lucency" (Fig. 1–3*A*) seen in the posterior fossa.[79] It is also the cause of the "apical" artifact[21] (higher attenuation values of upper cerebral brain tissue) and "cupping" artifacts seen at the brain periphery.

Partial-volume effects consist of inaccurate averaging of tissue attenuation values and result from imaging an object whose volume is less than the three-dimensional resolution of the imaging instrument. Partial-volume effects[35] commonly cause streaks emanating from sharp edges (Fig. 1–3*B*). As opposed to beam hardening artifacts, this type of artifact can be reduced by using thin sections.

Partial-volume effects can also be seen when two very different tissues in

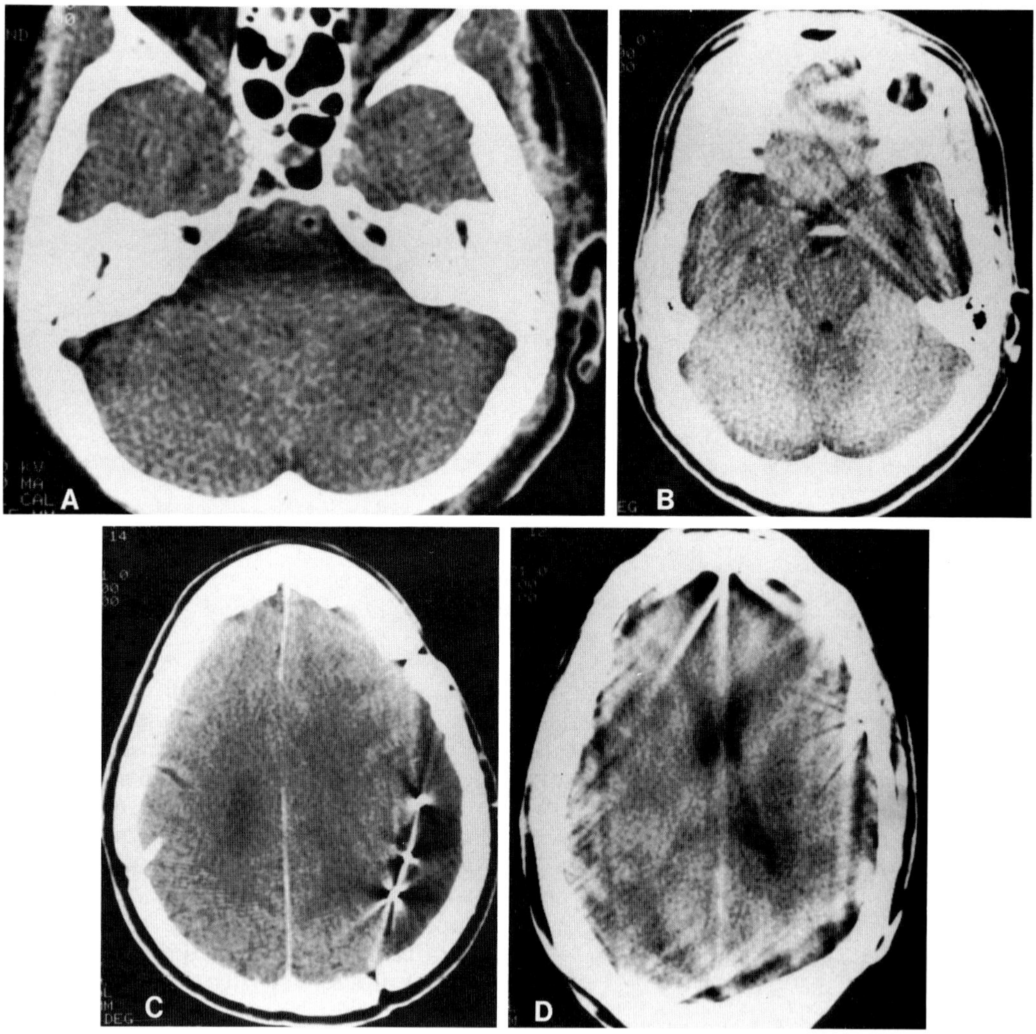

Figure 1–3. (*A*) Interpetrous lucency. Axial, 1.5-mm unenhanced x-ray CT image through the posterior fossa at the level of the petrous pyramids shows an area of relative lucency extending in a transverse direction between the apices of the pyramids. This is caused by beam hardening. (*B*) Nonlinear partial volume effect. 5-mm axial image in a patient whose head is slightly tilted demonstrates streaklike artifacts extending anteriorly from the left temporal bone. This is due to volume averaging of a sharp edge having high attenuation with adjacent brain tissue, which has relatively low attenuation. (*C*) Star artifact. Axial 10-mm x-ray CT image in a patient with prior surgery for a malignant glioma demonstrates multiple star artifacts from metallic clips. (*D*) Patient motion. 10-mm axial unenhanced image through the level of the lateral ventricles shows multiple linear alternating areas of lucency and increased density from side-to-side motion of the patient during the scan.

the same section volume are averaged. For example, a thick section may average part of the frontal bone and the inferior frontal lobe, giving the appearance of a contusion or subarachnoid hemorrhage, whereas thinner sections will demonstrate that the high-density material is bone.

A star pattern appears when foreign material with high density, such as aneurysm clips, dental prostheses, or pantopaque, is present (Fig. 1–3*C*). This is caused by the inability of the x-ray CT scanner to correct adequately for the dramatic difference in CT attenuation values in its reconstruction algorithm. The most practical method for eliminating this artifact is angling the gantry to exclude the high-density foreign material from the slice.

Machine-Related Artifacts

The accuracy of the CT number and hence the quality of the image will depend directly upon the accuracy of measurements by the x-ray CT scanner. If the machine is not properly calibrated, streaks or circular artifacts may appear. For example, the ring artifact is typical of a third-generation scanner in which either the detectors are poorly calibrated or one or more is nonfunctioning. Fourth-generation scanners do not produce this type of artifact. Detector malalignment can result in a centerpoint artifact (Fig. 1–3*A*).

Another source of machine-related artifact in x-ray CT results from an insufficiently high data sampling rate. This is termed *aliasing*. Bony edges having high CT numbers relative to adjacent tissue cause high-frequency components in the CT data set. If inadequate measurements are taken, artifacts with fine streaks of low frequency occur,[107] such as artifacts projected across the brainstem from the adjacent temporal bone. In regions of low contrast such as the abdomen, this is not clinically important, but in the head, where a high attenuator (the skull) is adjacent to a low attenuator (the brain), aliasing artifacts can be important. To avoid aliasing artifacts, an increased number of CT measurements is made so as to overlap adjacent projections.

PATIENT-RELATED ARTIFACTS

The most serious artifacts in x-ray CT result from patient motion. Side-to-side or rotary motion within the plane of scanning causes black and white vertical bands (Fig. 1–3*D*). When motion occurs in the z-axis, portions of the object move out of the scan plane and the images become uninterpretable. Artifacts related to patient motion have been reduced in recent years as scan times have been brought below the five-second range.

DOSIMETRY

Direct Radiation

With the evolution of x-ray CT scanners, spatial resolution has improved considerably, whereas contrast resolution has improved only minimally. The radiation dosage to the patient has increased. Several factors determine radiation dosage. The first and most important determinant is the desired image quality,[39] which depends on the combined factors of spatial and contrast resolution. For a given voxel size (pixel size × slice thickness), a certain number of photons are required to achieve statistical counting significance so that accurate CT numbers and hence good contrast resolution are produced. If spatial resolution is to be increased by diminishing either slice thickness or pixel size, then the radiation dose must be proportionally increased to maintain the same image quality.

The second determinant of patient dose in x-ray CT scanning is detector efficiency. Solid-state scintillation detectors are approximately 40% more efficient for x-ray detection than gaseous xenon detectors.[73] Thus, solid-state scintillation detectors such as bismuth germanate or cadmium tungstate will require a lower radiation dose than xenon detectors.

A third important factor in patient dose is scanner geometry. Second- and third-generation scanners, which use less than a 360° arc, cause a nonuniform dose distribution to the patient depending upon which side of the patient the x-ray beam enters. The variation may be as much as 25%.[72] In these scanners, a posterior transit of the x-ray beam is preferred to reduce the radiation dose to the orbit.

A final important variable affecting radiation dose is the use of a single scan versus multiple scans. Ideally, the dose profile of a single scan would represent a single rectangular slice of radiation and there would be no overlap to adjacent tissue. In practice, however, the dose distribution is more that of a parabolic curve. When multiple scans are performed, the overlapping radiation sums, so that the dose for a given area of tissue ranges from a value just slightly greater than the single-slice dose to 2.4 times it.[101] The effect of multiple scans is most pronounced with scanners that have poor axial radiation dose profiles. Studies involving high-resolution, thin-section images (such as for the orbit and pituitary gland) may result in a large dose to the patient, ranging as high as 15 to 20 rads. This will double if scanning is done both without and with contrast enhancement.[78]

Scatter Radiation

Dosage to the remainder of the body during head scanning arises from two sources: scattered radiation from within the patient, and leakage radiation from the x-ray tube housing.

CONTRAST AGENTS

Contrast agents for neurologic x-ray CT imaging include iodinated compounds for intravenous and intrathecal administration, air, and inhaled xenon.

Intravenous Contrast Agents

All currently used water-soluble contrast media are derivatives of tri-iodobenzoic acid.[2,15,33,84,93] The three iodine atoms in this compound have a high molecular weight and therefore an excellent x-ray stopping efficiency.

Ionic contrast agents have a free benzoic acid moiety that imparts water solubility to the benzene ring. The two other sites on the benzene ring are given various substitutions, the most common of which are the diatrizoate or the iothalamate groups (Fig. 1–4). A cation also must be supplied to neutralize the charge on the benzoic acid. This cation is usually sodium or an organic cation such as meglumine, or both in combination. The meglumine cation is somewhat less neurotoxic than the sodium and is thus preferred for cerebral studies, especially the intra-arterial injections made during cerebral arteriography.[15] There is no important difference in clinical contrast enhancement between the various agents and different cations, given an equal concentration of iodine.[84]

Nonionic contrast agents have been made by adding chains containing several alcohols to the tri-iodobenzoic acid ring. This allows the material to be water-soluble without the need for a cation. The first of these products was metrizamide (Amipaque [Nyegaard & Co.; Sterling-Winthrop in US and Canada]), which utilized a glucose moiety attached to the benzoic acid on the benzene ring. More recent agents use substituted alcohols. This eliminates the cation, decreasing the osmolality of the solution and hence its toxicity. A still different approach has been to attach two benzene rings together, obtaining six iodine atoms per molecule while requiring only one cation (e.g., Hexabrix [Mallinckrodt; St. Louis, MO]). Even more advanced nonionic compounds now utilize the same approach except that they have six atoms of iodine without any cation, even further increasing the ratio of iodine atoms per osmotically active molecule.[93] Table 1–2 lists representative intravenous contrast agents,[71a,125] the ratio of iodine atoms to osmotically active particles, and toxicity, as measured by LD_{50} in mice.

CONTRAST AGENT TOXICITY

Contrast media toxicity can be divided into two general categories: idiosyncratic and chemotoxic. Idiosyncratic reactions are poorly understood adverse reactions that can be classified into three general groups:[130] (1) vasomotor symptoms, including nausea, vomiting, flushing, numbness and tin-

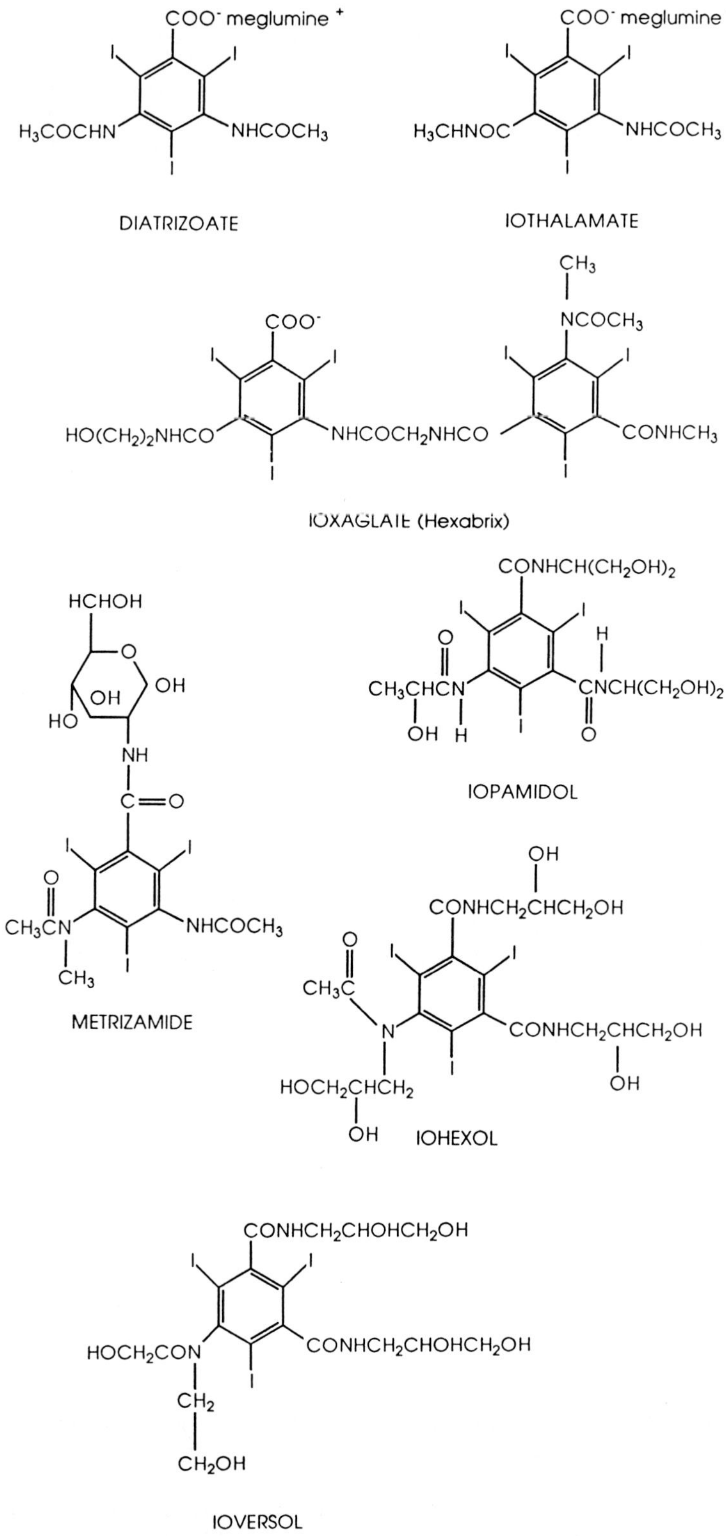

Figure 1–4. Chemical structures of iodinated contrast agents.

Table 1–2 OSMOTIC AND TOXIC PROPERTIES OF IODINATED CONTRAST AGENTS

*Agent**	*Atoms of Iodine/Particles*	*Intravenous Toxicity LD_{50} Iodine gr/kg in Mice*
Diatrizoate meglumine	1.5	7.6†
Hexabrix	3	11.2†
Metrizamide	3	18.1†
Iopamidol	3	17‡–22.1†
Iohexol	3	15‡–24.2†
Ioversol	3	17.0‡

*See Figure 1–4 for chemical structures.
†Package inserts.
‡"Optiray (Ioversol)." Formulary monograph. Mallinckrodt Medical, Inc., 1989.

gling of the extremities; (2) non–life-threatening skin rashes, including urticaria and papular or morbilliform skin eruptions accompanied by itching; (3) anaphylactoid reactions, which may include bronchospasm, hypotension, cardiac arrhythmias, laryngospasm, and syncope. In contradistinction to typical allergic reactions, a second adverse reaction occurs in only 30% to 60% of patients following repeated administration without premedication.[61,98,99] Prior sensitization to the contrast agent is not required for an adverse reaction to occur.[14] In general, if a patient has a repeat study and a contrast reaction occurs, then the reaction is unlikely to be worse than the initial reaction.[99] Also, unlike other types of allergic reactions, reliable screening tests are not available to predict which patients will have severe reactions.[34]

Several factors increase the likelihood that a patient will have a contrast reaction. These include a history of a prior reaction, cardiovascular disease, age greater than 60 years or less than 1 year, and a history of significant allergies or asthma.[99] Mortality rates for contrast administration are variably reported from 1 in 14,000 to 1 in 117,000 and for patients over 60 years of age, 1 in 12,500.[14] Approximately 5% of patients undergoing contrast administration will have some type of reaction, usually mild vasomotor symptoms. Approximately 0.03% of patients will require hospitalization and 1.6% of patients will require treatment.[98] Among 51,165 patients, 1.2% had mild reactions to iohexol (a nonionic agent), 0.9% had a reaction sufficient to require treatment, and 0.1% were hospitalized. No fatalities were recorded.[95]

A second major category of contrast agent toxicity is that related to the chemotoxicity of the agent. The osmolality of the contrast agent is directly related to its toxicity (see Table 1–2). For this reason, nonionic contrast agents are significantly less neurotoxic than ionic agents, whether given intrathecally or intravenously.[93] Contrast enhancement of brain in the pathologic state results from abnormal permeability of the blood-brain barrier (BBB). Leakage of a chemotoxic agent into areas of neuronal tissue that may be jeopardized but surviving can have a potentially deleterious effect on the injured tissue and thus on the clinical outcome. A retrospective study suggested that patients receiving contrast agent administration after cerebral infarction may have a worse prognosis than those who do not receive the agent.[53] In normal persons, the delivery of even large doses (80 g iodine) of intravenous contrast material does not appear to affect the BBB. Seizures occur in approximately 0.01% of patients receiving contrast material,[124] but can be significantly higher (1% to 10%) in patients with brain metastasis scanned with high dosages (80 g iodine).[96]

Contrast media have a direct chemotoxic effect on the renal tubules. In one study,[46] 1% of patients in the normal group with unrecognized renal disease and a precontrast serum creatinine level of less than 1.5 mg per dL underwent renal deterioration. In a second group, who had pre-infusion creatinine levels of 1.5 to 4.5 mg per dL, approximately 3% developed adverse renal effects. Among the patients with a serum creatinine level of less than 4.5 mg per dL, the degree of renal injury was unaffected by the dose of contrast medium in the 43- to 80-g iodine range. In a third group of patients who had a pre-infusion serum creatinine level of greater than 4.5 mg per dL, or in diabetic patients with an abnormal serum creatinine, however, the risk of nephrotoxicity was substantially greater, ranging from 31% to 87% for 43 g of iodine, with additional damage seen at higher doses. Additional risk factors for kidney damage include multiple myeloma (due to the precipitation of proteins in the renal tubules), sepsis, congestive heart failure, neonates, dehydration, and concomitant administration of other chemotoxic drugs such as aminoglycoside antibiotics and certain chemotherapeutic agents.[14]

THERAPY FOR CONTRAST-INDUCED REACTIONS

Given the potential gravity of contrast reactions, and their unpredictable nature, contrast media must be administered in a setting where a physician familiar with the treatment of such reactions is immediately available. Treatment is directed toward the specific nature of the reaction. For mild vasomotor symptoms and urticaria, reassurance and observation alone will usually suffice. For urticaria with significant pruritus, diphenhydramine (50 mg) should be given intravenously for the average 70-kg adult. With mild wheezing, the patient should be monitored closely, and an intravenous line should be started. If severe laryngospasm, angioedema, hypotension, or bronchospasm occurs, epinephrine (up to 1 mg, diluted 1:10,000) must be given intravenously. Administration of intravenous fluids for volume expansion should be started immediately in a patient with hypotension.[118] Electrocardiographic monitoring should be started whenever a suspected moderate-to-severe contrast reaction occurs or seems imminent. Hypotension due to a vasovagal reaction, which results in bradycardia, must be differentiated from hypotension due to anaphylactic shock, which results in tachycardia. In the former, atropine 0.5 mg IV is given in the average 70-kg adult. In the latter, prompt treatment for shock must be given.

Prevention of contrast reactions involves judicious decision making on the physician's part to ensure that contrast administration will provide additional information necessary for the patient's management and treatment. High-risk patients (those with a prior history of contrast reaction, or a significant history of allergy or asthma) should be pretreated with steroids. Some allergists consider urticaria a forme fruste of anaphylaxis and suggest pretreatment if such a history is obtained. Steroids must be given at least 12 hours prior to the examination for significant benefit to be achieved.[14,63] Although many different prophylaxis regimens have been proposed,[14,37,63] a simple two-dose schedule is effective.[63] In the adult, this involves the oral administration of methylprednisolone (Medrol) 32 mg 24 hours and 2 hours prior to the procedure. Diphenhydramine (Benadryl) 50 mg should also be given intravenously or intramuscularly 1 hour before the procedure. Pretreatment does not guarantee prevention of a second reaction, but the probability is significantly lessened. In one study, 3 of 37 patients experienced recurrent rashes and 1 of 9 patients with prior anaphylactoid reactions experienced urticaria.[130]

Anesthesiology assistance should be available if contrast administration must be performed on patients with a history of severe contrast reaction. Nonionic contrast agents have a significantly lower overall incidence of severe reactions than ionic agents.[52,86] Nonionic agents should be used in patients with a prior allergic history, based on the accumulated evidence of lower chemotoxicity (decreased enzyme inhibition, histamine release, and renal, cardiac, and neural toxicity) and decreased minor and severe reactions.[52,86,125]

Caution should be exercised in patients at risk for renal toxicity. The minimum amount of contrast material needed for the examination should be used and the patient should be well hydrated both before and after the procedure.

NONIONIC VERSUS IONIC AGENTS

Controversy exists regarding the use of nonionic versus ionic agents for intravenous use because of the difference in cost.[121] The current ionic contrast agents cost approximately $1.86 per examination, whereas nonionic agents cost approximately 25 times as much. Because of the rarity of "clinically significant" adverse effects such as renal failure, refractory arrhythmias, or anaphylaxis with either type of agent, however, it has been difficult to document the frequency of major side effects with these agents.[121] The data now available from the study of about 500,000 patients suggest that severe reactions will be less frequent with nonionic contrast agents.[52,86,95] In one study of patients at low risk, 0.09% of patients receiving ionic contrast media had a severe reaction, compared with 0% for patients receiving nonionic contrast media.[86] For high-risk patients, the rate was 0.36% for ionic and 0.03% for nonionic contrast media. The rate of death, however, has never been documented to be greater with ionic agents. The ability to produce contrast enhancement is the same with either agent. Thus, the type of agent used depends upon the clinician's view of the cost-benefit and risk-benefit ratios. One recent policy is that only patients in high-risk categories receive nonionic agents for intravenous use. This includes patients with a documented history of anaphylactic reaction to ionic contrast media, poorly compensated congestive heart failure, sickle cell disease, pulmonary hypertension, and diabetes with abnormal renal function.[74]

INTRAVASCULAR CONTRAST AGENT ENHANCEMENT

Normal Enhancement. Water-soluble intravenous contrast agents are cleared by the kidneys with a half-life in the body of approximately 3 hours. Contrast media also rapidly diffuse out of the capillaries into the extracellular interstitial space. When an infusion is given, the blood levels rise gradually until renal excretion equals the infusion rate. When the infusion is stopped, blood levels drop in proportion to the rate of renal clearance.[93] Thus, vascular structures will only be enhanced during the duration of the infusion and for a short while thereafter. The normal brain enhances only minimally. The slight increase in brain enhancement is due almost entirely to contrast agent within blood vessels, with almost none passing through the intact BBB. The gray matter, having four times the vascularity of white matter, enhances slightly more than white matter.[123] Thus, with an intact BBB, the brain parenchyma is affected little by contrast agents. Areas of the brain that have no BBB, such as the choroid plexus and the anterior lobe of the pituitary, normally enhance. Additionally, venous structures such as the epidural venous plexus in the spine and the venous sinuses demonstrate normal enhancement, as do the meninges (including the meninges surrounding the optic nerve).

Pathologic Enhancement. When the BBB is damaged, pathologic enhancement can occur. This enhancement is nonspecific and may be seen with neoplastic, inflammatory, infectious, and vascular disorders. Three types of abnormal enhancement occur.

The first is when contrast material is present within abnormal enlarged blood vessels without breakdown in the BBB. Examples include venous malformations, arteriovenous malformations, aneurysms, and certain neoplasms where the contrast agent pools within enlarged vascular spaces. With high-flow lesions such as aneurysms and arteriovenous fistulas, this abnormal enhancement will only be seen during the time that contrast material is in the blood vessel, unless there is coexisting damage to the BBB.

The second type of abnormal enhancement occurs when the BBB is disrupted and contrast material leaks into the interstitial space of the pathologic region and adjacent brain. In this situation, the contrast enhancement is not necessarily related to the vascularity of the tumor. Instead, contrast enhancement relates to a combination of the degree of abnormal capillary permeability, the vascularity of the disease process, and the concentration of the contrast agent in the blood.[19]

Cerebral neoplasms, both primary and metastatic, often have an abnormal capillary endothelium, which allows leakage of contrast material. The degree of enhancement is related to the degree of abnormality of the BBB. High-grade astrocytomas, glioblastoma multiforme, and primitive tumors such as medulloblastoma and pineal germinomas demonstrate intense enhancement because of BBB breakdown that is roughly correlated with their degree of malignancy.[68,113] Even low-grade cerebral adult astrocytomas that enhance have a poorer prognosis than those that do not.[90] Enhancement often is not uniform in the case of malignant astrocytomas, where tumor necrosis causes patchy, irregular, and even ring enhancement.[81]

Inflammatory lesions such as sarcoid, demyelinating lesions such as active multiple sclerosis (MS), and areas of infarction and infection also can be associated with BBB breakdown and enhancement. The time course of enhancement may be helpful. For example, abnormal enhancement due to ischemic endothelium will resolve over a period of weeks, whereas enhancement from tumor neovascularity will progress. Acute bacterial infections are distinguished by rapid suppuration and liquefaction followed by ring enhancement, as opposed to the slower evolution of more chronic inflammatory conditions.[30] The activity of MS plaques[119] can be suggested by their enhancement when active or lack thereof when inactive. Again, the demonstration of enhancement in and by itself is a nonspecific finding that must be correlated to the other imaging and clinical findings.

The generality that more enhancement equals a more malignant tumor[68,113] does not always hold, particularly for extra-axial tumors and tumors of the pituitary, choroid plexus, and vascular endothelium, which have no BBB. Malignant metastatic tumors likewise do not have a BBB. Also, the generality does not appear to apply uniformly in childhood neoplasms; many benign gliomas (e.g., optic nerve gliomas, cerebellar astrocytomas, and brainstem gliomas) demonstrate marked enhancement[1] and some malignant gliomas do not show enhancement (malignant brainstem gliomas[1]).

A third type of enhancement occurs in tissues that have no BBB. In this situation, the contrast material diffuses into the extracellular interstitial space of these tissues. Examples include extra-axial lesions such as meningiomas and acoustic neuromas,[127] as well as intra-axial lesions such as those of the choroid (choroid plexus papilloma) and pituitary gland (adenomas).

CLINICAL APPLICATIONS

Intravenous contrast media are currently used in x-ray CT scanning in several different ways: routine, high dose, delayed, and dynamic.

Routine. Most enhanced x-ray CT scans of the head are performed with an infusion of approximately 40 g of iodine.[47] For children, a dose of 1 mL per pound of 60% contrast agent is administered. Contrast material usually is administered as single intravenous bolus. For scanning areas requiring a longer period of vascular enhancement (such as the pituitary, head and neck, and orbit), a 25-mL bolus followed by an intravenous drip is used. This dose has been determined empirically to strike a balance between effective contrast enhancement and toxicity.

High Dose. For patients with normal renal function and no history of diabetes or kidney disorder, the dose of iodine can be increased safely to 80 g.[19,46] In studies employing the earlier-generation x-ray CT scanners, high iodine dose scans improved the sensitivity for detecting metastatic disease, demonstrated additional foci of demyelination in patients with MS, and better delineated the cystic components of primary brain tumors. This is not surprising, given that pathologic enhancement depends not only upon the abnormality of BBB but also on the concentration of the intravascular contrast agent. One group[19] found additional diagnostic information in 37% of patients by increasing the iodine dose from approximately 40 g to 80 g. In this study, scanning was performed on a 160 × 160 matrix second-generation x-ray CT scanner. Whether high doses are necessary with current third- and fourth-generation CT scanners has not been determined. For most routine studies, 40 g of iodine is adequate.

Delayed High Dose. Some central nervous system lesions are better seen on x-ray CT images obtained after a delay following contrast injection. This phenomenon relates to the degree of abnormality of the BBB, which may be minimal. A series of 94 patients[97] in which a comparison was made of immediate to delayed high-dose imaging demonstrated that additional lesions were observed in 44% of patients. The delayed scans were the only ones to demonstrate evidence of tumor in 11.5% of patients with intracranial metastases (lung cancer, breast cancer, and lymphoma). Delayed high-dose scanning also has been found useful in detecting active plaques of multiple sclerosis.[119] The advent of MRI[92] has lessened the need for delayed high-dose scanning. Studies comparing unenhanced MR and enhanced x-ray CT have been equivocal, with neither test showing clear superiority.[109] Comparative studies of delayed high-dose x-ray CT and contrast-enhanced gadolinium-DPTA (Gd-DTPA) MRI scanning in metastatic disease have been reported recently. Based upon the improved contrast sensitivity of MRI and its multiplanar capability, contrast-enhanced MRI is superior. If the index of clinical suspicion remains high, then MRI or delayed high-dose x-ray CT scanning should be used.

The dynamics of contrast wash-in and wash-out of CNS tumors may be helpful in differentiating types of tumors. On delayed x-ray CT scans, malignant gliomas tend to continue to accumulate contrast medium whereas some nonglial tumors demonstrate an initial peak followed by a decline in contrast enhancement. Because of the wide variation in individual blood concentrations of contrast medium, Takeda and colleagues[110] measured the tissue-blood contrast medium ratio to normalize for the variations in blood levels of contrast media. On the early enhanced scans, there was no difference between the tissue-blood ratios of various primary brain tumors, extra-axial tumors such as meningioma, pituitary adenoma, and metastatic disease. On delayed scans at 3 hours, however, all the meningiomas demonstrated diminished enhancement, the pituitary adenomas demonstrated only minimal increase in the tissue-blood ratio, and the gliomas, neurinomas, and metastatic tumors tended to show a significant rise in contrast accumulation over time. Taken with other information, delayed scanning may be helpful in the differential diagnosis of brain tumors (Fig. 1–5).

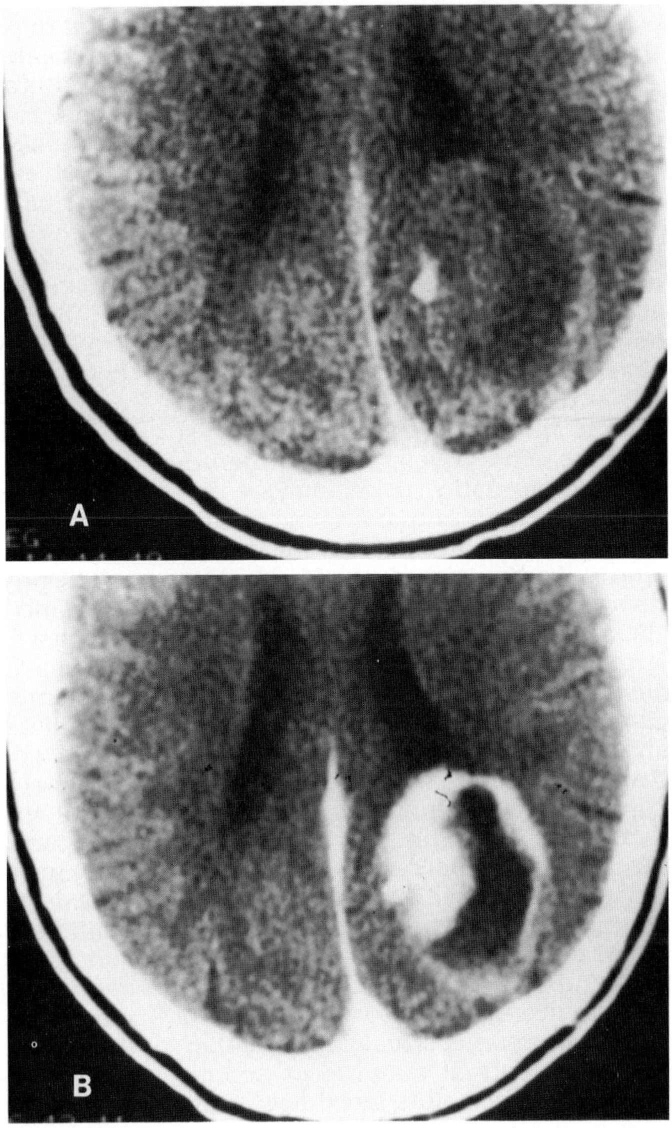

Figure 1–5. Contrast-enhanced x-ray CT scans of a case of malignant astrocytoma. (*A*) 10-mm axial image through the level of the lateral ventricles several minutes following the infusion of 40 grains of iodine demonstrates a ring-enhancing lesion with central low density. (*B*) A 2.5-hour delayed scan at the same level demonstrates a significant increase in the enhancement of the wall of this lesion with persistent central hypodensity that could represent either necrotic tumor or cavity formation.

Dynamic Scanning. True dynamic scanning now can be performed with the newer-generation x-ray CT scanners, which allow for rapid sequential acquisition of slices. Built-in software features allow the measurement of time-density curves of the enhancing area following a bolus administration of contrast agent. This measurement permits the recording of the physiologic process of contrast accumulation and vascularity. Although two lesions may appear to have identical contrast enhancement on a routine examination, they can be differentiated by their time-density curves on dynamic scanning. For example, an aneurysm can simulate the appearance of an intensely enhancing meningioma or neurinoma if the time course of enhancement is not known. Both intra- and extracranial lesions have been characterized by time-density curves.[75,104,105,123] In normal adults, the arm-to-brain transit time of the blood and, hence, of contrast media is approximately 8 seconds.[75] This, of course, is variable, since it is related to the patient's cardiac output and the origin and rapidity of the bolus given.

Tumors having an "arterial signature"[104,105] are highly vascular lesions such as aneurysms, arteriovascular malformations, hemangiomas, glomus vasculare tumors, and angiofibromas. With these lesions, there is a rapid wash-in, high peak, and rapid wash-out of contrast material. Meningiomas, however, typically have a rapid wash-in phase but a slow wash-out phase, giving a relative plateau region following the initial high peak in contrast enhancement. Hypovascular meningiomas, acoustic neurinomas, and other less vascular tumors tend to have a slower wash-in phase and wash-out phase. As mentioned earlier, certain tumors such as metastases, malignant gliomas, and neurinomas[110,127] demonstrate progressive contrast enhancement up to several hours after contrast administration. The differentiation of an arteriovascular lesion (e.g., an aneurysm) from an enhancing mass is perhaps the most helpful use of dynamic x-ray CT scanning, particularly in cases where preoperative angiography is not contemplated and such a distinction needs to be made. Alternative approaches include digital intravenous angiography and MRI.

Dynamic x-ray CT also has been used to assess cerebral perfusion, with either iodinated contrast material or xenon. Although the absolute blood flow to an area of brain tissue cannot be determined by iodinated contrast infusion, with rapid-sequence CT, a relative assessment of cerebral perfusion can be obtained.[4,83] This may be useful in follow-up of patients who have interventional procedures such as revascularization or bypass grafts. For calculations to be accurate, the BBB must be intact, or else iodinated contrast material will leak through the damaged capillaries into the interstitial tissues and a false elevation of regional blood flow will be estimated. The requirement for BBB integrity limits the scope and, in specific situations, the validity of the examination. In patients with ischemic disease, the peak concentration is low and delayed, and has an extended wash-out phase.[22,26] Dynamic x-ray CT also has been used to document brain death, in which case absence of brain perfusion is noted.[111]

Intrathecal Contrast

Traditional tri-iodinated ionic contrast media intended for intravenous enhancement cannot be used for intrathecal injection. At doses required for myelographic visualization, significant neurotoxicity occurs, inducing seizures and death.[49] At lower doses, severe arachnoiditis occurs.[43,44]

The physical density of oil-based contrast media (e.g., pantopaque) used in the past for myelography is far too great for use in x-ray CT scanning. Since these media have a lipid base, they do not diffuse in the CSF, and therefore give poor coating of the nerve roots and spinal cord.

The introduction of metrizamide[2,56] (Amipaque; Nyegaard & Co., Oslo, Norway) in the 1970s permitted the intrathecal injection of a contrast medium suitable for x-ray CT scanning. Second-generation nonionic contrast agents such as iohexol and iopamidol have replaced metrizamide for intrathecal use,[117] because of their lower cost and the lower incidence of seizures, arachnoiditis, and clinical side effects such as postprocedure nausea and vomiting. The toxicity of the nonionic agents in concentrations required for x-ray CT or lumbar myelography is roughly identical to that of diagnostic lumbar puncture with respect to the occurrence of arachnoiditis, seizures, headache, nausea, and other neurologic symptoms.[94] A recent prospective study of 110 patients demonstrated that postprocedural postural positioning in iohexol lumbar myelography did not significantly influence the frequency of adverse reactions.[60] A single seizure has been reported following iopamidol myelography;[38] no seizures have been reported following iohexol myelography. For this reason, pretreatment with antiepileptic medication is not warranted with these newer agents. CT myelography can be performed safely on an outpatient basis for most patients. Medications that lower the seizure threshold, such as phenothiazines and monoamine oxidase inhibitors, should be discontinued 2 days before the examination. The use of 25-gauge spinal needles has significantly reduced postprocedural headache as well.

PHARMACOLOGY OF INTRATHECAL CONTRAST MEDIA

Cerebrospinal fluid (CSF) resorption occurs in both the spinal arachnoid villi (15%) and the cranial arachnoid villi and granulations (85%).[93] Because contrast media are considerably more dense than CSF, they will pool in the lumbar region if the patient is in an erect position. Reabsorption of contrast media begins almost immediately via the spinal villi. It is accelerated by dispersion in the spinal column by supine positioning, which brings the media in contact with the more resorptive surface and also brings about faster mixing due to the greater degree of pulsations of the CSF in the upper spine.

In normal persons, water-soluble contrast media are rapidly cleared from the central nervous system.[29,122] Peak plasma levels are reached at 3 hours and return to baseline levels by 24–48 hours.[29] In patients with arachnoiditis or diminished CSF production from fluid depletion or drug therapy, however, this period may be prolonged.[29] The rate of clearance increases if media are administered via a C_{1-2} puncture or if the patient is in a supine position.

Intrathecal contrast material can be used to study CSF flow dynamics.[41] The usual dose is 10 mL of low concentration (180 mg iodine per milliliter) injected with the patient semierect. The patient then lies in a supine position with head and pelvis raised. Normally the cisterna magna and basal cisterns are visualized by 3 hours. As with isotope cisternography, filling of the fourth ventricle is not abnormal. By 6 hours, the sylvian cisterns and pericallossal cisterns can be visualized (Fig. 1–6). By 24 to 48 hours, the CSF is free of visible contrast material.

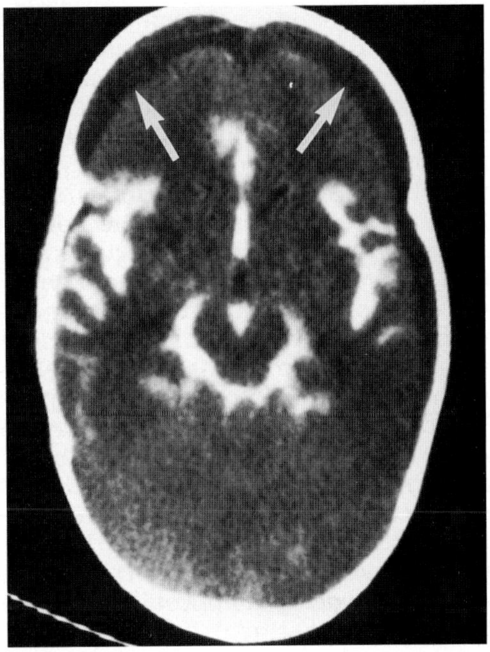

Figure 1–6. Axial x-ray CT scan through the level of the third ventricle in a patient who has had a recent myelogram performed with water-soluble intrathecal enhancement. The patient has capacious subarachnoid spaces as evidenced by enlarged Sylvian fissures and perimesencephalic cisterns. Of note are bifrontal subdural fluid collections, which do not communicate with the subarachnoid space (*arrows*). This fluid could not be appreciated on the nonenhanced x-ray CT.

Intrathecally administered water-soluble contrast material will spread through CSF pathways and also will penetrate both the brain and spinal cord. In normal persons, this occurs at the pial surface.[93] There is no BBB at this interface, as the extracellular fluid space of the brain and the cerebrospinal fluid comprise a single fluid compartment. In pathologic states, contrast material also can enter the brain substance via the ependymal surface, as in communicating hydrocephalus. In the brain, significant enhancement of the cortical gray matter, which can persist for a variable period of time, is seen on delayed x-ray CT scans following intrathecal administration of contrast material.[29] This enhancement causes accentuation of the relatively low density of the white matter. As the material clears from the brain substance, the normal appearance of the central nervous system is disturbed and can remain so for 48 to 72 hours. For this reason, if a head CT scan is contemplated for a patient, it should be performed prior to CT myelography. The pattern of enhancement is reversed in the spinal cord, where the white matter surrounding the deeper gray matter demonstrates significant enhancement. The density difference between gray and white matter then becomes reversed. This pattern can be used after a delay of approximately 6 to 8 hours to distinguish the internal structure of the spinal cord.[50]

CLINICAL APPLICATIONS

The primary use of intrathecal contrast in x-ray CT scanning is in the evaluation of cervical spondylosis and lumbar disc disease. Most often, it is used as an aid to diagnosis following myelography and is particularly valuable in patients with complex spinal degenerative disease, in postoperative patients with distortions of the thecal sac and nerve roots, and in patients who are technical failures with myelography. In one study comparing myelography and postmyelography CT, the postmyelography CT was superior in 68% of cases.[54] At the L_5-S_1 level, where the dural sac is at some distance from the disc, and in far lateral disc herniations, x-ray CT or MRI is helpful. Occasionally, arachnoiditis seen at myelography is difficult to discern with x-ray CT. The usual finding is clumping of the nerve roots and a featureless sac.

Intrathecal contrast has been used to evaluate abnormal CSF fluid dynamics for the demonstration of communicating hydrocephalus.[28] The same findings with radionuclide cisternography are replicated with CT cisternography in patients with normal-pressure hydrocephalus, including reflux of contrast material into the lateral ventricles, ventriculomegaly, and stasis of contrast material in the ventricular system on sequential scans. The stasis may persist for up to 48 hours. The pathophysiology and clinical significance of normal-pressure hydrocephalus remain controversial, but it is probably better evaluated by intrathecally enhanced x-ray CT than by radioisotope cisternography because of improved demonstration of anatomic details, lower radiation dose, and a lower technical failure rate.[41]

Intrathecal-enhancement CT can be used for the evaluation of arachnoid cysts, to define those that communicate with the CSF (and hence do not need shunting) and those that do not.[126] One caveat, however, is that noncommunicating arachnoid cysts may accumulate contrast medium over a period of time because of variable permeability of the wall. Thus, the scan must be timed so that contrast material will outline the CSF space surrounding the cyst, before internal permeation occurs. Subdural fluid collections are easily distinguished from prominent subarachnoid spaces secondary to atrophy (Fig. 1–6). Intrathecally enhanced CT also can be useful for identifying the location of CSF leaks[64] (Fig. 1–7).

In patients with pituitary adenoma and coexisting partially empty sella, CT cisternography can be useful, providing information valuable in operative planning, and in preventing the intraoperative development of a CSF fistula.[91] CT cisternography also has been used to evaluate suprasellar masses[27,28] and in the diagnosis of acoustic neurinomas. With the advent of thin-section x-ray CT and MRI, however, these applications have been greatly reduced.

INTRATHECAL AIR

X-ray CT with gas cisternography has been used to detect small intracanalicular acoustic neuromas. Usually, 5 mL of filtered O_2 or CO_2 are injected and directed into the cerebellopontine angle cistern with the patient

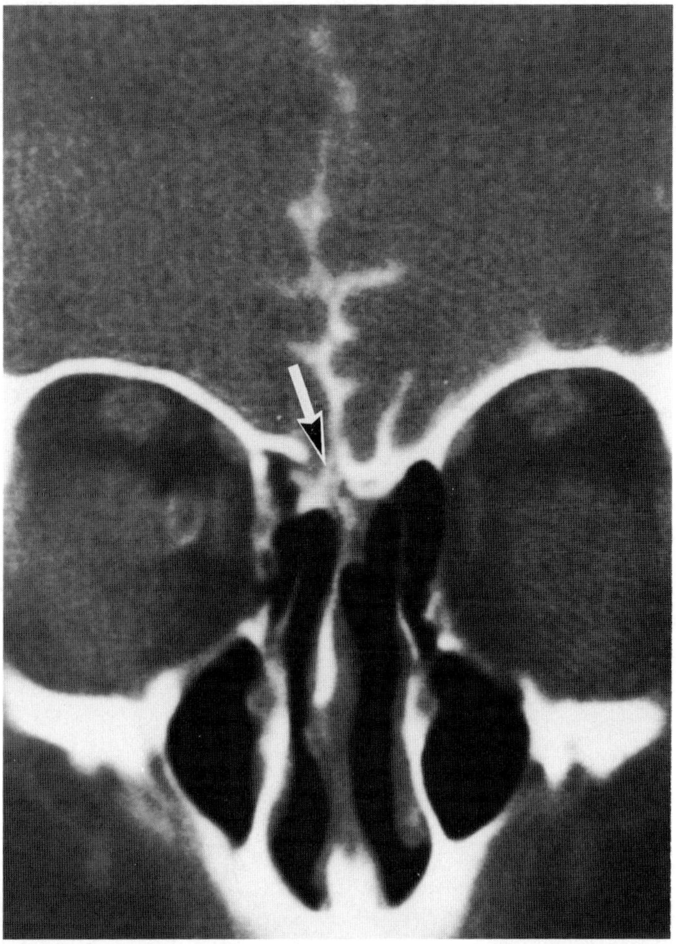

Figure 1–7. Coronal thin-section x-ray CT scan following instillation of water-soluble intrathecal contrast material. A CSF leak is identified in the cribiform plate with a small drop of contrast material (*arrow*) in one of the ethmoid air cells adjacent to the cribiform plate.

resting on one elbow.[6] The patient is scanned in the lateral decubitus position with thin (1.5-mm) CT sections using a bone reconstruction algorithm. The procedure is highly reliable in excluding tumor when gas completely fills the internal auditory canal.[5,58] Small (less than 1 cm) intracanalicular tumors can be reliably detected if the tumor protrudes into the cerebellopontine angle more than 5 mm. For tumors that protrude less than this, the false-positive rate becomes significant. Other conditions that can involve the internal auditory canal and obstruct the entrance of air into the canal, such as granulation tissue and arachnoid cysts, are pitfalls, as are the use of insufficient gas, partial-volume artifacts, and an air-fluid interface lock.[103] A helpful clue is the contour of the acoustic mass, which should have a convex medial surface. Rarely, an acoustic nerve tumor may have a relatively flat contour.[103] Because of the invasive nature of the examination, which requires a lumbar puncture, and because of diagnostic pitfalls in approximately 2% of cases, MRI with gadolinium enhancement is the procedure of choice if high-quality, thin-section, enhanced scans are available. If MRI is not available or is of poor quality, gas CT cisternography can be used (Fig. 1–8).

STABLE XENON CT

Xenon, one of the noble gases, is biochemically inert. It has significantly greater x-ray stopping ability than air, and has high lipid solubility which allows it to pass readily through the

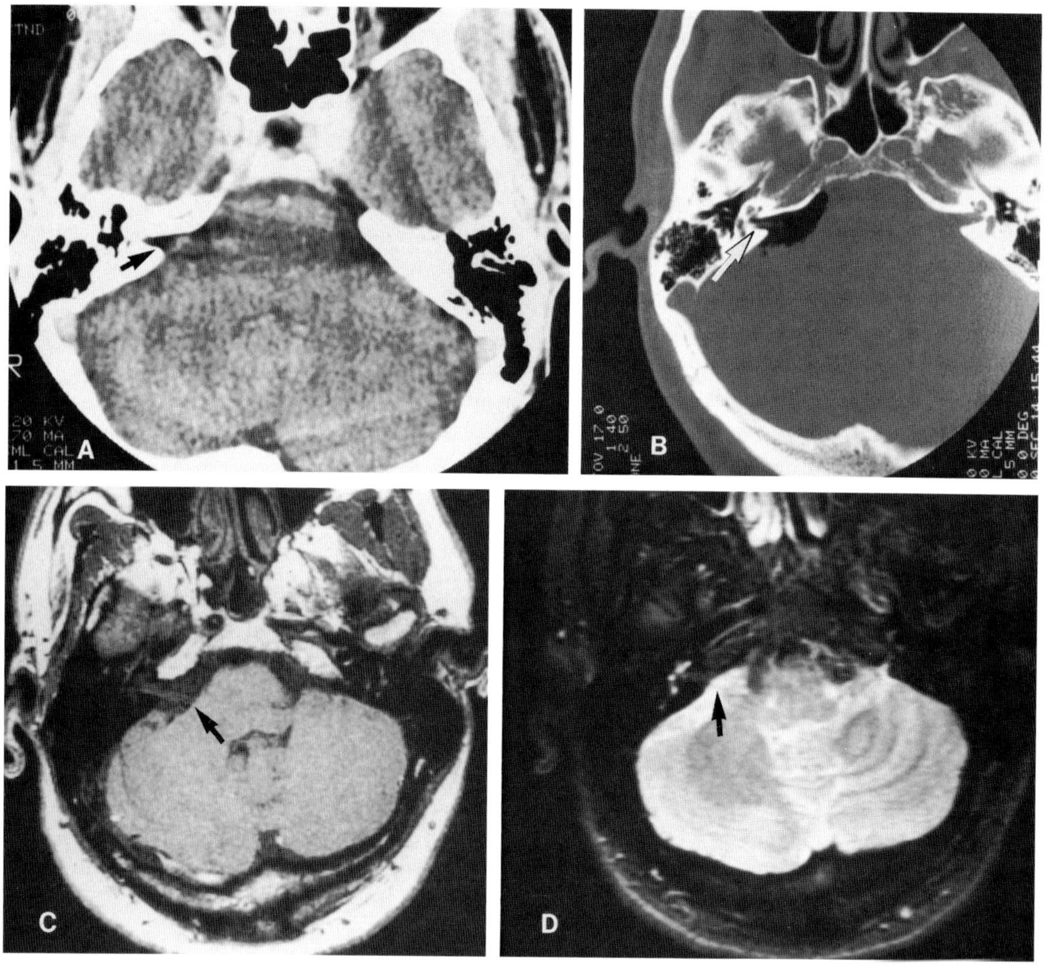

Figure 1–8. (*A*) 5-mm enhanced axial x-ray CT image through the level of the internal auditory canal (*arrow*). (*B*) 1.5-mm axial image through the level of the internal auditory canal following the instillation of intrathecal air. The eighth-nerve complex is outlined by air in this normal patient (*arrow*). (*C*) Axial, 3-mm thick, T_1-weighted (TR 600, TE 20) 1.5-T MR image through the eighth-nerve complex (*arrow*) in the same patient. (*D*) Axial, 5-mm thick, T_2-weighted (TR 2500, TE 80) 1.5-T MR image through the eighth-nerve complex (*arrow*) in the same patient.

BBB. The inhalation of nonradioactive xenon can be used to calculate two physiologic aspects of brain function with x-ray CT scanning: regional cerebral blood flow and local brain partition coefficients. This type of imaging has not achieved widespread clinical use, however, because of the difficulty of data interpretation, limits on the number of slice levels that can be scanned, the expense of the xenon itself and of additional equipment and software, and concern about high doses of radiation and the anesthetic effects of the gas. Nevertheless, it has been used for documentation of brain death[18,23] and to predict preoperatively which patients can safely undergo internal carotid artery ligation.[31] Other potential applications involve early stroke detection; the study of cerebral ischemia,[24,25] migraine headaches, and head trauma; and the evaluation of cerebral artery bypass surgery.

CLINICAL APPLICATIONS OF X-RAY CT

The technology of x-ray CT matured rapidly. Recently, only modest improvements in CT hardware and software have occurred, as opposed to the quantum leaps in image quality seen almost yearly with the early scanners. The task of determining whether x-ray CT should be used for a particular problem is complex, given the newer imaging modalities of MRI, PET, and high-resolution ultrasound. The choice of an imaging modality in a given clinical setting is determined not only by the efficacy of each as an imaging test, but also by the availability of other modalities, physician familiarity, and the population being examined. In many cases the application of various imaging tests is not mutually exclusive but complementary.

Brain

Comparative studies of intraparenchymal lesions imaged by either x-ray CT or MRI have demonstrated that MRI is superior in the evaluation of most disease entities.[10,11,45,129] By virtue of its high tissue contrast, MRI is more sensitive than x-ray CT for evaluation of demyelinating disease, metastatic disease,[109] primary intracerebral neoplasms, degenerative disease, hemorrhage,[36] and cerebral infarction. The multiplanar capability of MRI and the lack of bony artifacts also have contributed to its success.

MRI scanning cannot be performed in certain situations, notably upon patients who cannot remain immobile for 5 to 10 minutes per scan. These patients can be imaged by x-ray CT with scan times under 5 seconds per slice. The same applies to uncooperative patients, patients with movement and psychiatric disorders, and young children in whom sedation cannot be attained or is inadvisable. MRI cannot be used in patients with pacemakers, certain aortic valvular prostheses, or intracranial aneurysm clips, and in patients who are severely claustrophobic.

X-ray CT is the study of choice in patients suffering from trauma. In these patients, speed is important and MRI scanning is often not readily available. Also, monitoring of vital signs is usually less practical during MRI scanning, and scan times are prohibitively long. Many trauma patients require evaluation not only of their intracranial injuries but also of abdominal or pelvic injuries, for which x-ray CT scanning is the method of choice. The movement of life-support equipment (ventilators, monitoring devices, and life-support lines) into an MRI scanner requires time and planning often not easily available on short notice. Finally, MRI is inferior to x-ray CT in demonstrating subarachnoid hemorrhage[13] and craniofacial fractures. Conversion of oxyhemoglobin to deoxyhemoglobin is necessary for blood to be seen in CSF with MRI scanning. Because of the high oxygen tension of CSF, this conversion is delayed, making it difficult to demonstrate blood in the CSF even with high-field-strength magnets on long repetition time (TR) pulse sequences. In Figure 1–9, subarachnoid hemorrhage is demonstrated by x-ray CT but is invisible on the MRI scan obtained at the same time. Subacute head injury, on the other hand, can be evaluated more effectively with MRI than with x-ray CT because of its greater ability to demonstrate shearing injuries in the white matter as well as both hemorrhagic and nonhemorrhagic contusions. MRI is also superior in estimating the size of extra-axial fluid collections and in distinguishing chronic subdural hematomas from hygromas.[102]

Until very recently, x-ray CT has been superior to MRI for patients in whom the diagnosis is improved by the use of intravenous contrast material to evaluate BBB integrity. For example, x-ray CT is superior to MRI in demonstrating extra-axial meningiomas[10] (Fig. 1–10). In MRI scans, meningiomas[70] can be isointense with gray matter on both long and short TR images. Only subtle

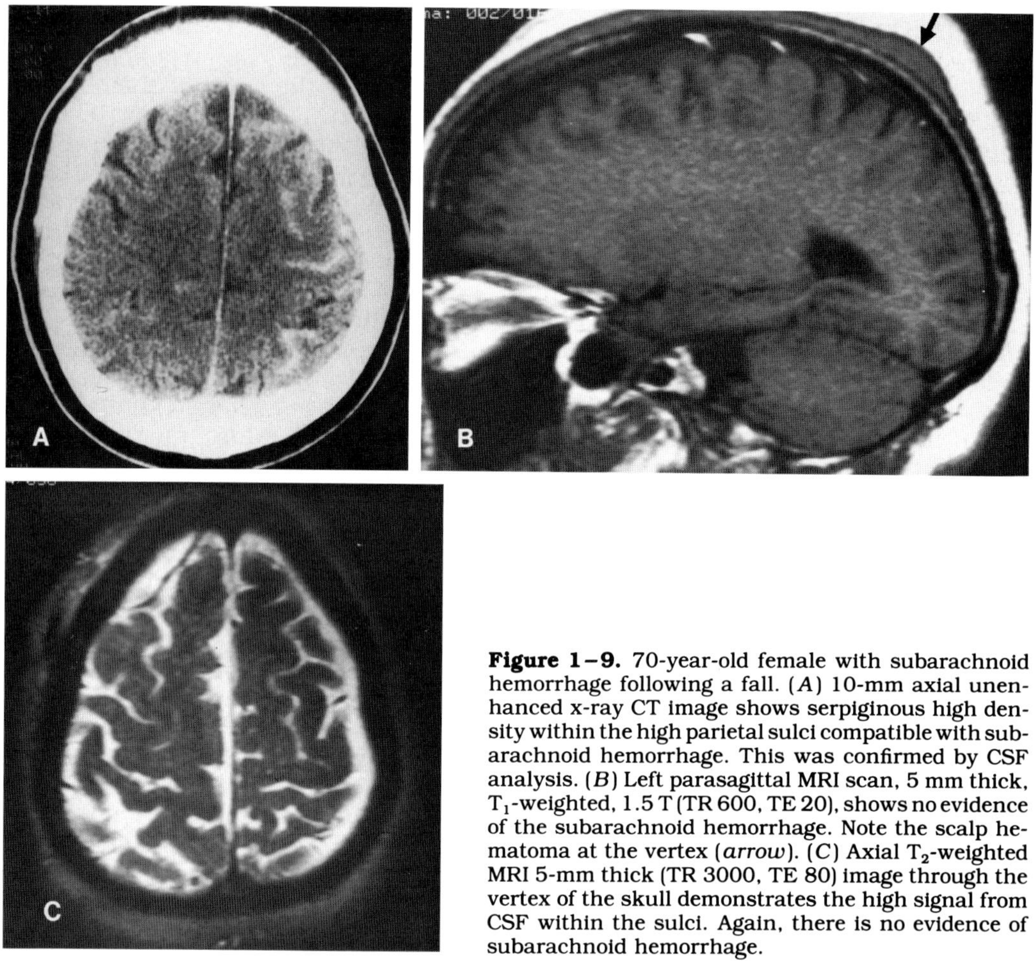

Figure 1–9. 70-year-old female with subarachnoid hemorrhage following a fall. (*A*) 10-mm axial unenhanced x-ray CT image shows serpiginous high density within the high parietal sulci compatible with subarachnoid hemorrhage. This was confirmed by CSF analysis. (*B*) Left parasagittal MRI scan, 5 mm thick, T_1-weighted, 1.5 T (TR 600, TE 20), shows no evidence of the subarachnoid hemorrhage. Note the scalp hematoma at the vertex (*arrow*). (*C*) Axial T_2-weighted MRI 5-mm thick (TR 3000, TE 80) image through the vertex of the skull demonstrates the high signal from CSF within the sulci. Again, there is no evidence of subarachnoid hemorrhage.

distortion of the gyral pattern can be seen, a finding that may be missed unless a careful search is made. This advantage of x-ray CT over MRI applies to other disorders in which enhancement contributes to diagnostic sensitivity. In Figure 1–11, the abnormality in Sturge-Weber syndrome (see Figs. 12–21, 12–22) is well demonstrated on x-ray CT but only seen with difficulty on MR images. With the increasing use of gadolinium-DTPA (Gd-DTPA), the advantage of x-ray CT over MRI in evaluating breakdown of the BBB has ended. In fact, the sensitivity to BBB abnormality is greater with MRI than CT, especially in the spinal cord, brainstem, and posterior fossa.

X-ray CT can add diagnostic specificity or improve the detection of lesions in patients in whom calcification is the dominant feature. If a calcified suprasellar mass is seen on x-ray CT, then the diagnosis is likely to be craniopharyngioma. MRI scans often fail to show calcification. While some calcifications can be seen with spin echo MRI, especially by certain limited flip angle techniques and gradient echo pulse sequences,[3] CT scanning remains the most sensitive and specific method for detection of calcification.

Finally, for some patients the improved spatial resolution of x-ray CT gives it a diagnostic advantage over MRI, particularly when CT scans are compared to MRI scans taken with lower-field-strength magnets. For ex-

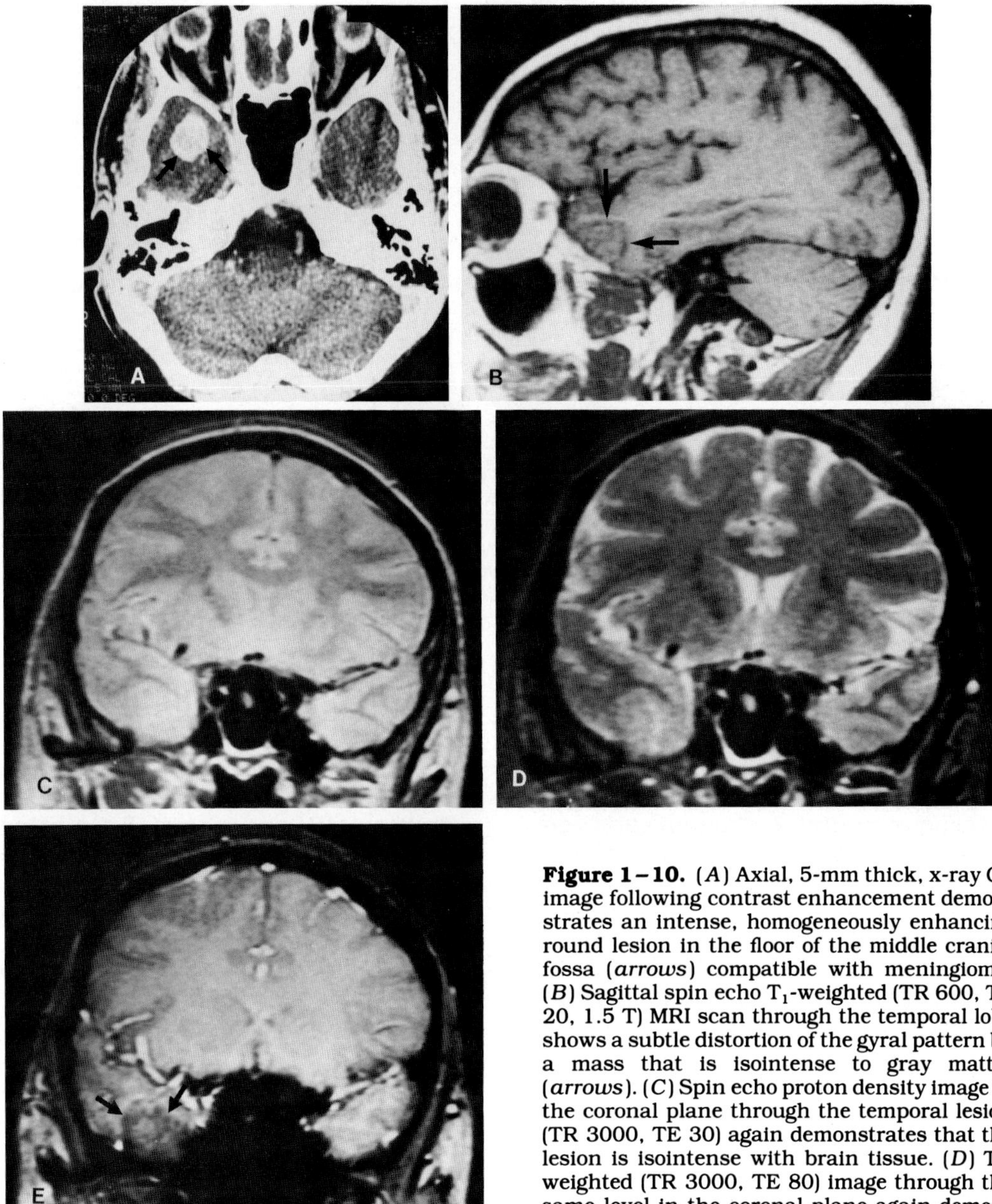

Figure 1–10. (*A*) Axial, 5-mm thick, x-ray CT image following contrast enhancement demonstrates an intense, homogeneously enhancing round lesion in the floor of the middle cranial fossa (*arrows*) compatible with meningioma. (*B*) Sagittal spin echo T_1-weighted (TR 600, TE 20, 1.5 T) MRI scan through the temporal lobe shows a subtle distortion of the gyral pattern by a mass that is isointense to gray matter (*arrows*). (*C*) Spin echo proton density image in the coronal plane through the temporal lesion (TR 3000, TE 30) again demonstrates that the lesion is isointense with brain tissue. (*D*) T_2-weighted (TR 3000, TE 80) image through the same level in the coronal plane again demonstrates that the patient's meningioma is essentially isointense with the underlying gray matter. (*E*) Coronal gradient echo image through the temporal fossa (TR 150, TE 15, flip angle 50°) shows the lesion somewhat better than other pulse sequences, possibly due to magnetic susceptibility effect from calcification within the lesion (*arrows*).

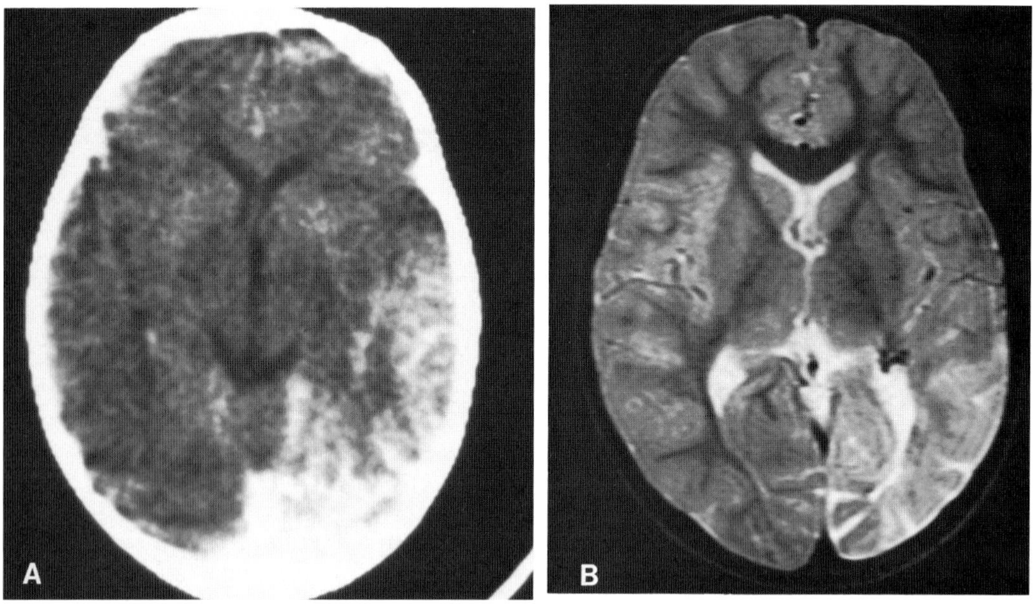

Figure 1–11. (*A*) 10-mm-thick, axial enhanced x-ray CT image through the level of the lateral ventricles in a patient with Sturge-Weber syndrome demonstrates diffuse gyral and cortical enhancement of the patient's known vascular malformation involving the left temporal-occipital lobes. (*B*) Axial spin echo (TR 2500, TE 80, 1.5 T) MR image through the same level shows a subtle area of hyperintensity of gray and white matter signal with slight prominence to the CSF spaces of the left occipital and parietal lobes. Dilated vascular structures present within the atria of the left lateral ventricle are an associated angioma (see Figs. 12–17, 12–21, and 12–22).

ample, macroadenomas are equally detected by MRI or thin-section x-ray CT, and MRI has the advantage of showing cavernous sinus extension and encroachment upon the optic chiasm with greater accuracy than does CT. In some series, however, microadenomas have been better demonstrated by x-ray CT than by MRI.[20,67] With technical improvements and high-field-strength imaging, however, one group[59] suggested that MRI was superior to CT in detecting microadenomas. Gd-DTPA can also improve the diagnostic efficacy of MRI for detecting microadenomas,[106] especially with dynamic scanning.

Orbit

Examination of the orbit is often best performed with thin-section, high-resolution CT using both the axial and coronal planes. The major reasons for the superiority of x-ray CT over MRI for this examination relate to decreased motion artifact. The orbits contain fat, muscle, and bone, giving this area high contrast with both MRI and x-ray CT scanning. With CT, bolus intravenous contrast is available, which can add diagnostic specificity. In addition, the ability to demonstrate calcification and bony destruction gives x-ray CT an advantage over MRI.

In some situations MRI may be complementary to x-ray CT, as when the relationship of a suspected lesion to the optic nerve is in doubt. In Figure 1–12, with high-resolution CT, both in the axial and coronal planes, with and without contrast, the lesion at this patient's orbital apex could not be clearly separated from the optic nerve. The differential considerations of a meningioma or hemangioma made it essential to know preoperatively whether this lesion was surgically resectable. A sagittal MRI scan demonstrated that the lesion was clearly separate from the optic

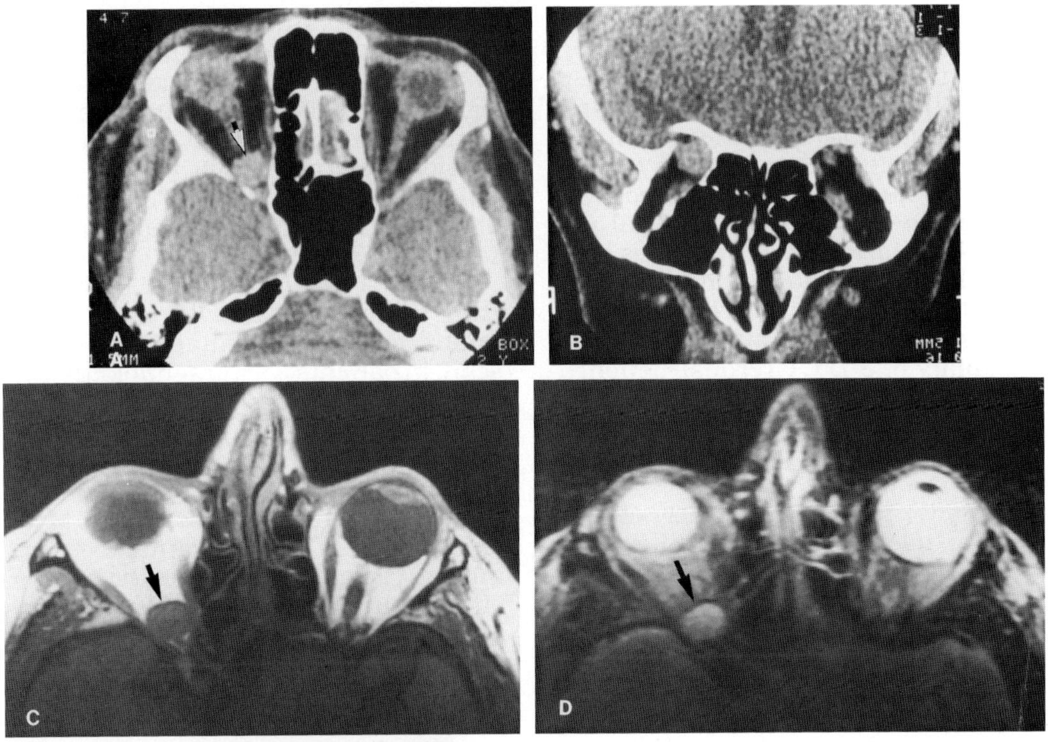

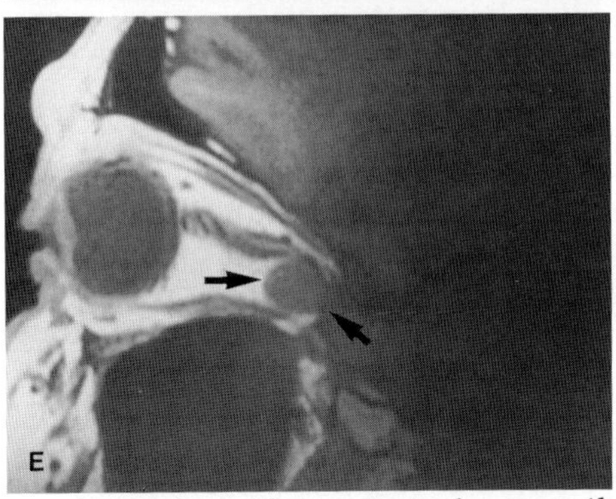

Figure 1–12. A 51-year-old male with progressive visual loss over several years. (*A*) With 1.5-mm-thick, axial enhanced x-ray CT image through the orbits, a small, rounded, 1-cm, slightly enhancing mass adjacent to or involving the proximal optic nerve (*arrow*) is seen. (*B*) With coronal, 1.5-mm-thick, axial enhanced x-ray CT image through the orbital apices, the lesion is again seen. It cannot, however, be separated from the optic nerve. (*C*) Axial, spin echo, surface coil, T_1-weighted MR image (TR 600, TE 20, 1.5 T) demonstrates a soft tissue mass in the orbital apex which is isointense with muscle (*arrow*). (*D*) Axial spin echo T_2-weighted (TR 2000, TE 80) image at the same level shows that the lesion (*arrow*) becomes brighter relative to muscle and brain. Again, however, the lesion cannot be distinguished from the optic nerve. (*E*) With sagittal T_1-weighted spin echo (TR 600, TE 20, 1.5 T) surface coil image, a plane of cleavage is present between the mass in the orbital apex and the optic nerve, which is draped over the lesion (*arrows*).

nerve and that the mass lay under the nerve. At surgery a small hemangioma was successfully removed.

New coil developments have vastly improved the spatial resolution of orbital MRI. This promises to provide fertile new areas of research into retinal lesions, tumors, and other space-occupying lesions.

Subacute hemorrhage is well demonstrated by MRI[36] and may add diagnostic specificity in cases of orbital lymphangioma, a mass that tends to bleed intermittently. Chronic orbital pseudotumor characteristically demonstrates low signal on both short and long TR pulse sequences.[7] Lesions such as lymphoma and metastatic disease, with which pseudotumor may be confused, have increased water content and demonstrate increased signal on long TR sequences. An additional advantage of MRI is that lesions affecting other portions of the visual pathways such as the chiasm and optic radiations can be seen optimally. When bony detail is needed, however, x-ray CT is the procedure of choice. The exquisite bony detail provided by thin-section CT provides more reliable evaluation of orbital fractures than MRI. Craniofacial reconstructive surgery is enhanced by the additional capability of 3-D CT reconstruction.

Otic Capsule

X-ray CT images can be degraded by bony artifacts, especially in the posterior fossa, which are absent with MRI. For lesions in which bony destruction or deossification are the hallmark, however, thin-section, high-resolution CT scan is superior to MRI. These include lesions of the otic capsule such as cholesteatoma, osteomyelitis, and otosclerosis.[65] Developmental abnormalities such as middle and external ear atresias are best evaluated with x-ray CT scan.[108] By virtue of contrast administration, glomus tumors often are better seen by x-ray CT scan.[62] While large acoustic neuromas can be equally identified with CT or MRI, smaller lesions are seen best by high-resolution MRI scan.[16,57] Although these can be identified with thin-section, intrathecally air-enhanced CT scans, because of occasional false positives and the invasive nature of air cisternography, MRI is preferred. Facial neuromas also are best seen with MRI.

Spine

Multiple approaches are now available for imaging the spine, including myelography with water-soluble agents, high-resolution x-ray CT scanning, and MRI. Algorithms for the evaluation of spinal disorders are shown in Figure 1–13. In the workup of radiculopathy, not only disc herniation, but also neural foramen encroachment and spinal canal stenosis must be considered. In a large blinded study[100] of lumbar disc disease, comparing nonenhanced x-ray CT and myelography, myelography was slightly more sensitive than CT (82% versus 73%), but the specificity was lower for myelography than for CT (67% versus 77%).

X-ray CT has limitations in visualizing the conus. Rarely are the upper lumbar segments examined in a routine scan. In patients with arachnoiditis and postoperative fibrosis, scar cannot be distinguished easily from recurrent disc by x-ray CT.[128] With myelography, the conus region and the upper lumbar disc segments are routinely visualized. Myelography has the disadvantage of permitting visualization only of the portion of the spinal canal that has a reasonably distendable thecal sac. At the L_5-S_1 level, the increased epidural fat provides a cushion between the thecal sac and the disc, making the visualization of a disc herniation at this level more difficult. Additionally, far lateral disc herniations can be difficult, if not impossible, to delineate by myelography.

For adequate evaluation of neuroforaminal encroachment in the lumbar spine, 3-mm contiguous or 5-mm overlapping thin sections should be obtained. With the aid of sagittal reconstructions, neuroforaminal stenosis usually can be adequately assessed. The loss of epidural fat surrounding nerve root sleeves, bony encroachment from facet joint disease, and ligamentum hypertrophy are best evaluated by x-ray CT scan. In addition, double dose IV-enhanced CT scans can be used to distinguish recurrent disc herniation from postoperative scarring.[32,66,114,128]

Surface coil MRI, with its improved resolution and soft-tissue contrast, compares favorably with x-ray CT and myelography for the diagnosis of spinal canal stenosis and herniated disc.[77] The advantages of MRI include the absence of ionizing radiation and the availability of direct sagittal and coronal scan planes. With new gradient echo pulse sequences, thin-section con-

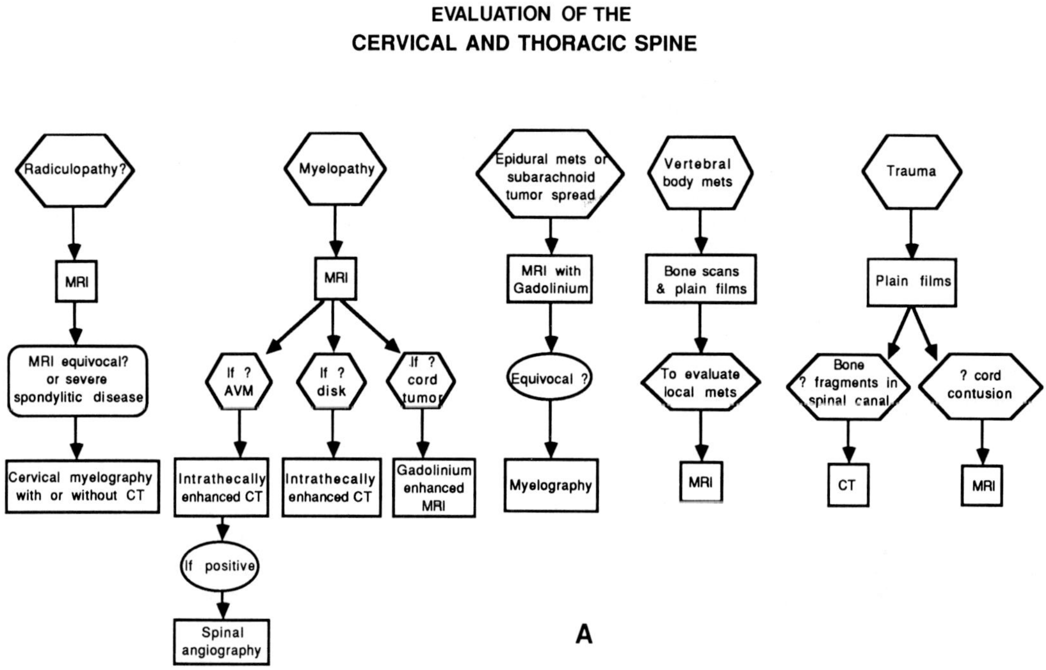

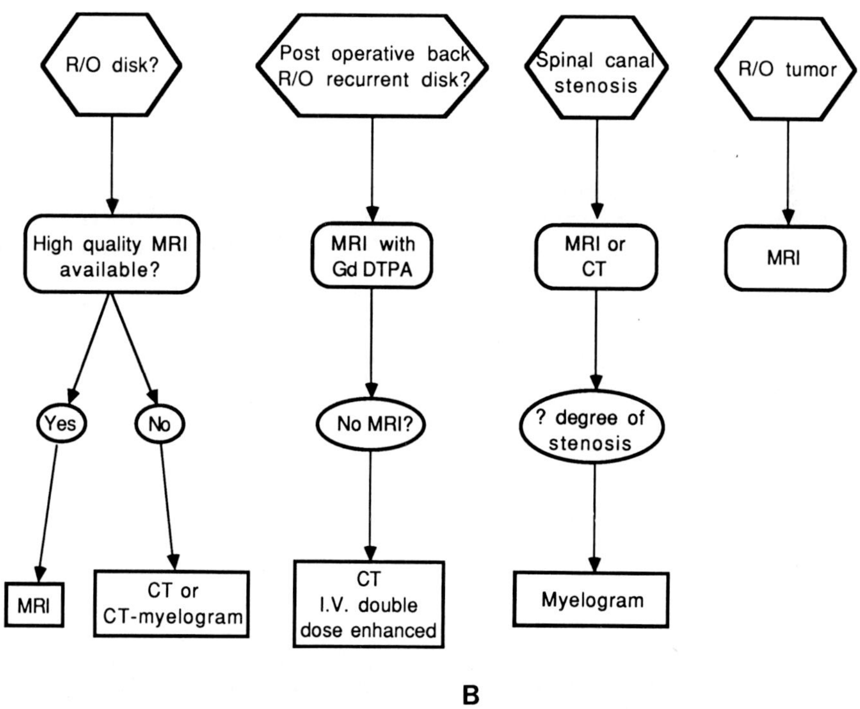

Figure 1–13. Algorithms for the neuroimaging evaluation of (*A*) the cervical/thoracic spine, and (*B*) the lumbar spine in specific clinical situations.

tiguous images can be obtained in a reasonable time period. The major disadvantage of MRI is the increased cost, which is approximately twice that of x-ray CT. Also, artifacts due to patient motion may occur, causing diagnostically uninterpretable studies. Facet disease is less well evaluated by MRI than by x-ray CT. Currently, we advocate a high-quality MRI scan for evaluation of patients with lumbar radiculopathy, followed by CT myelography if needed. If MRI is not available or is of poor quality, then high-resolution CT scanning or myelography with water-soluble contrast agents are excellent alternatives.

Not only are the discs in the thoracic spine smaller than those in the lumbar spine, but also less epidural fat is available for contrast with x-ray CT scanning. The difficulty of screening the thoracic spine is compounded by the fact that multiple levels must be examined with thin cuts. For this reason, surface coil MRI is the procedure of choice, complemented by plain or CT myelography.

In the cervical spine, nonintrathecally enhanced x-ray CT scanning is of limited value. With intravenous enhancement, the epidural plexus can be enhanced and the diagnosis of disc disease is facilitated. For disc herniation, thin-section, high-resolution surface coil MRI compares favorably with intrathecally enhanced thin-section CT scanning and with myelography.[42,48,51,69,76] A large percentage of patients suffer radiculopathy in the cervical spine due to neuroforaminal disease from osteophyte encroachment upon joints rather than just from disc herniation. In this subset of patients, myelography is the most sensitive means for detecting nerve root impingement. Thin-section, intrathecally enhanced x-ray CT scan using 1.5-mm slices gives an adequate evaluation, although it is time-consuming if used to evaluate a large portion of the spine. Figure 1–14 shows images from a patient in whom both x-ray CT and MRI demonstrate a disc bulge at C_5-C_6. A root cutoff secondary to Luska joint disease is less evident at the same level, however, a finding that the myelogram clearly demonstrates. Currently, we advocate high-quality surface coil MRI of the cervical spine in screening for disc disease. In most cases, disc herniations and neuroforaminal disease are adequately evaluated noninvasively. If the clinical findings are not explained on the basis of the MRI scan, then myelography complemented by postmyelography CT can be performed.

For other epidural processes such as abscess and tumor, both intrathecally enhanced x-ray CT and MRI are superior to myelography.[48,51,69] MRI, by virtue of its superior soft-tissue contrast discrimination, depicts soft-tissue extension of these processes better than x-ray CT. CT, on the other hand, can better demonstrate bony destruction, abnormal contrast enhancement, and, with intrathecal dye, displacement of the thecal sac.[71]

For lesions that are intradural and extramedullary, such as pial arteriovenous malformations, myelography is practical because of its ability to screen a large area of the spine rapidly. It also has greater sensitivity than the other techniques for depicting arachnoiditis. For other lesions such as tumors, however, MRI is the preferred method.

For intramedullary spinal disease, x-ray CT scans without intrathecal enhancement are extremely limited because of the lack of contrast between CSF and the cord. MRI is superior to myelography in depicting intraspinal pathology, including tumors, hemorrhage, and syrinx formation.[9,51,71,112]

In evaluation of spinal trauma, x-ray CT scanning is the method of choice for evaluating the integrity of the neural arch when plain films indicate a fracture or suspicion of fracture. Whereas MRI is useful in assessing spinal cord compression and contusion, it is the extradural components to the injury that need to be treated surgically. The principal disadvantage of MRI in evaluating spine injury is that it is not well suited to imaging patients with multisystem injuries in the acute setting. In the sub-

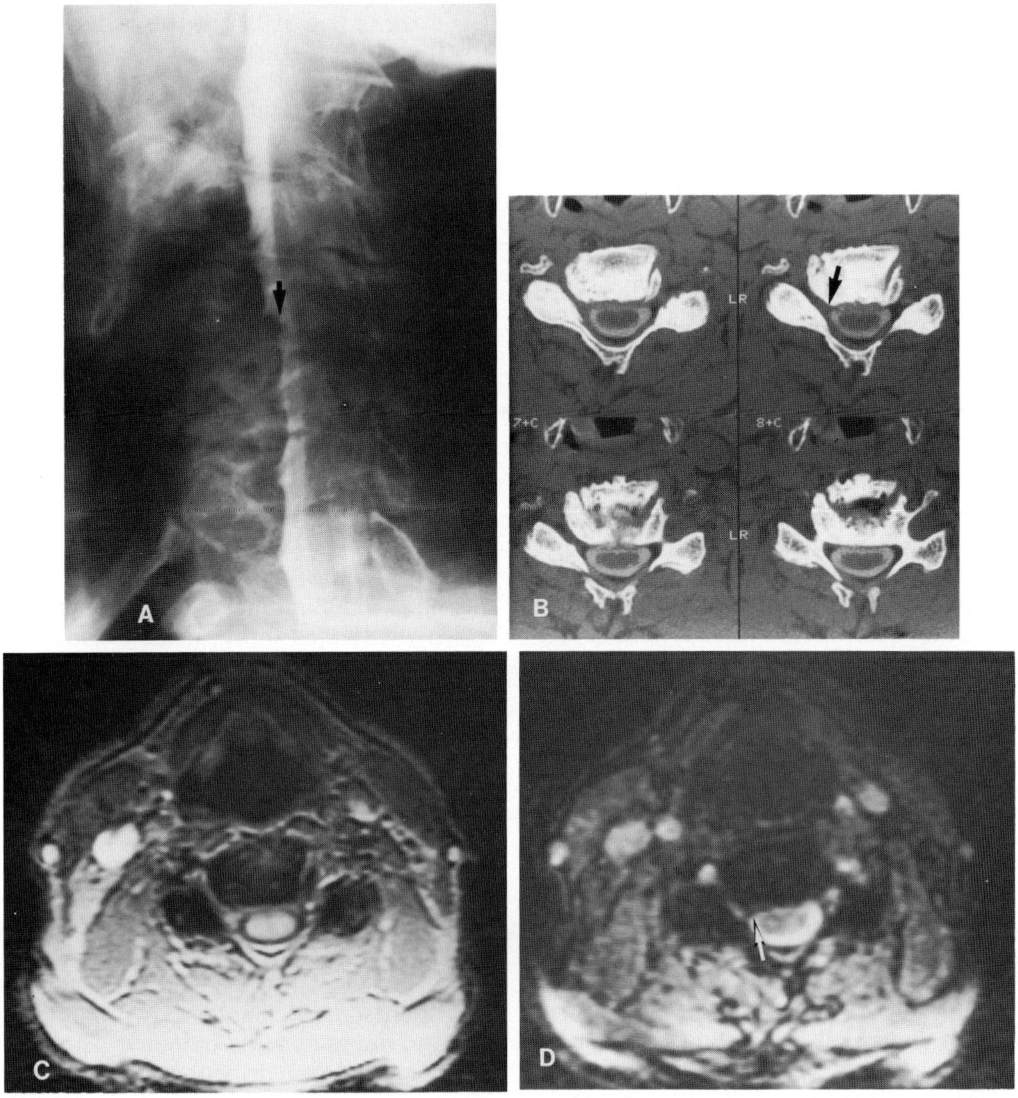

Figure 1-14. (*A*) Water-soluble myelogram in an LAO position shows a root cutoff at the $C_{5\text{-}6}$ level (*arrow*). (*B*) Thin section (1.5-mm) axial x-ray CT image at the $C_{5\text{-}6}$ level demonstrates narrowing of the $C_{5\text{-}6}$ neuroforamina due to degenerative disease of the apophyseal and uncovertebral joints (*arrow*). The root cutoff seen on the myelogram is not as well seen. (*C*) Axial T_1-weighted gradient echo image through the same level (TR 214, TE 10, flip angle 90°, slice thickness 3 mm, 1.5 T, 6 NEX [number of excitations]). The cord shadow is well delineated. The anterior aspect of the cord is minimally flattened from a bulging disk and osteophyte. The neuroforaminal disease is not seen. (*D*) Axial T_2-weighted gradient echo image (TR 40, TE 17, flip angle + 8°, 5 mm thick, 4 NEX) through the $C_{5\text{-}6}$ level shows slight effacement of the C_5 nerve root sleeve from anterior osteophytic disease (*arrow*). Owing to the thickness of the slice, effacement is less well seen than on the myelogram. Also noted is ventral indentation of the cord due to osteophyte and disk encroachment.

acute and chronic state, MRI can provide information regarding the sequelae of spinal cord injury, including myelomalacia and posttraumatic syrinx formation.[112]

Skull

The advantages of x-ray CT for imaging the skull arise from the capacity of this technique to distinguish subtle differences in density within bone. Thus, x-ray CT provides a better means of assessing skull base fractures[116] than do plain films. X-ray CT also can be used for 3-D bone reconstruction and optimum visualization of the bony defects that require repair after trauma.[120] With injuries of the face in particular, 3-D CT of the complex internal bony anatomy improves visualization of the pathologic anatomy, thus optimizing the surgical plan. By virtue of density measurements, x-ray CT can add specificity to bony lesions detected by plain film to determine whether the lesion contains fat, CSF, or soft tissue. In evaluation of metastatic disease, radionuclide bone scans provide greater sensitivity than x-ray CT, though CT is more sensitive than plain radiographs.[55] Tumor invasion of the base of the skull with bone destruction is easily observed on CT. The relationship of the tumor to brain, optic nerves, optic chiasm, and temporal lobes is better demonstrated with MRI than with x-ray CT.[85]

THE FUTURE

X-ray CT, the modality that revolutionized neurodiagnostic imaging, will remain a leading tool in the diagnosis of neurologic disease, particularly in anatomical regions where it presents advantages over other modalities in contrast and spatial resolution. These regions include the orbit, otic capsule, and bony features of the lumbar spine. As long as it is less expensive, more widely available, and more efficient in patient throughput, x-ray CT will continue to be used to image a large proportion of neurologic patients. Modest improvements in resolution and speed will undoubtedly continue. Further application of contrast techniques has the potential of increasing the range of applications of x-ray CT. For trauma patients, uncooperative postoperative patients, and patients with specific contraindications to MRI, CT will remain invaluable, despite the ever-increasing consciousness of our society about the hazards of ionizing radiation. Because of the utility of the other imaging modalities, the use of x-ray CT in the future will stabilize at a considerably lower level than at present.

REFERENCES

1. Albright, AL, Guthkelch, N, Packer, RJ, Price, RA, and Rourke, LB: Prognostic factors in pediatric brain-stem gliomas. J Neurosurg 65:751–755, 1986.
2. Almen, T: Angiography with metrizamide: Animal experiments and preliminary clinical experiences. Acta Radiol (Suppl) 355:419–430, 1977.
3. Atlas, SW, Grossman, RI, Hackney, DB, Gomori, JM, Campagna, N, Goldberg, HI, Bilaniuk, LT, and Zimmerman, RA: Calcified intracranial lesions: Detection with gradient-echo-acquisition rapid MR imaging. AJNR 9:253–259, 1988
4. Axel, L: Cerebral blood flow determination by rapid-sequence computed tomography: A theoretical analysis. Radiology 137:679–686, 1980.
5. Barrs, DM, Luxford, WM, Becker, TS, and Brackmann, DE: Computed tomography with gas cisternography for detection of small acoustic tumors. Arch Otolaryngol 110:535–537, 1984.
6. Bentson, JR, Mancuso, AA, Winter, J, and Hanafee, WN: Combined gas cisternography and edge-enhanced computed tomography of the internal auditory canal. Radiology 136:777–779, 1980.
7. Bilaniuk, LT, Atlas, SW, and Zimmerman, RA: Magnetic resonance imaging of the orbit. RCNA 25(3):509–528, 1987
8. Boris, P, Bundgaard, F, and Olsen, A: The CT (Hounsfield unit) number of brain tissue in healthy infants: A new reliable method for detection of possible degenerative disease. Child's Nerv Syst 3:175–177, 1987.
9. Bosley, TM, Cohen, DA, Schatz, NH, Zimmerman, RA, Bilaniuk, LT, Savino, PJ, and Sergott, RS: Comparison of metrizamide computed tomography and magnetic resonance imaging in the evaluation of lesions at the cervicome-

dullary junction. Neurology 35(4):485–492, 1985.
10. Bradley, WG, Waluch, V, Yadley, RA, and Wycoff, RR: Comparison of CT and MR in 400 patients with suspected disease of the brain and cervical spinal cord. Radiology 152:695–702, 1984.
11. Brant-Zawadzki, M, Davis, PL, Crooks, LE, Mills, CM, Norman, D, Newton, TH, Sheldon, P, and Kaufman, L: NMR demonstration of cerebral abnormalities: Comparison with CT. AJNR 4:117–124, 1983.
12. Brooks, RA and DiChiro, G: Theory of image reconstruction in computed tomography. Radiology 117:561–572, 1975.
13. Chakeres, DW and Bryan, RN: Acute subarachnoid hemorrhage: In vitro comparison of magnetic resonance and computed tomography. AJNR 7:223–228, 1986.
14. Cohan, RH and Dunnick, NR: Intravascular contrast media: Adverse reactions. AJR 149:665–670, 1987.
15. Cornell, SH and Fischer, HW: Comparison of mixtures of metrizoate and iothalamate salts with their methylglucamine solutions by the carotid injection technique. Invest Radiol 2:41–47, 1967.
16. Curati, WL, Graif, M, Kingsley, DPE, King, T, Scholtz, CL, and Steiner, RE: MRI in acoustic neuroma: A review of 35 patients. Neuroradiology 28:208–214, 1986.
17. Curry, TS III, Dowdey, JE, and Murry, RC: Christiansen's Introduction to the Physics of Diagnostic Radiology, ed 3. Lea & Febiger, Philadelphia, 1984,
18. Darby, JM, Yonas, H, Gur, D, and Latchaw, RE: Xenon-enhanced computed tomography in brain death. Arch Neurol 44(5):551–554, 1987.
19. Davis, JM, Davis, KR, Newhouse, J, and Pfister, RC: Expanded high iodine dose in computed cranial tomography: A preliminary report. Radiology 131:373–380, 1979.
20. Davis, PC, Hoffman, JC Jr, Spencer, T, Tindall, GT, and Braun, IF: MR Imaging of pituitary adenoma: CT, clinical, and surgical correlation. AJNR 8:107–112, 1987.
21. DiChiro, G, Brooks, RA, Dubal, L, and Chew, E: The apical artifact: Elevated attenuation values toward the apex of the skull. J Comput Assist Tomogr 2:65–70, 1978.
22. Dobben, GD, Valvassori, GE, Mafee, MF, and Berninger, WH: Evaluation of brain circulation by rapid rotational computed tomography. Radiology 133:105–111, 1979.
23. Drayer, BP, Dujovny, M, Wolfson, SK, Segal, R, Gur, D, Boehnke, M, Rao, G, and Cook, EE: Xenon- and iodine-enhanced CT of diffuse cerebral circulatory arrest. AJR 135:97–102, 1980.
24. Drayer, BP, Gur, D, Wolfson, SK, and Cook, EE: Experimental xenon enhancement with CT imaging: Cerebral applications. AJR 134:39–44, 1980.
25. Drayer, BP, Gur, D, Yonas, H, Wolfson, SK, and Cook, EE: Abnormality of the xenon brain : blood partition coefficient and blood flow in cerebral infarction: An in vivo assessment using transmission computed tomography. Radiology 135:349–354, 1980.
26. Drayer, BP, Heinz, ER, Dujovny, M, Wolfson, SK Jr, and Gur, D: Patterns of brain perfusion: Dynamic computed tomography using intravenous contrast enhancement. J Comput Assist Tomogr 3:633–640, 1979.
27. Drayer, BP, Rosenbaum, AE, Kennerdell, JS, Robinson, AG, Bank, WO, and Deeb, ZL: Computed tomographic diagnosis of suprasellar masses by elevated attenuation values toward the apex of the skull. J Comput Assist Tomogr 2:65–70, 1978.
28. Drayer, BP, Rosenbaum, AE, Kennerdell, JS, Robinson, AG, Bank, WO, and Deeb, ZL: Computed tomographic diagnosis of suprasellar masses by intrathecal enhancement. Radiology 123:339–344, 1977.
29. Duchin, KL, Drayer, BP, Ross, M, Allen, S, and Frantz, M: Pharmacokinetics of iopamidol after intrathecal administration in humans. AJNR 7:895–898, 1986.
30. Enzman, DR, Britt, RH, and Yeager, AS: Experimental brain abscess evolution, computed tomographic and neuropathologic correlation. Radiology 133:113–122, 1979.
31. Erba, SM, Horton, JA, Latchaw, RE,

Yona, H, Sekhar, L, Schramm, V, and Pentheny, S: Balloon test occlusion of the internal carotid artery with stable xenon/CT cerebral blood flow imaging. AJNR 9:533–538, 1988.
32. Firooznia, H, Kricheff, II, Rafii, M, and Golimbu, C: Lumbar spine after surgery: Examination with intravenous contrast-enhanced CT. Radiology 163:221–226, 1987.
33. Fischer, HW: Catalog of intravascular contrast media. Radiology 159:561–563, 1986.
34. Fischer, HW and Doust, VL: An evaluation of pretesting in the problem of serious and fatal reactions to excretory urography. Radiology 103:497–501, 1972.
35. Glover, GH and Pelc, NJ: Nonlinear partial volume artifacts in x-ray computed tomography. Med Phys 7(3):238–248, 1980.
36. Gomori, JM, Grossman, RI, and Goldberg, HI: High field magnetic resonance imaging of intracranial hematomas. Radiol 157:87–93, 1985.
37. Greenberger, P, Patterson, R, and Radin, RC: Two pretreatment regimens for high-risk patients receiving radiographic contrast media. J Allergy Clin Immunol 74:540–543, 1984.
38. Grunert, P and Pendl, G: Cerebral seizure following lumbar myelography with iopamidol. Radiology 26(11):526–527, 1986.
39. Haaga, JR, Miraldi, F, MacIntyre, W, LiPuma, JP, Bryan, PJ, and Wiesen, E: The effect of mAs variation upon computed tomography image quality as evaluated by in vivo and in vitro studies. Radiology 138:449–454, 1981.
40. Halliday, D and Resnick, R: Fundamentals of Physics. John Wiley & Sons, New York, 1974.
41. Hammer, B: Experiences with intrathecally enhanced computed tomography. Neuroradiology 19:221–228, 1980.
42. Haughton, VM: MR imaging of the spine. Radiology 166:297–301, 1988.
43. Haughton, VM and Ho, K: The risk of arachnoiditis from experimental nonionic contrast media. Radiology 136:395–397, 1980.
44. Haughton, VM, Ho, K, and Unger, GF: Arachnoiditis following myelography with water-soluble agents. Radiology 125:731–733, 1977.
45. Haughton, VM, Rimm, AA, Sobocinski, KA, Papke, RA, Daniels, DL, Williams, AL, Lynch, R, and Levine, R: A blinded clinical comparison of MR imaging and CT in neuroradiology. Radiology 160:751–755, 1986.
46. Hayman, LA, Evans, RA, Fahr, LM, and Hinck, VC: Renal consequences of rapid high dose contrast CT. AJR 134:553–555, 1980.
47. Hayman, LA, Evans, RA, and Hinck, VC: Delayed high iodine dose contrast computed tomography: Cranial neoplasms. Radiology 136:677–684, 1980
48. Hedberg, MC, Drayer, BP, Flom, RA, Hodak, JA, and Bird, CR: Gradient echo (GRASS) MR imaging in cervical radiculopathy. AJR 150:683–689, 1988.
49. Hilal, SK, Dauth, GW, Hess, KH, and Gilman, S: Development and evaluation of a new water-soluble iodinated myelographic contrast medium with markedly reduced convulsive effects. Radiology 126:417–422, 1978.
50. Jinkins, JR, Bashir, R, Al-Kawi, MZ, and Siquiera, E: The parenchymal CT myelogram: In vivo imaging of the gray matter of the spinal cord. AJNR 8:979–982, 1987.
51. Karnaze, MG, Gado, MH, Sartor, KJ, and Hodges, FJ III: Comparison of MR and CT myelography in imaging the cervical and thoracic spine. AJR 150:397–403, 1988.
52. Katayama, H: Report of the Japanese committee on the safety of contrast media. Scientific poster, Radiological Society of North America meeting, 1988.
53. Kendall, BE and Pullicino, P. Intravascular contrast injection in ischaemic lesions. II. Effect on prognosis. Neuroradiology 19:241–243, 1980.
54. Ketonen, L and Gyldensted, C: Lumbar disc disease evaluated by myelography and postmyelography spinal computed tomography. Neuroradiology 28:144–149, 1986.
55. Kido, DK, Gould, R, Taati, F, Duncan, A, and Schnur, J: Comparative sensitivity of CT scans, radiographs and radionuclide bone scans in detecting meta-

static calvarial lesions. Radiology 128:371–375, 1978.

56. Kieffer, SA, Finet, EF, Esquerra, JV, Hantman, RP, and Gross, CE: Contrast agents for myelography: Clinical and radiological evaluation of amipaque and pantopaque. Radiology 129:695–705, 1978.
57. Koenig, H, Lenz, M, and Sauter, R: Temporal bone region: High-resolution MR imaging using surface coils. Radiology 159:191–194, 1986.
58. Kricheff, II, Pinto, RS, Bergeron, RT, and Cohen, N: Air-CT cisternography and canalography for small acoustic neuromas. AJNR 1:57–63, 1980.
59. Kulkarni, MV, Lee, KF, McArdle, CB, Yeakley, JW, and Haar, FL: 1.5-T MR imaging of pituitary microadenomas: Technical considerations and CT correlation. AJNR 9:5–11, 1988.
60. Kuuliala, IK and Goransson, HJ: Adverse reactions after iohexol lumbar myelography: Influence of postprocedural positioning. AJNR 8:547–548, 1987.
61. Lalli, AF: Urography, shock reaction and repeated urography. Editorial. AJR 125:264–268, 1975.
62. Larson, TC, Reese, DF, and Baker, HL, McDonald, TJ: Glomus tympanicum chemodectomas: Radiographic and clinical characteristics. Radiology 163:801–806, 1987.
63. Lasser, EC: Pretreatment with corticosteroids to prevent reactions to IV contrast material: Overview and implications. AJR 150:257–259, 1988.
64. Luotonen, J, Jokinen, K, and Laitinen, J: Localisation of a CSF fistula by metrizamide CT cisternography. J Laryngol Otol 100 (8):955–958, 1986.
65. Mafee, MF, Aimi, K, Kahen, HL, Valvassori, GE, and Capek, V: Chronic otomastoiditis: A conceptual understanding of CT findings. Radiology 160: 193–200, 1986.
66. Mall, JC, Kaiser, JA, and Heithoff, KB: Postoperative spine: In Newton, TH, Potts, DG, (eds): Computed Tomography of the Spine and Spinal Cord. Clavedel Press, San Anselmo, Calif, 1983, pp 187–204.
67. Marcovitz, S, Wee, R, Chan, J, and Hardy, J: Diagnostic accuracy of preoperative CT scanning of pituitary somatotroph adenomas. AJNR 9:19–22, 1988.
68. Marks, JE and Gado, M: Serial computed tomography of primary brain tumors following surgery, irradiation, and chemotherapy. Radiology 125: 119–125, 1977.
69. Masaryk, TJ, Modic, MT, Geisinger, MA, Standefer, J, Hardy, RW, Boumphrey, F, and Duchesneau, PM: Cervical myelopathy: A comparison of magnetic resonance and myelography. J Comput Assist Tomogr 10(2):184–194, 1986.
70. Mawhinney, RR, Buckley, HJ, Holland, IM, and Worthington, BS: The value of magnetic resonance imaging in the diagnosis of intracranial meningiomas. Clin Radiol 37:429–439, 1986.
71. McAfee, PC, Bohlman, HH, Han, JS, and Salvagno, RT: Comparison of nuclear magnetic resonance imaging and computed tomography in the diagnosis of upper cervical spinal cord compression. Spine 11(4):295–304, 1986.

71a. McClennan, BL: Low-osmolality contrast media: Premises and promises. Radiology 162:1–8, 1987.

72. McCullough, EC, Baker, HL Jr, Houser, OW, and Reese, DF: An evaluation of the quantitative and radiation featues of a scanning x-ray transverse axial tomograph: The EMI scanner. Radiology 111:709–715, 1974.
73. McCullough, EC and Payne, T: Patient dosage in computed tomography. Radiology 129:457–463, 1978.
74. McLean, GK: Personal communication. Ad Hoc Committee on Prophylaxis for Patients. University of Pennsylvania, Philadelphia, Pa,
75. Michael, AS, Mafee, MF, Valvassori, GE, and Tan, WS: Dynamic computed tomography of the head and neck: Differential diagnostic value. Radiology 154:413–419, 1985.
76. Modic, MT, Masaryk, T, Boumphrey, F, Goormastic, M, and Bell, G: Lumbar herniated disk disease and canal stenosis: Prospective evaluation by surface coil MR, CT, and myelography. AJNR 7:709–717, 1986.
77. Modic, MT, Masaryk, TJ, Ross, JS,

and Carter, JR: Imaging of degenerative disk disease. Radiology 168:177–186, 1988.

78. Moseley, RD and Linton, OW: 1984 conference on CT dosimetry. Editorial. AJR 144:1087–1088, 1985.

79. Mostrom, U and Ytterbergh, C: Artifacts in computed tomography of the posterior fossa: A comparative phantom study. J Comput Assist Tomogr 10(4):560–566, 1986.

80. Mull, RT: Mass estimates by computed tomography: Physical density from CT numbers. AJR 143:1101–1104, 1984.

81. Murovic, J, Turowski, K, Wilson, CB, Hoshino, T, and Levin, V: Computerized tomography in the prognosis of malignant cerebral gliomas. J Neurosurg 65:799–805, 1986.

82. New, PFJ, Scott, WR, Schnur, JA, Davis, KR, and Taveras, JM: Computerized axial tomography with the EMI scanner. Radiology 110:109–123, 1974.

83. Norman, D, Axel, L, Berninger, WH, Edwards, MS, Cann, CE, Redington, RW, and Cox, I: Dynamic computed tomography of the brain: Techniques, data analysis, and applications. AJR 136:759–770, 1981.

84. Norman, D, Enzmann, DR, and Newton, TH: Comparative efficacy of contrast agents in computed tomography scanning of the brain. J Comput Assist Tomogr 2:319–331, 1978.

85. Paling, MR, Black, WC, Levine, PA, and Cantrell, RW: Tumor invasion of the anterior skull base: A comparison of MR and CT studies. J Comput Assist Tomogr 11(5):824–830, 1987.

86. Palmer, FJ: The RACR survey of intravenous contrast media reactions: Final report. Australasian Radiology 32: 426–428, 1988.

87. Peters, TM and Lewitt, RM: Computed tomography with fan beam geometry. JCAT 1(4):429–436, 1977.

88. Phelps, ME, Gado, MH, and Hoffman, EJ: Correlation of effective atomic number and electron density with attenuation coefficients measured with polychromatic x-rays. Radiology 117: 585–588, 1975.

89. Phelps, ME, Hoffman, EJ, and Ter-Pogossian, MM: Attenuation coefficients of various body tissues, fluids, and lesions at photon energies of 18 to 136 KeV. Radiology 117:573–583, 1975.

90. Piepmeier, JM. Observations on the current treatment of low-grade astrocytic tumors of the cerebral hemispheres. J Neurosurg 67:177–181, 1987.

91. Pompili, A, Iachetti, M, Bianchini, AL, Crecco, M, Giannini, P, and Mastrostefano, R: CT iopamidol cisternographic diagnosis of coexisting partial empty sella and pituitary adenoma. Report of two cases. Neuroradiology 29:93–94, 1987.

92. Reese, L, Carr, TJ, Nicholson, RL, and Lepp, EK: Magnetic resonance imaging for detecting lesions of multiple sclerosis: Comparison with computed tomography and clinical assessment. CMAJ 135:639–643, 1986.

93. Sage, MR: Kinetics of water-soluble contrast media in the central nervous system. AJR 141:815–824, 1983.

94. Sand, T, Stovner, LJ, Dale, L, and Salvesen, R: Side effects after diagnostic lumbar puncture and lumbar iohexol myelography. Neuroradiology 29: 385–388, 1987.

95. Schrott, KM, Behrends, B, Clauss, W, Kaufmann, R, and Lehnert, J: Iohexol in excretory urography. Fortschritte der Medizin 104:153–156, 1986.

96. Scott, WR: Seizures: A reaction to contrast media for computed tomography of the brain. Radiology 137:359–361, 1980.

97. Shalen, PR, Hayman, LA, Wallace, S, and Handel, SF: Protocol for delayed contrast enhancement in computed tomography of cerebral neoplasia. Radiology 139:397–402, 1981.

98. Shehadi, WH: Adverse reactions to intravenously administered contrast media. Am J Roentgenol 124:145–152, 1975.

99. Shehadi, WH: Contrast media adverse reactions: Occurrence, recurrence, and distribution patterns. Radiology 143: 11–17, 1982.

100. Shipper, J, Kardaun, JWPF, Braakman, R, van Dongen, KJ, and Blaauw,

G. Lumbar disk herniation: Diagnosis with CT or myelography? Radiology 165:227–231, 1987.

101. Shope, TB, Gagne, RM, and Johnson, GC: A method for describing the doses delivered by transmission x-ray computed tomography. Med Phys 8(4):488–495, 1981.

102. Snow, RB, Zimmerman, RD, Gandy, SE, and Deck, MDF. Comparison of magnetic resonance imaging and computed tomography in the evaluation of head injury. Neurosurgery 13(1):45–52, 1986.

103. Solti-Bohman, LG, Magaram, DL, Lo, WWM, Witten, RM, Shimizu, FH, McMonigle, EM, and Rao, AKR: Gas-CT cisternography for detection of small acoustic nerve tumors. Radiology 150: 403–407, 1984.

104. Som, PM, Lanzieri, CF, Sacher, M, Lawson, W, and Biller, HF: Extracranial tumor vascularity: Determination by dynamic CT scanning. Part I: Concepts and signature curves. Radiology 154:401–405, 1985.

105. Som, PM, Lanzieri, CF, Scher, M, Lawson, W, and Biller, HF: Extracranial tumor vascularity: Determination by dynamic CT scanning. Part II: The unit approach. Radiology 154:407–412, 1985.

106. Steiner, E, Imhof, H, and Knosp, E: Gd-DTPA enhanced high resolution MR imaging of pituitary adenomas. Radiographics 9(4):587–598, 1989.

107. Stockham, CD: A simulation study of aliasing in computed tomography. Radiology 132:721–726, 1979.

108. Swartz, JD, Glazer, AU, Faerber, EN, Capitanio, MA, and Popky, GL: Congenital middle-ear deafness: CT study. Radiology 159:187–190, 1986.

109. Sze, G, Shin, J, Krol, G, Johnson, C, Liu, D, and Deck, MDF: Intraparenchymal brain metastases: MR imaging versus contrast-enhanced CT. Radiology 168:187–194, 1988.

110. Takeda, N, Tanaka, R, Nakai, O, and Ueki, K: Dynamics of contrast enhancement in delayed computed tomography of brain tumors: Tissue-blood ratio and differential diagnosis. Radiology 142: 663–668, 1982.

111. Tan, WS, Wilbur, AC, Jafar, JJ, Spigos, DG, and Abejo, R: Brain death: Use of dynamic CT and intravenous digital subtraction angiography. AJNR 8:123–125, 1987.

112. Tarr, RW, Drolshagen, LF, Kerner, TC, Allen, JH, Partain, CL, and James, AE: MR imaging of recent spinal trauma. J Comp Assist Tomogr 11 (3):412–417, 1987.

113. Tchang, S, Scotti, G, Terbrugge, K, Melancon, D, Belanger, G, Milner, C, and Ethier, R: Computerized tomography as a possible aid to histological grading of supratentorial gliomas. J Neurosurg 46:735–739, 1977.

114. Teplick, JG and Haskin, ME: Intravenous contrast-enhanced CT of the postoperative lumbar spine: Improved identification of recurrent disk herniation, scar, arachnoiditis, and diskitis. AJR 143:845–855, 1984.

115. Ter-Pogossian, MM: Computerized cranial tomography: Equipment and physics. Semin Roentgenol XII(1):13–15, 1977.

116. Terrier, F, Raveh, J, and Burckhardt, B: Conventional tomography and computed tomography for the diagnosis of fronto-basal fractures. Ann Radiol 27:391–399, 1984.

117. Valk, J, Crezee, FC, de Slegte, RGM, Hazenberg, GH, Wolbers, J, and Rach-Gansmo, T: Iohexol 300 mg I/ml versus iopamidol 300 mg I/ml for cervical myelography double blind trial. Neuroradiology 29:202–205, 1987.

118. van Sonnenberg, E, Neff, CC, and Pfister, RC: Life-threatening hypotensive reactions to contrast media administration: Comparison of pharmacologic and fluid therapy. Radiology 162:15–19, 1987.

119. Vinuela, FV, Fox, AJ, Debrum, GM, Feasby, TE, and Ebers, GC: New perspectives in computed tomography of multiple sclerosis. AJR 139:123–127, 1982.

120. Virapongse, C, Shapiro, M, Gmitro, A, and Sarwar, M: Three-dimensional computed tomographic reformation of the spine, skull, and brain from axial images. 18(1):53–58, 1986.

121. White, RI Jr, and Halden, WJ Jr:

Liquid gold: Low-osmolality contrast media. Radiology 159:559–560, 1986.
122. Wilcox, J, Evill, CA, and Sage, MR. Rate of clearance of intrathecal iopamidol in the dog. Neuroradiology 28:359–361, 1986.
123. Wing, SD, Anderson, RE, and Osborn, AG: Dynamic cranial computed tomography: Preliminary results. AJR 134: 941–945, 1980.
124. Witten, DM, Hirsch, RD, and Hartman, GW: Acute reactions to urographic contrast medium: Incidence, clinical characteristics and relationship to history of hypersensitivity states. AJR 119:832–840, 1973.
125. Wolf, GL: Safer, more expensive iodinated contrast agents: How do we decide? Radiology 159:557–558, 1986.
126. Wolpert, SM and Scott, RM: The value of metrizamide CT cisternography in the management of cerebral arachnoid cysts. AJNR 2:29–35, 1981
127. Wu, E, Tang, Y, Bai, R: CT in diagnosis of acoustic neuromas. AJNR 7: 645–650, 1986.
128. Yang, PJ, Seeger, JF, Dzioba, RB, Carmody, RF, Burt, TB, Komar, NN, and Smith, JR: High-dose IV contrast in CT scanning of the postoperative lumbar spine. AJNR 7:703–707, 1986.
129. Zimmerman, RA, Bilaniuk, LT, Johnson, MH, Hershey, B, Jaffe, S, Gomori, JM, Goldberg, HI, and Grossman, RI: MRI of central nervous system: Early clinical results. AJNR 7:587–594, 1986.
130. Zweiman, R, Mishkin, MM, and Hildreth, EA: An approach to the performance of contrast studies in contrast material–reactive persons. Ann Intern Med 83:159–162, 1975.

Chapter 2

MAGNETIC RESONANCE IMAGING

Robert B. Lufkin, M.D.

PHYSICAL PRINCIPLES OF MRI SCANNING
FORMATION OF THE MR IMAGE
MRI INSTRUMENTATION
MRI CONTRAST AGENTS
THE UTILITY OF MRI IN NEUROLOGIC STUDIES

Magnetic resonance imaging (MRI) exploits the principles of nuclear magnetic resonance (NMR) to produce clinically exquisite images of human anatomy and pathology. MRI has been extremely useful in the evaluation of patients with a wide variety of neurologic disorders. It has been particularly effective in the evaluation of patients suspected of having multiple sclerosis (MS), in patients soon after a cerebrovascular event, and in the evaluation of tumors of the central nervous system. MRI has the advantage of allowing visualization of human anatomy without the risk of ionizing radiation. This chapter will review the physical principles of MR scanning, the methods of forming the MR image, the use of contrast agents in MRI, and the strengths and weaknesses of MRI.

PHYSICAL PRINCIPLES OF MR SCANNING

The Nucleus of the Atom

Unlike x-ray images, which are produced by attenuation of x-ray photons by orbital electrons, NMR signals arise in the nuclei of atoms. The nuclei of all atoms except hydrogen contain two basic types of particles (or nucleons): protons and neutrons. These two particles, along with the planetary electrons, make up the atom. Although the number of positively charged protons and negatively charged orbiting electrons are usually the same in order to maintain electrical neutrality, the numbers of protons and neutrons are often unequal.

The balance between the number of protons and neutrons in an atom determines the angular momentum of the nucleus. *Angular momentum* refers to the rotational motion of a body. If a nucleus contains either unpaired protons or unpaired neutrons or both, then it has *net spin* and angular momentum. If the nucleus has no unpaired nucleons, the nuclear angular momentum is zero. Any other combination of unbalanced nucleons results in a nonzero nuclear angular momentum.

If it has angular momentum, a nucleus will precess (wobble) when placed in a magnetic field. Without precession, there will be no resonance (that is, internal motion) and no NMR signal. Thus, angular momentum must be nonzero for the NMR phenomenon to occur.

Only the subset of atoms with unpaired protons, neutrons, or both (such as hydrogen, sodium 23, phosphorus 31, carbon 13, and others) may be used to produce a signal in NMR. Although roughly one third of the almost 300 stable nuclei have unpaired nucleons and therefore have angular momentum, only a select subset of these are of interest for biological systems.

Of all the atoms with unpaired nucleons, hydrogen is the simplest in that it has only one nucleon, a proton. It is also the most important atom for medical MRI currently. Hydrogen is a particularly good material to examine with MRI in humans because it makes up two thirds of all atoms in human beings. In addition to its abundance in the human body, it is also highly magnetic, producing a high MR sensitivity (Table 2–1).

MRI with nuclei other than hydrogen is possible in humans but results in images with at least an order of magnitude poorer signal because of the lower abundance and sensitivity (see Table 2–1). The remainder of this chapter will concentrate on proton or hydrogen MRI. Unless otherwise mentioned, the word *proton* will refer to the nucleus of the hydrogen atom.

Magnetic Properties of the Nucleus

As indicated above, the nucleus of the hydrogen atom consists of a proton, a small, positively charged particle with angular momentum or spin. The spinning atom has a current loop, causing the formation of a magnetic field (or moment) with two poles (north and south). This is also referred to as a *magnetic dipole moment* (Fig. 2–1). MRI requires this property.

When a material has a magnetic dipole moment, the material tends to align with externally applied magnetic fields, acting like small bar magnets. An arrow or "vector" is often used to describe the orientation and magnitude of the north and south poles of the magnetic dipole moment. In the absence of any great externally applied magnetic field, the vectors of the magnetic dipole moments of protons are oriented randomly.

Table 2–1 MR PROPERTIES OF SELECTED NUCLEI

Nucleus	*Nuclear Spin*	*Relative Abundance*	*Relative Sensitivity*
^{1}H	1/2	99.98	1.0
^{2}H	1	0.015	0.0096
^{13}C	1/2	1.11	0.016
^{23}Na	3/2	100	0.093
^{31}P	1/2	100	0.066
^{19}F	1/2	100	0.830

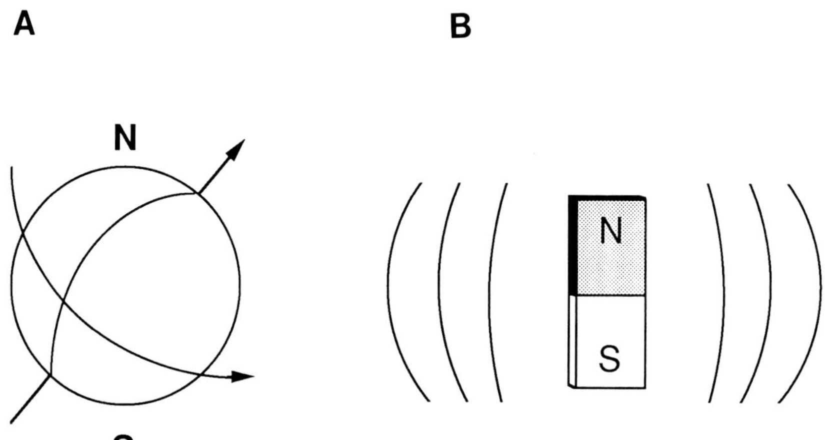

Figure 2–1. Magnetic dipole moment of the spinning proton (*A*) is similar to the fields produced by the bar magnet (*B*).

To produce an MR image, the patient is placed in a large, powerful, uniform magnetic field. Magnetic field strength is measured in units of tesla. The international unit of tesla (T) is the preferred term for medical MRI applications. One T is equal to 10,000 gauss. A gauss (G) is a unit of magnetic induction equal to the magnetic flux density that will induce an electromotive force of one one-hundred-millionth of a volt in each linear centimeter of a wire moving laterally with a speed of one centimeter per second at right angles to a magnetic flux. The magnetic field strength of most systems for medical MRI ranges from 2 T (20,000 G) to 0.02 T (200 G) in strength.

When protons are placed in a large external magnetic field, they line up with the applied field like tiny bar magnets or compasses. Protons can have only one of two discrete orientations or states, either parallel or antiparallel to the applied field.

The protons oriented parallel to the applied field are in a low-energy condition called the ground state. The orientation antiparallel to the applied field is a high-energy condition termed the excited state. When placed in the magnetic field, slightly more than half the protons orient in the ground state because of the effect of the applied field.

The difference in numbers in each state depends on the strength of the applied magnetic field, but is small in all cases. Approximately one additional proton out of one million will be in the ground state. Although this is an incredibly small difference, it is still sufficient to produce an MR signal.

The actual total number of protons in a given patient or sample is very large; every milliliter of water has approximately 10^{23} protons. Because of these extremely large numbers, it is more convenient to think of the sum of all the spin magnetic orientations as a single arrow or vector known as the *net magnetic field vector*. The population of protons placed in the static magnetic field would have a net magnetic field vector whose direction is parallel to the applied field because of the slightly greater number of protons in the parallel orientation.

The degree to which a material responds to the applied magnetic field is called its *magnetic susceptibility*. While most soft tissues of the body have similar susceptibilities, certain substances with unpaired electrons, which are said to be paramagnetic or ferromagnetic, have significantly different susceptibilities.

Resonance of the Nucleus

When placed in an applied magnetic field, protons do not line up precisely with the axis of the applied magnetic field, but precess (wobble) a few degrees off the central axis (Figs. 2–2, 2–3). The "hourglass" convention is used to combine the concepts of low and high energy states and proton precession in one drawing (see Fig. 2–3). The sum of this energy and precessional information is represented by the magnetization vector. This precession may be thought of as analogous to how a spinning gyroscope or top wobbles in the earth's gravitational field. The frequency of precession is known as the resonant or Larmor frequency, after the British physicist Sir Joseph Larmor. The resonant frequency is proportional to the strength of the applied magnetic field.

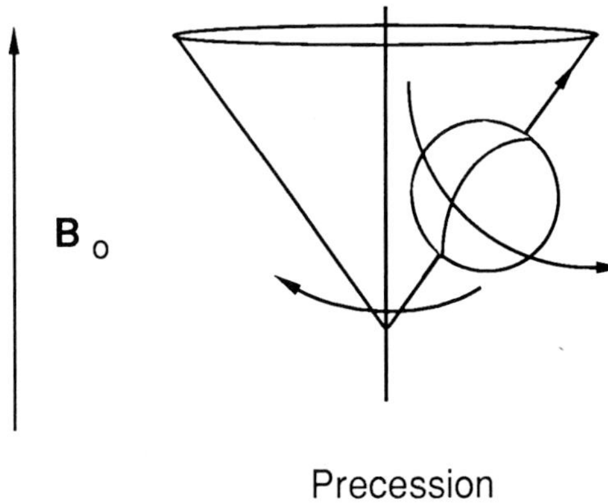

Figure 2–2. Precession of spinning proton about the axis of the applied field.

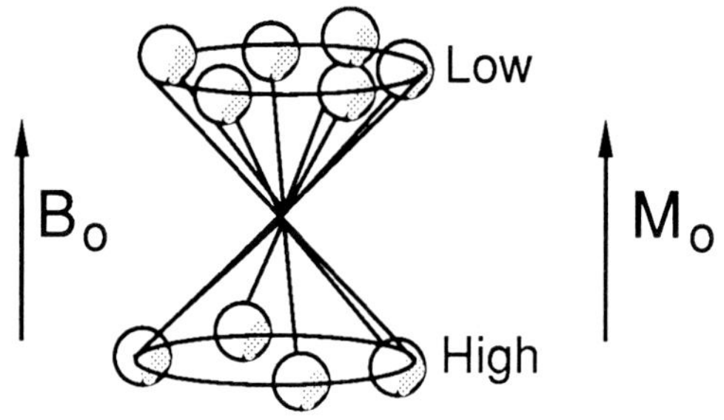

Figure 2–3. Hourglass representation of precession of protons and net magnetization (M_O). Slightly more protons are in the lower energy position and thus the magnetization vector (M_O) is directly parallel to the main field vector, B_O. Because the protons are out of phase or spread all around their orbital path, no component of the magnetization occurs in the transverse plane. Note that the protons are only allowed two possible orientations (high or low).

The fundamental relationship between precessional frequency and magnetic field strength is the basis for spatial encoding of the NMR signal, which makes all MR imaging possible:

$$W = B_o \times \text{Gyromagnetic Ratio}$$

W = Precessional frequency, B_o = static magnetic field strength, Gyromagnetic Ratio = constant for given nucleus.

To produce an MR signal, the net magnetization vector must be moved from the equilibrium longitudinal plane (parallel with the main magnetic field) into the transverse plane (perpendicular to B_o), where the magnetization vector causes a signal in radiofrequency (RF) receiver coils. To do this, a second magnetic field is applied (Fig. 2–4). In addition, protons must be brought into phase so they are all spinning together. When this is done, energy is added to the system and some of the nuclei move to the higher energy state. The effect is that the net magnetization (M_o) is now in the transverse plane for detection by RF coils.

The applied second magnetic field must be synchronized with the resonant frequency of the precessing spins to move the net magnetization into the transverse plane. This is analogous to pushing a child on a swing. A child and swing have a natural resonant frequency of oscillation based on their weight and length. To add energy effectively and increase the amplitude of the swinging motion, the frequency of pushing must be the same as (or in resonance with) the natural resonant frequency of the system.

The oscillating applied second magnetic field is the same as an RF pulse. The frequency of the oscillation is thus the resonant frequency of the system. The RF pulse in NMR changes the direction of the net magnetization to the transverse plane. This is necessary because the transverse orientation is the only one that can be detected by receiver RF coils. The amplitude and duration of the RF may be controlled to produce a range of angulations in the vector toward the transverse plane. The amount of angulation of the magnetization vector following the RF pulse from the parallel-antiparallel (B_o) axis toward the transverse plane is referred to as the tip or flip angle (θ).

The amount of angulation of the vector may be varied by using different amounts and durations of RF energy. A 180° RF pulse causes the magnetization to rotate 180° to the antiparallel direction. A 90° RF pulse moves the longitudinal magnetization into the transverse plane. RF pulses with flip angles of less than 90° result in a smaller magnetization vector in the transverse plane but are sometimes useful for fast scanning applications with gradient refocusing or field echoes.

In addition to moving the protons to a higher energy level, the RF pulse rephases the protons so that they are precessing in synchrony; that is, they are coherent. This has the effect of moving the net magnetization vector into the transverse plane (see Fig. 2–4). *Only when the protons are precessing in phase is it possible to detect a signal with the RF receiver coils.*

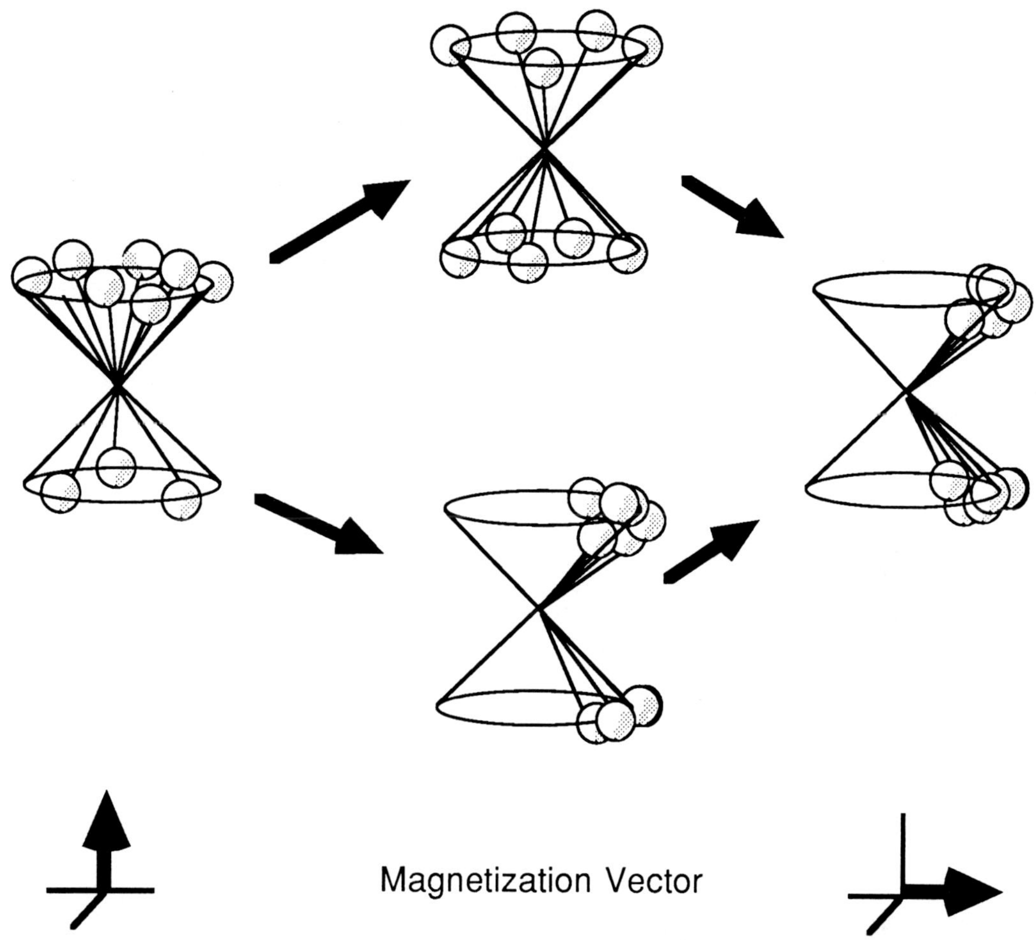

Figure 2–4. Following a 90° RF pulse, the net magnetization vector moves to the transverse plane. For this to occur, two processes must take place simultaneously. First, protons are moved to the higher energy state until there is an equal number of protons in the higher and lower energy states. Second, the protons are brought into coherence (all protons are precessing in phase). Although the protons can be in only one of two orientations, the resulting magnetization vector may be in a variety of directions.

Transverse Magnetization and the MR Signal

Following the RF pulse, the component of the magnetization in the *transverse plane* (that is, transverse magnetization) induces a current in RF receiver coils. The detected signal actually oscillates at the same frequency as the spin vector passes by it. This is analogous to creating a current in a generator by moving a magnet past a coil of wire. The detected RF output is the MR signal. All MRI contrast effects manifest themselves as alterations in the transverse magnetization detected by the RF coil.

The amplitude of the signal after a 90° pulse rapidly decays to zero. This damped oscillation is called a *free induction decay* or FID. The amplitude of the FID is proportional to the number of protons present in the sample, or proton density. The rate of decay is characterized by the exponential decay term T2* (pronounced "tee-too-star") (Fig. 2–5). This decay occurs because all magnetic fields are imperfect and protons in the sample in slightly different areas of the magnet all experience

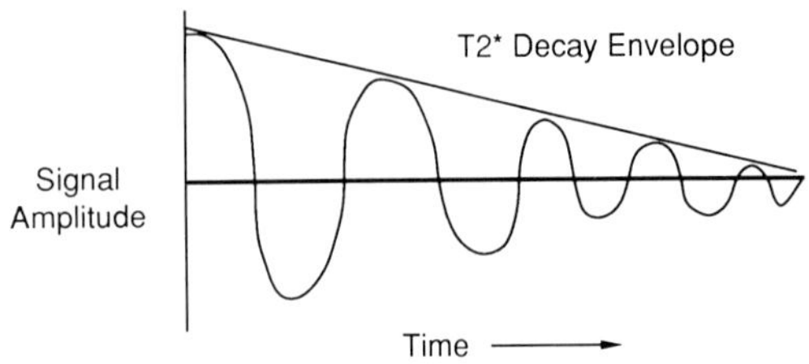

Figure 2–5. Free induction decay detected by the RF coil following a 90° pulse.

slightly different magnetic fields. The Larmor relationship states that the local magnetic field experienced by the protons determines the frequency of precession. Thus the variation in magnetic field translates into a variation in precessional frequency, which results in loss of coherence, or transverse dephasing (Fig. 2–6).

The loss of coherence results in loss of induced current in the RF receiver coil. Protons that are in phase produce a high-amplitude RF signal. If the same number of protons are precessing out of phase, the RF signal detected by the coil will be much less. Because this decay depends on the magnetic field imperfections rather than the patient, T2* contains little useful information about the *sample* and must be eliminated (see Fig. 2–6). In order to cancel out the spurious T2* information from the signal, the protons must be brought back into coherence. This recovery of the signal is referred to as an "echo" and is accomplished by the application of a 180° RF pulse (Fig. 2–7).

Although the echoes cancel out T2* effects due to magnetic field nonuniformities, *the recovered signal at the echo is still less than its original height as determined by the proton density* (Fig. 2–8). This important decrease in transverse magnetization results from irreversible losses in the sample itself due to T_1 and T_2 relaxation effects. These relaxation effects depend on the local environments of the pro-

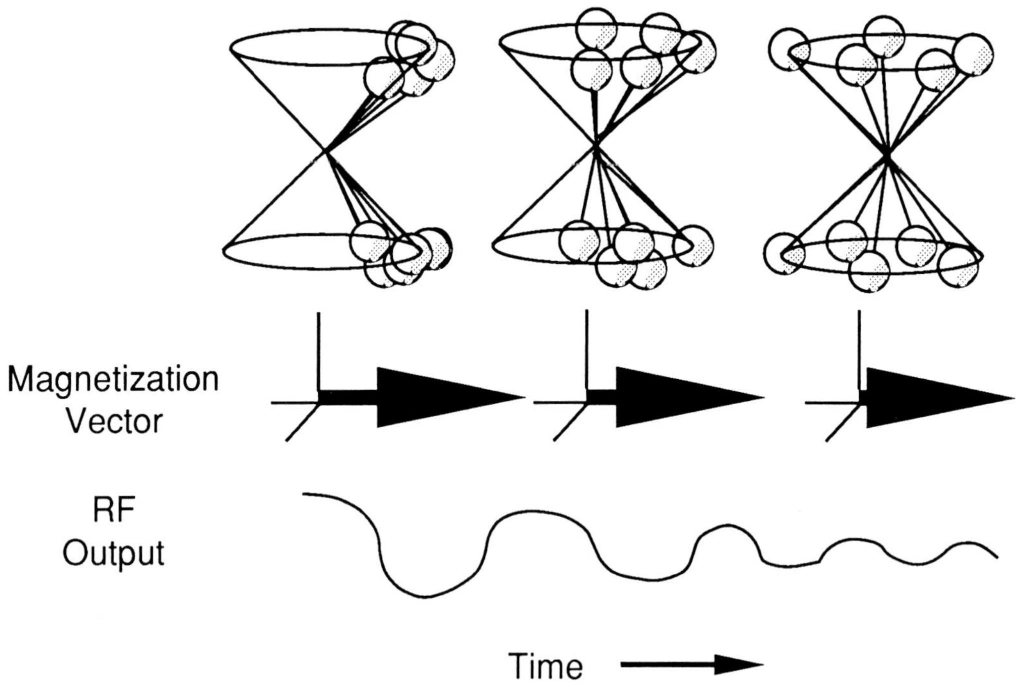

Figure 2–6. Dephasing of protons due to magnetic field inhomogeneities (T2* effects). As dephasing occurs, the transverse vector decreases, resulting in a smaller RF signal. Similar dephasing of protons (T_2 relaxation) occurs as a result of varying intrinsic magnetic fields created by adjacent nuclei.

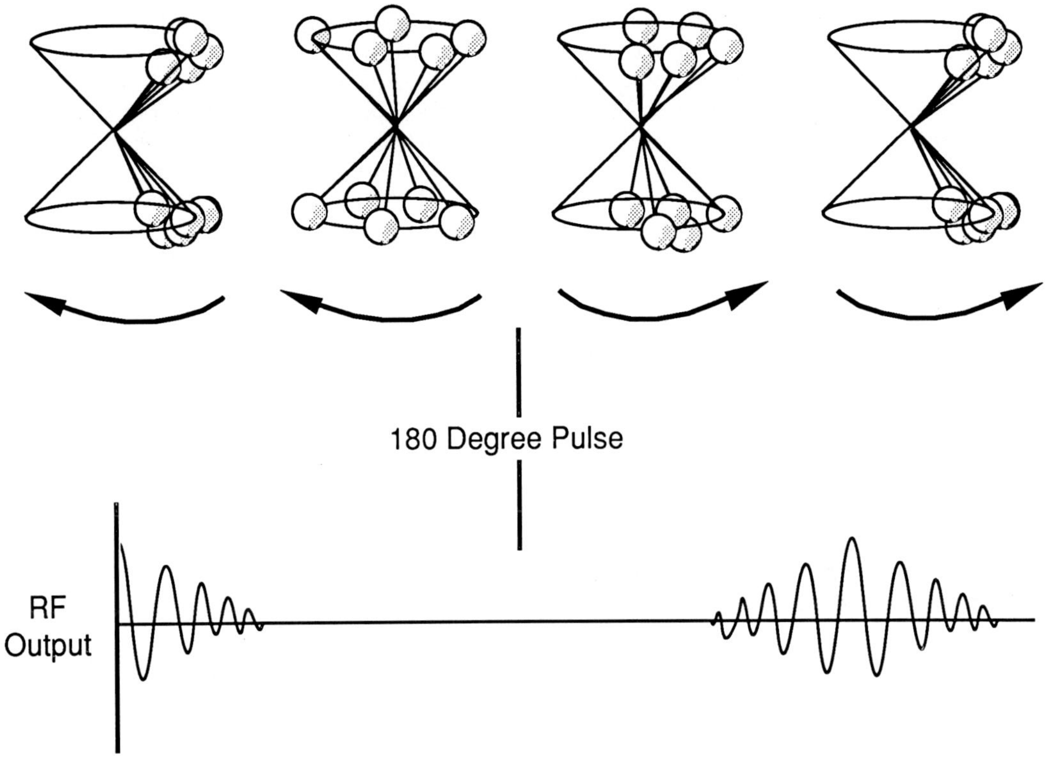

Figure 2–7. Diagram showing rephasing of the protons with a 180° RF pulse to produce a spin echo. As the protons regain coherence, the signal is again generated in the RF coil.

tons in the sample, which reflect chemical structure and ultimately human anatomy.

T_2 Relaxation

T_2 relaxation time is also known as spin-spin or transverse relaxation

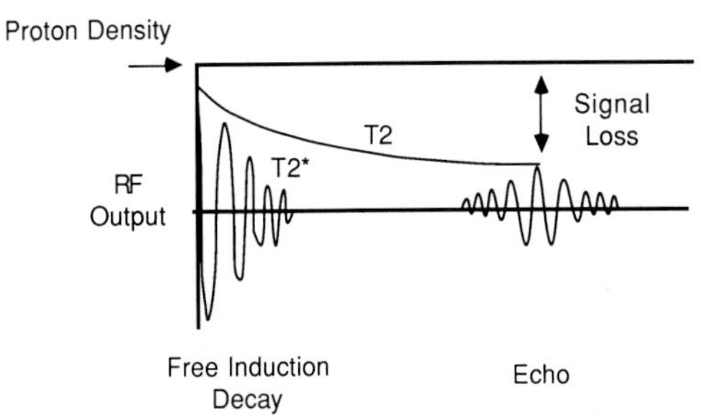

Figure 2–8. Despite the correction for T_2* effects through the use of the echo, there remains a signal loss due to tissue relaxation effects.

time. T_2 (like T2*) results from magnetic field inhomogeneities. Unlike the reversible dephasing that occurs due to static field T2* effects, however, T_2 dephasing is due to *randomly* varying intrinsic magnetic fields created by adjacent nuclei in the patient. For this reason, these effects are essentially irreversible and are not corrected by the spin echo or gradient echo. The term *spin-spin* refers to the fact that interactions between proton spins determine the rate of T_2 relaxation. No energy is actually lost, but rather energy is exchanged between spins. The term *transverse relaxation* is used because the T_2 dephasing effects occur in the transverse plane (see Fig. 2–6).

T_2, which is measured in milliseconds, may be thought of as the time necessary to reduce the transverse magnetization to 37% of its original value following the RF pulse. The relationship of signal intensity (I) to time for T_2 relaxation depends on the time from the 90° pulse until the echo (known as the echo time or TE), as well as on the T_2 of the tissue.

Unlike T2*, T_2 is the time constant for irreversible spin dephasing due to *intrinsic sample* properties. Typical values for T_2 in biological tissues are in the range of 50–500 milliseconds (always $\leq T_1$). T_2, unlike T_1 (discussion follows), is also essentially independent of magnetic field strength.

T_1 Relaxation

RF stimulation adds energy to the system and causes protons to move to a higher energy state. The dissipation of this energy to the lattice and the returning of protons to the lower energy state is known as T_1 relaxation (Fig. 2–9). The word *lattice* is a throwback to the days when NMR was used to investigate molecules in a crystalline lattice. Today the definition has been broadened to mean the surrounding magnetic environment. The lattice fields result from other nuclei and paramagnetic molecules. Just as the rate of oscillation of the RF affects the efficiency of stimulation, so the frequency of lattice field fluctuations affects the efficiency of T_1 relaxation.

T_1 in milliseconds is the time required for 63% of the longitudinal magnetization to recover following the RF pulse. The relationship of signal intensity (I) to time for T_1 relaxation depends on the time between 90° RF pulses (repetition time or TR) as well as the T_1 of the tissue.

Like T_2, T_1 is dependent on the sample and therefore provides useful medical information. Typical T_1 values for biological materials are 200–2000 millisecond ($>T_2$). While tissue T_2 values show very little dependence on field strength, T_1 tissue values actually increase slightly with increasing magnetic field strength. This is because the precessional frequencies, and thus the efficiency of T_1 relaxation, depend on the strength of the applied external magnetic field (B_o).[13] Although T_1 and T_2 relaxation occur simultaneously and each affects the image quality, they are essentially independent of one another.

Pulsing Sequence

The MR signal intensity (I) due to transverse magnetization is represented as pixel brightness on MR

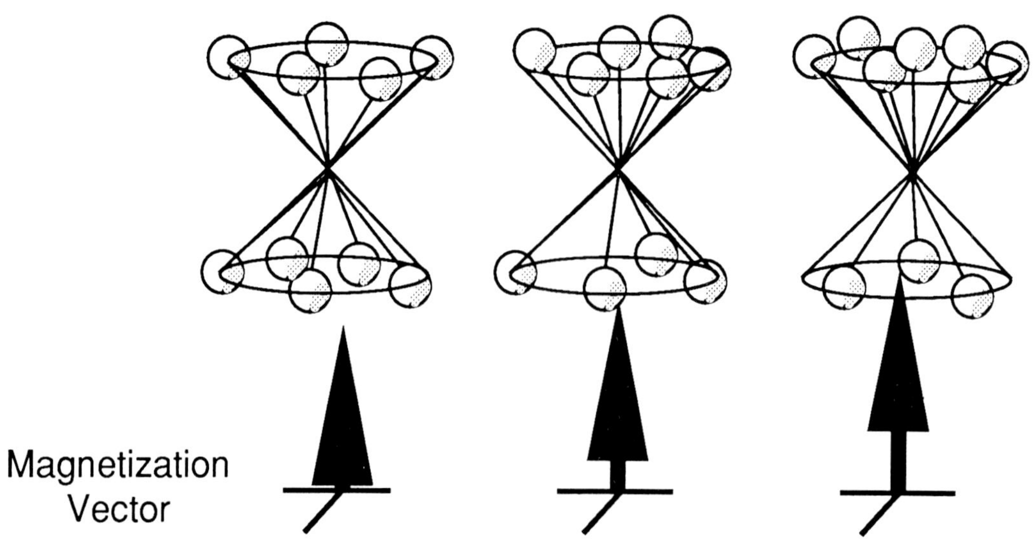

Figure 2–9. Recovery of longitudinal magnetization with time (T_1 relaxation).

images. This signal intensity reflects T_1 and T_2 relaxation times and several other factors. These factors include proton density, flow (both blood and CSF), magnetic susceptibility, and RF pulse characteristics. The relative contributions of some of these factors to the transverse magnetization can be manipulated by controlling the timing of the RF pulses (known as a pulsing or pulse sequence) to form the image. The timing values are the repetition time (TR) and echo time (TE).

MRI Contrast Mechanisms

MRI contrast arises from a complex relationship of many different factors, including proton density, T_1, T_2, magnetic susceptibility, and flow. The only variable directly measured is the transverse magnetization or signal intensity. Consequently, it is difficult to segregate from a single image the relative contribution to image contrast for each of these factors.[10,15,16,27,28]

The main approach to MRI tissue characterization through contrast effects is by rescanning the patient with different combinations of pulse sequences (TR and TE). A short TR, TE sequence produces what is referred to as a "T_1-weighted" image and a long TR, TE sequence, a "T_2-weighted" image. The change in signal intensity in each sequence permits the tissue characteristics (long T_1, short T_2, low proton density, and so forth) to be inferred.[25] In addition, changing the pulse sequence parameters permits the manipulation of image contrast with MRI in ways not possible with x-ray CT. The effects on signal intensity for T_1 and T_2 prolongation are opposite and thus tend to offset one another. This can be a problem because the majority of pathological conditions that affect the cell, whether neoplasia, inflammation, or edema, all tend to prolong T_1 and T_2 due to increased free water. Thus, the effects on the image of T_1 and T_2 tend to cancel each other out and may even cause an area of abnormality to be undetectable in an image. The use of various pulse sequences with different degrees of T_1 and T_2 weighting will help to avoid this situation.

Proton Density

Proton density in a sample determines the initial NMR signal amplitude (i.e., the height of the free induction decay). A large number of mobile protons results in a strong signal. This strong signal will then be further affected by T_1 and T_2 to produce either a strong or weak signal, depending on the entire set of other factors. Materials with high proton density include fat, CSF, blood, and other fluids.

If there are relatively few mobile protons in the tissue, the effects of T_1 and T_2 and the other parameters are negated. Therefore, regardless of how the pulse sequence is changed, if there are few mobile protons, the image will be low in intensity (black) (Fig. 2–10).

T_1 and T_2 Contrast Mechanisms

The proton density of tissue varies only about 10% throughout soft tissues of the body. Consequently, if proton density were its sole source of contrast, MRI would not be any better than x-ray CT in contrast resolution. Fortunately, proton density is not the main source of contrast in NMR. Instead, the remarkably superior soft-tissue contrast resolution in MRI compared with CT results from *T_1 and T_2 relaxation effects*. Many substances with similar proton and electron densities give different signal intensities as a result of marked differences in T_1 and T_2 values (Table 2–2).

Effects of T_1 and TR on Image Contrast

T_1 relaxation times allow for the differentiation of certain types of tissue. Substances with a short T_1 (high signal) can be fat, lipid-containing molecules, or proteinaceous fluid. Subacute hem-

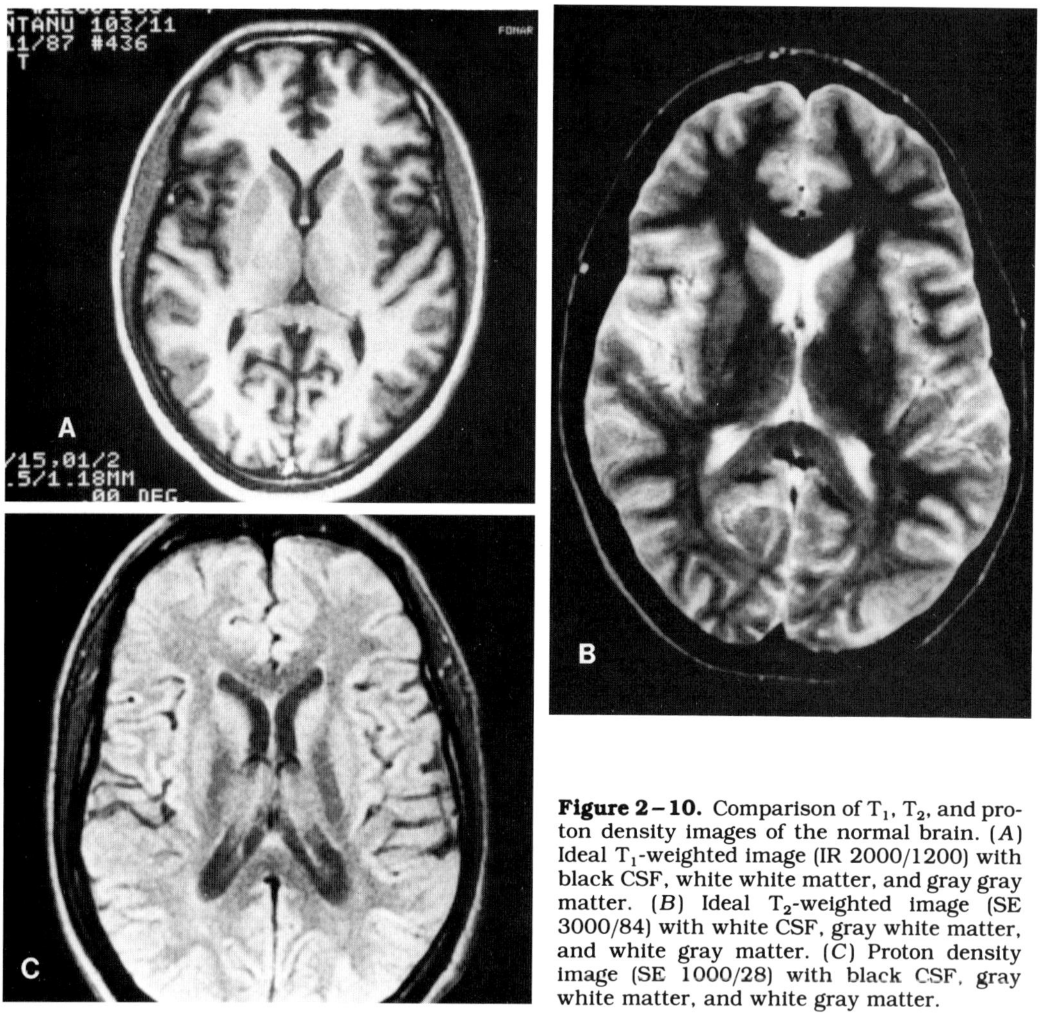

Figure 2–10. Comparison of T_1, T_2, and proton density images of the normal brain. (*A*) Ideal T_1-weighted image (IR 2000/1200) with black CSF, white white matter, and gray gray matter. (*B*) Ideal T_2-weighted image (SE 3000/84) with white CSF, gray white matter, and white gray matter. (*C*) Proton density image (SE 1000/28) with black CSF, gray white matter, and white gray matter.

Table 2–2 COMPARISON OF REPRESENTATIVE PROTON DENSITY, T_1 AND T_2 VALUES*

Tissue	*Proton Density*	*T_1 (ms)*	*T_2 (ms)*
CSF	10.8	2000	250
Gray matter	10.5	475	118
White matter	11.0	300	133
Fat	10.9	150	150
Muscle	11.0	450	64
Liver	10.0	250	44

*Values at midfield strength (0.5 T)

orrhage, melanin, or other paramagnetic substances in low concentration (such as chelated gadolinium) may also shorten the T_1. Substances with long T_1 (low signal) include neoplasms (both benign and malignant), inflammation, and any kind of cellular alteration that opens cell membranes and increases bulk water. The differences in image intensity due to T_1 relaxation values (T_1 contrast) (Fig. 2–11) can be increased by the use of certain pulse sequences (Table 2–3).

To maximize the difference in signal intensity based on tissue T_1 times (T_1 contrast), the TR time in the pulse sequence is shortened. This results in a "T_1-weighted image." With longer TR time, both tissues have fully recovered their longitudinal magnetization and have similar signal intensities and little contrast.

Shortening the TR sequence (for ex-

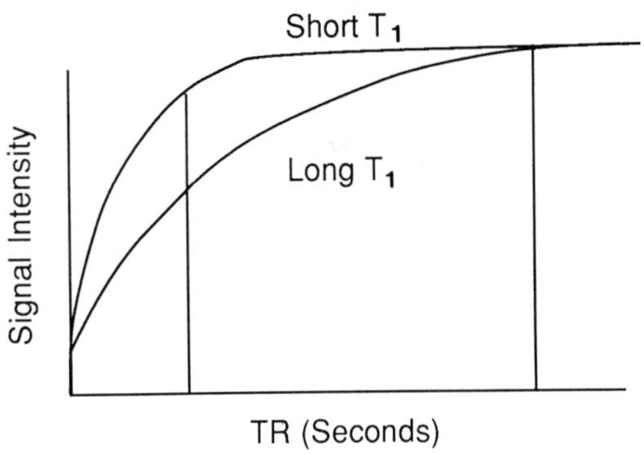

Figure 2–11. Effects of TR and tissue T_1 values on image intensity and contrast. The material depicted in the upper curve has a short T_1 and the one in the lower curve a longer T_1. T_1 contrast is maximal with a short TR and signal-to-noise ratio (S/N) is highest with a long TR.

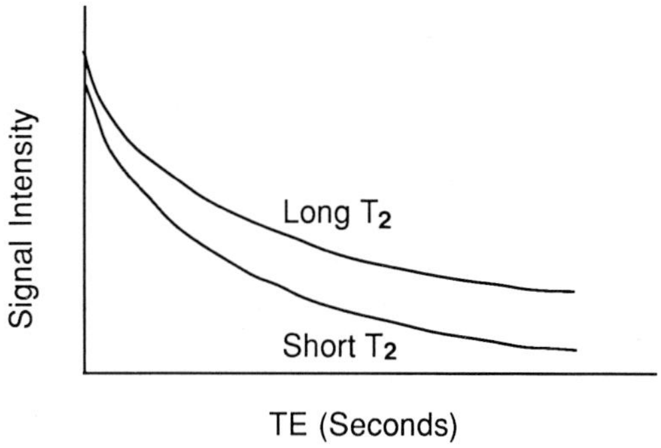

Figure 2–12. Effects of TE and tissue T_2 values on image intensity and contrast. The substance in the upper curve has a long T_2 compared to that in the lower curve. T_2 contrast is maximized with a long TE, and SNR is highest with a short TE.

ample, TR 300 milliseconds, TE 30 milliseconds) affects other aspects of image quality. As the TR is shortened, although the T_1 contrast increases, the overall signal to noise ratio (S/N) decreases. Thus, in order to optimize S/N, it is necessary to use a relatively long TR compared to the T_1 of the tissues (that is, TR 2000–3000 milliseconds).

Effects of TE and T_2 on Image Contrast

T_2 relaxation times (like T_1 and other tissue parameters) allow certain types of tissues to be distinguished (Fig. 2–12). Substances with a short T_2 (low signal) are often iron-containing, such as blood breakdown products and nonheme forms of iron such as ferritin. Substances with long T_2 (high signal) include neoplasms (both benign and malignant), inflammation, and practically any kind of cellular alteration that opens cell membranes to increase the intracellular water content (Table 2–4).

To maximize the difference in signal intensity based on T_2 times, the TE time in the pulse sequence is lengthened. This results in a "T_2-weighted image." With a shorter TE time, the tissues have similar signal intensities and little contrast, because sufficient time has not elapsed for differences in T_2 to cause dephasing of the spins.

In producing a heavily T_1-weighted image, a short TR is used to maximize

Table 2–3 T_1 EFFECTS ON IMAGE APPEARANCE (T_1-WEIGHTED IMAGE; SHORT TR, SHORT TE)

SHORT T_1 (WHITE)
Fat
Proteinaceous fluid
Subacute bleed (methemoglobin)
Other paramagnetic substance with proton-electron dipole-dipole interaction in low concentration (gadolinium, melanin?)
LONG T_1 (DARK)
Neoplasm
Edema
Inflammation
Pure fluid
CSF

Table 2–4 T_2 EFFECTS ON IMAGE APPEARANCE (T_2-WEIGHTED IMAGE; LONG TR, LONG TE)

SHORT T_2 (DARK)
Iron deposition in the liver
Magnetic susceptibility effect (hemosiderin, deoxyhemoglobin, ferritin)
LONG T_2 (WHITE)
Neoplasm
Edema
Inflammation
Gliosis
Pure fluid
CSF

T_1 contrast and a short TE to minimize T_2 contrast. Conversely, a heavily T_2-weighted image requires use of a long TE to maximize T_2 contrast and a long TR to minimize T_1 contrast.

Finally, a short-TE and long-TR sequence maximizes the S/N in the image. This is accomplished at the expense of T_1 and T_2 contrast. Because of the lack of strong T_1 or T_2 contrast, these high-S/N images are sometimes referred to as *proton density* or spin density images (see Fig. 2–10C).

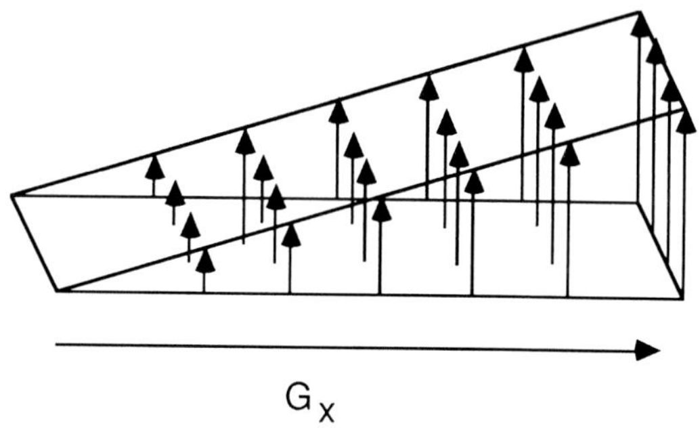

Figure 2–13. The magnetic field (indicated by arrows) varies in a linear fashion along G_X to produce a gradient.

FORMATION OF THE MR IMAGE

The application of NMR technology to the production of medical images is based on the ability to localize the NMR signal accurately. The technique of MR image formation is different from all other computed tomographic imaging techniques. The concept of imaging with magnetic resonance is to measure the NMR signal from various points in the human body nondestructively and noninvasively.[4,17]

Currently, most clinical magnetic resonance imagers use *sequential plane (2-D) imaging*, which allows clinically practical scan times (for example, 2–10 minutes per image set acquisition). *Volume imaging (3-D)* techniques are under investigation and are promising for certain clinical applications.

Magnetic Field Gradients

Magnetic field gradients are the key tools that allow MR imaging to occur. They allow the signal to be localized in space. A gradient is a variation in magnetic field with distance (Fig. 2–13), and specifically a linear variation in magnetic field from weaker to stronger along one dimension of the patient. The amount of variation is actually very small, typically two to three orders of magnitude less than the static magnetic field of the system.

When a magnetic field gradient is superimposed on the existing static magnetic field, the resonant frequency of the protons varies along the gradient according to the local magnetic field. Thus, the frequency of the protons varies with spatial location along the axis of the applied gradient.

Slice Select Gradient (G_{ss})

To select a slice, a linear magnetic field gradient is applied during presentation of the 90° RF pulse in order to stimulate a plane of finite thickness. With a patient in the tomograph, an axial slice may be selected by turning on the gradient, runs from head to toe. This has the effect of speeding up the resonant frequency from the top of the head and slowing down the frequency which runs near the feet. Concomitant with this gradient, the 90° pulse is applied. Because this gradient allows the selection of the image slice, it is termed the slice select gradient (G_{ss}) (Fig. 2–14). The location of the slice along the gradient is determined by the center frequency of the 90° RF pulse.

The slice thickness can be determined by controlling the range of frequencies used in the 90° pulse. This range of frequencies is called the bandwidth. A larger bandwidth will result in a thicker slice and a smaller bandwidth, a thinner slice.

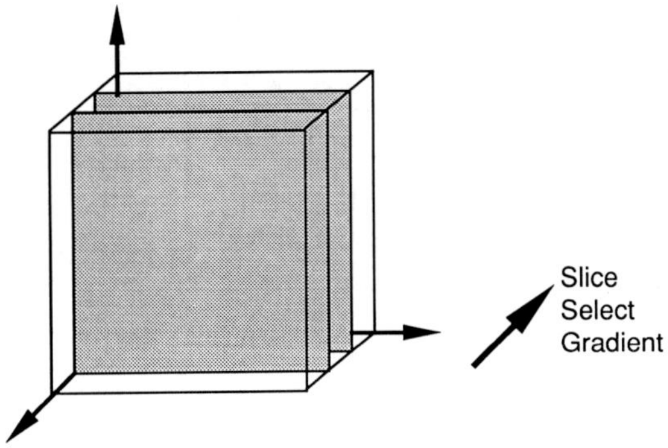

Figure 2–14. The slice select gradient is turned on during the application of the 90° RF pulse to allow selective stimulation of a plane of protons (gray area).

Two-Dimensional Fourier Transformation (2D-FT) Imaging

Most modern MR scanners use a method of image reconstruction called two-dimensional Fourier transformation reconstruction (2D-FT).[11]

Three steps are used in 2D-FT imaging technique: slice selection, phase encoding, and frequency encoding. Slice selection in 2D-FT imaging is similar to projection reconstruction. One gradient is activated during the 90° pulse and this gradient, whichever it is, becomes the slice select gradient. The next step uses phase encoding, a concept not entirely familiar from x-ray CT experience. One gradient has already been used to select the tissue slice. Two gradients are left with which to encode the remaining two spatial dimensions and make the image.

At this point, as shown by step 1 of Figure 2–15, all the protons have the same phase angles following the 90° RF pulse (T2* effects are ignored for now because they are handled by the echo.) The frequency is also the same for all nine protons because all are experiencing the same magnetic field, as determined by the main magnet. Activating one of the two remaining gradients has the effect of changing the magnetic field strength slightly along its axis. This in turn changes the Larmor frequencies of the protons according to their position in the gradient. This is shown in step 2 of Figure 2–15. Now the locations of the protons along the axis are mapped with their frequencies. When the gradient is first activated, the protons are still in phase. After a few milliseconds, because the protons have different frequencies according to their location along the gradient, they no longer stay in phase. The dephasing that occurs, however, takes place in a very specific manner according to the protons' location along the gradient, as shown in step 3. After a period of time, the protons at the lower field end have a lower frequency and a phase angle of 3 o'clock. The intermediate protons have a higher frequency and a phase angle of 6 o'clock. The protons at the high field end then have the highest frequency and a phase angle of 9 o'clock.

The last step in the process is shown in step 4. At this point, the gradient is turned off and all the protons return to a constant frequency, as determined by the main magnetic field strength. The spatial locations of the spins along the gradient were encoded briefly by their frequency. When the gradient was turned off, though, all the protons returned to uniform frequency and the spatial information encoded by frequency was lost.

Actually, the "memory" of that gradient was preserved by the proton spins in the form of their phase angles. Although the frequencies all returned to a constant, the phase angles remained different according to the location along that axis. If a proton has a phase angle of 3 o'clock, then the proton is somewhere in the left column. For a phase angle of 9 o'clock, that proton is somewhere in the right column. Thus, location has been encoded with phase. For this reason, this gradient is called the *phase encoding gradient* and the image axis along the gradient is called the phase encoding axis. Unlike the slice select gradient, which must be activated during the 90° RF pulse, the phase encoding gradient is turned on

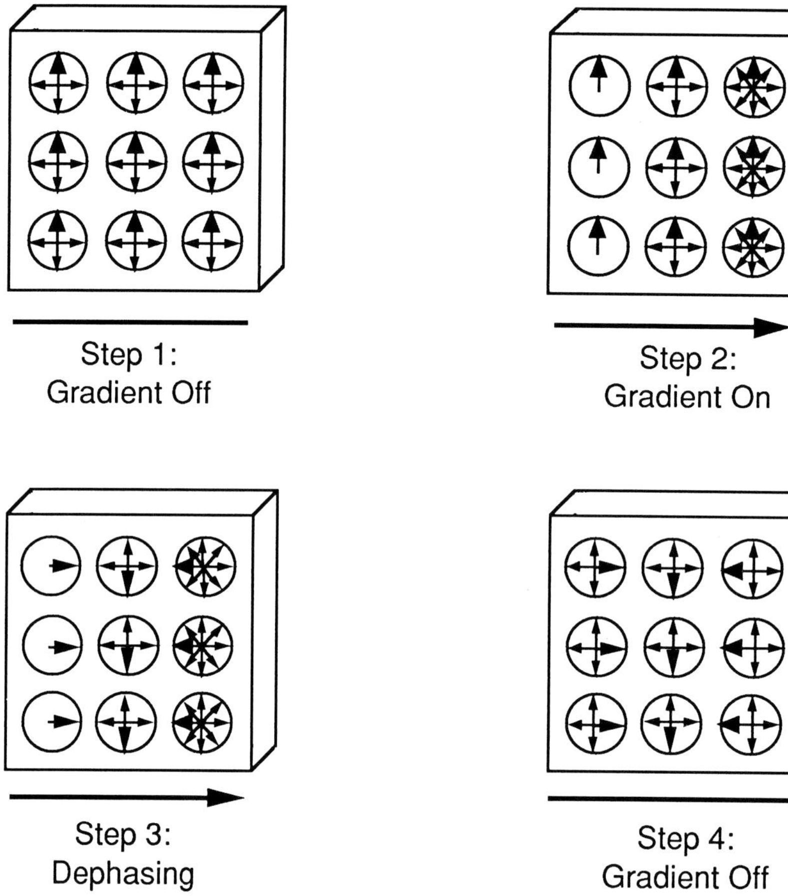

Figure 2–15. Phase encoding. Frequency is indicated by the number of arrows present and phase is indicated by the direction of the large arrow. With the gradient turned off (step 1), all protons are at the same frequency and phase. When the gradient is turned on (step 2), the protons immediately change frequency according to their position along the gradient. After a few milliseconds, the protons also dephase along the gradient (step 3). Finally (step 4), the phase-encoding gradient is turned off and all the protons return to precessing at the same frequency. The phase angles, however, remain changed according to the position along the gradient that was turned on moments before.

and off in the absence of any RF stimulation.

Frequency encoding is the last spatial dimension to encode and the last gradient to use. Before this last gradient is turned on, the spins are all at the same frequency, as shown in step 1 of Figure 2–16. The phase angles are different depending on the locations of the spins along the other axis, from the prior application of the phase encoding step.

When the third gradient is activated, just as before, the magnetic field changes along the gradient and the frequencies of the protons also change according to their spatial location. The only thing different is that this gradient is turned on *during the echo collection*. Therefore, this frequency-encoded spatial information is detected in the RF output of the echo. For this reason, the last gradient is referred to as the *frequency encoding gradient* and the image axis along the gradient is the frequency encoded or readout axis. The frequency encoding gradient thus creates a one-to-one correspondence between the frequency of the return signal and the position of the source along the readout direction. Again, the location of the proton along the frequency-encoded axis can be determined completely from the strength of the readout gradient and the difference between the

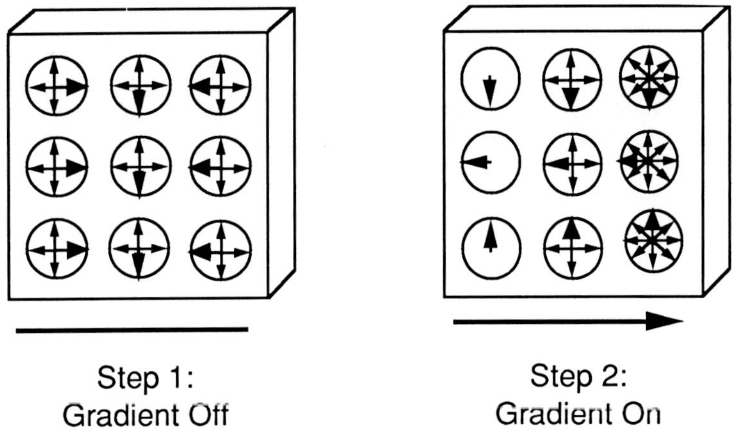

Figure 2–16. Frequency encoding. With the gradient turned off (step 1), all protons are precessing at the same frequency. The phase angles are different due to the effects of the prior phase-encoding step. When the gradient is turned on (step 2), the spin frequencies change according to the location along the gradient.

return signal frequency and the resonant frequency of the background field.

Pulse Sequence Timing Diagram

Split-second timing is required for turning on and off the slice select, phase encoding, and frequency encoding gradients and coordinating them with the 90° RF pulse and the echo. The pulse sequence timing diagram is a graphic display that includes each of the events activated (Fig. 2–17).

Image Formation Matrix

Despite the complexity of gradient actions necessary to encode spatially the signal that is detected in the echo, that

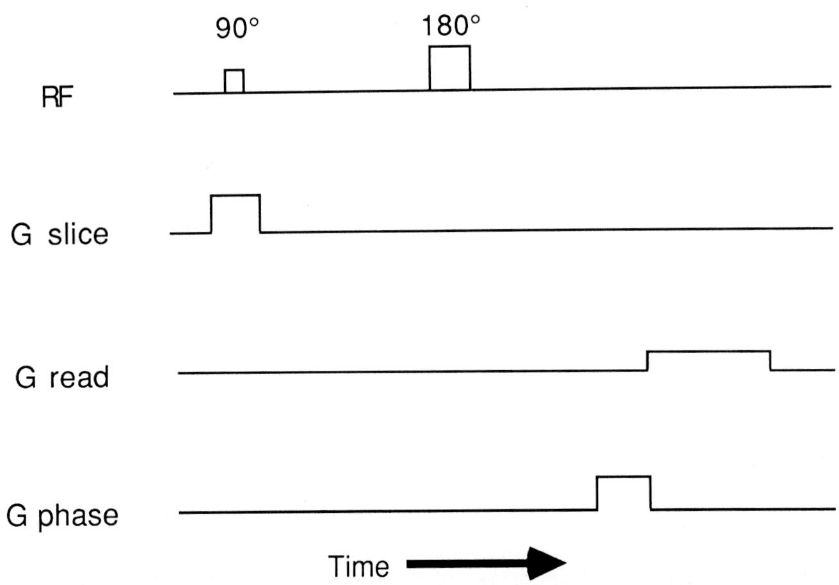

Figure 2–17. Standard spin echo pulse sequence timing diagram. The slice select (G slice), readout (G read), and phase-encoding (G phase) gradients must be activated at specific times.

single signal is not enough to make an entire image. Instead, the process of producing the signal must be repeated many times. Each repetition of this process is referred to as a view (level, or phase encoding step). Modern MR imagers typically require from 128 to 384 of these steps to form an image.

The slice select gradient is turned on the same amount with each view. This is necessary to select the same slice repetitively. The readout gradient also remains the same with each of these steps. The only change is in the phase encoding gradient, which varies through many different steps from shallow to steep. The shallow-gradient acquisitions sample low-spatial-frequency information in the image, and steeper portions sample the high-spatial-frequency aspects of the image. Each time the phase encoding gradient is turned on, an echo is collected. The echoes are then digitized and loaded into a two-dimensional data acquisition matrix (Fig. 2–18). This display is referred to as *k space*. The data are then Fourier transformed in two dimensions (2D-FT), the phase-frequency information is mapped onto the image by location, and the signal amplitude information for each pixel is displayed as brightness.

Spatial Resolution

The boundaries of diseased tissue are often recognized by subtle alterations in normal anatomy or slight blurring of fascial planes. Consequently, spatial resolution in MR imaging is important. A complete discussion of the issues of spatial resolving power for MRI is beyond the scope of this chapter. Such a discussion involves S/N, image contrast, motion, and other factors addressed in detail elsewhere.[7,10,15,16,18,26–28]

Spatial resolution in MR images is set by how finely the image is divided into pixels (i.e., image matrix size). The other factor that affects the size of each pixel, and thus spatial resolution, is the size of the image or field of view (FOV). Both factors must be considered in determining pixel size.

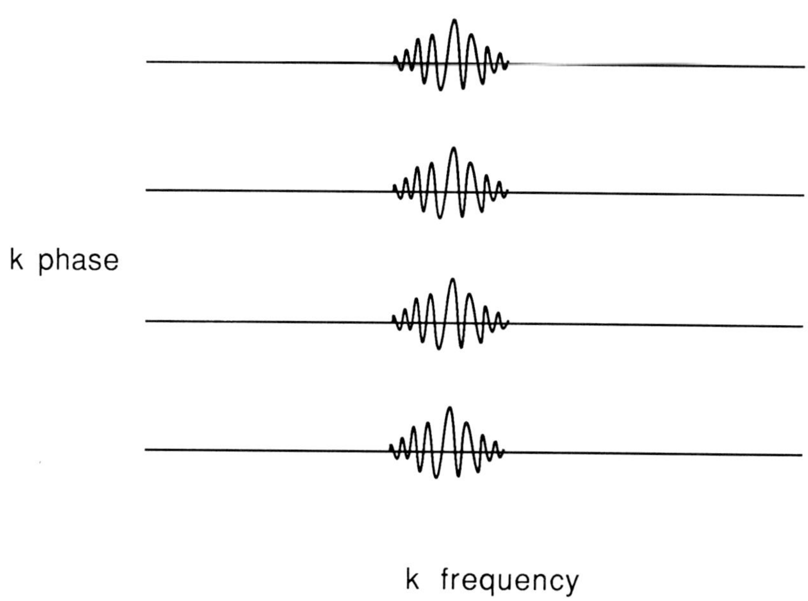

Figure 2–18. Normal spin echo k-space data acquisition. Each frequency axis line contains the signal from one echo. This information is digitized and stored in the acquisition matrix. This process is repeated until the matrix is filled.

$$\text{Pixel Size} = \frac{\text{Field of View}}{\text{Matrix Size}}$$

For example, a 4 × 4 image matrix acquired using a 4 × 4-cm field of view will result in 1 × 1-cm pixels. Spatial resolution can be increased in either of two ways. The data matrix can be increased to 8 × 8 with a constant FOV and the pixel size will decrease to 0.5 × 0.5 cm (Fig. 2–19). This approach requires an increase of acquisition time because of the greater number of phase encoding steps with the larger matrix size. Alternatively, the matrix size can be kept constant and the field of view decreased to 2 × 2 cm. This also results in a 0.5 × 0.5-cm pixel. This approach decreases the S/N and increases certain types of aliasing artifacts.

Multiecho Pulse Sequence

The time between 90° pulses (repetition time or TR) is sometimes termed the *duty cycle* because it represents the total amount of time required for each view or phase encoding step in image formation. The time in each duty cycle from the 90° pulse until the echo is collected is referred to as the echo time or TE. This time is typically ten to one hundred times shorter than the TR for many pulse sequences. Therefore, most of the time in the duty cycle is spent in waiting and not in collecting data. This inefficiency occurs because the long TR ultimately determines scan time.

Long TRs are costly in scan time and patient throughput. Shortening the duty cycle by decreasing the TR results

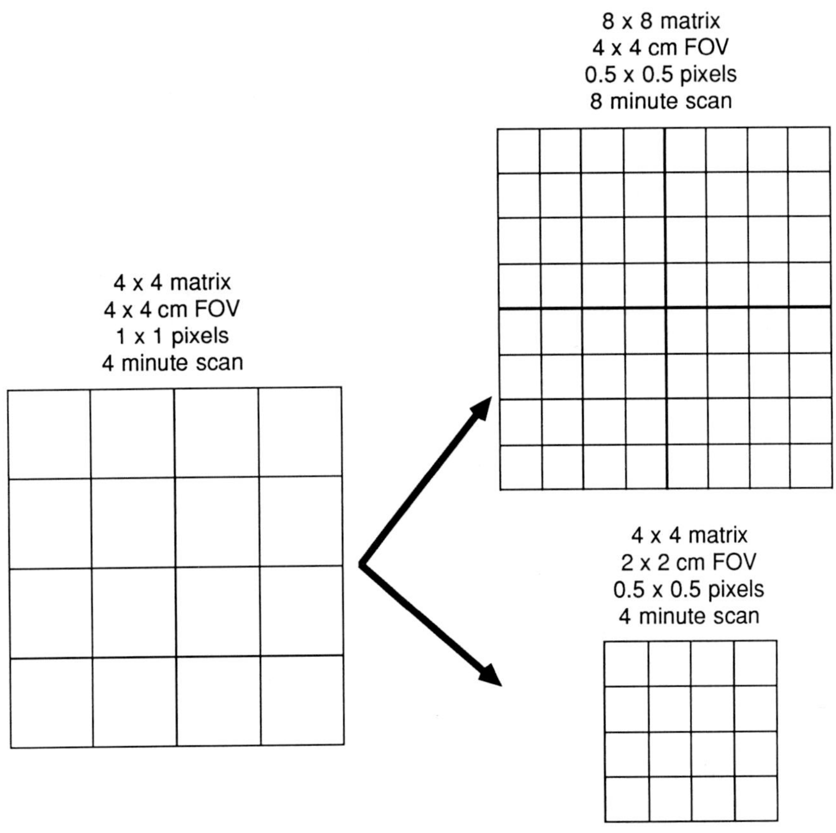

Figure 2–19. Field of view (FOV) demonstration showing spatial resolution–time trade-offs. Spatial resolution can be increased by using a larger matrix at the expense of increased acquisition time. Spatial resolution may also be increased while preserving acquisition time by using a smaller FOV at the expense of increased aliasing artifacts and decreased S/N.

in faster image formation times, but also affects image quality by lowering the S/N and increasing T_1-weighting of the image. Consequently, although data are not being collected during most of the cycle, a long dead time is necessary for T_1 recovery to occur, and is especially necessary for T_2-weighted images.

The *multiecho technique* provides one means of using the dead time effectively. With this technique the first echo is collected and, after a brief delay (for example, $\frac{1}{2}$ TE), another 180° pulse is given and a second echo is collected a short time later (for example, TE) (Fig. 2–20). Data are then collected onto a separate matrix and transformed into a second image. This can be done repeatedly to produce third, fourth, and fifth echoes. In general, the longer the TR relative to the TE (that is, the greater the dead time), the more echoes can be collected. For practical reasons, only a first and second echo are obtained in most situations. Both the first and second echo images are obtained in the same amount of total image acquisition time required for just the first echo.

Both the first and second echo images will have the same TR time and will involve the same slice, since they both have the same 90° pulse and slice select gradient. The second image will be more T_2-weighted than the first because of the longer TE. Initially the TEs used were multiples of each other for multiecho sequences such as TR 2000 millisecond with TEs of 28–56 or 56–112 millisecond. These are called *symmetrical multiecho* acquisition because the TEs are symmetrical. As described below, asymmetrical multiecho acquisition was developed later.

Multiecho sequences are efficient in that two image sets are obtained in the amount of time it takes to acquire only one; however, the contrast separation between the two sequences is small. This is because both sequences must have the same TR. Thus, the short-TE sequence may not be particularly T_1-weighted and the long-TE sequence may not be particularly T_2-weighted.

To improve this situation, *asymmetric multiecho* acquisition sequences were developed. These allow greater separation of TEs for improved contrast distinction. Instead of a TR 2000 millisecond, TE 28–56 millisecond double echo, a 2000/20–90 double echo can be performed. In many cases this provides sufficient contrast separation of the images, but occasionally, when heavy T_1- and T_2-weighting are required, two separate pulse sequences must be acquired; this involves a greater cost of time.

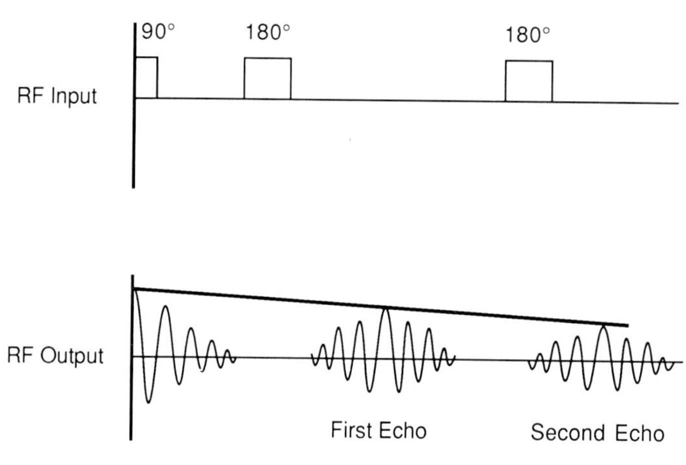

Figure 2–20. Multiecho pulse sequence. After the first echo is collected following the 180° RF pulse, a second 180° pulse is given to refocus the protons and form a second echo.

Multislice Pulse Sequence

Another option for reducing dead time in the duty cycle is to obtain multiple slices. Instead of just stimulating a single slice and then waiting, after the echo another 90° – 180° pulse train can be delivered to select a second slice. This results in the acquisition of multiple slices in the same amount of time it takes to obtain a single slice. For this to work, a change in the slice select gradient or the 90° RF pulse frequency is needed for each new slice. Thus, a new slice is selected in a different location from the first so that the relaxation processes do not interfere with one another (Fig. 2–21).

Either multislice or multiecho techniques may be used in MR imaging to take advantage of the "dead time" in the duty cycle. Often both multislice and multiecho procedures are performed in the same sequence. The only constraint is the finite time from the TE until the next 90° pulse (that is, TR-TE). Consequently, one slice can be obtained with 10 echoes, or 10 slices with one echo, or, most commonly, 5 slices with 2 echoes.

Orthogonal Scan Plane Selection

MRI systems have three separate physical magnetic field gradient coils, each capable of creating a gradient field along one of three orthogonal directions. These are usually chosen to coincide with the principal axes of the patient: superior to inferior (z axis); anterior to posterior (y axis); and left to right (x axis). If each of the three physical coils is assigned a separate gradient function (slice selection, phase encoding, or frequency encoding), images in the three principal planes may be obtained. For each of these three planes, there are two choices for the phase encoding direction. When an axial scan is desired, Gz becomes the slice select gradient and there is a default assignment for the phase encoding and readout gradients. Selection of the scan plane is thus the assignment of function to these physical gradients (see Fig. 2–17).

A given gradient becomes the slice select gradient if it is turned on during the 90° slice select pulse. Another gradient becomes the readout gradient if it is

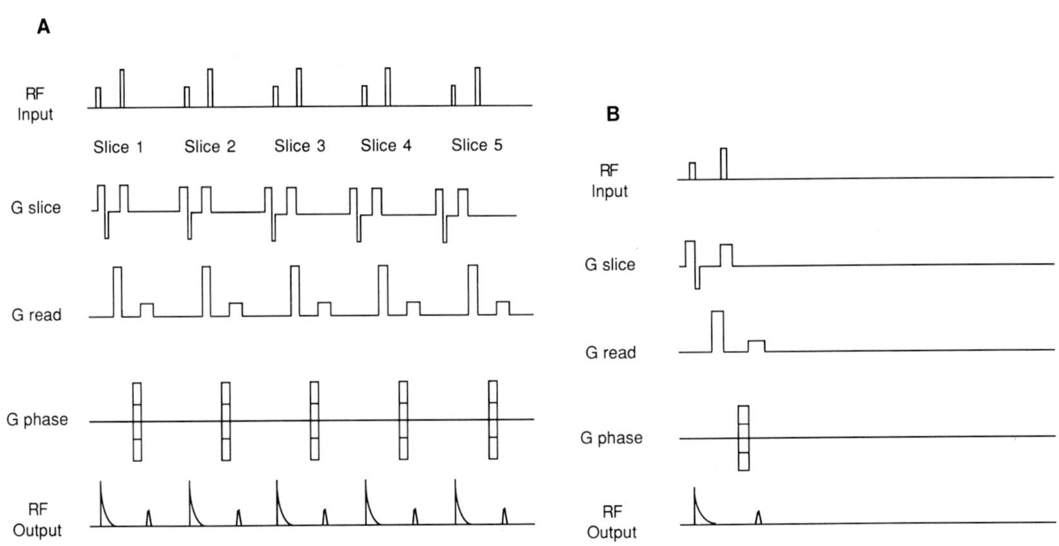

Figure 2–21. (*A*) Multislice pulse sequence timing diagram for a five-slice acquisition. The slice select gradient (G slice) changes for each 90° pulse in order to specify a new slice. (*B*) Comparable single-slice acquisition timing diagram.

turned on during the readout. Timing is key to image formation and this is why the representation of these choices is termed a pulse sequence timing diagram.

Effects of Varying TE

Varying TR and TE has many effects on MR image quality in addition to changes in contrast. TR and TE determine slice thickness, degree of slice contiguity, imaging time, S/N and the number of echoes or slices in a simultaneous acquisition. As TE is increased, the weighting of the image is increased and the overall signal-to-noise ratio is lowered. The S/N effect is somewhat offset because with longer TEs, greater bandwidth reduction is possible for S/N improvement. Since the dead time decreases as TE increases with a constant TR, the number of slices or echoes possible in multimode decreases. Lengthening TE has no effect on overall scan time.

Effects of Varying TR

Decreasing TR results in an increase in T_1 weighting and a decrease in S/N. This S/N loss is somewhat offset by the decreased overall scan time with shorter TRs. This allows some improvement in S/N through signal averaging in the same scan time. As TR decreases with a constant TE, the dead time decreases and the number of slices or echoes possible in multimode decreases.

MRI INSTRUMENTATION

All MRI instruments have the same basic subsystems. If the computer, data storage, image display, and keyboard (which are similar to those found in other cross-sectional imaging machines such as x-ray CT) are excluded, MR imaging instrumentation can be divided into three main component subsystems: (1) main magnetic field, (2) gradient magnetic field generators, and (3) radiofrequency (RF) transmitter and receiver.

For each of these components, specific performance parameters and options are available. For each choice, close attention must be paid to the equipment-performance tradeoffs. Any improvement in S/N, contrast, or spatial resolution is usually offset by longer scan times, increased cost, or increased sensitivity to artifacts.

Main Magnetic Field

The key component in any MR imager is the main magnet.[20] This component produces a uniform static magnetic field (also known as the B_0 field) upon which is superimposed magnetic field gradients and radiofrequency pulses as necessary for imaging.

Four different types of magnets are available for generation of the main magnetic field: permanent, air core resistive, iron core resistive, and superconductive. The type of magnet used to generate the B_0 field is in many ways irrelevant as far as the individual protons are concerned. Just as the electric current that flows from a wall outlet is the same whether it is generated from a nuclear, hydroelectric, or coal-burning electric power plant, the protons respond to the B_0 field of the magnet regardless of the type of magnet used to produce it. There are, however, considerable differences in site considerations, operating costs, main field axis, and other factors with the different types of magnets (Table 2–5).

PERMANENT MAGNET

The permanent magnet design constitutes the simplest approach to creating a magnetic field. Permanent magnets consist of large blocks of ferromagnetic materials similar to those used in simple horseshoe magnets (Figs. 2–22, 2–23). The magnetic field is generated between the two poles of

Table 2–5 MAGNET TYPES

Magnet Technology	*Fringe Magnetic Fields*	*Field Axis*	*Installation*	*Upper Limit Field Strength*	*Operating Cost ($ million)*
Permanent	Low	Vertical	Unassembled	0.3 T	0.5→
Air core resistive	Medium	Horizontal	Preassembled	0.2 T	1.0→
Iron core resistive	Low	Vertical	Unassembled	0.6 T	1.0→
Superconductive	High	Horizontal	Preassembled	4.0 T+	1.5→

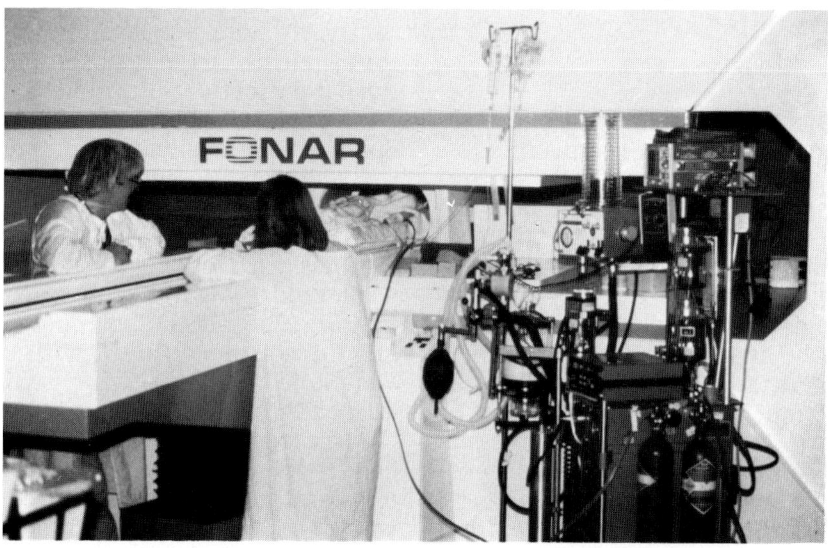

Figure 2–22. Permanent magnet system. The vertical field and contained flux return path allow the use of ferromagnetic life-support equipment in close proximity to the magnet.

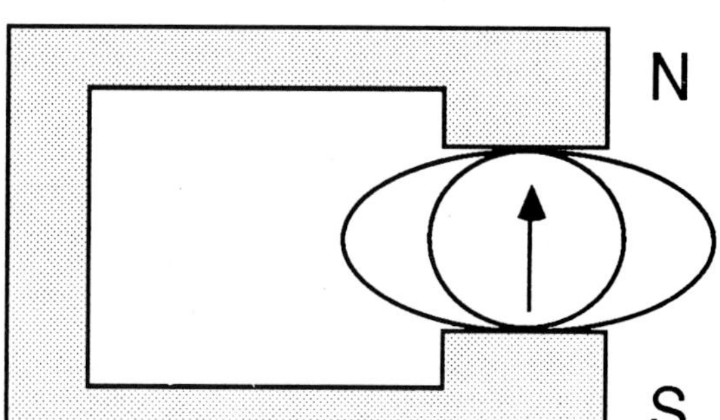

Figure 2–23. Permanent magnet. The vertical field is produced between the two magnet end plates.

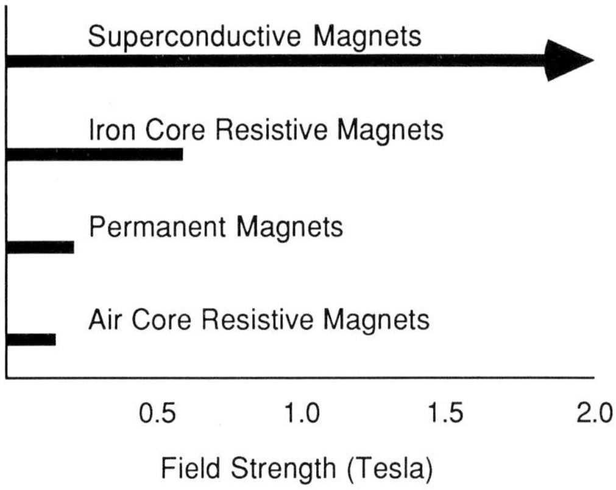

Figure 2–24. Field strength versus magnet design.

the magnet without any additional power supply or cooling requirements. This design is the most efficient of the four magnet configurations to be discussed.

A limitation of permanent magnet technology is that the upper practical field strength is around 0.3 T for purely permanent magnet–design whole-body imagers (Fig. 2–24). The theoretical problems of field stability with temperature change do not present practical problems with permanent magnets, probably because of the significant thermal stability associated with a 200,000-lb mass. The field strength and uniformity of current permanent systems do not allow spectroscopy.

AIR CORE RESISTIVE MAGNET

Air core resistive and superconductive magnets are based on the phenomenon that wires carrying electrical current create magnetic fields proportional to the amount of current. If a wire carrying current is wrapped into the form of a coil, a magnetic field will be generated along the coil's axis. This is known as an electromagnet.

Air core resistive and superconductive magnets are sometimes termed solenoidal-design magnets because the field is generated from loops of wire forming a solenoid. This design is based on the theoretically ideal configuration for an electromagnet necessary to produce a perfectly uniform field, which is a wire conductor wound to form a sphere. This design is not practical for medical imaging because patients cannot, of course, enter or leave a sphere. A workable approximation is to simulate a sphere with four coils of wire that form a solenoid, allowing patient access (Fig. 2–25). The term "solenoid" magnet should not be confused with the term "solenoid" RF coils, which will be discussed later.

Air core resistive magnets typically consist of four coaxial coils of copper or aluminum with associated cooling water jackets. Because current must be maintained in the wire to generate the magnetic field, this type of magnet has a large electrical power requirement (20 kW at 0.12 T). Since current flowing in

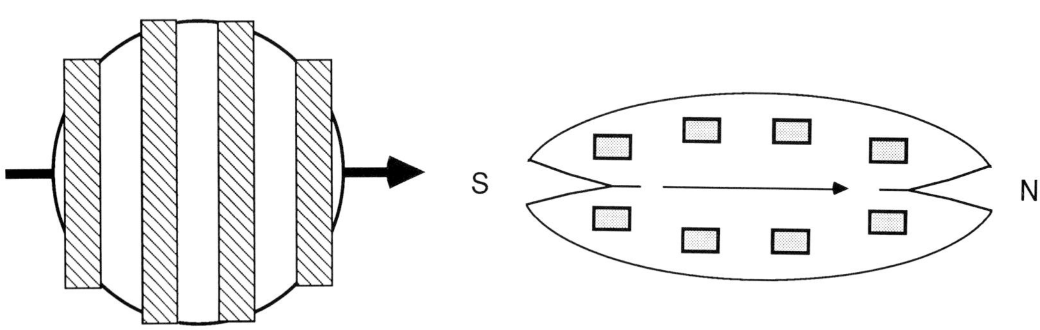

Figure 2–25. (*A*) Practical approximation of the ideal electromagnet sphere with coils in an air core resistive magnet allows patient access, yet still has good spatial field uniformity. (*B*) Most air core resistive magnet installations are oriented so that a horizontal magnetic field axis is produced.

the wire at normal temperatures encounters resistance and produces heat, significant water cooling is needed to remove this thermal load.

IRON CORE (HYBRID) RESISTIVE MAGNETS

A new type of hybrid magnet called the iron core resistive system has been created by combining the features of permanent and air core resistive magnet systems. This is done by forming blocks of iron or other materials into large magnetic endplates on poles, like the permanent magnet, and then adding coils of wire to each endplate, as in the air core resistive magnets. This type of magnet design affords many of the advantages of the first two types, but with relatively few of their disadvantages (Figs. 2–26, 2–27).

The iron core resistive component results in lower power and cooling requirements than the air core design system of similar field strength. The result is lower operational costs. Because the iron core aspect of the system is supplemented with resistive components, iron core resistive magnets can be made much smaller and lighter than pure permanent magnet systems of the same field strength. Because the magnetic field does require power to be maintained, the field may be turned off, as with air core resistive magnets.

SUPERCONDUCTIVE MAGNETS

Superconductive magnets are similar to air core resistive magnets in that they are electromagnets of the solenoidal design. Both types use large coils of wire to generate the electromagnetic field. Unlike the air coil resistive design, which uses water to remove heat generated by the resistance encountered by the current, however, superconducting magnets exploit the fact that the electrical resistance of most metals is proportional to their temperature. Thus, the resistance can be reduced dramatically by cooling the wires to near absolute zero (−459.67° F) with liquid helium to maintain a superconducting state. The current in a superconductive wire en-

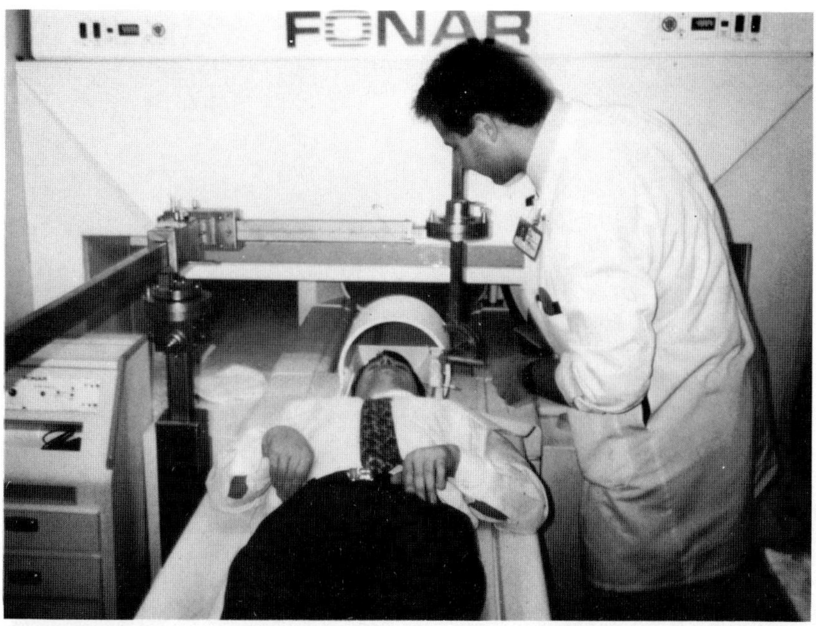

Figure 2–26. Iron core resistive (hybrid) system. The metal stereotaxic system is being used for an MR-guided needle aspiration biopsy.

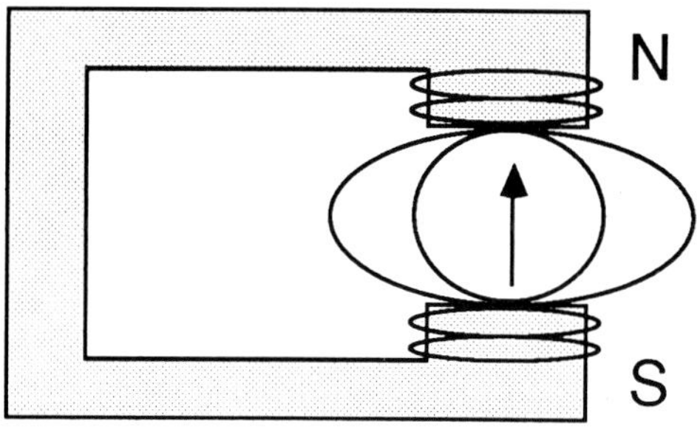

Figure 2–27. Iron core resistive magnet. Like the permanent magnet, the vertical field is produced between the magnet end plates.

counters practically no resistance and circulates nearly perpetually.

A superconductive magnet requires a large vacuum cryostat or Dewar (similar to a thermos bottle) that contains the conducting wires. Instead of copper, niobium and titanium or similar alloys that are superconductive at 10–20 K are combined in a copper matrix to create the superconducting environment (Figs. 2–28, 2–29).

Unlike the air core resistive electromagnet system, in which only four coils are used to approximate the ideal sphere to minimize heat production, most superconductive magnets are wound around aluminum or fiberglass cylinders with the ideal spherical condition simulated by varying numbers of turns of the coils (see Fig. 2–29).

A jacket of liquid helium maintains the temperature of the wires at near absolute zero (4.2 K). Because liquid helium is expensive, boiloff of the helium is reduced with an insulating layer of liquid nitrogen, which is less expensive and boils at around 70 K. The liquids placed in the cryostat to maintain superconduction are referred to as *cryogens*.

A superconductive system can fail if either the temperature or current density becomes too high. At that point the magnet goes from superconductive to resistive mode and is said to "quench." Quenching results in rapid collapse of the magnetic field, release of heat and sudden boiling off of the cryogens. The collapse of the field usually occurs over 20–60 seconds and does not constitute a risk to the patient; however, the sudden release of gas can jeopardize patient safety because of the rapid displacement of breathable oxygen. For this reason, most superconductive magnet

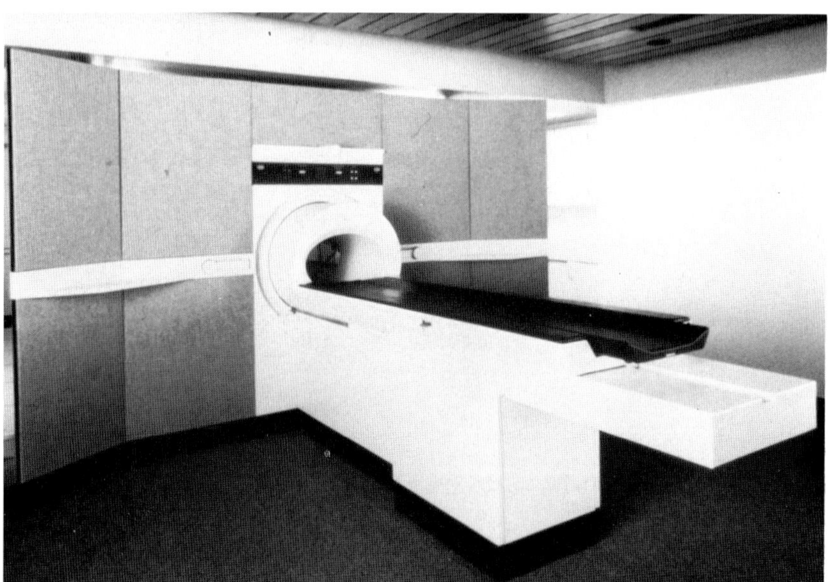

Figure 2–28. Superconductive system. (Photo courtesy of M Anselmo, MD)

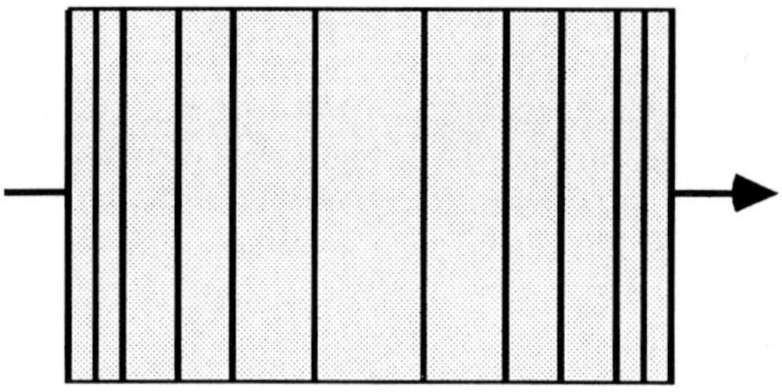

Figure 2–29. Superconductive magnet. The ideal spherical electromagnet is simulated by varied spacing of the magnetic coils. As with other solenoidal electromagnets, a horizontal field is produced.

scanner suites have a large space over the magnet for gas collection in the event of a quench. Boiling of the cryogens constitutes an expensive loss.

Gradient Magnetic Field Generators

A magnetic field gradient subsystem is used to create linear variations in the uniform main magnetic field to allow spatial localization of the MR signal. This is accomplished by superimposing relatively weak gradient magnetic fields on the stronger uniform main magnetic field. The resulting field influencing the patient results from the sum of the two applied fields. Although the main magnet type is important in machine performance, the gradient subsystem in many ways defines the limits of imaging performance.

For the majority of pulse sequences, the gradient amplitude is small compared to the main field strength because gradients merely modify the field created by the primary magnet. Gradient fields must be strong enough to overcome nonuniformity of the main magnetic field and to keep chemical shift misregistration errors at an acceptable level. This strength is approximately two to three orders of magnitude lower than the main field strength. As with the main magnetic field, gradients are measured in units of mT/m (millitesla per meter), so that a typical strength gradient for a 0.5-T system is 1.0 mT/m (0.1 G/cm).

The gradients are produced in all types of MR imagers by current flowing in wires in the form of electromagnets. Typical gradient systems consist of three coaxial sets of coils corresponding to three physical gradients Gx, Gy, and Gz. The imaging software assigns one or more of the physical gradients to the image formation functions of slice selection, phase encoding, and frequency encoding.

In practice, when the gradients are rapidly pulsed on and off with current, as they are in normal MR image production, they may produce a slight click or thump. With steep gradients in higher-field systems, this sound may be loud. Manufacturers now go to great lengths to shield the gradient coils acoustically to avoid this problem. In some machines with particularly loud pulse sequences, patients are routinely given ear plugs to protect the auditory system.

Radiofrequency (RF) Subsystem

Although the hardware devices producing the gradients are sometimes referred to as coils, they must be distinguished from the type of hardware known as the RF coil subsystem. This system delivers RF pulses (at the Larmor frequency) to the patient, and detects the emitted RF signal from the transverse magnetization of the patient in the form of an FID (free induction decay) or echo.

The first function of the RF subsystem is to synthesize and transmit the RF signal to the patient at the resonant frequency. In general, transmitter coils are large and have high RF uniformity for excitation. Because fine control of frequency is not needed for transmission, high amplifier gains can be used. In general, transmitter coils have a low Q (quality factor), which is ideal for broad excitation.

After the signal is detected by the receiver coils, it passes to a preamplifier to increase its strength. A demodulator then subtracts the detected signal from a reference signal at the Larmor frequency so that the image signal information may be processed in the kilohertz rather than the megahertz range.

The receiver coil has a dramatic effect on the S/N of the system. Since one of the major sources of noise in MR imagers is the patient, it is critically important to optimize the function of the RF receiver coil, which is the interface between the machine and the patient. Coil loading and filling factors are measures of how well the patient is matched to and fills the coils. In routine brain imaging, these factors, which determine the S/N for the standard head coil, are generally high because of the favorable anatomy of the region. For many areas of the body such as the knee or neck, however, it is difficult to maneuver RF coils close to the body part being imaged. Thus, the S/N of many areas imaged with standard head and body coils is often poor. When they are positioned close to a patient, surface coils dramatically improve image quality, achieving 4-fold to 10-fold improvements in the S/N compared to standard head or body coils.

The S/N is a critical factor in MR image quality. An improvement in this ratio may translate to shortened scan times (fewer excitations), improved spatial resolution (steeper gradients and smaller pixels), or decreased volume-averaging errors (thinner slices). Surface coils are designed to improve two important terms that affect S/N, the filling factor and coil loading by the patient. In addition, surface coils provide other benefits because of their localizing design. Unlike conventional body or head coils with broad regions of sensitivity in the body, surface coils generally have a markedly limited region of sensitivity. This localized sensitivity is often maximal for superficial or surface structures; hence the name "surface coils."

Most manufacturers allow all standard pulse sequences to be used with surface coils. Since the magnetic field gradients are not affected by the coils, all gradient options (field-of-view and slice-thickness change) and nonorthogonal imaging are available with surface coils. Surface coils were initially used for in vivo phosphorus spectroscopy to localize the volume of tissue to be studied.[1,14] Now surface coils are being applied to an increasing variety of clinical MR imaging situations with dramatic results, and are already considered essential for certain studies.[2,3,9,12,19,22–24]

One disadvantage of planar surface coils is that, because of the loss of signal with depth, the coils work best for superficial structures. Deep structures are best imaged with circumferential coils (Fig. 2–30). Also, the drop-off in signal with depth from the surface results in images that have a large dynamic range of signal intensities in the image. This range may make display and photography of the images difficult. Strategies for dynamic range compression are being developed to eliminate this problem.[21]

MRI CONTRAST AGENTS

Gadolinium is a lanthanide (one of the rare earth elements) metal with unpaired electrons. Gadolinium is paramagnetic (that is, when placed in a magnetic field, it possesses magnetization in direct proportion to field strength) and therefore results in T_1 shortening.[6] Although as a free metal gadolinium is toxic, when bound to DTPA or other chelates, it is safe for human use. It is the first major paramagnetic intravenous contrast agent to be approved for MRI use. Gadolinium has similar pharmacokinetics to iodinated contrast agent in x-ray CT; it has a similar volume of distribution and is cleared by the kidneys. It appears to be much safer, however. Lower doses are used and as yet no idiopathic anaphylactoid reactions to gadolinium-DTPA have been reported.

MRI contrast agents provide an important means of evaluating the blood-

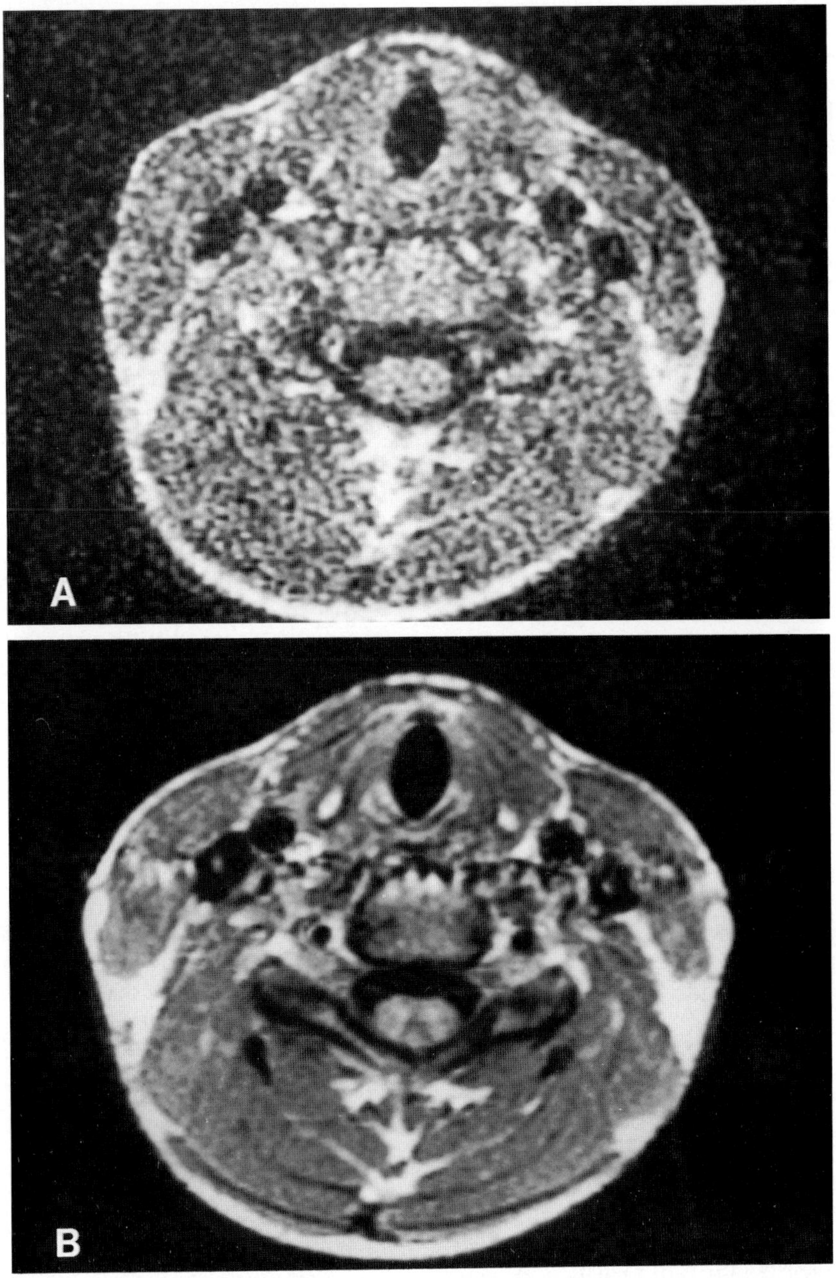

Figure 2–30. Normal neck imaged with body coil and solenoidal surface coil. The same imaging parameters were used in both studies. (*A*) The images obtained using the body coil have good signal uniformity, but rather poor S/N. (*B*) Using the circumferential surface coil, the S/N is dramatically improved while reasonable signal uniformity is maintained.

brain barrier (BBB). On T_2-weighted images, gliosis or edema is visible, but BBB disruption cannot be seen separately. Contrast-enhanced MRI is also valuable in the evaluation of leptomeningeal disease. Since gadolinium contrast affects T_1 primarily, higher-S/N T_1-weighted images may be used to show the contrast enhancement optimally.

Newer, low-osmolality gadolinium complexes such as gadolinium-DOTA and gadolinium-D03A are currently under investigation for human uses. Other chelates, as well as ferromagnetic and superparamagnetic materials, are also being investigated and may soon be available for general MRI use. (Ferromagnetic substances possess magnetization in the absence of an external magnetic field.) Researchers are trying to tag monoclonal antibodies with paramagnetic substances or ferromagnetic substances for more specific contrast enhancement.

THE UTILITY OF MRI IN NEUROLOGIC STUDIES

MRI has dominated imaging of the central nervous system in the few years since its introduction. MRI has had a major impact on x-ray CT and myelography, and a lesser impact on angiographic studies. Nevertheless, in some situations MRI does not provide a specific diagnostic answer and a more invasive study is indicated. The role of MRI in imaging the central nervous system can be considered by reviewing the strengths and weaknesses of this technique compared with other imaging techniques, especially x-ray CT.

Strengths

LACK OF IONIZING RADIATION

The fact that the MR images are produced using only magnetism and radio waves is an advantage over other studies that require ionizing radiation, particularly in individuals requiring many examinations, in the pediatric patient, or during pregnancy.

SENSITIVITY TO FLOW

MRI is exquisitely sensitive to flow because any change in location of protons due to arterial, venous, or CSF pulsations during the NMR process results in a change in signal, allowing visualization of flowing material. This obviates the need for intravenous contrast material (as in the case of x-ray CT) to demonstrate vascular structures. Usually MRI without contrast is superior to x-ray CT with contrast for the definition of fine vascular anatomy. As noted above, intravenous contrast material is valuable in MRI in the central nervous system as a method of showing BBB disruption, but it is not necessary for the demonstration of flow.

The inherent sensitivity of MRI to flow can be used to create projection images of flowing blood in patients, in a technique referred to as MR angiography. Although the spatial resolution of this technique is lower than with conventional angiography, MR angiography is performed without contrast material or ionizing radiation (Fig. 2–31).

MULTIPLANAR CAPABILITIES

MRI possesses a remarkable ability to perform multiplanar studies. With x-ray CT, the scan plane is defined by the x-ray tube–detector axis through the gantry. Consequently, scanning is limited to the axial or, in some cases, the coronal plane. In MRI, the scan plane is defined by the selection of radiofrequencies and magnetic field gradients, which are completely variable under electronic rather than physical control.

IRON SENSITIVITY

Many forms of iron have paramagnetic and ferromagnetic properties because of their unpaired electrons. As a result, these substances have a special effect on the MR image. Many types of iron cause subtle alterations in the local magnetic field environment of the protons, which in turn cause relaxation, enhancement, or shortening of either T_1 or T_2 relaxation times. The type and amount of shortening reflects the form and quantity of the iron-containing compound. As a result of the high sensitivity of MR to iron, it has been said that

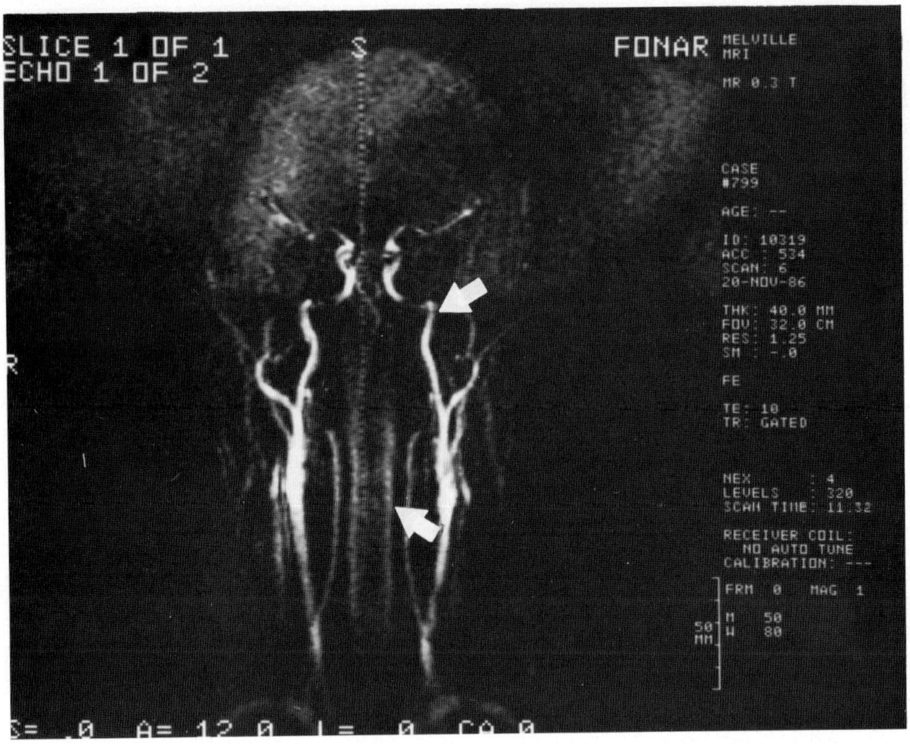

Figure 2–31. Normal MRI angiogram obtained in the coronal plane of the neck shows the internal carotid arteries (arrowhead). Signals from CSF pulsations in the spinal canal also appear in the image (*arrow*).

"iron is to MRI as calcium is to x-ray CT."

Accumulation with aging of nonheme brain iron in the form of ferritin has been demonstrated on MRI in otherwise normal individuals.[8] This form of iron results in a loss of signal due to preferential T_2 shortening (see Chapter 10). It is found most commonly in the globus pallidus, red nucleus, and substantia nigra (Fig. 2–32).

Heme iron has a characteristic appearance on MRI due to the changing form of iron as hemoglobin passes through several breakdown stages. Although the iron in oxyhemoglobin has no significant relaxation, the reversible transformation to deoxyhemoglobin results in preferential T_2 shortening on MR images. After 72–90 hours, the deoxyhemoglobin is irreversibly converted to methemoglobin, which has a characteristic high signal on T_1-weighted images due to the T_1 shortening effect. Gradually this breakdown product is converted to hemosiderin, which appears as a low signal due to T_2 shortening. Whereas x-ray CT is sensitive to acute hemorrhage due to the protein content of the blood, MRI is far more sensitive to the later phases (>72 hours) following hemorrhage, after much of the protein has broken down (see Chapter 7).

HIGH SOFT-TISSUE CONTRAST RESOLUTION

The high sensitivity of MRI to differences in proton density and T_1 and T_2 relaxation times is extremely valuable for imaging CNS pathology. All forms of cerebral edema are generally better seen with MRI than with x-ray CT. The lack of beam hardening artifact, a common problem in x-ray CT (see Chapter

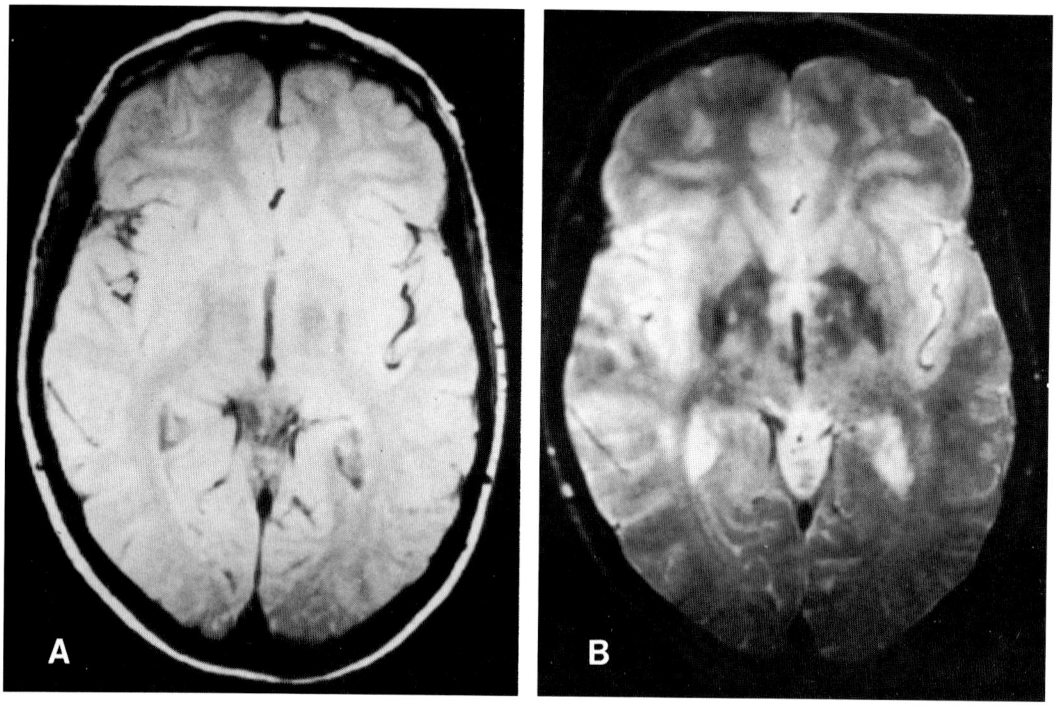

Figure 2–32. Normal brain iron deposition. (*A*) On the proton density image (SE 1000/30), the ferritin in the basal ganglia is poorly seen. (*B*) The preferential T_2 shortening of the ferritin results in decreasing signal with heavier T_2 weighting (SE 2000/90).

1), results in superior MR imaging of the vertex, posterior fossa, floor of middle fossa, skull base, and vertebrae.

Weaknesses

LOW CALCIUM SENSITIVITY

MRI is inferior to x-ray CT for the detection of calcification in masses and associated hyperostosis. Newer gradient echo pulse sequences, which have a higher T2* sensitivity, may improve the sensitivity of MRI to calcium, but MRI will probably not surpass x-ray CT in this area even with these new techniques.

SUBOPTIMAL EVALUATION OF ACUTE HEMORRHAGE

Although MRI is clearly superior to x-ray CT in the evaluation of subacute (>72 hours) and chronic hemorrhage, the high sensitivity of x-ray CT to the protein in acute hemorrhage has made it the study of choice for patients with recent hemorrhage. New field echo pulse sequences with high T2* sensitivity are under investigation for detection of acute hemorrhage with MRI.

CONTRAINDICATIONS

Exposure to the magnetic fields and RF required for MR scanning is contraindicated in certain patients. These patients are best studied with other techniques, such as x-ray CT.

The operation of cardiac and other forms of pacemakers may be adversely affected by MR scanning, so patients with these devices are generally excluded from examination with MRI. Metal intracranial aneurysm clips can develop torque from the changing magnetic fields and actually twist off vessels, so patients with these clips are also excluded. New nonferromagnetic clips that allow MR scanning are available for aneurysm clipping.[5] MRI studies of patients with skull plates, wires, other surgical clips, or even large orthopedic implants may contain small image artifacts but are otherwise safe for the patient. These devices are fixed in tissue and resistant to torque from magnetic fields.

SLOW IMAGE ACQUISITION

Conventional MR scanning is generally slower than comparable x-ray CT studies. Critically injured patients or those who are too ill to be placed in the MR magnet for scan times in excess of 10 minutes are best studied with other techniques.

The slow rate of data acquisition and the high sensitivity of MRI to moving protons can result in artifacts due to motion. While periodic motion such as that from the heart can be removed with gating, other types of physiologic motion can degrade image quality, even with special motion-supression pulse sequences. These motion artifacts are particularly troublesome at high field strengths.

The problem of slow data acquisition with MRI may change in the future as newer pulse sequence strategies are developed with gradient echoes or echo planar technique. This approach may allow scan times comparable to or shorter than x-ray CT scanning. MR fluoroscopy may be developed in the future.

HIGH COST

MRI generally is more expensive than x-ray CT. This is a relative disadvantage for MRI when both techniques provide similar information. The high cost of MRI limits its application to studies that justify the expenditure. With the introduction of newer, more efficient, lower-cost MR scanners in the near future, the cost per MRI examination will decrease and central nervous system applications will continue to increase.

REFERENCES

1. Ackerman, JJH, Grove, TH, Wong, GG, Gadian, DG, and Radda GK: Mapping of metabolites in whole animals by ^{31}P NMR using surface coils. Nature 283: 167–170, 1980.
2. Axel, L: Surface coil magnetic resonance imaging. J Comput Assist Tomogr 8:381–384, 1984.
3. Bernardo, ML, Cohen, AJ, and Lauterbur PC: Radiofrequency coil designs for nuclear magnetic zeugmatographic imaging. IEEE Proceedings of the International Workshop on Physics and Engineering in Medical Imaging, 277:284, March 1982.
4. Bottomley, PA: NMR imaging techniques and applications: A review. Rev Sci Instrum 53:1319–1337, 1982.
5. Brothers, M, Fox, AJ, and Lee, DH: MR of postoperative cerebral aneurysm (abstr). AJNR (in press).
6. Carr, DH, Brown, J, and Leung, AWL: Iron and gadolinium chelates as contrast agents in NMR. J Comput Assist Tomogr 8:385–389, 1984.
7. Christianson: Nuclear magnetic resonance. In Christianson (ed): Introduction to the Physics of Diagnostic Radiology. Lea & Febiger, 1984.
8. Drayer, B, Burger, P, and Darwin R: MRI of brain iron. AJR 147:103–110, 1986.
9. Edelman, RR, McFarland, E, Stark, DD, Ferrucci, JT Jr, Simeone, JF, Wismer, G, White, EM, Rosen, BR, and Brady, TJ: Surface coil MR imaging of abdominal viscera. Part I. Theory, technique and initial results. Radiology 157(2): 425–430, 1985.
10. Edelstein, WA, Bottomley, PA, Hart, HR, and Smith LS: Signal, noise, and contrast in nuclear magnetic resonance (NMR) imaging. J Comp Assist Tomogr 7:391–401, 1983.
11. Edelstein, WA, Hutchinson, JMS, Johnson, G, and Redpath T: Spin warp NMR imaging and applications to human whole-body imaging. Phys Med Biol 25:751–756, 1980.
12. Fitzsimmons, JR, Thomas, RG, and Mancuso, AA: Proton imaging with surface coils on a 0.15-T resistive system. J Mag Res Med 2:180–185, 1985.

13. Fullerton, GD, Cameron, IL, and Ord, VA: Frequency dependence of magnetic resonance spin lattice relaxation of protons in biological materials. Radiology 151:135–138, 1984.
14. Gadian, DG: Nuclear magnetic resonance and its applications to living systems. Clarendon Press, Oxford, 1982.
15. Hendrick, RE, Nelson, TR, and Hendee, WR: Optimizing tissue contrast in magnetic resonance imaging. Mag Res Imag 2:193–204, 1984.
16. Hendrick, RE, Newman, FD, and Hendee, WR: MR imaging technology: Maximizing the signal to noise from a single tissue. Radiology 156:749–752, 1985.
17. Kumar, A, Welti, D, and Ernst, R: NMR zeugmatography. J Magn Reson, 18: 69–85, 1985.
18. Lufkin, R: The MRI Manual. Mosby-Yearbook Publishers, Chicago, 1990.
19. Lufkin, R and Hanafee, W: Application of surface coils to NMR anatomy of the larynx. AJR 6:491–497, 1985.
20. Lufkin, R and Hanafee, W: Comparison of superconductive, resistive, and permanent magnet MR imaging systems. In Viamonte M (ed): NMR Update Series. Vol 1, Book 4, Continuing Professional Education Center, Princeton, 1984.
21. Lufkin, R, Sharples, T, Flannigan, B, and Hanafee, W: Dynamic range compression of surface coil MRI. AJR 147(2):379–382, 1986.
22. Lufkin, R, Hanafee, W, Wortham, D, Hoover, L: High resolution surface coil MRI of the tongue and oropharynx. (Abstract) Radiology 157(P), 1985.
23. Schenck, JF, Foster, TH, and Henkes, JL: High field surface coil MR imaging of localized anatomy. AJNR 6:181–186, 1985.
24. Schenck, JF, Hart, HR, and Foster, TH: Improved MR imaging of the orbit at 1.5 T with surface coils. AJNR 6:193–196, 1985.
25. Smyth, WR: Static and Dynamic Electricity. McGraw-Hill, New York, 1968.
26. Stark, D and Bradley, W: Magnetic Resonance Imaging. CV Mosby, St. Louis, 1987.
27. Wehrli, F, Macfall, JR, and Shutts, D: Mechanisms of contrast in NMR imaging. J Comp Assist Tomogr 8:369–380, 1984.
28. Wehrli, FW, MacFall, JR, and Newton, TH: Parameters determining the appearance of NMR images. In Newton TH and Potts DG (eds): Advanced Imaging Techniques. Clavedel Press, San Anselmo, Calif, 1983.

Chapter 3

POSITRON EMISSION TOMOGRAPHY (PET)

Michael E. Phelps, Ph.D.

POSITRON DECAY
PRODUCTION OF LABELED COMPOUNDS
PET SCANNERS
TRACER KINETIC MODELING
THE VALUE OF PET IN NEUROLOGIC AND PSYCHIATRIC DISORDERS

Positron emission tomography (PET) has enhanced our understanding of the biochemical basis of normal and abnormal functions of the brain, and permitted biochemical examination of patients as part of their clinical care. These capabilities are important because:

1. The basis of all functions of the brain is chemical.
2. Diseases of the brain result from errors introduced into its chemical systems by viruses, bacteria, genetic abnormalities, drugs, environmental factors, aging, and behavior.
3. The most selective, specific, and appropriate therapy is one chosen from a diagnostic measure of the basic chemical abnormality.
4. Detection of chemical abnormalities provides the earliest identification of disease, even in the presymptomatic stages before the disease process has exhausted the chemical reserves or overridden the compensatory mechanisms of the brain.
5. Assessment of restoration of chemical function provides an objective means for determining the efficacy of therapeutic interventions in the individual patient.
6. The best way to judge whether tissue is normal is by determining its biochemical function.

Another principle relates to the value of examining these biochemical processes with an imaging technology. Because in most cases the location and extent of a disease is unknown, the first objective is an efficient means of searching throughout the brain to determine its location. Imaging is an extremely efficient process for accomplishing this aim, because data are presented in pictorial form to the most efficient human sensory system for search, identification, and interpretation — the visual system. Recognition depends upon the type of information in the image, both in terms of interpreting what it means and how sensitive it is to identifying the presence of disease.

PET provides the means for imaging the rates of biologic processes in vivo. Imaging is accomplished through the integration of two technologies, the tracer kinetic assay method and computed tomography (CT) (Fig. 3–1). The tracer kinetic assay method employs a radiolabeled biologically active com-

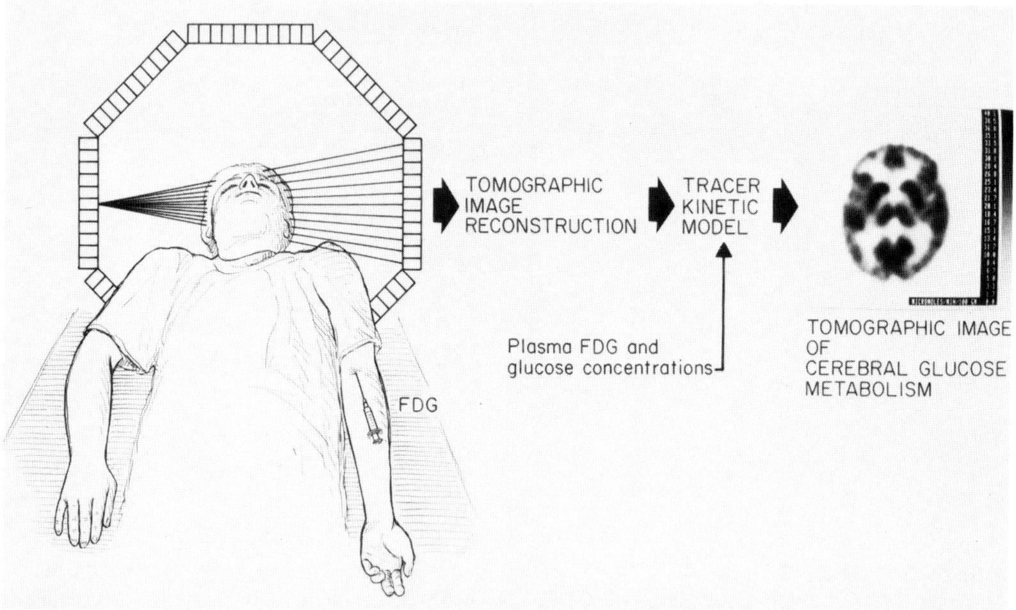

Figure 3–1. Schematic illustration of processes involved in tracer kinetic assays with PET. Particular example is the use of 2-[^{18}F]fluoro-2-deoxy-D-glucose (FDG) for the tomographic imaging and measurement of the cerebral metabolic rate for glucose. Units of image are μmole/min/g. (With permission from Annals of Internal Medicine, 98:339–359, 1983.)

pound (tracer) and a mathematical model that describes the kinetics of the tracer as it participates in a biological process. The model permits the calculation of the rate of the process. The tissue tracer concentration measurement required by the tracer kinetic model is provided by the PET scanner, with the final result being a three-dimensional (3-D) image of the anatomic distribution of the biological process under study.

Radiolabeled tracers and the tracer kinetic method are employed throughout the biological sciences to measure such processes as blood flow, membrane transport, metabolism, synthesis, and ligand-receptor interactions; for mapping axonal projection fields through anterograde and retrograde diffusion; measurement of cell birth dates; marker assays using recombinant DNA techniques; radioimmunoassays; and the study of drug interactions with chemical systems of the body. The tracer technique continues to be one of the most sensitive and widely used methodologies for performing assays of biological systems. PET allows the transfer of the tracer assay methodology to the living subject, particularly humans. PET builds a bridge of communication and investigation between the basic and clinical sciences, based upon a commonality of methods used and problems studied.

The transfer of tracer methods from the basic biological sciences to humans with PET is made possible by the unique nature of the radioisotopes used in PET to label compounds: ^{11}C, ^{13}N, ^{15}O, and ^{18}F. These are the only radioactive forms of the natural elements (^{18}F is used as a substitute for hydrogen) that emit radiation that will pass through the body for external detection. Natural substrates, substrate analogs, and drugs can be labeled with these radioisotopes without altering their chemical or biological properties. This allows the methods, knowledge, and interpretation of results from tracer kinetic assays used in the basic biological sciences to be applied to humans by the quantitative measurement abilities of the PET scanner.

POSITRON DECAY

Positrons (β^+) are positively charged electrons. They are emitted from the nucleus of some radioisotopes that are unstable because they have an excessive number of protons and a positive charge. Positron emission stabilizes the nucleus by removing a positive charge through the conversion of a proton into a neutron. In doing this, one element is converted to another, the latter having an atomic number one less than the former. For radioisotopes commonly used in PET, the element formed from positron decay is stable (i.e., not radioactive).

After emission, the positron collides with electrons until it comes to rest (Fig. 3–2). The positron then combines with an electron to form positronium. Since

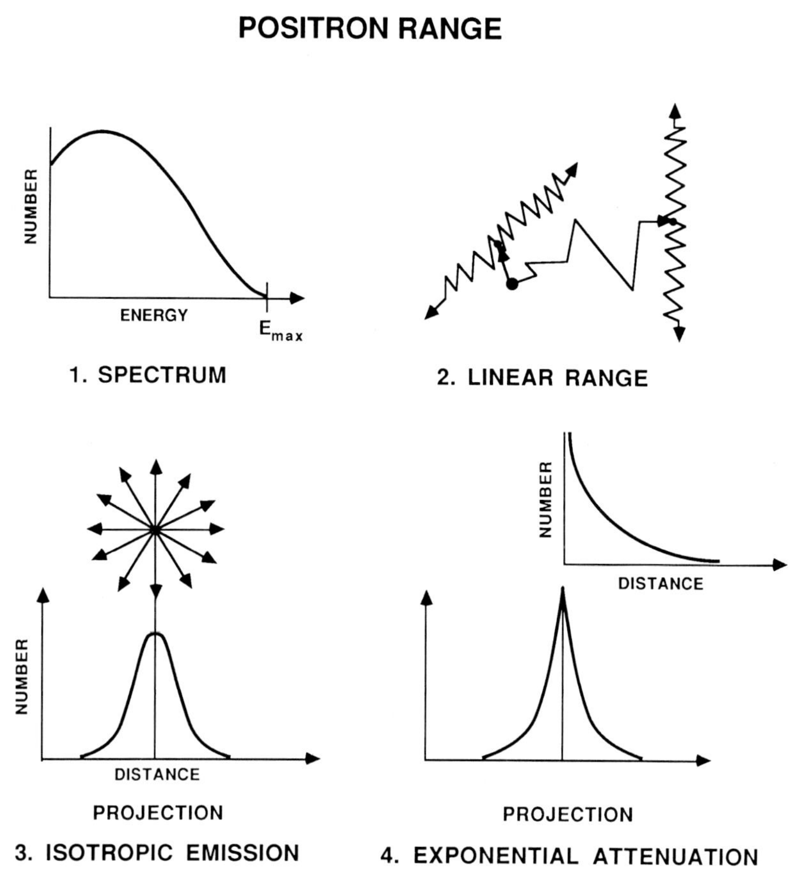

Figure 3–2. Effect of positron range on spatial resolution. (*1*) The energy spectrum of positrons emitted from the nucleus. Energy of positrons has a continuous range from near zero to a maximum value, E_{max} (Table 3–1). (*2*) Pathway of the positron after emission from the nucleus as it collides with electrons, changing its pathway. The positrons finally come to rest and annihilation occurs with emission of two 511-keV photons. The distance traveled from the nucleus to the site of annihilation is proportional to the energy of the emitted positron. (*3*) The isotropic emission of positrons produces a gaussian response in the projection data recorded by the scanner. (*4*) The attenuation of positrons by tissue as they travel to the point of annihilation is approximately exponential, as seen in the graph of the number of positrons annihilating versus distance. The projection data are, therefore, exponentially weighted to the origin. All of these factors together weight the data to the origin of emission and produce a very small effect of positron range on image resolution (Table 3–1).

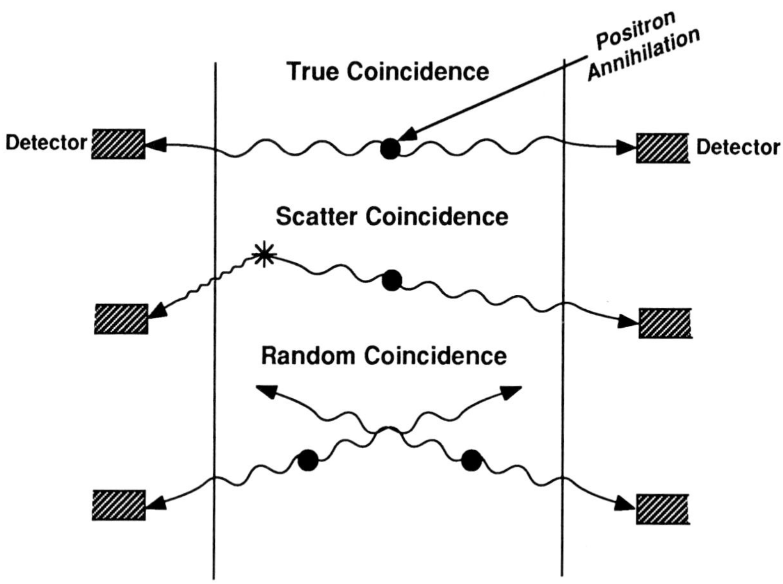

Figure 3–3. Annihilation coincidence detection of the 180° photon emission. True coincidences restrict the origin of radioactivity to a well-defined region between detectors. Scatter coincidences produce misplacement of information, as do random coincidences. Random coincidences occur when photons from two different annihilation events strike two coincidence detectors simultaneously.

the positron is an "anti-electron," the positron and electron annihilate, and their masses are converted to electromagnetic energy. The mass of the electron and positron are equal and equivalent to 511.006 electron volts (keV) of energy. This annihilation process produces the simultaneous emission of two 511-keV photons 180° apart (Fig. 3–3). These photons easily escape from the human body and can be recorded by external detectors.

The properties of positron-emitting radioisotopes commonly used in PET are shown in Table 3–1.

PRODUCTION OF LABELED COMPOUNDS

Positron-emitting isotopes for PET are produced with charged particle accelerators. The two general classes are linear accelerators and cyclotrons. Currently, cyclotrons are used because they are compact devices.

Cyclotron

Cyclotrons are electronic devices for accelerating charged particles to high velocity and energy. These high-energy particles are used to induce nuclear reactions that yield positron-emitting radioisotopes. The basic principle of a cyclotron is illustrated in Figure 3–4. Cyclotrons for PET typically accelerate protons (H^+) or deuterons (heavy hydrogen, D^+). Proton acceleration is described here; recent newer concepts for PET employ cyclotrons that accelerate only protons.

A conventional cyclotron consists of a pair of hollow, semicircular metal electrodes called "dees" because of their semicircular shape. The dees are positioned between the poles of an electromagnet (see Fig. 3–4) and separated from one another by a narrow gap. Near the center of the dees is an ion source in which hydrogen gas is passed through a hot filament to ionize it to positively charged protons.

Table 3–1 PROPERTIES OF COMMON POSITRON-EMITTING RADIOISOTOPES

Radioisotope	*Half-life (min)*	*% β^+ Emission (% 511 KeV)*	*γ-ray Emission Energy (%)**	*Maximum β^+ Energy (MeV)*	*FWHM(mm)†*	*FWTM(mm)†*
^{18}F	109.7	97% (194%)	None	0.635	0.22	1.09
^{11}C	20.4	99% (198%)	None	0.96	0.28	1.86
^{13}N	9.96	100% (200%)	None	1.19	0.60*	2.8
^{15}O	2.07	99.9% (200%)	None	1.72	1.1*	5.3
^{68}Ga	68.3	90% (180%)	1.08 MeV (3%)	1.90	1.35	5.92
^{82}Rb	1.25	96% (192%)	0.777 MeV (13.6%)	3.35	2.6	13.2

*Some positron-emitting radionuclides also emit γ-rays.

†FWHM and FWTM refer to the full width at half the maximum and one tenth the maximum height of a line-spread function of the resolution measurement due to finite positron range. The shape of the line-spread function for positron range is not gaussian. It is sharply peaked toward the origin of annihilation. For a gaussian function, FWTM equals approximately 2 FWHM. The * refers to estimated values. The others are measured values (Derenzo, SE: Proceeding of the 5th International Conference on Positron Annihilation. Sendai, Japan, 1979, pp 819–824, with permission).

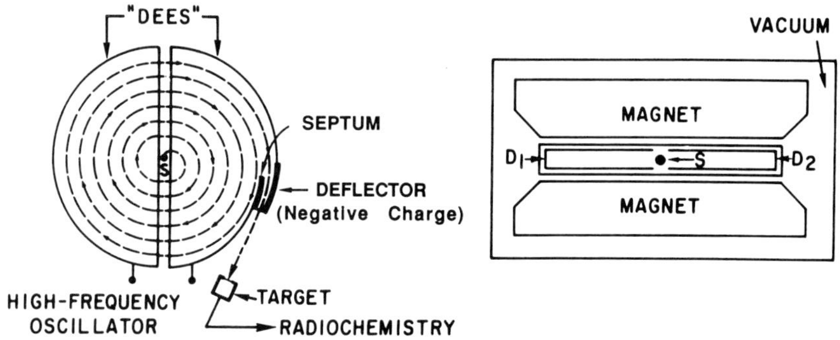

Figure 3–4. Schematic description of a positive-ion cyclotron. S is ion source where H_2 gas is ionized to H^+. D_1 and D_2 are the two "dees."

During operation of the cyclotron, protons are generated in bursts by the ion source, and a high-frequency alternating current (AC) voltage generated by a high-frequency oscillator (e.g., 200 kV, 5 MHz) is applied across the dees. The positively charged protons are injected into the gap and immediately accelerated toward the negatively charged dee by the electrical field generated by the applied voltage. Inside the dee there is no electrical field, but because the protons are within a magnetic field they follow a circular path around to the opposite side of the dee. The AC voltage frequency is such that the protons arrive at the gap just as the voltage across the dees reaches its maximum value (200 kV) in the opposite direction (i.e., the opposite dee is now negative). The protons are accelerated across the gap, gaining about 200 KeV of energy in the process, and then continue on a circular path within the opposite dee. The dees are contained in a vacuum tank so that the accelerated protons do not collide with gas particles in the machine.

Each time the protons cross the gap they gain energy and velocity, so the orbital radius continuously increases and the protons follow a spiraling path of increasing radius. The increasing speed of the protons exactly compensates for the increasing distance travelled per half orbit, so they continue to arrive back at the gap exactly in phase with the AC voltage. This condition applies so long as the charge-to-mass ratio of the accelerated protons remains constant. This is the case for the low energy required to make ^{15}O, ^{13}N, ^{11}C, and ^{18}F. When the protons reach the maximum orbit they are extracted from the cyclotron and aimed at a target chamber. The target chamber is where the nuclear reactions take place to produce the positron-emitting radioisotopes.

A modern self-shielding cyclotron especially designed for PET is shown in Figure 3–5.

The common nuclear reactions used to produce ^{15}O, ^{13}N, ^{11}C and ^{18}F are shown in Table 3–2. The nomenclature for nuclear reaction is

$$^{18}_{8}O\ (p,n)\ ^{18}_{9}F \qquad (3\text{-}1)$$

where ^{18}O is the target material (i.e., H_2O enriched in ^{18}O), *p* is the energetic proton that enters the target and reacts with ^{18}O by expelling a neutron (*n*) to yield radioactive ^{18}F. The subscripts are the atomic numbers.

Labeled Compounds

Over 500 compounds have been labeled with ^{15}O, ^{13}N, ^{11}C and ^{18}F for PET.[1,3] These compounds range from simple labeled molecules such as $H_2{}^{15}O$, $C^{15}O$ and $^{15}O_2$ to many forms of sugars, amino acids, fatty acids, carboxylic acids, alcohols, numerous substrate analogs, and drugs. Examples of these labeled compounds and their uses are listed in Table 3–3. Excellent reviews of the labeled compounds and their

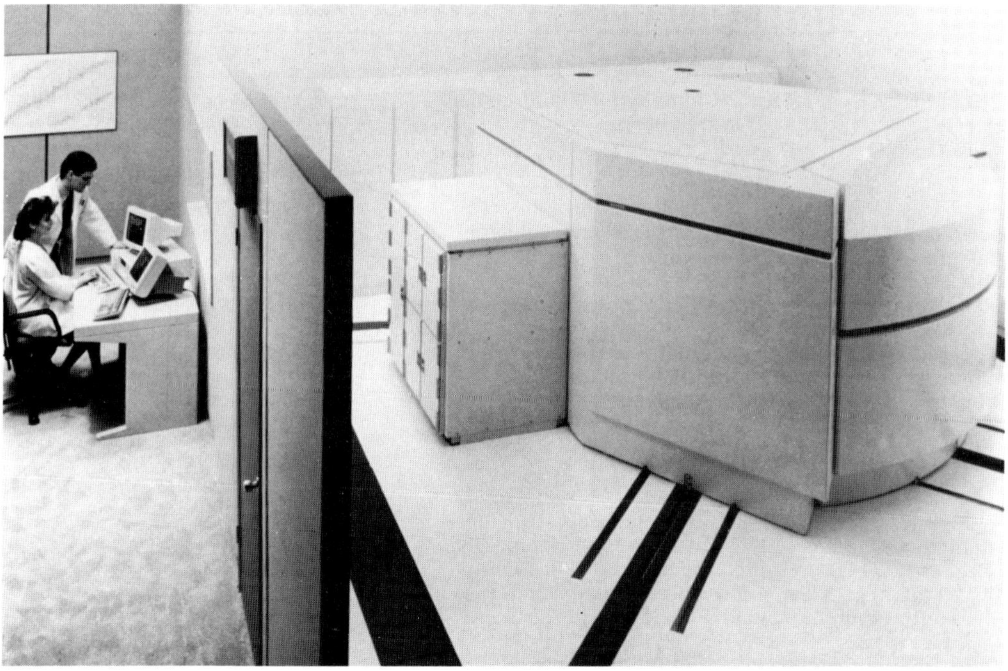

Figure 3–5. Photograph of a self-shielded negative-ion cyclotron. The cyclotron is located inside the shields. The rectangular cabinet on the left of the shield contains the automated chemical synthetic systems for producing labeled compounds. The cyclotron and chemical synthesis are controlled by a personal computer station shown to the left. (Courtesy of Siemens Corporation.)

methods of synthesis for PET have been compiled.[1,3]

Because of the short half-life of the positron-emitting radioisotopes, the chemical synthesis has to be rapid. Usually, the synthesis must be accomplished in less than one or two half-lives in a research environment and in much less time in a clinical setting. The self-contained and automated production of labeled compounds with cyclotrons is now designed to produce repeated doses as needed for patient studies. The ^{18}F-labeled compounds are made in larger batches and stored, thus making patient doses available throughout the day.

The *specific activity* (SA) of a labeled compound is defined as the ratio of radioactivity (A) to mass of the compound (stated in curies per gram [Ci/g] or curies per millimole [Ci/mmol]). Thus, SA determines the mass of a compound that is given to a patient to achieve the desired radioactivity to be injected. In some cases low specific activity is required because of chemical conditions in the target or to improve yields of

Table 3–2 COMMON NUCLEAR REACTIONS FOR PRODUCING ^{15}O, ^{13}N, ^{11}C, AND ^{18}F

Radioisotope	*Nuclear Reaction**
^{18}F	$^{18}O\ (p,n)^{18}F$; $^{20}Ne\ (d,\alpha)^{18}F$
^{11}C	$^{14}N\ (p,\alpha)^{11}C$
^{13}N	$^{13}C\ (p,n)^{13}N$; $^{16}O\ (p,\alpha)^{13}N$; $^{12}C\ (d,n)^{11}C$
^{15}O	$^{15}N\ (p,n)^{15}O$; $^{14}N\ (d,n)^{15}O$

*p, d, n and α refer to proton, deuteron, neutron, and alpha particles, respectively. ^{18}O, ^{13}C, and ^{15}N are target materials enriched in these stable isotopes.

Table 3–3 PARTIAL LIST OF POSITRON-LABELED COMPOUNDS*

Labeled Compound	*Application*
$H_2{}^{15}O$, $C^{15}O_2$, $CH_3{}^{18}F$, ^{77}Kr, [^{11}C]butanol, [^{18}F]fluoroethanol	Cerebral blood flow
^{11}CO, $C^{15}O$, [^{68}Ga]EDTA, ^{68}Ga-transferrin	Cerebral blood volume
[^{11}C]DMO, $^{11}CO_2$	Tissue pH
$^{15}O_2$	Oxygen extraction and metabolism
	TRANSPORT AND METABOLISM
2-deoxy-2-[^{18}F]fluoro-D-glucose, 2-[^{11}C]deoxy-D-glucose, -lactate, -pyruvate, -acetate, -succinate, 3[^{11}C]-O-methyl-D-glucose, [^{18}F]-fluoroacetate	Glucose and metabolites
[^{13}N]-L-glutamate, -glutamine, -alanine, -aspartate, -leucine, -valine, -isoleucine, -methionine, -tyrosine, -phenylalanine	Amino acids [^{13}N]
[^{11}C]-L-aspartate, -valine, -glutamate, -tryptophan, -phenylalanine, -L-DOPA, -α-aminoisobutyric	Amino acids [^{11}C]
[^{11}C]-palmitic, -oleic, -heptadecanoic, -octanoic, -β-methylheptadecanoic	Free fatty acids
[^{11}C]-L-leucine, -methionine, -phenylalanine, 3-[^{18}F]fluorotyrosine	**PROTEIN SYNTHESIS**
	NEUROTRANSMITTER SYSTEMS
[^{11}C]-methylspiperone, -raclopride, -pimozide, [^{18}F]spiperone, -fluoromethyl, -fluoroethyl and -fluoropropylspiperone, -haloperidol, [^{76}Br]-p-bromospiperone, [^{11}C]-L-DOPA, 6-[^{18}F]-fluoro-L-DOPA, 4-[^{18}F]fluorometatyrosine	Dopaminergic
[^{11}C] and [^{18}F]fluoronitrazepam, [^{18}F]fluorodiazepam, [^{11}C]-diazepam, [^{11}C] RO-15-1788, [^{11}C]-PK11195	Benzodiazepine
[^{11}C]-carfentanil, -etorphine, -morphine, -heroin	Opiate
[^{11}C]-norepinephrine, -propanolol	Adrenergic
[^{11}C]-imipramine, -QNB	Cholinergic
[^{11}C]-valproate, -diphenylhydantoin	Anticonvulsants

*Selected examples from about 500 compounds labeled with positron radioisotopes. See Reference 21. DMO is dimethyloxazolidinedione, EDTA is ethylenediaminetetraacetic acid, QNB is quinuclidinylbenzilate.

chemical synthesis, or is purposely reduced to examine the mass effects of the compound on a biological system.[1,3] Examples of the specific activity of several common labeled compounds are shown in Table 3–4.

Dosimetry

The ultimate limiting factor in image quality in PET is determined by the dose of the radioisotope given to the patient. In an imaging study, one would like to

Table 3–4 EXAMPLES OF SPECIFIC ACTIVITY OF LABELED COMPOUNDS

Compound	*Typical Specific Activities (SA)*
2-Deoxy-2-[^{18}F]fluoro-D-glucose*	10 Ci/μmol
2-[^{14}C]-deoxy-D-glucose	50 μCi/μmol
6-[^{18}F]fluoro-L-DOPA*	2 mCi/μmol
[^{3}H]spiperone	30 mCi/μmol
[^{11}C]methylspiperone	5 Ci/μmol
[^{18}F]fluoroethylspiperone	10 Ci/μmol

*Specific activity of FDG is from synthesis employing high-specific-activity [^{18}F]fluoride ion. Earlier FDG synthesis employed low-specific-activity [^{18}F]F_2, which is currently used for 6-[^{18}F]fluoro-L-DOPA.

Table 3–5 RADIATION DOSE FOR SELECTED COMPOUNDS*

Compound	Radiation Absorbed Dose (mrad/mCi administered) Whole Body	Critical Organ (organ, dose)	Brain	Typical Amount Administered per Study (mCi)
2-deoxy-2-[^{18}F]fluoro-D-glucose	6	bladder, 320†	60	5–10
6-[^{18}F]fluoro-L-DOPA	33	kidney, 257	22	5–10
[^{18}F]fluoroethylspiperone	36	small intestine, 360	10	5–10
[^{18}F]fluoromethylspiperone	40	kidney, 300	6	5–10
CH_3[^{18}F]	2	lung, 4	2	50
2-[^{11}C]-deoxy-D-glucose	9	bladder, 111	8	7.5–15
[^{11}C]L-leucine	8	small intestine, 32	4	20
[^{11}C]acetate	4	small intestine, 83	2	20
[^{11}C]methylspiperone	15	bladder, 75	30	20
[^{11}C]CO	19	spleen, 91	5	20
[^{15}O]O_2	2	lungs, 5	1	30–60
H_2[^{15}O]	3	whole body, 3	1	30–60
C[^{15}O]	2	spleen, 8	1	20–30
[^{15}O]CO_2	2	lungs, 6	1	30–60
[^{13}N]H_3	5	bladder, 50	16	20
[^{13}N]glutamate	3	heart, 80	28	20

*Average values from literature. Includes voiding at 1 hr after injection.
†Assumes voiding urine at 2 hr postinjection. Earlier voiding will reduce dose significantly.

be able to deliver the dose to the patient only when data are being collected. This is rarely the case in nuclear medicine studies. In fact, in conventional nuclear medicine, the overwhelming amount of the dose to the patient occurs when data are not being collected because of the long half-lives of the isotopes used. With the short half-lives used in PET, this is not the case; there is a much higher ratio of imaging time to total exposure time.

With positron-emitting radioisotopes, the majority of the absorbed dose originates from ionization produced by the positively charged positron and not the 511-keV photons. For example, with FDG the dose to the brain is 77% from positrons and 23% from the 511-keV annihilation photons. Although dosimetry is determined for organs throughout the body, the common reporting format is to list the critical organ and whole-body dose. The unit of dose is the radiation absorbed dose rated as rads or grays (Gy) (1 rad = 0.01 Gy) which equals 100 ergs of energy deposited per gram of tissue.

The dosimetry for some of the common positron-labeled compounds is shown in Table 3–5. The maximum allowable doses in research studies are typically set by local human-protection committees and generally follow the guidelines set by the National Council on Radiation Protection.

PET SCANNERS

The objective of the PET scanner is to provide both a tomographic image and analytical measurement of the tissue concentration of the injected tracer and its labeled products. This objective is achieved using the principles of computed tomography (CT).

The Principle of Computed Tomography in PET

CT techniques are based on rigorous mathematical algorithms for forming tomographic images from projections of an object. They provide an intrinsically high signal-to-noise ratio (S/N) as well as a quantitative representation of the actual radioactivity tissue-concentration distribution. The tomographic planes usually are oriented perpendicular to the long axis of the body; however, other orientations of the planes also can be obtained. In contrast to x-ray CT, which uses transmitted radiation, PET uses emitted radiation from labeled compounds that have been administered to the patient.

The data for reconstructing tomographic images in PET consist of a set of standard two-dimensional (2-D) projection images taken at many angles around the body. Reconstruction of tomographic images mathematically requires a sufficient number of scan projection profiles at specific angles over a 180° arc. Consider the scan profiles for the simple case of a point source of activity within an object (Fig. 3–6). Each profile maps the location of the point source in the direction parallel to the scan profile; however, the source could lie at any point along the line perpendicular to that profile. For a point source, this ambiguity is easily resolved by inspection of profiles from other angles, but with distributed sources such a judgment becomes more complex. Because the location of the activity in the field of view is unknown, a first approximation for the source distribution can

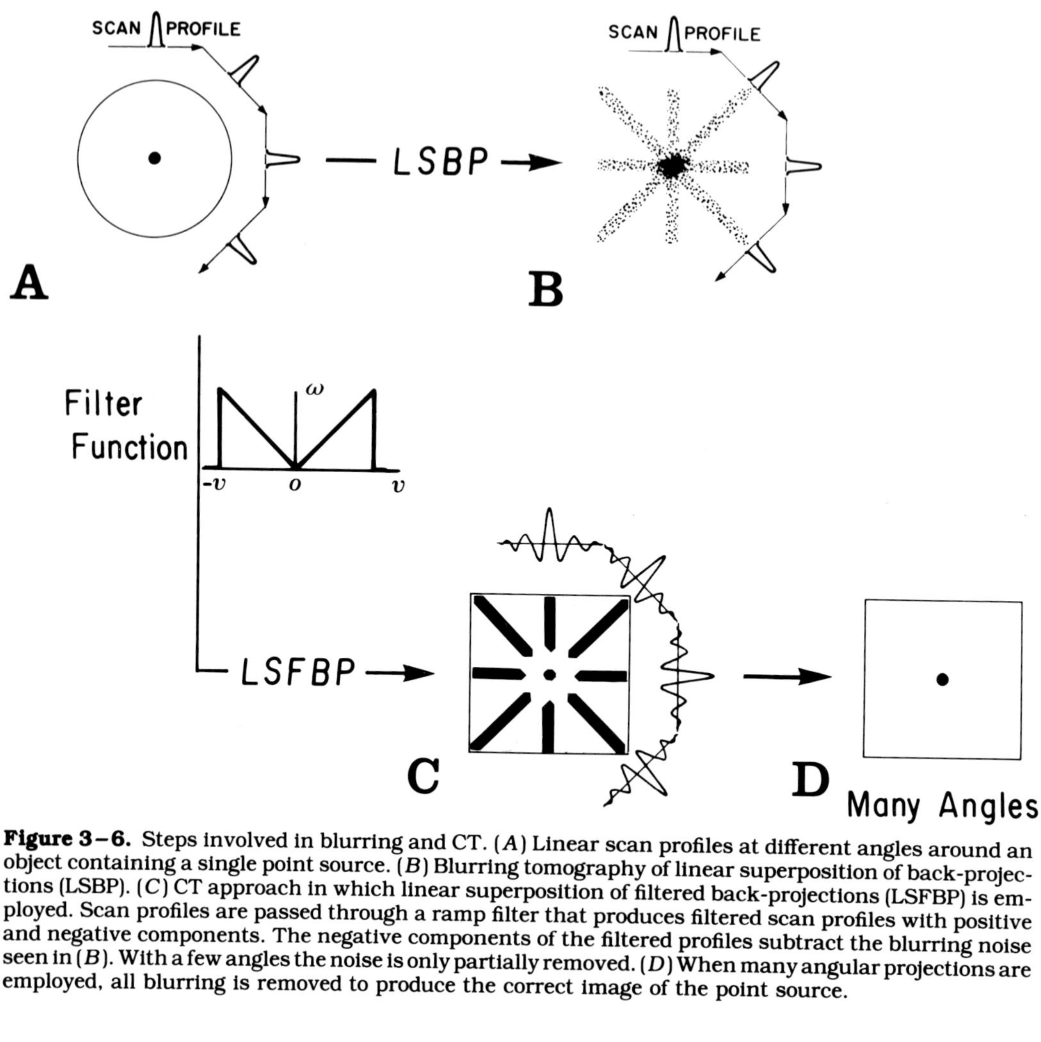

Figure 3–6. Steps involved in blurring and CT. (*A*) Linear scan profiles at different angles around an object containing a single point source. (*B*) Blurring tomography of linear superposition of back-projections (LSBP). (*C*) CT approach in which linear superposition of filtered back-projections (LSFBP) is employed. Scan profiles are passed through a ramp filter that produces filtered scan profiles with positive and negative components. The negative components of the filtered profiles subtract the blurring noise seen in (*B*). With a few angles the noise is only partially removed. (*D*) When many angular projections are employed, all blurring is removed to produce the correct image of the point source.

be obtained by projecting the data from each scan profile back across the entire image grid. That is, equal values are assigned to all points in the object plane contributing to the scan profile. This operation is known as *back-projection*. If the back-projections of scan profiles at different angles are then added together (linear superposition), an approximation of the original object distribution results (Fig. 3–6*B*). The complete operation, using simple addition of uncorrected scan profiles, is called *linear superposition of back-projections* (LSBP). This is commonly referred to as "blurring" tomography.

Sampling Requirements

Scan profiles or projections are not continuous functions but collections of discrete points. The distance between these points is the *linear sampling distance*. In addition, scan profiles are obtained only at a finite number of *angular sampling intervals* around the object. The choice of linear and angular sampling intervals and the maximum frequency of the reconstruction filter (i.e., the cutoff frequency), in conjunction with the detector resolution, determine the reconstruction image resolution.

In PET, image resolution depends on detector resolution and on the cutoff frequency (V_{max}) used for the reconstruction filter. Figure 3–7 illustrates the trade-offs between these variables. If the filter cutoff frequency is low compared with the detector resolution, then the reconstruction filter determines the tomographic image resolution. As the filter cutoff frequency is increased, tomographic image resolution initially increases in proportion to the cutoff frequency (Fig. 3–8). As the cutoff frequency is further increased, improvements in image resolution become disproportionately smaller and eventually reach the limit determined by the detector resolution. Beyond this point, no improvements in image resolution

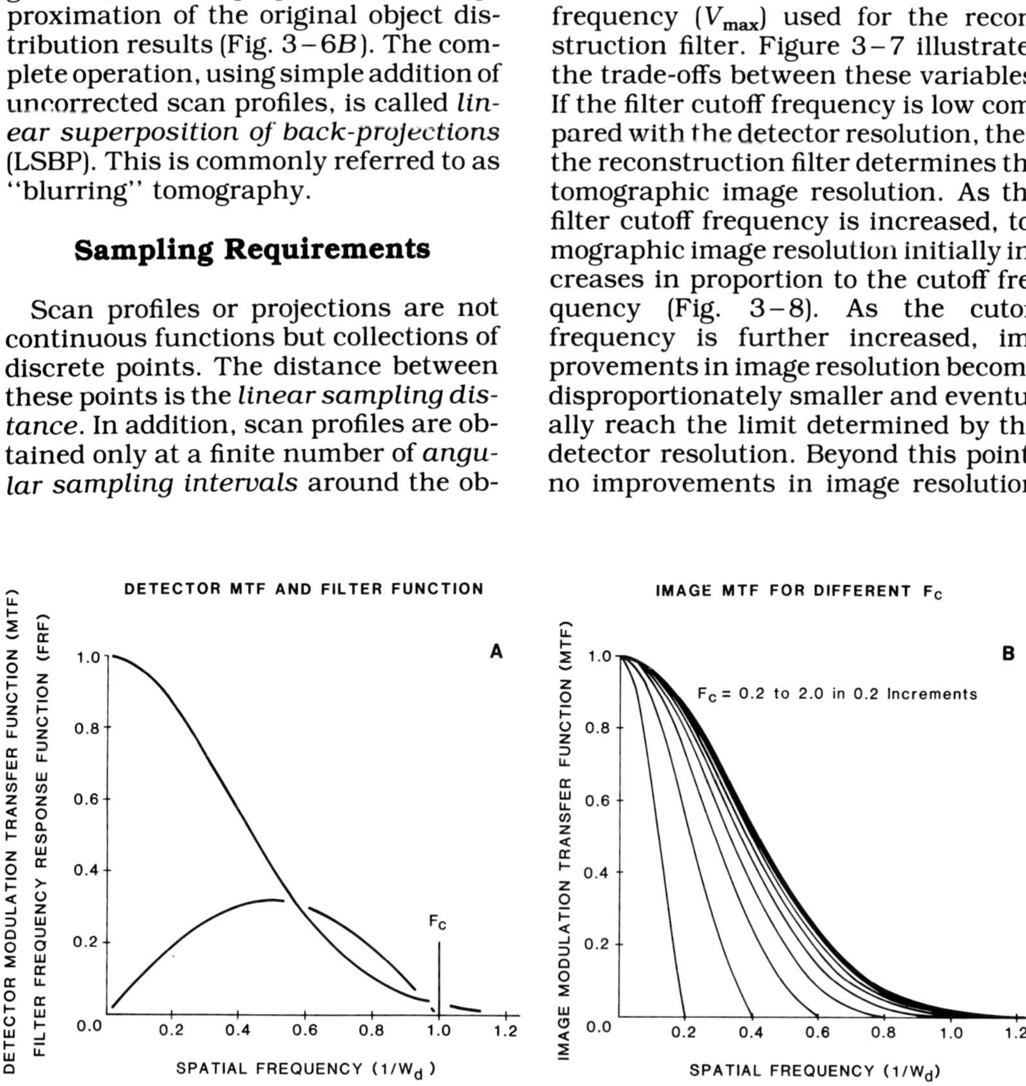

Figure 3–7. Relationship between detector resolution, reconstruction filter function, and image resolution. (*Left*) Detector resolution shown by the modulation transfer function (MTF; see Fig. 3–11) and a rounded version of a reconstruction filter function with a cutoff frequency, V_m. (*Right*) MTF of image resolution as the cutoff frequency of the reconstruction filter is increased in linear increments. Note that initially the image resolution increases linearly with increases in the cutoff frequency. Progressive constant incremental increases in the cutoff frequency produce a diminishing increase in image resolution. When the cutoff frequency of the reconstruction filter is low, it is the dominant factor in determining the image resolution. As the cutoff frequency is increased, the detector resolution dominates the image resolution.

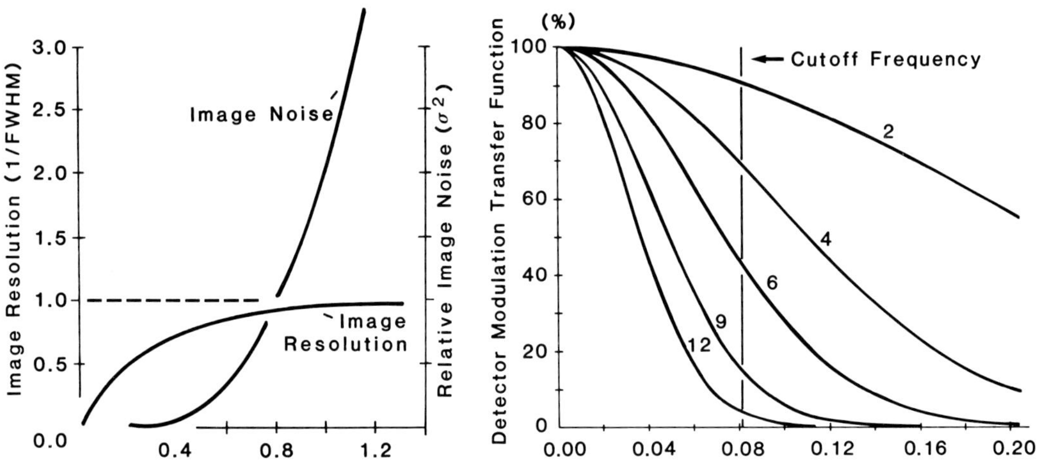

Figure 3–8. Principle of the signal amplification technique (SAT). (*Left*) Image resolution as the reconstruction filter cutoff frequency is increased (see Fig. 3–8). The response is initially linear, becomes nonlinear, and then asymptotic. Image noise (in terms of variance) increases by the third power of the cutoff frequency. Common reconstruction cutoff frequencies are around 0.9 in units of 1/FWHM. Thus, in the nonlinear portion of the response, small increases in image resolution are obtained at the expense of large increases in image noise. (*Right*) Detector modulation transfer function for detectors with FWHM resolutions of 12, 9, 6, 4, and 2 mm. Conventional reconstruction cutoff frequency for a 12-mm resolution detector system is shown as a vertical line. Note the increase in MTF amplitude in the region between 0 and the conventional cutoff frequency for a 12-mm detector. In this region, small high-resolution detectors provide signal amplification and increased image resolution without increasing image noise. (From Reference 16, Phelps, Huang, Hoffman, et al.,[16] with permission.)

can be achieved unless the detector resolution is increased. Once the limiting resolution, as determined by detector resolution and filter cutoff frequency, has been established, the linear sampling distance should be selected to recover this resolution properly.

For proper reconstruction of the image, a number of requirements must be met:[5,14]

1. Data must originate from well-defined lines through the body (i.e., spatial resolution is essentially depth-independent).
2. Data represent the linear sum of radioisotope concentrations along these lines. Thus, corrections must be applied for attenuation of 511-keV photons by the body.
3. Data are properly sampled in the linear and angular directions.

All of these conditions are easily met with the unique detection system used in PET.[5,14]

Annihilation Coincidence Detection (ACD)

In traditional nuclear medicine imaging, the location in the body of emitted radiation is determined with lead collimators, as shown in Figure 3–9. Several limitations result from this approach:

1. Most of the radiation emitted from the body (about 99%) is absorbed by the collimator and not used to form the image.
2. Each collimated location on the detector can only "look" in one direction at a time.
3. Attenuation corrections are complex and inaccurate.

Criteria 1 and 2 reduce detection sensitivity and criterion 3 limits quantitation and produces artifacts in tomographic imaging.

Annihilation coincidence detection (ACD)[5,14] in PET provides solutions to

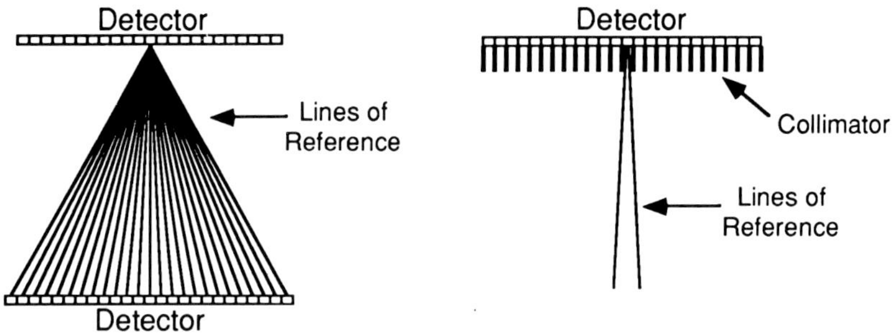

Figure 3–9. Lead collimation used in single photon imaging (*right*) versus annihilation coincidence detection (ACD) (*left*) used in PET. Each detector resolution element collects data from one region in single photon imaging, versus many regions with ACD.

each of these problems. Lead collimators are not required in ACD. The location of emitted radiation is determined by using the simultaneous detection of the two 511-keV photons emitted in positron decay (see Figs. 3–3 and 3–9). In a PET scanner, a circumferential array of detectors surrounds the patient. When a 511-keV photon strikes a detector, an electronic circuit checks to see if one of the detectors on the opposite side of the detector array was simultaneously hit. The simultaneous or coincident recording of events in opposing detectors indicates that the radiation originated somewhere along a line between the two detectors because of the 180° emission of the two 511-keV photons. Because this approach employs the identification of coincident photons from the annihilation of a positron and an electron, it is referred to as annihilation coincidence detection.[14]

Many coincident combinations of detector pairs are employed in PET scanners to yield "fan beam" fields of view for each detector (Figs. 3–9 and 3–10). In modern PET scanners there can be 1,000,000 or more of these coincident detector combinations collecting data simultaneously. Thus, each detector in a PET scanner can "look" in many different directions at once. This concept provides high detector efficiency, or what is commonly referred to as sensitivity.

The time resolution of ACD is determined by the particular detector material used (see next section). Time resolution determines how well ACD can discriminate between "true coincident events" (TC) and "random coincidences" (RC). Only true events contain valid spatial information about the radioisotope distribution. Random coincidences occur when two unrelated 511-keV photons accidentally strike two opposing detectors simultaneously (see Fig. 3–3). This produces information that is randomly distributed in space and therefore contributes noise to the image. Photons can also be scattered by the body and still occur in true coincidence (see Fig. 3–3). These scatter coincidences (SC) also contribute noise to the image. Thus, scanner designs attempt to maximize true coincidences and minimize random and scatter coincidences.

Detectors and Geometric Configuration

The desired properties of detectors for PET are:

1. High stopping power for 511-KeV photons. This requires material with high density and high atomic numbers.
2. Fast response time, to minimize random coincidences and allow high count rates. Detectors used in PET (scintillation detectors) produce light when struck by radiation. Thus, detectors should have high light yield and fast decay times for the light.

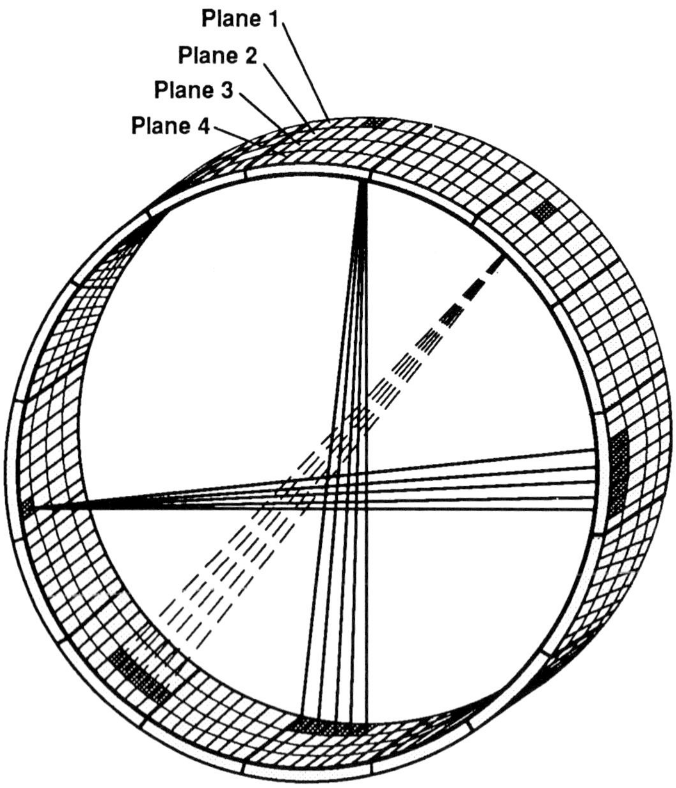

Figure 3-10. Schematic illustration of fan beam coincidences between detectors in a detector ring and between detector rings of a multidetector-ring PET scanner.

3. Good energy resolution. This requires high scintillation light yield.
4. Nonhygroscopic (i.e., do not absorb water), so that detectors do not have to be placed in vacuum-sealed containers. This allows detectors to be closely packed together to maximize geometric efficiency.

The properties of different detector materials are shown in Table 3-6. Although the first PET scanners employed sodium iodide NaI(Tl) detectors, almost all commercial scanners presently use bismuth germanate (BGO), because of its high density, high atomic number, nonhygroscopic properties, and relatively low cost. Its disadvantages include a relatively low light yield

Table 3-6 PROPERTIES OF DETECTOR MATERIALS

	Materials				
Property	***NaI(Tl)***	***CsF***	***BGO***	***GSO***	***BaF_2***
Density (g/cm^3)	3.67	4.61	7.13	6.71	4.89
Atomic numbers	11,53	55,9	83,32,8	58,64,14,8	56,9
Effective atomic number	50	53	74	59	54
Scintillation decay time (ns)*	230	2.5	300	60	0.8;620†
Relative scintillation light yield	100	6.3	12	16	5;16.3†
Hygroscopic	yes	very	no	no	very little

BGO = $Bi_3Ge_4O_{12}$.
GSO = $Ge_2SiO_5(Ce)$.
*Time required for emission of 67% of the light.
†The decay of BaF_2 has two components. The one with the lower light yield (5) has a decay time of 0.8 nanoseconds, while the one with the highest light yield (16.3) has a decay time of 620 nanoseconds.

and slow decay time. These factors have not been a significant negative issue in system performance. One commercial scanner uses BaF_2 because its fast decay time produces very good coincidence time resolution. Its lower stopping power compared to BGO is a disadvantage.

Spatial Resolution

Two important measures of spatial resolution are the intrinsic resolution of the detector and the reconstructed image resolution. Both are determined by measuring the spatial response to a thin line source of radioactivity to yield a *line spread function* (LSF) (Fig. 3–11). The Fourier transform of the LSF produces what is called the *modulation transfer function* (MTF), as shown in Figure 3–11. The LSF shows the amplitude of signal as a function of distance. The MTF shows the amplitude of signal as a function of spatial frequency (i.e., cycles per unit distance). The most common term used to describe spatial resolution is the *full width at half maximum* (FWHM) of the LSF. The MTF is the most informative of the two types of resolution measurements because it shows what fraction of the signal at each spatial frequency will be recorded by the system. The MTF in Figure 3–11 shows that at low spatial frequency (i.e, low spatial resolution), all of the signal is recorded. With increasingly high frequencies (i.e., high spatial resolution), there is a progressive loss in the fraction of the signal that the system can faithfully record. Thus, the MTF provides a measure of how much detail can be seen and quantitatively measured in structures of varying sizes with a particular scanner.

Spatial resolution in the tomographic image is determined by a number of physical factors, including:

1. Intrinsic detector resolution and its uniformity with distance from the detector surface,
2. The distance the positron travels before it annihilates,
3. Errors that occur because there is some variation in the 180° angle at which the two 511-keV photons are emitted (i.e., angulation error),
4. Random and scatter coincidences, and
5. Image reconstruction algorithm.

The intrinsic detector resolution is determined primarily by detector size, although to a lesser degree the shape and type of detector material contribute as well. In general, the FWHM of the LSF ranges from about 45%–70% of the detector width; the smaller the detector, the larger the fraction (i.e., 10- and 3-mm wide BGO detectors have FWHMs of 5 and 2.1 mm). Annihilation coincidence detection also provides resolution that is very uniform in depth across the image field of view of the scanner (Fig. 3–12), as required by the image reconstruction algorithm.

The magnitude of spatial resolution

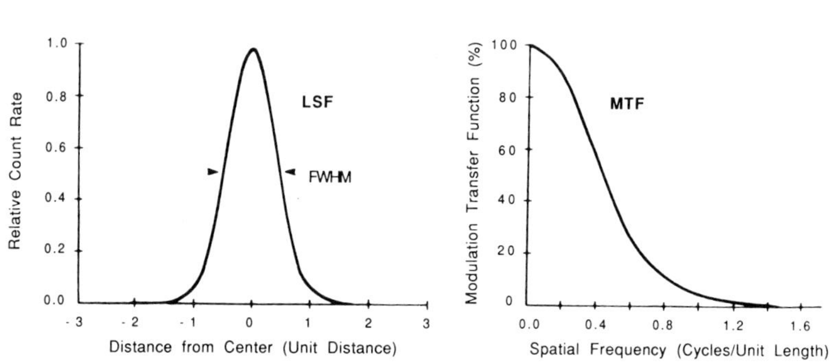

Figure 3–11. A line spread function (LSF) and the Fourier transformation of the LSF combine to yield a modulation transfer function (MTF). The full-width at half-maximum (FWHM) resolution is illustrated on the LSF.

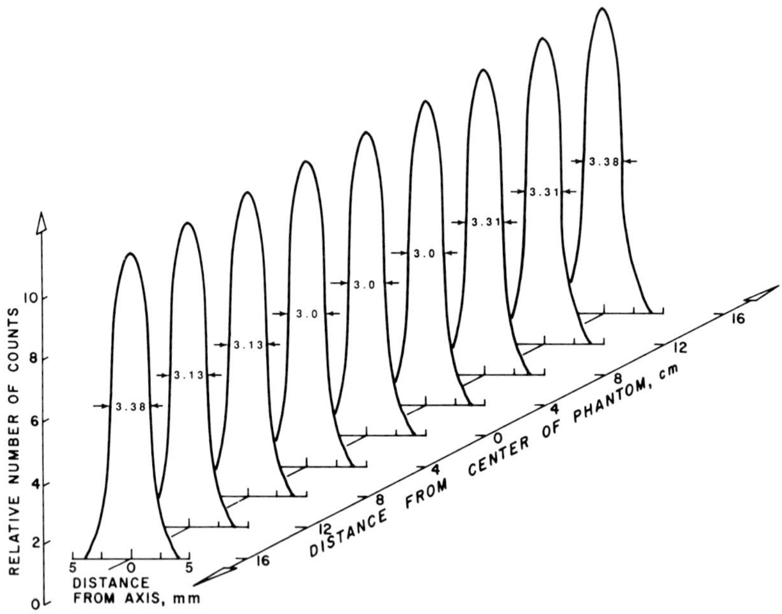

Figure 3–12. LSF to illustrate the small variation of resolution with depth for the ACD technique. The detector separation distance is 60 cm. Numerical values are the FWHM resolutions in mm.

due to positron range depends upon how far the $\beta+$ travels before annihilation—in other words, on its energy. Measured resolution values from the effect of positron range for specific radioisotopes are shown in Table 3–1. Positron range is normally not a limiting factor in the image resolution of a PET scanner.

Statistical Noise

Statistical sources of noise also affect spatial resolution; in fact, this is the determining factor of resolution in PET, as well as in all other medical imaging technologies. The mathematical algorithm for forming the image in all forms of computed tomography generates large amounts of image noise. This can be intuitively understood from several perspectives. The process for producing the tomographic images involves an enormous number of arithmetic operations, with their corresponding error propagation. Another way to appreciate the particular pathway error propagated in computed tomography is by comparison of 2-D imaging as shown in Figure 3–13.

The "statistical resolution" of structures is illustrated in Figure 3–14. Even though these two images have the same physical resolution of 6 mm, the resolution of structures is much less in the image with fewer counts and, hence, higher statistical noise.

Resolution of structures in an image is dependent on:

1. Physical resolution,
2. Object size,
3. Object contrast (i.e., radioactivity ratio of a structure to its surrounding), and
4. Statistical noise.

Generally, object contrast must be ≥ 1.5 times statistical noise for the object to be reliably identified. Thus, the higher the object contrast, the higher the resolving power in the image for a given number of image counts. The statistical accuracy also sets confidence limits on the absolute accuracy of concentration measurements of structures in the image.

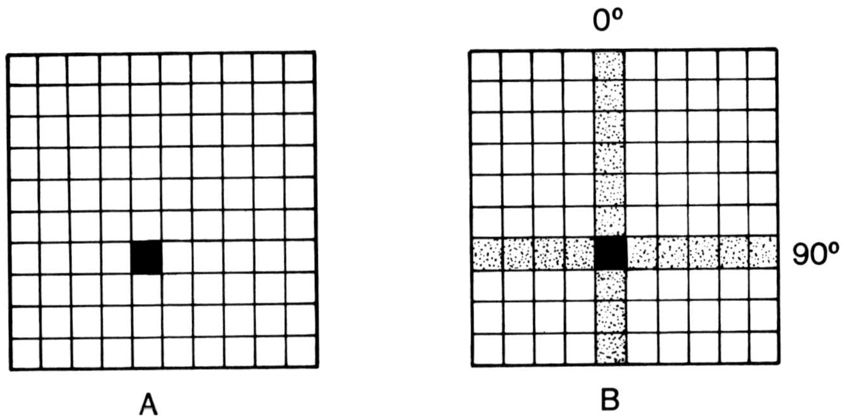

Figure 3–13. Error propagation in planar versus computed tomography imaging. (*A*) In two-dimensional imaging, signal and noise are restricted to each individual picture element. (*B*) In x-ray computed tomography, data are collected as projections of an object. Example shows 0° and 90° projection angles. Data in the black pixel are collected by looking through all of the pixels along the line involving it. Thus, error from data in the black pixel is propagated into all those through which it is examined.

Partial-Volume Effect

The partial-volume effect describes the relationship between object size and physical image resolution.[5,11] Tomographic systems have a characteristic "resolution volume" determined by the combination of their in-plane and axial resolutions. This volume has an approximately cylindrical shape of

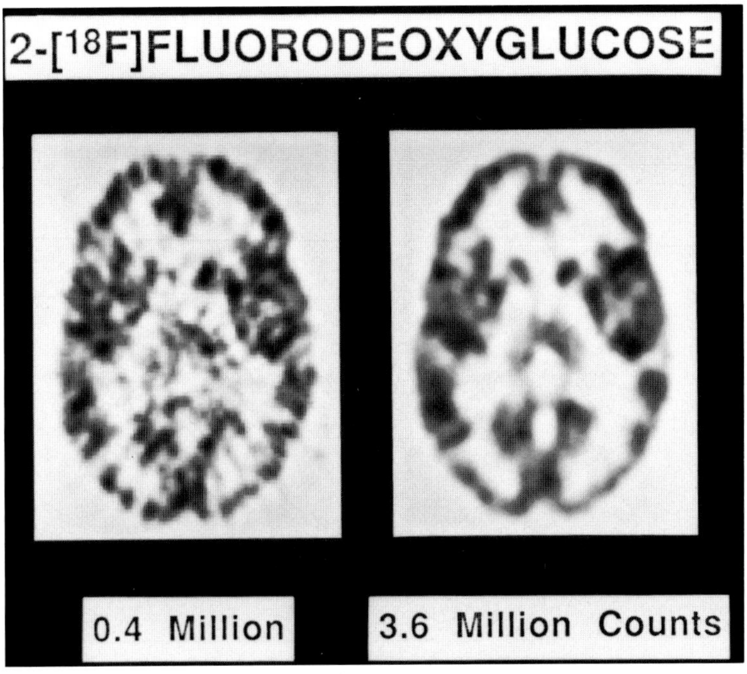

Figure 3–14. Statistical components of resolution in PET. Patient study of cerebral glucose metabolism. Frames were added to result in 400,000 counts (*left*) and 3.6 million counts (*right*) per image and reconstructed to the same physical resolution of 6 mm. These images demonstrate that the actual image resolution is not necessarily equal to the physical resolution of a scanner.

height = 2 × FWHM of the axial resolution and diameter = 2 × FWHM of the in-plane resolution. The images produced by a PET scanner reflect the amount of activity within these individual volume elements. For a structure equal to the resolution volume or larger, the image correctly reflects both the absolute amount and concentration of activity. Smaller objects only partially occupy the characteristic volume. In this case, the system response reflects the amount, but not the concentration, of activity within the object. Thus, if the concentration of radioactivity within an object is held constant, the apparent concentration in the image decreases as object size decreases, if the object is small compared with image resolution (Fig. 3–15). Total counts are conserved for smaller objects, but the counts are distributed over a volume larger than the physical dimensions of the object and thus appear to represent a larger object with a radioactivity concentration lower than its true value.

This partial-volume effect is important for both qualitative and quantitative interpretation of PET data. The ratio of the apparent concentration to true concentration is called the *recovery coefficient* (RC). The RC for a 3-D object is a product of the RCs in each dimension. RC gives the fraction of information that can be recovered for different-sized structures in an image of a specific resolution. In principle, if a PET system has a known and uniform spatial resolution and if the size of the object is known, a "recovery coefficient correction factor" can be applied to correct the partial-volume errors for small objects. Although this approach works well in phantom studies in which object sizes are well characterized, the sizes of in vivo objects are usually too poorly defined for this method to be useful. MRI definition of structure size does provide one means to make partial-volume corrections for small structures in PET images. The concept of RC is important in understanding the quantitative re-

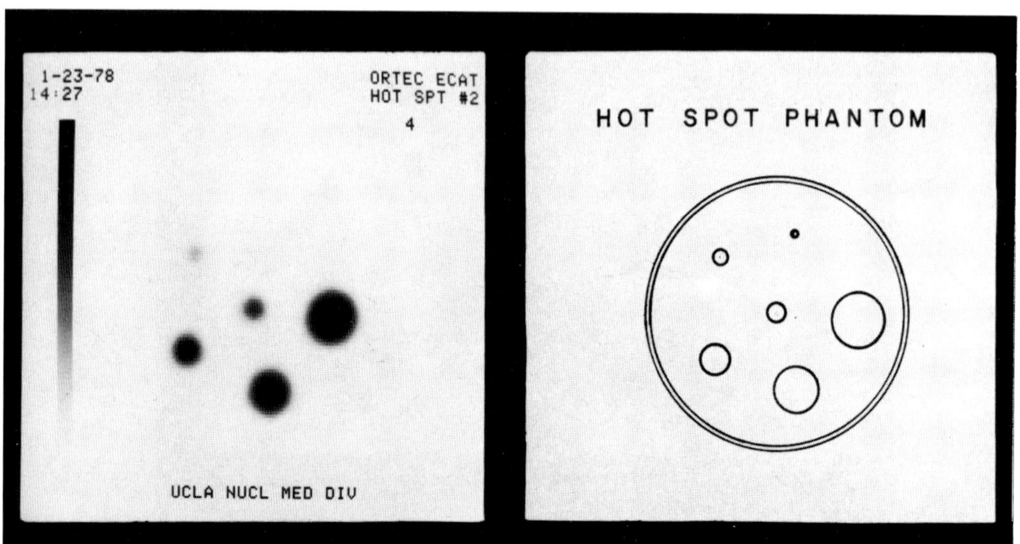

Figure 3–15. Phantom images illustrating partial volume effect. Phantom is a 21-cm diameter, water-filled cylinder containing six cylinders, 6.35, 9.53, 15.9, 22.2, 31.8, and 38.1 mm in diameter. Each of the small cylinders has the same concentration of positron-emitting activity. The image resolution in this example was 13 mm FWHM. The decreased intensity in the smaller cylinders results from the fact that the recovery coefficient is less than 1. (From Hoffman and Phelps,[5] with permission.)

covery of information in PET as a function of structure size and spatial resolution.

RCs for various neuroanatomic structures are given in Table 3–7. With improving spatial resolution there is clearly an increase in the number of structures seen, as well as in their image contrast and the accuracy of their tissue radioactivity concentration measurement.

Axial Resolution and Sampling

The greatest focus of attention in all tomographic imaging techniques is on in-plane image resolution, with less attention paid to the axial resolution (i.e., thickness of the tomographic image) or sampling distance between images. This naturally occurs because the in-plane image resolution is what one sees. Three-dimensional structures are being imaged, however, so the accuracy and magnitude of image contrast are determined by the relationship between the size of the structure and the volumetric resolution, as discussed earlier.

Full coverage of the brain can be achieved with PET in several ways. If the axial field of view of the tomograph does not cover the entire brain (which is the case for all existing scanners), then either the patient or the gantry is moved so that multiple sets of scans are required to cover the full axial extent of the brain. Although this is the current practice, it has several disadvantages. First, in dynamic studies this procedure requires movement back and forth to collect temporal information for each image set. Such movement produces time gaps in the data. Second, as opposed to x-ray CT and MRI, where radiation dose can be restricted in time and limited to selected tissue for collecting data, in PET all the tissue is receiving radiation dose whether data are being collected or not. Since radiation dose poses the ultimate limit, as well as for the other reasons given above, PET scanner designs are evolving with axial fields of view that cover the entire brain. These designs also provide proper axial sampling. The objective of these tomographic designs is to provide high inplane and axial resolution with proper sampling in all three dimensions without any patient or gantry motion.

Efficiency and Temporal Resolution

Efficiency of a PET scanner is typically measured by counting a 20-cm-diameter uniform cylinder of known activity concentration (for example, μCi/mL) of a pure positron emitter. The units of efficiency are counts per second per μCi/mL. The counts in this case refer only to true coincidences. Thus, the random and scatter coincidences must also be measured and subtracted from the total counts recorded by the scanner.

Temporal resolution is determined by the efficiency and count rate capability of the tomograph. The limit in temporal resolution is the number of true image counts that can be collected per unit of time. Besides efficiency, the primary factors affecting temporal resolution are random coincidences and deadtime.

Deadtime refers to the fraction of time over which the tomograph is processing an event and cannot accept another. Deadtime limitations can occur in the detector, associated electronics, data buffers, and data transfer lines. The rate-limiting step depends upon the particular tomograph design and detector material. These factors are described in detail elsewhere.[5]

TRACER KINETIC MODELING

Tracer kinetic models are mathematical descriptions of dynamic processes. They allow formal quantitative descriptions and measurements of a process. Extensive descriptions of tracer kinetic modeling as applied to PET are provided elsewhere.[9] This description will be lim-

Table 3–7 RECOVERY COEFFICIENTS OF NEUROANATOMIC STRUCTURES FOR SPECIFIC VOXEL SIZE*

Structure[b]	*Volume*	Voxel Size (mm)				
		5 × 5 × 5	*5 × 5 × 10*	*10 × 10 × 10*	*10 × 10 × 15*	*15 × 15 × 15*
Corpus callosum	11.6	1.0	0.98	0.94	0.90	0.83
Caudate	5.2	1.0	0.90	0.73	0.50	0.24
Putamen	5.1	1.0	0.95	0.86	0.76	0.59
Thalamus	5.0	1.0	0.89	0.70	0.48	0.23
Internal capsule	2.7	1.0	0.91	0.75	0.62	0.42
Globus pallidus	1.8	1.0	0.89	0.70	0.55	0.34
Hippocampus	1.7	1.0	0.64	0.26	0.16	0.06
Cerebellar vermis	1.2	1.0	0.77	0.51	0.42	0.29
Substantia nigra	0.7	0.94	0.69	0.42	0.37	0.20
Amygdala	0.4	0.75	0.42	0.13	0.07	0.02
Dentate	0.3	0.61	0.33	0.09	0.04	0.01
Anterior commissure	0.2	0.55	0.37	0.13	0.09	0.05
Red nucleus	0.2	0.51	0.21	0.04	0.02	<0.01
Lateral geniculate	0.1	0.22	0.10	0.01	0.01	<0.01
Medical geniculate	0.1	0.22	0.10	0.01	0.01	<0.01
Mammillary body	0.06	0.08	0.04	<0.01	<0.01	<0.01

*From Mazziotta, JC and Phelps, ME[11], with permission.

ited to the definitions, principles, and examples of approaches. In general, the tracer kinetic models in PET are used to convert tissue and plasma data into quantitative measurements of a biological process (see Fig. 3–1).

Definition of Terms

TRACER

A tracer is a substance that follows (traces) a process under study. In this chapter the term *tracer* refers to the use of compounds labeled with a positron-emitting radioisotope. The tracers used in PET consist of labeled natural substrates, substrate analogs, inert compounds, and drugs (see Table 3–3). A tracer must satisfy the following criteria:

1. The behavior of the tracer should, in a known and predictable manner, be identical or related to that of the natural compound or process being traced.
2. The mass of the tracer used should not alter the process being studied. The mass of the tracer should be small compared to the mass of the endogenous compound being traced. In general, the mass of the tracer should be less than 1% of that of the endogenous compound.
3. Any difference between the tracer and the natural compound should be negligible, or a correction should be applied to the effect.

ANALOG TRACERS

Analog tracers are compounds that possess many of the properties of natural compounds, but with differences that change the way the compound behaves in biological systems. For example, analogs that participate in only a limited number of steps in a sequence of biochemical reactions have been developed in biochemistry and pharmacology to simplify and increase specificity in a tracer study. For example, analogs can be formed by slightly modifying a natural compound so that it will proceed through several steps of a complex reaction sequence to a point where the product is no longer a substrate for the remainder of the pathway. Analogs are also used to bind, irreversibly or reversibly, to enzymes or receptors to assay their concentration and distribution in tissue.

With the use of analogs, correction terms must be developed so that measurements of the analog can be converted to the natural substrate or process. The measurement of the local cerebral metabolic rate for glucose with the glucose analog 2-[^{18}F]fluoro-2-deoxy-D-glucose (FDG) is an example of the use of such an analog.

COMPARTMENTAL MODELS

These are the most common form of tracer kinetic models used in PET. In compartmental models, physical spaces or steps in a reaction sequence are divided into separate compartments and the model is designed to measure transport of tracer between compartments (Fig. 3–16).

A *compartment* is a volume or space within which the tracer rapidly becomes uniformly distributed (that is, it contains no significant concentration gradients). The kinetics of a compartment can be described by a single rate constant (i.e., single exponential clearance). In some cases a compartment has an obvious physical interpretation, such as the intravascular blood pool, reactants and products in a chemical reaction, or spaces bounded by membranes. For other compartments the physical interpretation may be less obvious. For example, a tracer may be metabolized or trapped by one of two different cell populations in an organ, defining two populations of cells as separate compartments. Additionally, while the definition of a particular compartment may be appropriate for one tracer (e.g., the distribution of labeled red blood cells in the intravascular blood pool), it might not apply for a different tracer (e.g., the distribution of ox-

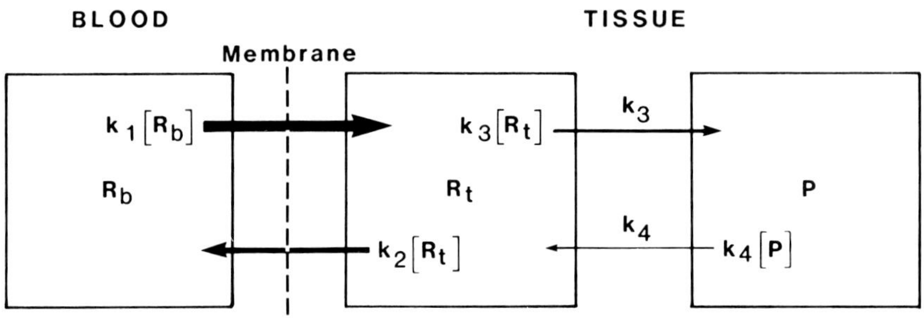

Figure 3–16. A three-compartment model consisting of reactants in blood (R_b), tissue (R_t), and product (P) in tissue. The fluxes between the compartments, indicated by arrows, are products of the first-order rate constants (k_1, k_2, k_3, k_4) and the respective compartmental concentrations.

ygen, which has both an intravascular and an extravascular distribution). Thus, the number, interrelationship, organization, and definition of compartments in a compartmental model must be developed from knowledge of biological and biochemical principles.

DISTRIBUTION VOLUME AND PARTITION COEFFICIENT

A compartment may be *closed* or *open* to a tracer. A closed compartment is one from which the tracer cannot escape, whereas an open compartment is one from which it can escape to other compartments. Whether a compartment is closed or open depends on both the compartment and the tracer. Indeed, a compartment may be open to one tracer and closed to another.

If a tracer enters a closed compartment, such as a nondiffusible tracer in the vascular system, conservation of mass requires that after the distribution of the tracer reaches equilibrium, or steady-state conditions, the amount of tracer injected, *A* (in millicuries or other units of activity), must equal the concentration of the tracer in the compartment, *C* (in μCi/mL), multiplied by the *distribution volume*, V_d, of the compartment. Thus,

$$V_d(\text{mL}) = [A/C] \text{ at equilibrium} \quad (3\text{-}2)$$

This is the basis for the *dilution principle*, which provides a convenient method for determining the distribution volume of a closed compartment.

More commonly, a compartment will be open (that is, the tracer will be able to escape from it). This applies, for example, to tracers that are distributed and exchanged between blood and tissue. In this case, after the tracer reaches its equilibrium distribution, the concentration in blood will typically be different from that in the tissue. Equilibrium in this case means that the concentration of the tracer in the compartment has reached a constant value with time. It does not imply equilibrium in the thermodynamic sense (i.e., that there is no further transport of tracer between tissue and blood). Thus, tracer equilibrium is synonymous with the term "steady state" (see p. 93). The ratio of tissue to blood concentration, at equilibrium, is called the *partition coefficient*, λ, defined by

$$\lambda \text{ (mL/g)} = C_t(\mu\text{Ci/g})C_b(\text{mCi/mL}) \quad (3\text{-}3)$$

In PET studies the blood concentration, C_b, is usually measured by taking blood samples, whereas the tissue concentration is obtained from PET image data. Assuming that the concentration of tracer in tissue is the same as the concentration in blood, equation 3-2 leads to an apparent distribution volume in tissue given by $V_1 = A_t/C_b$, where A_t is the activity in the tissue. Also, $A_t = C_1 \times V_t$, where V_d (Eq. 3-2) is the volume (or mass) of tissue; therefore, combining these relationships and Equation 3-3, yields:

$$\lambda = V_1/V_t \qquad (3\text{-}4)$$

Thus, another interpretation of the partition coefficient is that it is the distribution volume per unit mass of tissue for a diffusible substance or tracer. This interpretation is employed in some models for estimating blood flow and perfusion.

FLUX

Flux refers to the amount of a substance that crosses a boundary or surface per unit time (e.g., mg/minute or μmol/minute) (see Fig. 3–16). It can also refer to the transport of a substance between different compartments in terms of flux/unit volume or mass of tissue (e.g., mg/minute per mL or μmol/minute per gram.

Flux is a general term that can refer to a variety of processes. For example, the total mass of red blood cells moving through a blood vessel per unit time is a flux. The "boundary" or "surface" in this case could be any transverse plane through the vessel. The amount of glucose moving across a cell membrane per unit time is also a flux. The primary objective of PET is to measure fluxes such as the flow of blood through tissue; of substrate through a biochemical pathway; or drug interactions with receptors, substrates or enzymes.

RATE CONSTANTS

Rate constants describe the relationships between the concentrations and fluxes of a substance between two compartments. For simple *first-order processes*, the rate constant, *k*, multiplied by the amount or concentration of a substance in a compartment, determines the flux:

$$\text{Flux} = \text{k} \times \text{Amount of Substance} \qquad (3\text{-}5)$$

For first-order processes, the units of k are reciprocal time (time^{-1}). If "amount" refers to the mass of tracer in the compartment, the units of flux are mass/time (e.g., mg/minute). If "amount" refers to concentration of tracer in the compartment, the units of flux are mass/time per unit of compartment volume (e.g., mg/minute per mL), or mass/time/unit of compartment mass (e.g., mg/minute per gram or μmol/minute per gram.) As illustrated by Figure 3–16, different directions of transport between two compartments are characterized by different rate constants.

Figure 3–16 illustrates a three-compartment system consisting of a blood compartment separated by a membrane barrier (e.g., capillary wall) from two sequential tissue compartments consisting of chemical reactants and products. The widths of the arrows are proportional to the magnitude of the corresponding flux. In this example, the fluxes into and out of tissue are larger than corresponding fluxes between the reactant and product compartments in tissue. Thus, the majority of the substance initially transported into the tissue space is transported back into blood without undergoing any biochemical reactions. This is a common occurrence in real biochemical systems and provides a reserve capacity in the system that can accommodate changes in metabolic supply and demand.

STEADY STATE

The term *steady state* refers to a condition in which a process, parameter, or variable is not changing with time. For example, a flux through a biochemical pathway is said to be in steady state when the concentration of reactants and products remains unchanged with time. Even though the concentrations are not changing, however, there is continual transport of substances between compartments. In all tracer kinetic models, it is assumed that the underlying process being measured by the tracer is in a steady state. Because of biorhythms, steady states almost never exist in the body; however, if the magnitude or temporal period of change is small compared with the process being measured, then the steady-state assumption is reasonable. In many cases, the experimental temporal sampling rate is slow compared with the biorhythm (e.g., blood sampling rate versus pulsatile nature of vascular blood flow) and it is not detected in the measured data. In these cases, the measured parameter represents an average value of the function measured. If the period of the biorhythm is large compared with the temporal sampling rate or the average rate of the process observed, significant errors in the model calculations may result. In this case, the calculated parameters typically do not represent a simple average of the non–steady-state values.

Steady state of a process should not be confused with steady state of the tracer. Measurements of the tracer commonly are made when the tracer itself is not in steady state, but rather while it is distributing through the process under study. Some tracer kinetic models are used in which measurements are made when both the tracer and process studied are in that steady state. These methods usually are referred to as "equilibrium" models.[9,10]

An important and useful property of a steady-state condition is that the rates (fluxes) of all steps in a nonbranching transport or reaction sequence are equal. Thus, if a tracer technique is used to measure one step in a sequence, the rate for each step in the entire sequence is equal and known. If the reaction branches into two or more separate pathways, then the sum of the rates in each pathway must equal the rate of the preceding step. In this case, if one determines the rate of any of the preceding steps and also knows the branching fraction, then the rate of each branch can be determined by multiplying the rate of the preceding step by the branching fraction (Fig. 3–17).

BLOOD FLOW AND PERFUSION

These terms are often confused. Blood flow refers to the volume of blood flowing through vessels per unit time (i.e., mL/minute). Perfusion refers to blood flow per mass of tissue (i.e., mL/minute per gram). Perfusion is measured with PET. By convention, cerebral perfusion is referred to as cerebral blood flow (CBF). Because the tracer techniques used in PET measure blood flow at the capillary vessel level, they provide a measure of the blood flow where nutrients or metabolic substrates are exchanged between blood and tissue.

CEREBRAL BLOOD FLOW

Measurement of blood flow per mass of tissue (i.e., perfusion) is performed by a number of different approaches in PET. Only two of these approaches will be illustrated, the clearance and the equilibrium techniques. The desirable properties for such a tracer are that it:

1. Is chemically inert,
2. Is freely diffusible through the BBB, and
3. Has a known partition coefficient

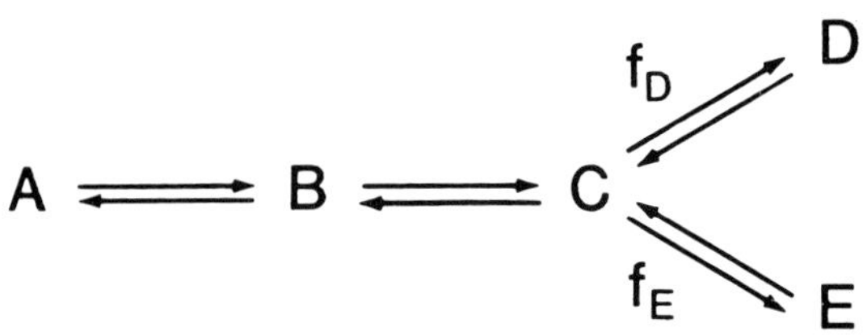

Figure 3–17. Example of a multistep reaction sequence that branches into two pathways. The terms f_D and f_E are the branching fractions for the corresponding pathways. If this reaction sequence is in a steady state, and the rate of disappearance of A is R_A, the rates of formation of B, C, D, and E are R_B, R_C, R_D, and R_E, respectively, and f_D and f_E are the branching fraction down the corresponding pathways, then

$R_A = R_B = R_C = (R_D + R_E)$; $R_D = f_D \times R_C$; $R_E = f_E \times R_C$; and $f_D + f_E = 1$.

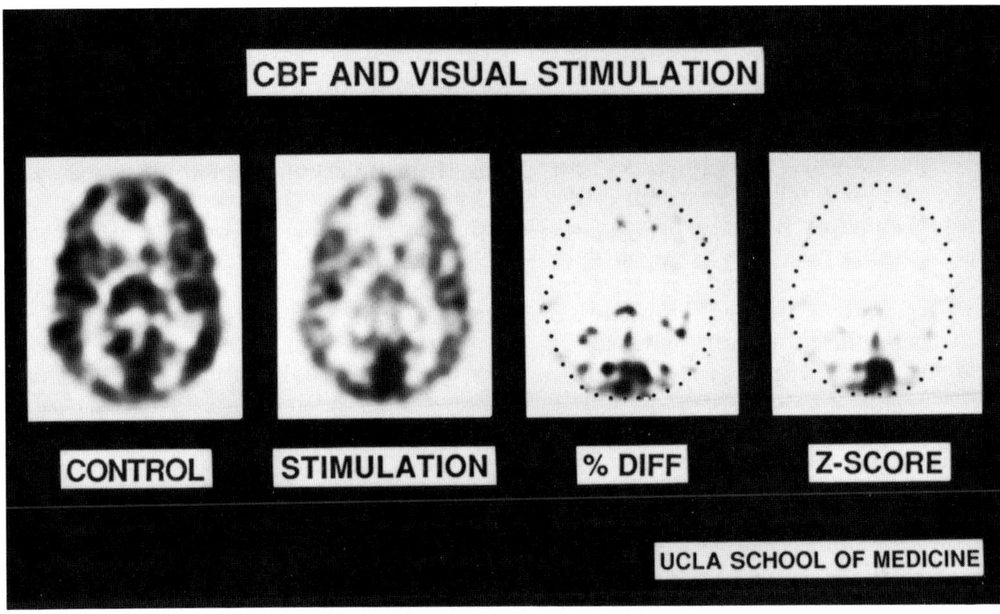

Figure 3–18. Cerebral blood flow studies performed with PET and ^{15}O labeled water. The same subject was studied twice in this illustration, first with his eyes closed in the "Control" state and 10 minutes later with central field black-and-white checkerboard stimulation ("Stimulation"). Note the activation of the calcarine cortex at the bottom of the images when one compares the "Stimulation" to the "Control" state. The third image represents the percent difference between the stimulation and control studies. Note that most cerebral blood flow activity is eliminated and only the area of the brain activated by the stimulus remains. The rightmost image is the "z-score" statistical map showing areas of maximal statistical difference between the stimulation and control states. Although it is similar to the percent difference image, there is a smaller zone of cortical activity constrained by the more stringent statistical criteria. (Provided by S Grafton and JC Mazziotta, UCLA School of Medicine.)

that does not vary significantly between different types of normal tissues or between normal and pathologic tissues.

The most commonly used tracers that meet these requirements are $H_2{}^{15}O$ (Fig. 3–18) and $CH_3{}^{18}F$.

Clearance Technique. Clearance techniques for the measurement of perfusion in the brain are based on the *central volume principle*:

$$F = V/\tau \qquad (3\text{-}6)$$

where F is blood flow, V is the volume in which the tracer is distributed and τ is the mean transit time of the tracer through the volume, V. Freely diffusible tracers are extracted from blood into tissue almost exclusively at the capillaries, because of the large capillary surface area. Since the tracer is inert, it will distribute through and clear from the tissue in proportion to blood flow. Flow can then be determined using Equation 3-6. The specific volume of tissue into which the tracer distributes depends upon the specific diffusion and solubility properties of the tracer. If this volume, denoted as V, is substituted into a rearranged form of Equation 3-6 and both sides of the equation are multiplied by V_1/V_t, where V_t is the total tissue volume, then

$$F/V_1\,(V_1/V_t) = (1/\tau)\,(V_1/V_t) \qquad (3\text{-}7)$$

$$F/V_t = \lambda/t$$

where λ is the partition coefficient given by Equation 3.4. F/V_t is the blood flow per volume or mass of tissue, and is appropriately termed perfusion. Although the usage is confusing, F/V_t is commonly referred to as "cerebral blood flow" (CBF). Thus,

$$CBF = \lambda/t \tag{3-8}$$

The value of λ for a tracer is either measured in vitro by determining the tracer equilibrium concentration ratio between plasma and tissue, or in some cases is measured in vivo from the actual kinetic measurements with PET.[7]

Clearance techniques for determining CBF with PET employ either intravenous bolus injections of $H_2{}^{15}O$ or $CH_3{}^{18}F$, or inhalation of a bolus of $C^{15}O_2$, which is rapidly converted to $H_2{}^{15}O$ in the lungs by carbonic anhydrase. The short half life of ^{15}O (2 minutes) and rapid tissue clearance of $H_2{}^{15}O$ allow measurements of CBF to be performed in time intervals of 40–300 seconds, depending on the method employed.[9] Measurements can be repeated every 8–10 minutes. This allows rapid sequences of multiple measurements to be performed in a single setting as the functional states of the brain are varied by behavior tasks (Fig. 3–19) or sensory (see Fig. 3–18) and drug stimuli. The short half life of ^{15}O also is associated with a low radiation dose to the

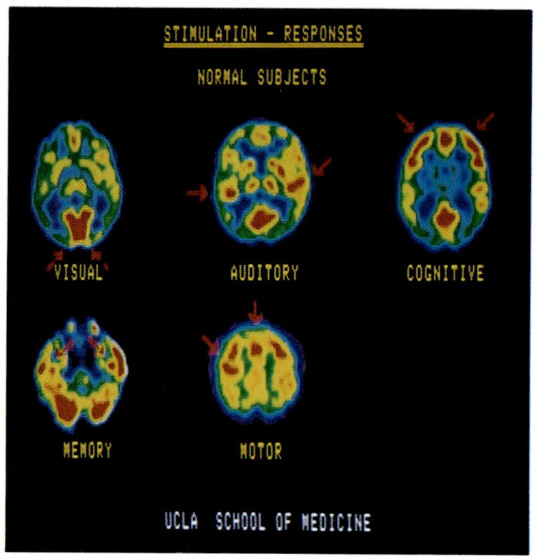

Figure 3–19. Five states of behavioral activation demonstrated with PET and FDG as increments in glucose metabolism. The Highest metabolic rates are shown as red, the lowest rate as blue, and intermediate values are yellow and green. The arrows indicate the stimulus-induced metabolic responses appropriate to the behavioral tasks. In the "Visual" task the subject was asked to look at full-field checkerboard stimulation, which activated the entire anterior-posterior extent of the calcarine cortex. The "Auditory" stimulus was a combination of verbal and nonverbal material played binaurally, producing bilateral activations of the transverse temporal cortex, which are seen in the appropriate anatomically asymmetric distributions in the two hemispheres. The "Cognitive" task required subjects to remember and solve problems, with resultant bilateral prefrontal cortex activations in glucose utilization. The "Memory" task required that the subjects listen to a long narrative passage and remember as many details about the passage as possible. They were told they would be paid in proportion to the amount of factual information they could recall. Bilateral mesial temporal activations were seen in all subjects performing this paradigm. These activations were in the region of the hippocampus and parahippocampal gyri. The "Motor" task required subjects to sequentially touch fingers to the opposing thumb of the right hand. Note the activation of the contralateral sensory motor cortex as well as the midline supplementary motor cortex. These studies demonstrate that PET can be used to map the neuronal networks that subserve normal behavioral tasks and, by extrapolation, can be used to look at the compensatory rearrangements of such networks in response to acute or chronic injury to the brain. (From Phelps, M and Mazziotta, J: Positron emission tomography: Human brain function and biochemistry. Science 228:799–809, 1985, with permission.)

patient, allowing multiple studies in the same patient (see Table 3–6).

Equilibrium Technique. The short radioactive half-life of ^{15}O-labeled water provides another convenient tracer technique for measuring blood flow quantitatively with PET, using an equilibrium method. The constant-infusion method originally developed by Jones and co-workers[10] is a good example of an approach that simplifies data acquisition because it produces a flat input function and a constant tissue concentration of the tracer, once tracer steady state has been reached. The novel aspect of this approach is that the steady state is one between the blood flow delivery of $H_2{}^{15}O$ to tissue and removal by venous outflow, plus the radioactive decay of the short half life of ^{15}O ($t_{1/2}$ = 2 minute). This method works for any diffusible tracer with a very short radioactive half-life (short, that is, compared with the diffusion time of the tracer out of tissue).

CEREBRAL BLOOD VOLUME

Cerebral blood volume (CBV) is the volume of blood per mass of tissue (units of mL/g). CBV can be measured with a red-blood-cell or plasma tracer. The most common method employs either ^{15}O- or ^{11}C-labeled CO, which is given by inhalation. Labeled CO is bound tightly to hemoglobin. After about 3 or 4 minutes of equilibration time, images of the tissue concentration are recorded with PET and a venous blood sample is drawn. The local CBV is then calculated by:[15]

$$\text{CBV (mL/g)} = \frac{C_t}{C_b 0.85\ d} \qquad (3\text{-}9)$$

where C_t is the local tissue activity concentrations, C_b is the peripheral venous blood activity concentration, 0.85 is a correction factor for the difference between peripheral and central hematocrit, and d is the density of brain tissue (1.04 g/mL).

DEOXYGLUCOSE MODEL

The deoxyglucose model represents a number of principles employed in biochemistry and also in PET. The 2-deoxy-D-glucose (DG) or its positron-labeled version 2-[^{18}F]fluoro-2-deoxy-D-glucose (FDG) are competitive substrate analogs of glucose.[9,18] The tracer kinetic model for the measurement of the local cerebral metabolic rate for glucose metabolism (LCMRGlc) is based upon the principle of competitive substrate kinetics.

FDG competes with glucose for the carrier-mediated transport sites in the BBB. After entering the cerebral tissue, FDG and glucose then compete for hexokinase for respective phosphorylation to FDG-6-PO_4 and glucose-6-PO_4. At this point, glucose-6-PO_4 either proceeds down the glycolytic pathway or is converted to glycogen. FDG-6-PO_4 is not a significant substrate for either of these pathways. FDG-6-PO_4 does not diffuse through membranes, so it is trapped and accumulates in cells in proportion to LCMRGlc. The compartmental model description for these processes is shown in Figure 3–20.

The tracer measurement yields the transport and metabolic rate of the brain for FDG. What is desired, however, is to know these rates for glucose. This is accomplished by knowing the relationship between FDG and glucose for transport and phosphorylation. Based on the principles of competitive substrate kinetics, a correction term can be applied to the FDG measurement, converting it to the corresponding value for glucose. The correction factor is called the "lumped constant" (LC). The FDG model requires the measurement of the temporal course of plasma FDG (input function) after intravenous injection, the value of the plasma glucose concentration and the tissue ^{18}F concentration. It assumes the end product of the reaction (FDG-6-PO_4) is trapped in the tissue. The model calculation uses average values of the rate constants and a standard value of LC. The average values of the rate constants are obtained from separate ki-

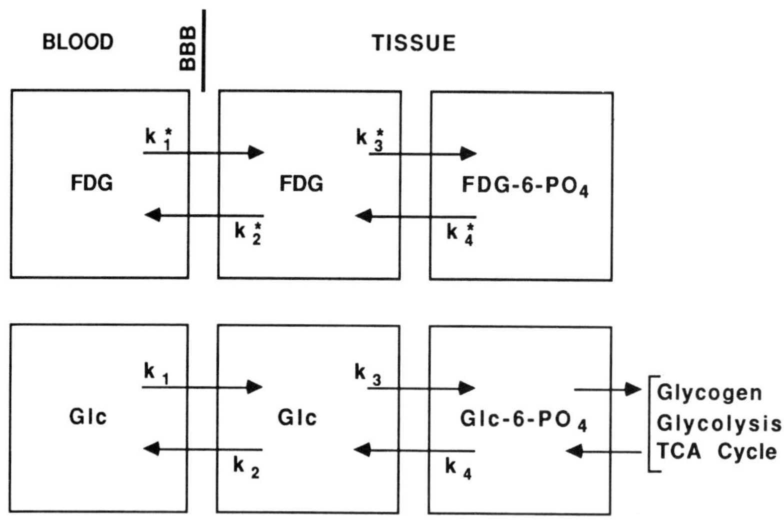

Figure 3–20. Three-compartment model for FDG with the four first-order rate constants describing transport between the compartments. Model illustrates the competition of transport, phosphorylation, and dephosphorylation between the competitive substrates FDG and glucose to the point of phosphorylation. TCA = tricarboxylic acid.

netic studies in a population of subjects. Because these are not the exact values of the rate constants for a particular study, they produce some error. The tissue measurement is performed at late times after injection (30–40 minutes), when these terms become small and the inaccuracies of using average values for the rate constants are minimized.

The published values of LC for FDG in the human brain range from 0.42 to 0.56. Since LC represents the net ratio of extraction by the brain of FDG to glucose, the value of LC implies that FDG is normally used by the brain at about one half the rate of glucose.

The descriptive formulation of the FDG model is shown at the bottom of the page.

The total ^{18}F activity minus free FDG equals the tissue concentrations of the reaction end product, namely, FDG-6-PO_4. Thus, the term in square brackets represents the fraction of FDG delivered to tissue that is metabolized to FDG-6-PO_4. Dividing this term by LC converts it to the fraction of glucose that would be metabolized to glucose-6-PO_4. Multiplication by the plasma glucose value converts this figure to the amount of glucose metabolized.

CEREBRAL PROTEIN SYNTHESIS

A model for the measurement of protein synthesis in the brain with PET illustrates an approach to simplify the tracer kinetic model by the specific selection of the radioactive label and its position in the labeled compound. The purpose of this model is to estimate the

---

$$\begin{pmatrix}\text{Local Glucose}\\ \text{Metabolic Rate}\end{pmatrix} = \left(\frac{\text{Plasma Glucose}}{\text{LC}}\right)\left[\frac{\begin{pmatrix}\text{Total }^{18}\text{F}\\ \text{in Region}\end{pmatrix} - \begin{pmatrix}\text{Free FDG}\\ \text{in Region}\end{pmatrix}}{\begin{pmatrix}\text{Total Net FDG Concentration}\\ \text{Transported to the Region}\end{pmatrix}}\right]$$

rate of protein synthesis in the brain or, more specifically, the rate of incorporation of amino acids into proteins.

Desirable properties of a tracer for measuring protein synthesis in the brain include a high BBB permeability, a rapid turnover rate of the amino acid in the brain precursor pool (i.e., rapid incorporation into protein), and a rapid clearance of the labeled amino acid from the blood pool. [^{11}C]-L-leucine satisfies these requirements reasonably well.

A difficulty is encountered because leucine is both incorporated into proteins and metabolized through an alternate pathway as shown in Figure 3–21. The two branching pathways cannot be differentiated by simply measuring the total rate at which the brain uses leucine. To remove this confounding factor, Smith, Sokoloff, and colleagues used leucine labeled with ^{14}C in the carboxyl (i.e., number-1) position.[17] In the metabolic pathway, leucine is transaminated to α-ketoisocaproic acid, which then is decarboxylated in the mitochondria with release of the label in the form of $^{14}CO_2$. The labeled $^{14}CO_2$ diffuses through the brain tissue and then is removed by blood flow. As the

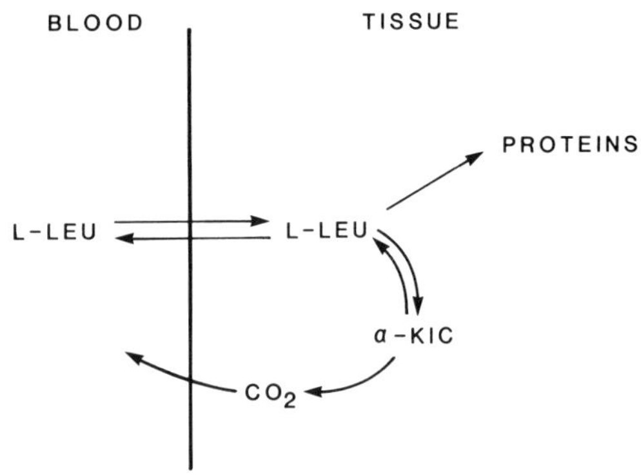

Figure 3–21. Schematic illustration of leucine transport through the blood-brain barrier (BBB), its incorporation into proteins, and metabolism by deamination to α-ketoisocaproic acid (α-KIC) followed by decarboxylation with the release of CO_2. When leucine is labeled in the carboxyl group with radioactive carbon, it is incorporated into proteins or metabolized to the decarboxylation step and the label is removed from tissue as CO_2.

decarboxylation process and clearance of labeled $^{14}CO_2$ proceeds, there is an increasing fraction of the label remaining in the protein pool relative to the metabolic pool (see Fig. 3–21). Thus, labeling with ^{14}C, or in the case of PET, with ^{11}C in the carboxyl position[1] effectively produces a "shunt" that removes the label in the metabolic pathway by de-

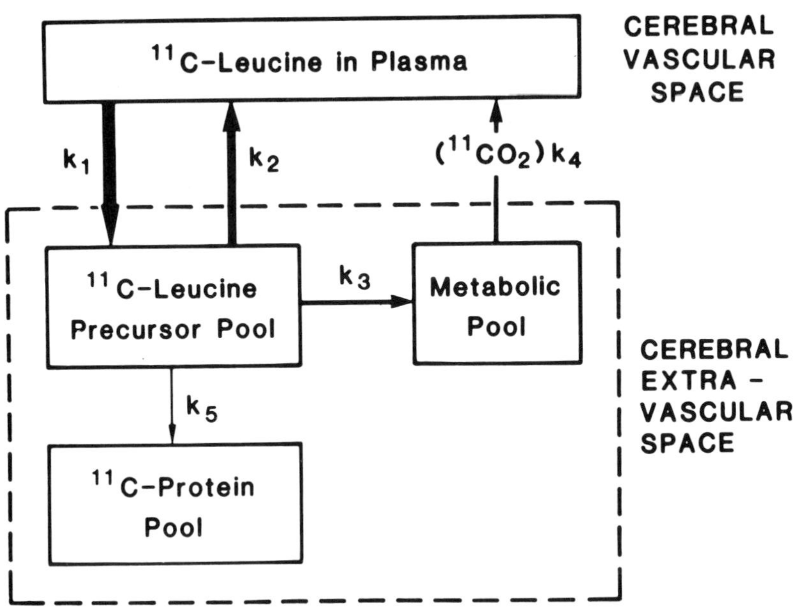

Figure 3–22. Leucine compartmental model corresponding to Figure 3–21.

carboxylation and clearance from the tissue by diffusion and blood flow.

The compartmental model shown schematically in Figure 3–22 can be used to estimate the various rate constants if the tissue time activity curve and input functions (i.e., plasma time activity curve for [^{11}C]-L-leucine and plasma concentration of leucine) are measured. Because both protein synthesis and metabolism originate from the same tissue precursor pool, both the protein synthesis rate (PSR) and metabolic rate (MR) can be measured.

NEUROCHEMICAL SYSTEMS

The study of neurotransmitters and receptors is currently a very active area of development in PET. Examples of the different ligands and substrate analogs for studying the pre- and postsynaptic processes of neurotransmission are listed in Table 3–3. Methods are being developed to study most of the neurotransmitter systems. The methods for estimating ligand binding to postsynaptic receptor systems employ many of the principles of saturation binding using Schatchard and Hill plots[2,4,8] as well as novel new kinetic methods.[4,6,8,12,13,19,20]

Figure 3–23 illustrates the different aspects of dopaminergic neurotransmission for which PET assay methods are being developed. The principles of competitive substrate analogs and ligands that bind to enzymes in their active state are being developed to investigate the presynaptic system (see Table 3–3).

The multiple processes involved in such a tracer study are illustrated in Figure 3–24. The labeled ligand initially appears in the vascular system. It then diffuses into cerebral tissue. In the later images, one sees the differential

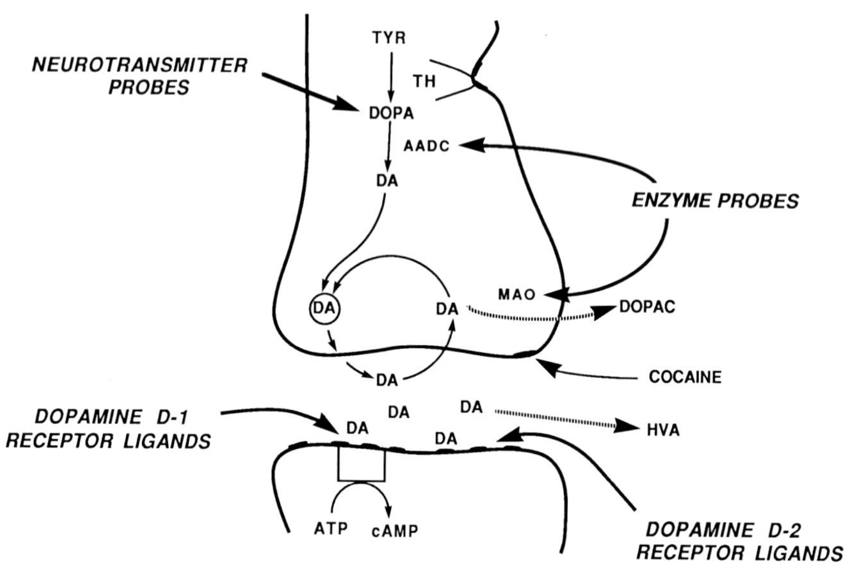

Figure 3–23. Schematic illustration of the neurotransmitter presynaptic probes and ligands for the postsynaptic receptors of the cerebral dopaminergic system. Examples of probes for the presynaptic biosynthetic pathway are: 6-[^{18}F]fluoro-L-DOPA and 4-[^{18}F]fluoro-metatyrosine as substrate analogs for L-DOPA; and α-fluoromethyl-4-[^{18}F]fluorometatyrosine and (E)-β-fluoromethylene-4-[^{18}F]fluorometatyrosine, which employ the principles of enzyme suicide inactivation for assaying the enzyme activities of AADC and MAO, respectively. [^{11}C]-cocaine is shown as an example of a drug that binds to the dopamine re-uptake sites. An example of a dopamine D_1 subtype receptor ligand is [^{11}C]SCH23390. Dopamine D_2 subtype receptor ligand examples are [^{11}C]-methylspiperone, [^{11}C]-raclopride, and [^{18}F]-fluoroethylspiperone. TYR is tyrosine, TH is tyrosine hydroxylase, DA is dopamine, AADC is aromatic amino acid decarboxylase, MAO is monoamine oxidase, DOPAC is dihydroxyphenylacetic acid, and HVA is homovanillic acid.

kinetics of specific versus nonspecific localization. All of these processes must be taken into account in the model for the formulation of the estimate of such parameters as receptor density and affinity for the labeled ligand.

Assays of receptor systems with PET have required the synthesis of very high specific-activity–labeled ligands and illustrate the high sensitivity of the technique for assays of the brain involving very low (e.g., picomolar) chemical concentrations.

THE VALUE OF PET IN NEUROLOGIC AND PSYCHIATRIC DISORDERS

A number of examples demonstrate the clinical utility of PET. For example, consider the studies shown in Figure 3–25. Relative to the normal subject, the Parkinson's patient has normal glucose metabolism but a profound putamenal dopamine deficiency. The Huntington's patient has a profound

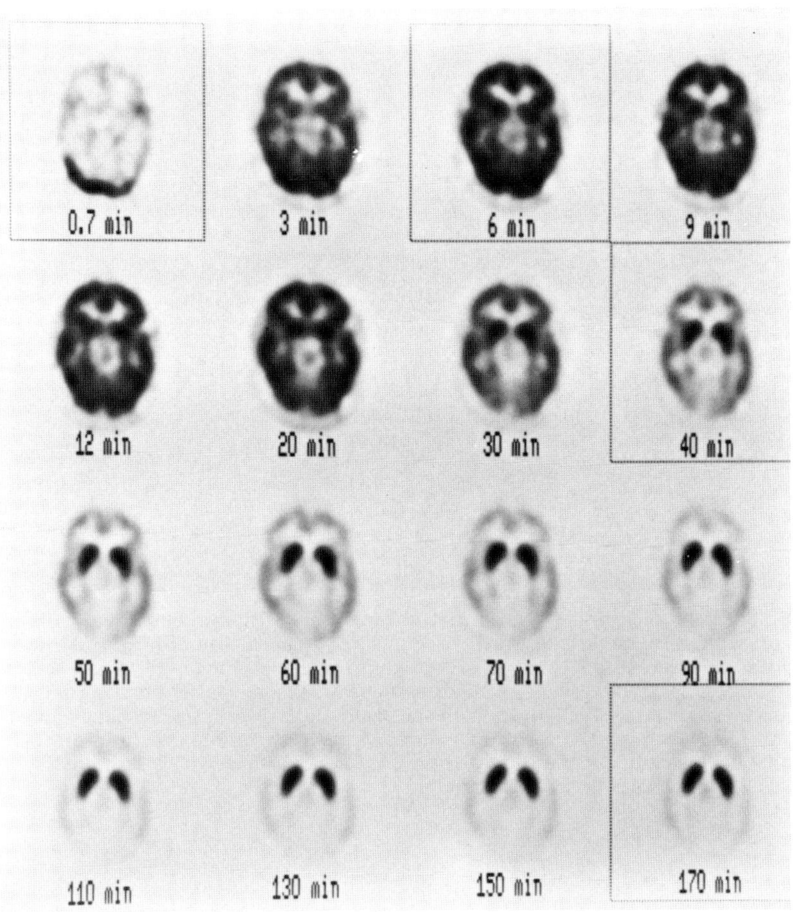

Figure 3–24. Changing temporal distribution of [^{18}F]fluoroethylspiperone in the brain. The elapsed time after intravenous injection is shown with each image. The temporal sequence of images illustrates the different kinetics for this ligand in different structures of the brain. Initially, the labeled ligand appears prominent in the vascular system and subsequently diffuses into the brain with a dependence on blood flow and the ligand's permeability to the BBB. Subsequently, the ligand is seen to clear more rapidly from nonspecific sites and those with low-affinity serotonergic S_2 subtype receptors and accumulate in the high-affinity (D_2) receptors of the caudate and putamen.

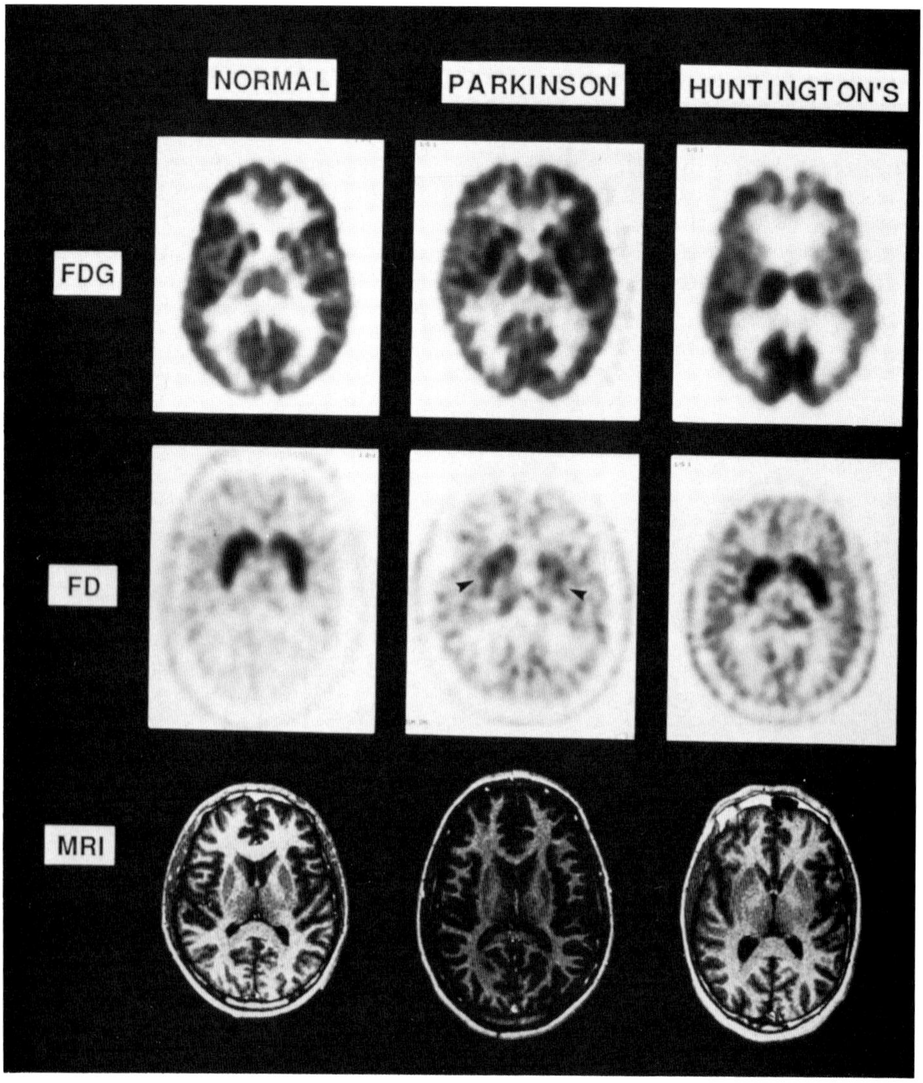

Figure 3–25. The relationship between structural imaging (MRI) and two chemical imaging assays (PET) in patients with different disorders. FDG denotes PET images of cerebral glucose metabolism with fluorodeoxyglucose; FD denotes PET images of dopamine synthesis using 6-[^{18}F]fluoro-L-DOPA, and MRI denotes magnetic resonance imaging (T_1 weighted). The Parkinson's patient has normal glucose metabolism and structure (as seen by MRI) throughout the brain, but a dopamine deficiency, most pronounced in the putamen. The Huntington's patient has normal striatal dopamine synthesis and structure, but a profound metabolic deficiency in the caudate and putamen. (Courtesy of S Grafton, JC Mazziotta, JR Barrio, and ME Phelps, UCLA School of Medicine.)

deficiency in striatal glucose metabolism but normal striatal dopamine synthesis. All the MRI studies are normal. There are several conclusions:

1. Chemical abnormalities exist in these patients and precede gross structural degeneration.

2. The dopamine deficiency of Parkinson's disease is profound (85% in putamen; see Chapter 8) and easily

seen, but does not produce a significant abnormality in glucose metabolism of the striatum. Although about 80% of the brain's dopamine is in the striatum, it is a minority neurotransmitter and energy consumer in this structure; hence, glucose metabolism appears unaffected.

3. Huntington's disease is associated with profound reductions in glucose metabolic function of the striatum, but with sparing of the presynaptic dopamine system (see Chapter 8).

4. The appropriate chemical assay must be used to identify a particular disease.

Multiple types of PET studies can be used to identify and separate overlapping disease processes, such as that shown in Figure 3–26. The undemented Parkinson's patient has a nor-

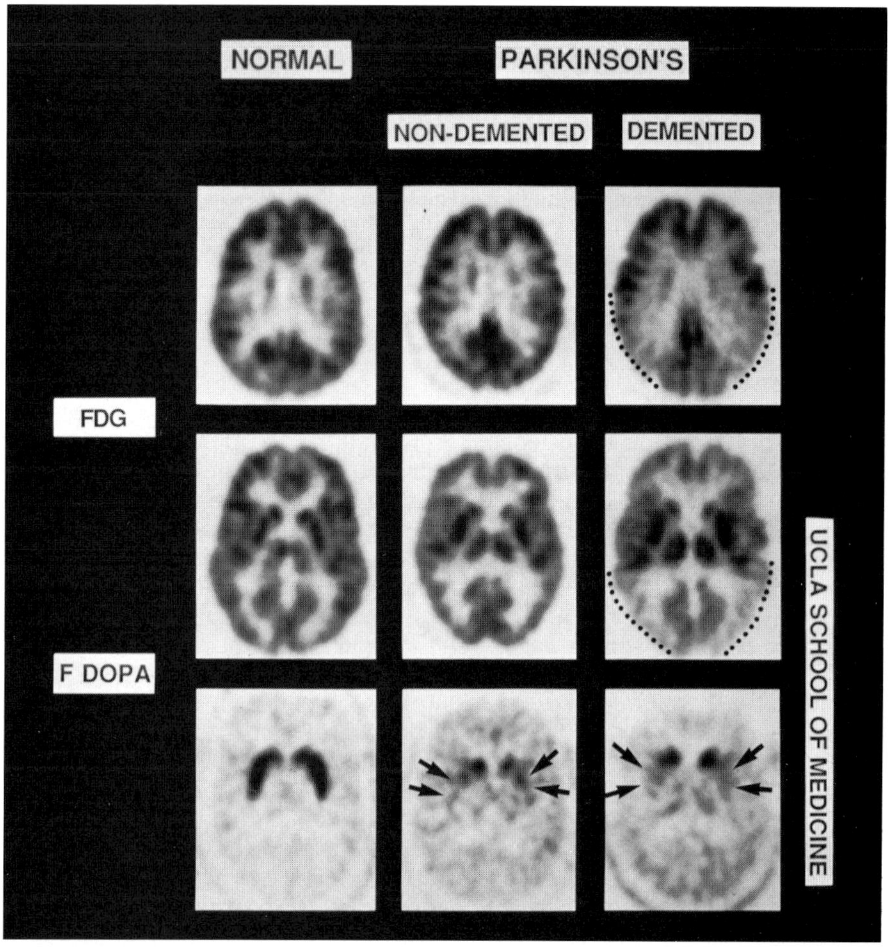

Figure 3–26. PET studies with two different chemical assays to delineate two different disease processes (Parkinson's and Alzheimer's disease). Nondemented Parkinson's patient exhibits normal glucose metabolism and a profound dopamine deficiency in the striatum, particularly the putamen. The demented Parkinson's patient has the dopamine deficiency of Parkinson's disease and, in addition, the classic PET findings of Alzheimer's disease, with hypometabolism bilaterally in the parietotemporal cortex (Courtesy of S Grafton, JC Mazziotta, JR Barrio, and ME Phelps, UCLA School of Medicine.)

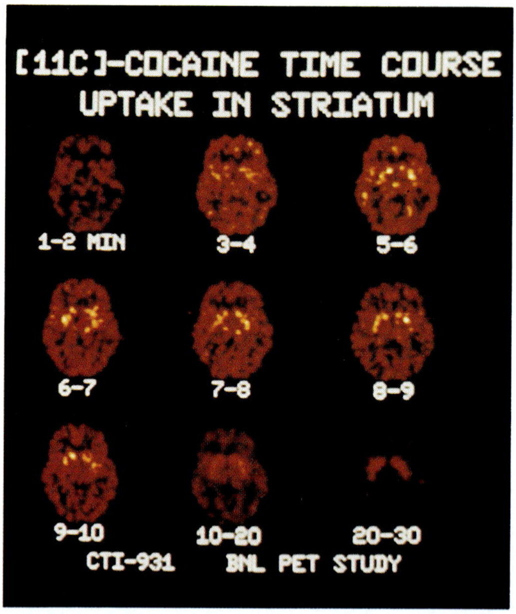

Figure 3–27. PET study illustrating the anatomical distribution of [^{11}C]-cocaine in the human brain as a function of time after injection. Red indicates the highest tissue concentration. Initially cocaine is distributed throughout the brain, with a progressive differential localization of the basal ganglia. (Courtesy of AP Wolf and J Fowler, Brookhaven National Laboratory).

mal anatomical distribution of glucose metabolism and a striatal dopamine deficiency. The Parkinson's patient with a confounding Alzheimer's syndrome demonstrates a striatal dopamine deficiency associated with his Parkinson's disease and, in addition, the characteristic biparietal metabolic abnormality in the cortex (see Chapters 8 and 9). Two assays with PET are used to delineate two disease processes.

Drugs are chemicals that are used to restore deficient, block overactive, accelerate underactive, or destroy chemical systems deranged by disease or injury. PET provides two ways to study and monitor drug therapy. One is to label the drug itself, identify its sites of action in the brain and study the mechanisms of interaction. This can be done with high-specific-activity–labeled drugs as shown in Figure 3–27 where ^{11}C-cocaine is shown to target the striatum. This approach can be expanded to include the use of the labeled drug to examine changes under conditions where pharmacologic doses are given to the patient. The second part of the study is to use a PET assay of the dopamine system to examine the effect of the drug on the endogenous system, as shown in Figure 3–28.

Once a patient is characterized in terms of biochemical pathophysiology, these same markers can be used to objectively monitor therapeutic interventions. For example, ischemia in cerebral vascular disease is, by definition, a problem of an insufficient blood supply of nutrients to meet normal metabolic demand. PET provides a means to assess the status of both blood flow and metabolism, as well as the effectiveness of therapies to correct deficiencies in them. Figure 3–29 illustrates the use of PET in objectively assessing therapeutic response to a drug intervention.

In diseases of the brain, it is impor-

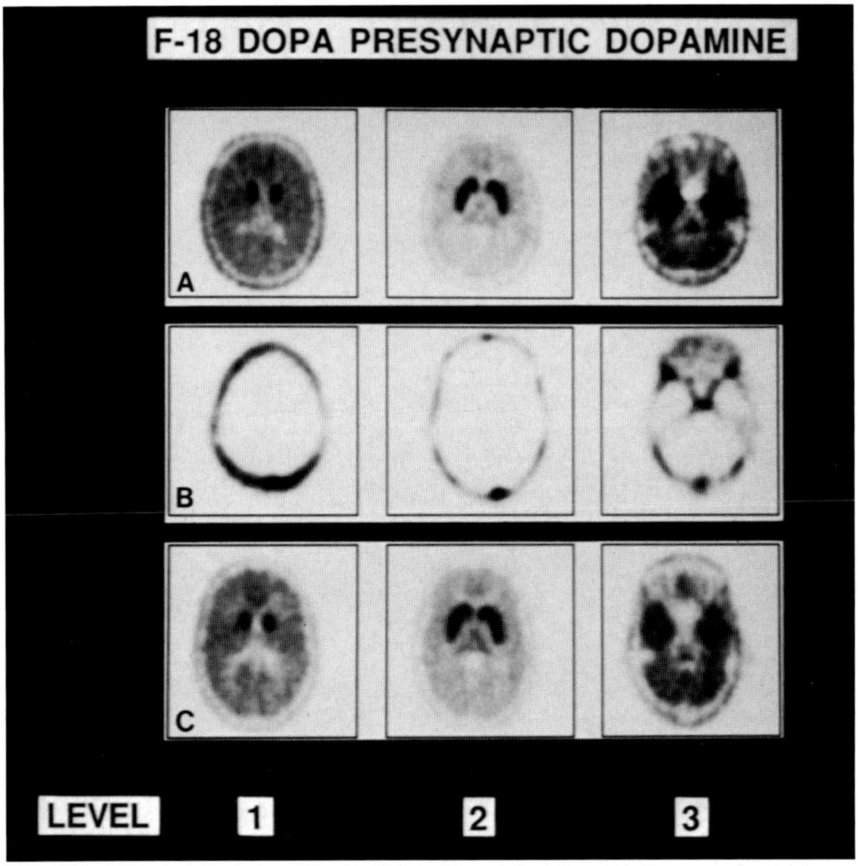

Figure 3–28. PET study of dopamine synthesis in a heavy cocaine user (1 g per day IV for 4 years). Images represent relative tissue concentrations, with black being the highest and white the lowest. The left column shows levels at the superior portion of the caudate. The center column is at the level of the caudate and putamen. The right column shows the level of the inferior temporal lobes and cerebellum. A normal subject is shown in row A. Four days after withdrawal (*row B*), the cocaine abuser has a profound lack of dopamine synthesis in the caudate and putamen. One month after withdrawal (*row C*) there is an apparent return of dopamine synthesis. (Courtesy of LR Baxter, J Schwartz, J Barrio, and ME Phelps, UCLA School of Medicine.)

tant not only to identify abnormalities but also to determine the amount and distribution of normal brain function. It is particularly important in planning surgical interventions to define an area for cerebral resection, guide the route of entry, identify the functional status of adjacent and remote structures, and predict recovery of function.

Diagnosis is by its very nature a process of exclusion and identification. A commonly sought examination is one that excludes the presence of disease. The degree of certainty of exclusion is determined by the sensitivity of the examination. Biochemical markers used in combination with the clinical examination should provide the most sensitive and specific exclusionary criteria. When disease is present, they should also provide the most accurate way to identify and characterize the biological alterations of the disease process.

Studies with PET to advance our knowledge of the fundamental biological basis of cerebral function in humans during development, adult life, and aging will also expand the opportunities to use this knowledge and associated techniques to develop new approaches to improved care of patients with cerebral disorders.

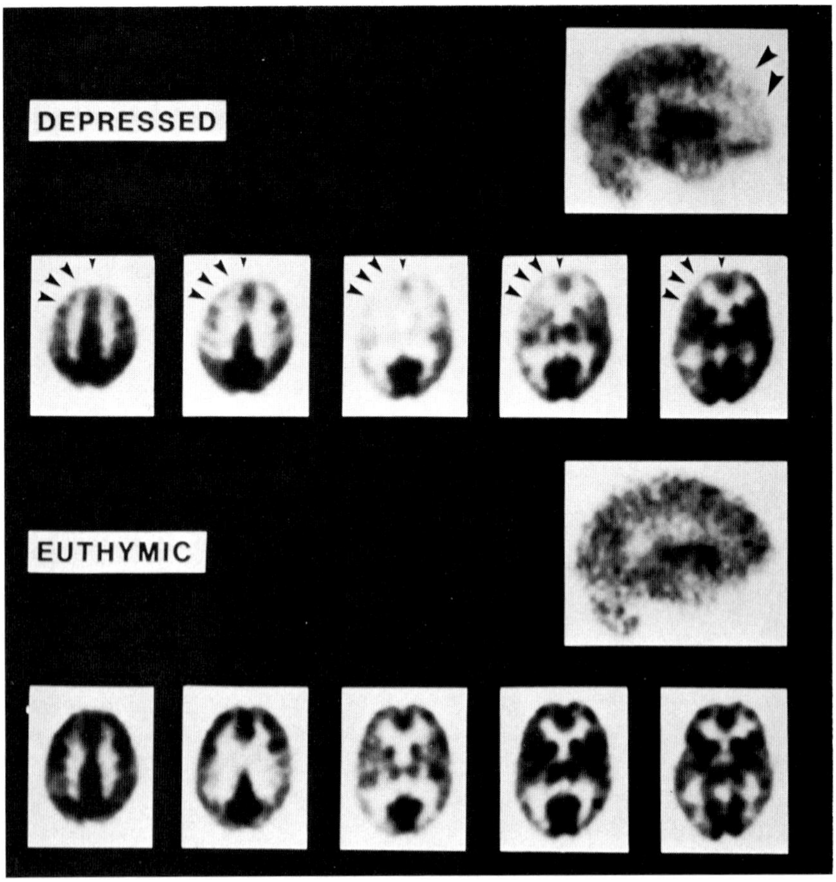

Figure 3–29. Use of PET studies of cerebral glucose metabolism to objectively assess therapeutic drug response in a patient with obsessive-compulsive disorder and unipolar depression. (*Top*) Lateral view showing depressed glucose metabolism in the frontal cortex. Tomographic images from superior to inferior (left to right) show that the hypometabolic deficit is primarily in the left frontal cortex and cingulate. (*Bottom*) After treatment with an MAO inhibitor, the patient's mood is normal (euthymic). The PET study illustrates that the metabolic deficiencies have resolved. (Courtesy of L Baxter, J Schwartz, JC Mazziotta, and ME Phelps, UCLA School of Medicine.)

REFERENCES

1. Barrio, JR: Biochemical principles in radiopharmaceutical design and utilization. In Phelps, ME, Mazziotta, JC, and Schelbert, HR (ed): Positron Emission Tomography and Autoradiography Raven Press, New York, 1986, pp 451–492.
2. Farde, L, Hall, H, Ehrin, E, and Sedvall, G: Quantitative analysis of dopamine-D2 receptor binding in the living human brain using positron emission tomography. Science 231:258–261, 1986.
3. Fowler, JS and Wolf, AP: Positron emitter-labeled compounds: Priorities and problems. In Phelps, ME, Mazziotta, JC, and Schelbert, HR (eds): Positron Emission Tomography and Autoradiography. Raven Press, New York, 1986, pp 391–450.
4. Frost, JJ: Pharmacokinetic aspects of the in vivo, noninvasive study of neuroreceptors in man. In Eckelman, WC (ed): Receptor Binding Radiotracers, Vol II. CRC Press, Boca Raton, Fla, 1982, pp 25–39.
5. Hoffman, EJ and Phelps, ME: Positron emission tomography: Principles and quantitation. In Phelps, ME, Mazziotta,

JC, and Schelbert, HR (eds): Positron Emission Tomography and Autoradiography, Raven Press, New York, 1986, pp 237–286.

6. Huang, SC, Bahn, MM, Barrio, JR, Hoffman, JM, Satyamurthy, N, Hawkins, RA, Mazziotta, JC, and Phelps, ME: A double-injection technique for in vivo measurement of dopamine D2 receptor density in primates with 3-(21[^{18}F]-fluoroethyl)spiperone and dynamic PET. J Cereb Blood Flow Metabol 9:850–858, 1989.
7. Huang, SC, Carson, RE, and Phelps, ME: Measurement of local blood flow and distribution volume with short-lived isotopes: A general input technique. J Cereb Blood Flow Metab 2:99–108, 1982.
8. Huang, SC, Barrio, JR, and Phelps, ME: Neuroreceptor assays with positron emission tomography: Equilibrium vs dynamic approaches. J Cereb Blood Flow Metabol 6:515–521, 1986.
9. Huang, SC and Phelps, ME: Principles of tracer kinetic modeling in positron emission tomography. In Phelps, ME, Mazziotta, JC, and Schelbert, HR (eds): Positron Emission Tomography and Autoradiography. Raven Press, New York, 1986, pp 287–346.
10. Jones, T, Chelser, DA, and Ter-Pogossian, MM: The continuous inhalation of oxygen is for assessing regional oxygen extraction in the brain of man. Br J Radiol 49:339–343, 1976.
11. Mazziotta, JC and Phelps, ME: Positron emission tomography studies of the brain. In Phelps, ME, Mazziotta, JC, and Schelbert, HR (eds): Positron Emission Tomography and Autoradiography. Raven Press, New York, 1986, pp 493–579.
12. Mintun, MA, Wooten, DF, and Raichle, ME: A quantitative model for the in vivo assessment of drug binding sites with positron emission tomography. Ann Neurol 15:217–227, 1984.
13. Perlmutter, JS, Larson, RB, Raichle, ME, Markham, J, Mintum, MA, Kilbourn, MR, and Welch, MJ: Strategies for in vivo measurement of receptor binding using positron emission tomography. J Cereb Blood Flow Metab 6: 154–169, 1986.
14. Phelps, ME, Hoffman, EJ, Mullani, NA, and Ter-Pogossian, MM: Applications of annihilation coincidence to transaxial reconstruction tomography. J Nucl Med 16:210–224, 1975.
15. Phelps, ME, Huang SC, Hoffman, EJ, Selin, C, and Kuhl, DE: Tomographic measurement of cerebral blood volume with C-11-labeled carboxy hemoglobin. J Nucl Med 20:328–334, 1979.
16. Phelps, ME, Huang, SC, Hoffman, EJ, Kuhl, DE, and Carson, RE: An analysis of signal amplification using small detectors in positron emission tomography. J Comput Assist Tomogr 6:551–565, 1982.
17. Smith, CB, Davidsen, L, Deibler, G, Patlak, C, Pettigrew, KA, and Sokoloff, L: A method for the determination of local rates of protein synthesis in brain (abstr). Trans Am Soc Neurochem 11: 94, 1980.
18. Sokoloff, L, Reivich, M, Kennedy, C, Des Rosiers, MH, Patlak, CS, Pettigrew, KD, Sakurada, O, and Shinohara, M: The (^{14}C)-deoxyglucose method for the measurement of local cerebral glucose utilization: Theory, procedure and normal values in the conscious and anesthetized albino rat. J Neurochem 28:897–916, 1977.
19. Wong, DF, Gjedde, A, and Wagner, HN, Jr: Quantification of neuroreceptors in the living human brain. I: Irreversible binding of ligands. J Cereb Blood Flow Metab 6:137–146, 1986.
20. Wong, DF, Gjedde, A, Wagner, HN Jr, et al: Quantification of neuroreceptors in the living human brain. II: Inhibition studies of receptor density and affinity. J Cereb Blood Flow Metab 6:147–153, 1986.

Chapter 4

SINGLE PHOTON EMISSION COMPUTERIZED TOMOGRAPHY (SPECT)

Niels A. Lassen, M.D., Ph.D. and Søren Holm, Ph.D.

SPECT IMAGING SYSTEMS
RADIOISOTOPES USED IN SPECT
SPECT IMAGING OF CEREBRAL BLOOD FLOW
RECEPTOR LIGANDS LABELED WITH IODINE 123

Single photon emission computerized tomography (SPECT) is a technique for studying radioactive tracers introduced into the body, usually by intravenous injection or inhalation. SPECT is particularly useful for studies involving the brain, and the development of SPECT for the brain is currently ahead of the development of SPECT for other organs. Depending upon the tracer used, SPECT can provide information about cerebral blood flow, cerebral blood volume, and cerebral neurotransmitter receptors.

As indicated in Chapter 1, with x-ray CT scanning, the signal used for reconstruction is the photons, transmitted from an x-ray source, that have passed through the body. In emission CT (ECT), the signal detected is the decay of radioactive nuclides inside the body, introduced by injection or inhalation of a radioactive (labeled) tracer and distributed primarily by the blood stream. The kind of information obtained depends on the fate of the tracer substance.

The types of radioactive decay and the consequent differences in detection equipment divide emission tomography into two separate fields: positron emission tomography (PET) and single photon emission (computerized) tomography, SPE(C)T. The term "single photon" refers to the fact that in SPECT the photons are detected one at a time, not in coincidence pairs like the photons detected with PET. Because the photons are detected one at a time, when many photons emerge they will not have any simple spatial correlation. Consequently, the origin of photons in SPECT must be traced by collimation with lead structures having carefully designed openings that allow only photons from well-defined regions to enter. Collimation refers to a process whereby electromagnetic radiation can be made into parallel beams.

ECT images in general have much less detail than transmission CT images. An x-ray beam can be turned on and off. It can be shaped and directed towards a particular field of interest and it can be well focused and very intense. Therefore a high degree of photon utilization is obtained with respect to the dose of radiation absorbed by the subject. In ECT, the decay providing the photons is a random and isotropic process (exhibiting properties such as velocity with the same values when measured along axes in all directions), and only a limited fraction of the decays can be registered as events in the counting detector system. The tracers used with ECT are distributed throughout the entire body, not only to the target organ. Therefore, the non–target organ radiation exposure is high relative to that of transmission CT. The overall or total radiation exposure is expressed in terms of the whole-body dose equivalent.

In *static* studies of a stationary distribution, the effective half-life of the tracer often can be an order of magnitude greater than the time actually used for imaging. In *dynamic* studies of a physiologic process, the imaging time needed may be dictated by the time constants of the process, which cannot be controlled. In either case, ECT images are generally collected over much longer time and with many fewer photons (three orders of magnitude less) than transmission CT, and therefore with more random noise and less resolution.

SPECT IMAGING SYSTEMS

SPECT instrumentation has been separated into two categories: systems based on standard gamma cameras, and dedicated SPECT systems (Fig. 4–1). This distinction has become less clear, since dedicated systems now exist that are based upon camera principles. A second distinction is between three-dimensional (3-D) volume-sampling (camera type) and discrete slice-sampling devices. A third distinction is between head and body devices. Hybrids now exist that have sufficient flexibility to study both the head and the body without loss of performance.

For any system, the data are usually organized as slices and the slices are reconstructed separately from projections spaced over a full 360° arc of rotation around the subject. The sampling requirements and the reconstruction methods for SPECT are almost identical to those for PET described in Chapter 3 and are not described in detail here. Almost all algorithms, including the most frequently employed "linear superposition of filtered back-projection" method, assume that the observed projection data repre-

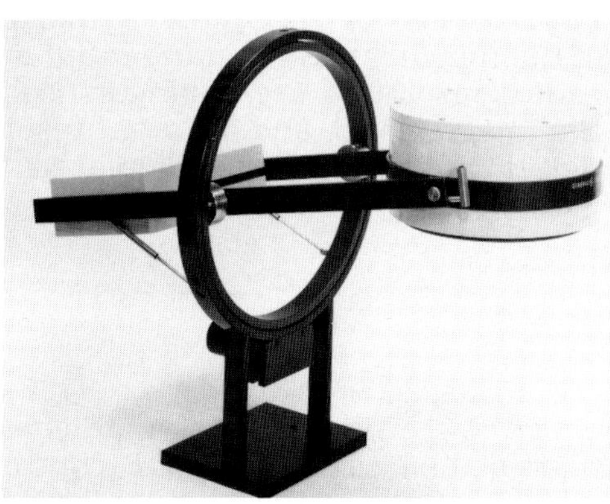

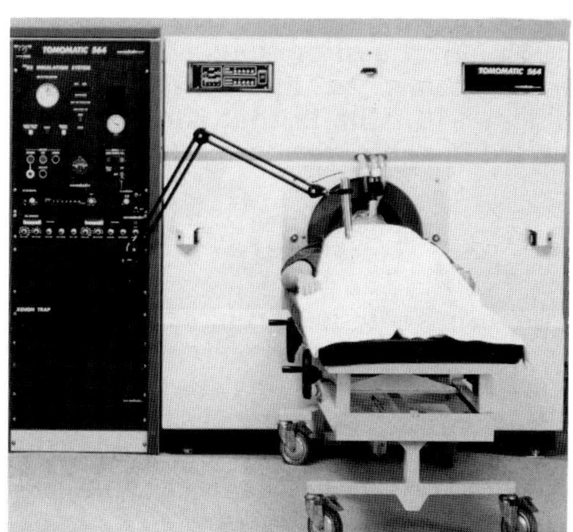

Figure 4–1. (*A*) A rotating gamma camera system. (*B*) An example of a dedicated brain SPECT instrument (Tomomatic 564) with gas administration system and external detector. (*A* Courtesy of General Electric, *B* courtesy of Medimatic.)

sent a complete set of ideal integrations along the detector axis. Thus, any element of a projection should be a measure of the tracer substance contained within a narrow cylinder through the body. No SPECT system can fully comply with this assumption; the degree to which a system actually does so is of major importance for its image quality and its potential for quantitative measurement.

With one exception,[45] all existing SPECT systems use lead collimators to define the sample. Each collimator hole accepts photons from only a certain solid angle, usually a narrow cone or pyramid, while photons arriving at the collimator surface through any other angles are absorbed by the lead, so that most of the photons go undetected. The detecting system behind the collimator is, in almost all systems, sodium iodine crystals with standard photomultiplier tubes (PMT).

Camera systems generally use a single, large crystal covered by many PMTs. Other systems use multiple crystals, either with one PMT each or with different encoding schemes for localizing the individual photons in the crystal. Multiple detector systems usually have higher count-rate capability suitable for dynamic studies, but less energy resolution than large, single crystals. With the use of a suitable focused collimation on a multiple detector system, the ideal assumptions of uniform sampling may be approached. The problem with this is that the volume sampled in each scan is reduced.

Sensitivity

The term *sensitivity* refers to the degree to which a system responds to incoming signals. Typically, sensitivity in a SPECT system is defined as the number of recorded counts per second (cps) per slice for a 20-cm-diameter cylinder with an aqueous solution of the nuclide containing a unit activity concentration (mBq/L or mCi/L).[28] Usually values are quoted for ^{99m}Tc, but values for other nuclides may be found in the literature. The sensitivity is determined by the geometric configuration of the system (the number and kind of detectors, their distance from the object, and so on), the collimation, and the energy window settings. If the measured sensitivity is compared with the total number of decaying nuclei within a properly defined slice volume, an efficiency index is obtained.

Resolution

SPECT images, like other nuclear medicine images, are usually described in terms of their resolution, contrast, and noise. The term *resolution* refers to the capability of making distinguishable the individual parts of an object. Spatial resolution can be determined in SPECT systems by the response of the system to a point source of radioactivity. The most commonly used index of resolution is the full-width-half-maximum (FWHM) of a point spread function (PSF) at the center of the image—that is, the width of the spot in the image plane measured at half the maximum intensity. This is a convenient measure because it approximates the minimum distance that allows two points to be separated in the image, although this depends strictly on the form of the total PSF. Because of the circular symmetry of the imaging process, *tangential* and *radial* resolution are distinguished in the image plane, and an *axial* resolution is determined perpendicular to the plane.

Contrast

Contrast refers to the degree of difference between the darkest and lightest parts of a picture. For SPECT, contrast can be defined by the modular transfer function (MTF), which gives the response of the imaging system to any spatial frequency in the object (see Chapter 3). This is meaningful insofar as the whole tomographic process is linear and stationary. MTF can be calculated from the PSFs (and vice versa) and therefore carries the same information.

Attenuation and Scatter

When a beam of photons passes through matter, some of the photons are removed by scattering and absorption processes (Fig. 4–2). Traditionally, in SPECT, attenuation and scatter are treated as separate problems, although the first is caused mainly by the second. The term *attenuation* is used to describe the apparent lack of photons in the projection due to absorption or deflection away from the detector. The term *scatter* indicates that some photons are deflected from their initial path and appear as false information in detectors.

ATTENUATION CORRECTION

Several methods have been proposed for attenuation correction in SPECT. Most are based on the assumption that the linear attenuation coefficient at a given energy is a constant for all body tissues. This assumption is incorrect for the head, where the subtle differences in photon attenuation between gray and white matter are unimportant, but the varying thickness of the skull and its higher density (1.8 times that of the brain tissues) are significant.

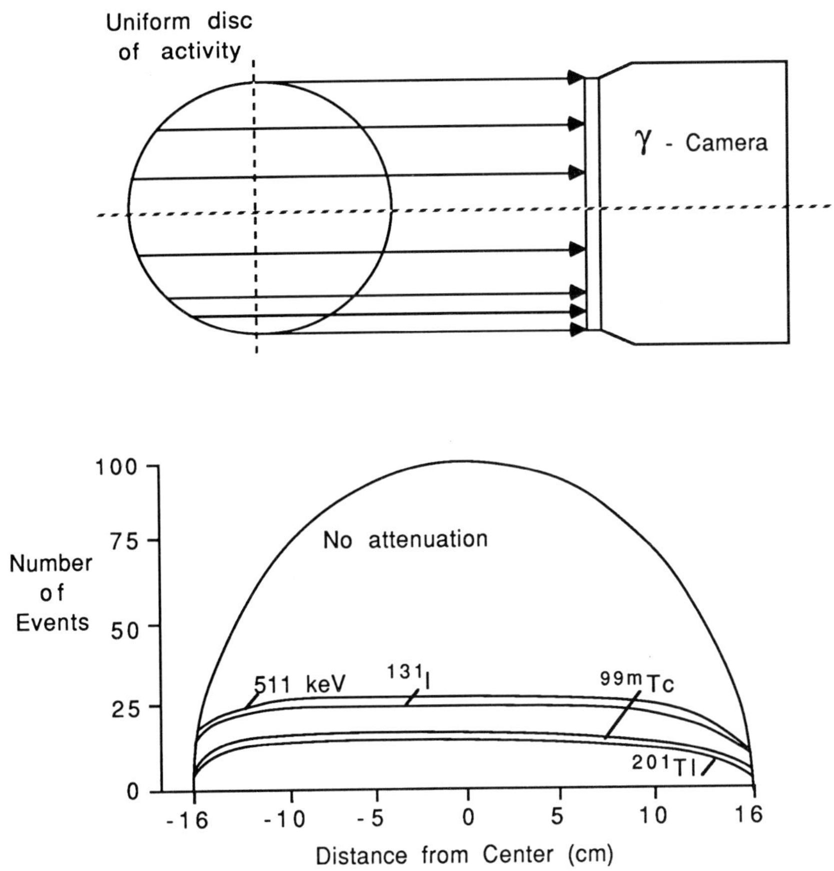

Figure 4–2. Distortion of projection data due to attenuation. (*Top*) A simulated measurement of uniform radioactivity in a cylinder in front of the gamma camera. (*Bottom*) The projection data obtained with various radionuclides in the cylinder. (From Larsson,[28] p. 29, with permission.)

In a simple after-correction method that is in widespread use, an initially uncorrected image is multiplied by a correction matrix, in which the value for each pixel depends on the average attenuation for that position.[8] Another simple and widely used approach is to combine—point by point—all pairs of opposed projections (180° apart) either by using the arithmetic mean or the geometric mean. To each element of these so-called logical projections, a factor is applied that depends on the length of the ideal ray (chord) through the object at that position.[28] This length or thickness of object can be estimated either from an uncorrected image, or by applying a threshold procedure to the projections.

SCATTER: EFFECTS AND CORRECTION

For the energy range and tissue elements considered in SPECT, Compton scattering is by far the most important attenuation process. In Compton scattering the photon transfers part of its energy to an electron and is deflected a certain angle (see Chapter 1). Since the energy of the scattered photons is less than that of the unscattered photons (Fig. 4–3), the scattered photons might be eliminated from the measurement process by rejecting those of lower-than-expected energy. Unfortunately, the energy resolution of the detector systems, measured as FWHM in the spectra, is typically on the order of

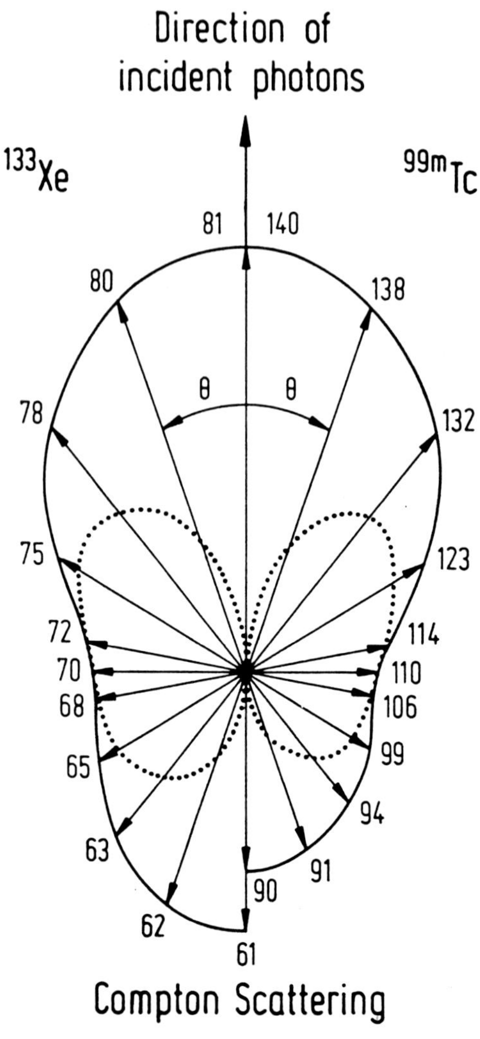

Figure 4–3. Compton scattering of photons from ^{133}Xe (81 KeV) and ^{99m}Tc (140 KeV). In this polar diagram, the incident photons are directed upwards with their original energy. When they hit a "scatter center," they are deflected at a certain angle θ and come out with an energy dependent on the angle, as shown on the figure. The length of the vectors (*arrows*) at the angle θ is proportional to the probability of scattering into a unit solid angle element in that direction; that is, it is proportional to the measured count rate in a small detector. To get the fraction of all photons scattered through an angle θ, this probability must be integrated on the cone of angle θ around the axis of incidence, leading to a factor of $|\sin\theta|$ (dotted curves). With higher energy, forward scatter predominates and the relative energy loss increases, making scatter discrimination more efficient.

10%–20% at 140 KeV, so that scatter rejection cannot be very effective. Currently, several different approaches are used for scatter correction, including iterative computations. This results in more correct image reconstruction than the conventional single-step back-projection algorithm.[5,18]

NOISE AND RESOLUTION

SPECT images generally are limited in quality by statistical fluctuations in the number of counts that can be obtained with acceptable radiation absorbed doses to the subject and reasonable acquisition times. Improvement in resolution by a factor p requires an increase in registered counts by p^3 to maintain the level of variance among pixels that are scaled to match the improved resolution.

The basic goals of scanner design, high sensitivity and high resolution, are mutually exclusive and must be balanced by the purpose for which the scanner is designed. The coupling between sensitivity and resolution is an unavoidable characteristic of SPECT (Fig. 4–4). Axial resolution is depen-

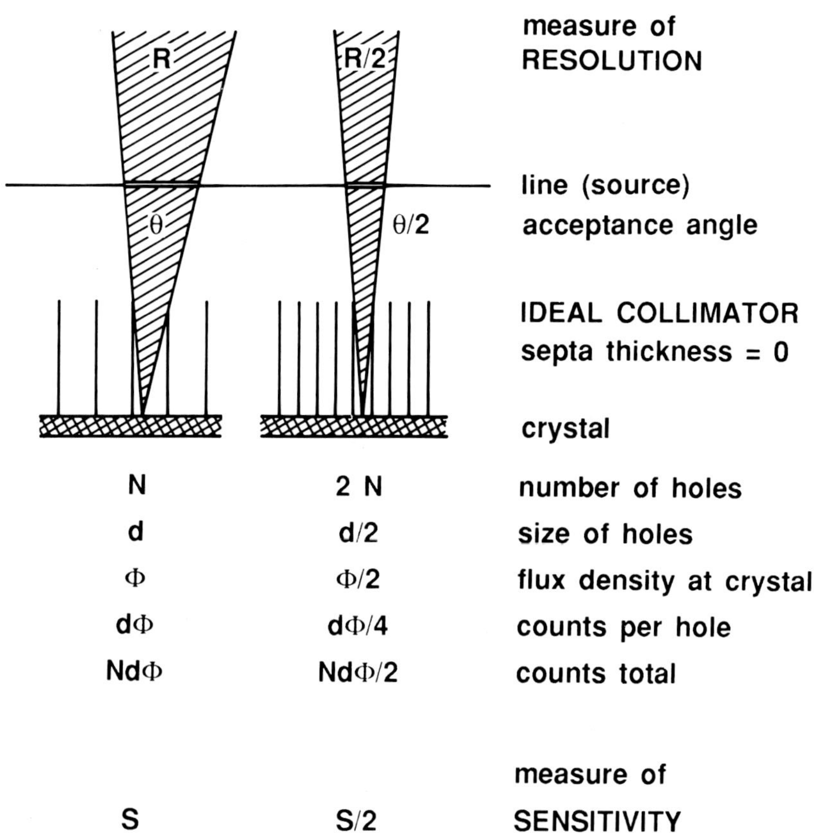

Figure 4–4. A simple, one-dimensional example is used here to illustrate the coupling between resolution and sensitivity in SPECT. The system consists of an ideal collimator (zero septa thickness) with an ideal detector (perfect intrinsic resolution) behind. If a change is made only in septa distance, any resolution measure R will certainly scale linearly with this distance, since the whole geometry is similar. The sensitivity (to an extended source) will also scale linearly; At any point of the detector surface the number of incident photons per unit length (photon flux density Φ) will be proportional to the angle extended by the collimator opening (that is, the septa distance). Since the septa are assumed to be infinitely thin, the total area for detection is unchanged. Therefore, the total sensitivity is proportional to Φ and hence to R. If in a physical two-dimensional collimator changes are made in both directions, the result in sensitivity is the product of the two. In any realistic collimator, the loss of counts with improved resolution is greater than the ideal, since septa tend to cover a larger part of the crystal surface area.

dent on the type of instrument and its collimators. For a camera where the complete crystal area is already in use, an improvement in axial resolution by a factor p is accompanied by a reduction in sensitivity per slice of approximately p^2, and by an increase in the number of slices by p. For discrete-slice machines, the number of recordings to get full coverage must in principle be increased by p. The influence on sensitivity ranges from p to p^2 depending on the utilization of the crystal area (Table 4–1).

Improvement by a factor of 2 for the in-plane as well as the axial resolution requires that the imaging time, for a given dose of activity, must be prolonged by a factor of 64–128. Thus, the desirability of using high spatial resolution must be tempered by the need to use short imaging durations. In a sensitive SPECT system with a spatial resolution of 2 cm, using approximately 0.7 GBq of ^{99m}Tc-propylene-amine-oxime PnAO (which has an initial or "first-pass" brain distribution proportional to CBF), it is possible to image CBF in only *10 seconds* for three slices of brain tissue simultaneously.[20] With the same system and the same amount of ^{99m}Tc-d,1-hexamethyl-propylene-amine-oxime (HMPAO), 0.8–1.0-cm resolution requires *20 minutes* of acquisition. Within 20 minutes, a standard gamma camera would allow only 15 mm resolution at the same noise level.

The immediate conclusion from Table 4–1 is that improvements beyond the present limits of about 8 to 9 mm resolution are impossible. This, however, is too pessimistic in that it inherently assumes that the pixel variance must be kept at a fixed level for improvements in resolution to be useful. This is not necessarily true.

Table 4–1 NOISE AND RESOLUTION IN SPECT*

If resolution in the plane is improved by a factor p, and statistical noise is to be kept constant:
Increase number of counts per slice by p^3
As sensitivity drops by (at least) p:
*Increase (time*activity) by p^4*
If axial resolution is also improved by p:
*Increase (time*activity) by $p^5 - p^6$*
If all slices shall still be recorded:
*Increase (time*activity) by $p^6 - p^7$*

Camera-Based Systems

Most SPECT systems still use a standard-type rotating gamma camera. The camera is suspended so that it can slowly rotate around the body, either continuously or in a "step-and-shoot" mode. Sampling from the whole volume in one rotation allows the reconstruction of a contiguous stack of slices in one setting, and facilitates the construction of coronal, sagittal, or even oblique planes. The latter are of particular interest in studies of the heart (Fig. 4–5).

A standard camera is not an optimal instrument for SPECT. Tomography necessitates a much higher accuracy of positioning of the individual events (counts) than ordinary planar imaging, and uniformity corrections better than 1% are required to avoid artifacts in the image. Other important and difficult factors are the precision of the collimator, the influence of magnet fields changing with orientation, knowledge of the center of rotation, and the absence of any motion other than the presumed circular orbit. This requires a rigid suspension system. In new cameras designed for use with SPECT, considerable effort has been put into correction procedures, including on-line adjustments of amplification on the individual PMTs.

Dedicated SPECT Systems

With one exception, the ASPECT, all systems designed specifically for SPECT utilize multiple discrete scintillation detectors that view the head from several angles simultaneously. Each detector has a converging collimator that increases the crystal surface area

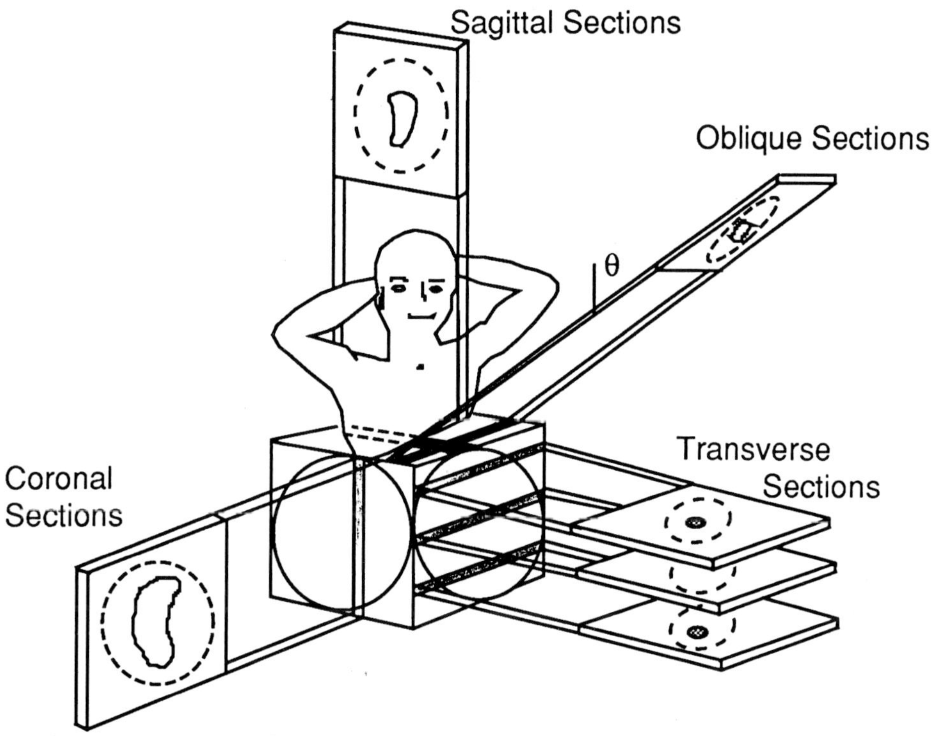

Figure 4–5. The stack of image sections in a body scan showing the image capability of a volume-sampling camera-type system. If the camera is circular, it sweeps only a sphere inside the cube. (From Larsson,[28] p. 40, with permission.)

looking at a given slice, thus increasing the sensitivity. Multidetector systems now available commercially are based on three different principles (Table 4–2). They are designed to achieve high sensitivity per slice at the cost of the number of slices (1 to 6) that can be obtained in each recording. With repeated examinations and shifting the position of the head between each, a contiguous stack of slices can be obtained, allowing image reconstruction also in the coronal and sagittal planes.

The Tomomatic scanner[31,49] follows the design of Kuhl and Edwards[25] but has been extended to multiple slices (Fig. 4–1*B*). The Headtome scanner[22,50] has 64 stationary scintillation detectors arranged in a ring. A circular collimator rotates inside the ring (Fig. 4–6). The Harvard Brain Scanner[48] is based on the use of 12 large crystals equipped with heavily converging collimators (Fig. 4–7). Recently a dedicated brain scanner, ASPECT (A = annular), has been described.[19,20a] It is based on a single crystal ring equipped with 36 large PMTs and positioning circuits analogous to the standard planar camera.

RADIOISOTOPES USED IN SPECT

There are more than 1000 known radioactive nuclides, naturally occurring or man-made, and many have been used as tracers in nuclear medicine. For radioisotopes to be useful in SPECT, a number of conditions must be fulfilled:

1. The nuclide must have a half-life (hours to days) that is long enough to allow its production and administration, but short enough to allow its use with a justifiable radiation load to the subject or the environment.

2. The decay of the nuclide must yield photons of high-enough energy to

Table 4–2 COMPARISON OF SPECT SYSTEMS AT APPROXIMATELY THE RESOLUTION* ACHIEVED WITH A WELL-TRIMMED ROTATING GAMMA CAMERA

System Studied	*Number of Crystals*	*Number of Slices*	**Resolution in cm**		*Sensitivity to ^{99m}Tc in cps/(MBq/L)/slice*	*Duration (min) of a ^{99m}Tc-HMPAO Study (0.5×10^6 counts)*
			In Plane	*Axially*		
Camera systems						
Single head*	1	6	1.6–1.9	1.6–2.0	40	15
Dual head†	2	6	1.6–1.9	1.6–2.0	80	7.5
Triple head†	3	6	1.6–1.9	1.6–2.0	120	5
Multidetector systems						
Four heads (*Tomomatic*)	64	3	1.5–1.9	1.9–2.0	1000	0.5
Ring (Shimadzu) (*Headtome*)	64	3	1.2–2.0	3.4	1500	0.3
Moving detectors (*Harvard*)	12	1	1.6	1.6	3000	0.5

*Cutoff camera for brain SPECT

†Extrapolating from the single-head performance

Data compiled from the literature and from the systems vendors by S. Holm (Ph.D. thesis, Copenhagen 1987).

Comparing the various types of brain SPECT systems at about the same spatial resolution as in this table, the marked difference in sensitivity and aquisition time is apparent. In routine use, the multidetector instruments are usually employed at their highest spatial resolution of about 1.0 cm, with correspondingly longer data aquisition times on the order of 5–20 min.

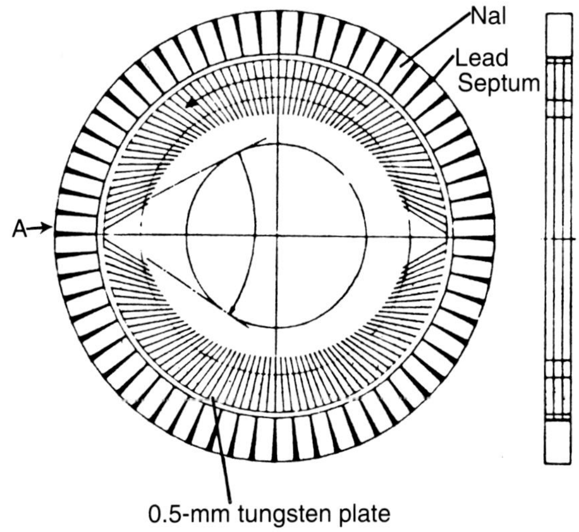

Figure 4–6. Basic principle of the Headtome II turbofan collimator. Detectors are stationary outside the rotating lead collimator. The mapping of the field of view onto the detectors can be traced by selecting a fixed point (for example, A on the figure) and imagining that the collimator turns; during rotation the angle of the collimator septa changes relative to the detector surface, so that each detector sweeps the whole field of view twice during one rotation. (From Tanaka et al.,[50] with permission.)

escape the body, but not so high that penetration of detector systems precludes localization.

3. The number of useful photons must be high relative to the number of low-energy photons and particles locally absorbed in the tissue, to keep the absorbed radiation dose reasonably low.

4. The nuclide must be a chemically inert tracer or it must be attachable chemically to a tracer substance of biological interest without an important change in properties.

These requirements limit the isotopes of interest in SPECT to ^{133}Xe, ^{127}Xe, ^{99m}Tc, ^{123}I, and ^{201}Tl. Krypton 81m, with its 13-second half-life, has been used with limited success. Bromine 77, which is of potential interest for labeling receptor ligands, contains too many high-energy emissions to be suitable for imaging patients with standard equipment. Problems in brain studies arise

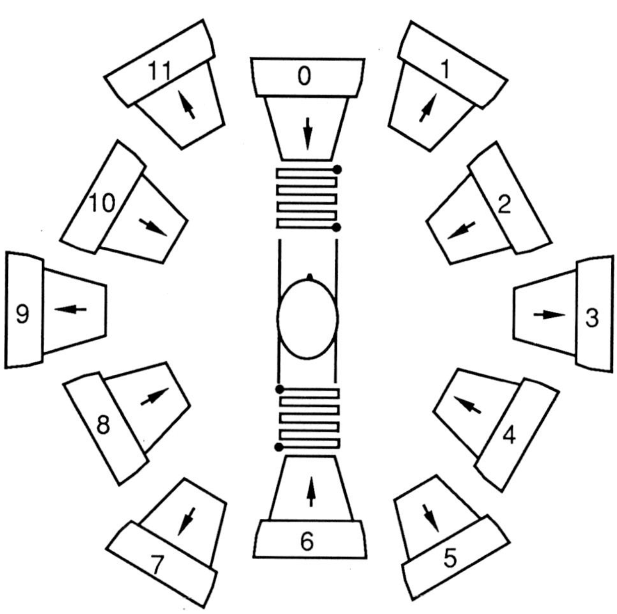

Figure 4–7. Basic scanning principle of the multidetector brain scanner of Stoddart and Stoddart. Each of the 12 strongly focused detectors scans half the total field of view in a rectilinear motion. Neighboring detectors are moving in opposite directions radially in order to maximize the solid angle of detection.

Table 4–3 THE MOST IMPORTANT RADIONUCLIDES USED FOR BRAIN SPECT

Nuclide	*Half life*	*Decay**	*Energy in KeV of Most Important Photon*	*Higher Energy Photons*
Technetium 99m	6.02 h	i.t.	140 in 89% of decays	none
Iodine 123	13.2 h	e.c.	159 in 83% of decays	529 in 1.4% of decays
Xenon 127	36.4 d	e.c.	203 in 68% of decays	375 in 18% of decays
Xenon 133	5.25 d	e.e.	81 in 36% of decays	None of significance
Thallium 201	73.1 h	e.c.	68–82 in 95% of decays	157–167 in 13% of decays

*i.t. = isomeric transition; ^{99m}Tc decays to ^{99}Tc, having extremely slow decay rate.
e.c. = electron capture
e.e = electron emission
} In all cases listed, the decay product is not radioactive.

because 95% or more of the total activity is located in the body outside the imaging field of view, with large amounts of scatter and penetration as a result.

Technetium 99m has excellent properties for SPECT because its monoenergetic 140-KeV gamma radiation is well suited for collimation and because the isotope's short physical half-life results in low radiation exposure (Tables 4–3 and 4–4). Moreover, ^{99m}Tc is inexpensive and available in all major hospitals, supplied weekly in the form of a generator containing its longer-lived precursor, molybdenum 99. Technetium 99m-labeled red cells allow tomographic imaging of the blood volume of the brain, and ^{99m}Tc-pertechnetate or ethylene-diaminetetra-acetate (EDTA) can be used to image the permeability of the blood-brain barrier (BBB).

Iodine 123 is not as suitable as ^{99m}Tc because it is more costly and must be supplied several times weekly to be available every day. Also, the dosimetry is less favorable than for ^{99m}Tc. High-energy photons arising in 2% of the radioactive decays tend to blur the images (see Tables 4–3 and 4–4). Impurities with other iodine isotopes constitute another problem. Iodine 123-labeled amines such as isopropyl-iodo-amphetamine, IMP, allow measurement of cerebral blood flow (CBF) by SPECT. As ^{99m}Tc-labeled CBF imaging compounds become clinically available, the use of ^{123}I for CBF tomography is about to become outdated. Yet ^{123}I continues to be of considerable interest for SPECT since receptor ligands labeled with ^{123}I can be used for studying cerebral neurotransmitter receptors.

Xenon 127 and ^{133}Xe can be used to study CBF with SPECT. The image quality obtained is practically the same with either agent. With ^{133}Xe, scattered

Table 4–4 RADIATION EXPOSURE WITH SOME TRACERS USED FOR BRAIN SPECT

Radionuclide	*Tracer* and Activity*	**Radiation Absorbed Dose in mGy per Examination Dose** *Highest Exposure*		*Gonads*	*Reference*
Technetium 99m	^{99m}Tc-HMPAO, 500 mBq	Lacrimal gland	35	3.0	14
Iodine 123	^{123}I-HIPDM, 85 mBq	Lung	28	2.0	56
Xenon 127	Rebreathing for 1.5 min from 5 L of air with 3 GBq	Airway mucosa	6	0.4	4
Xenon 133	same as for ^{127}Xe	Airway mucosa	50	0.6	4
Thallium 201	^{201}Tl-DDC, 130 mBq	—		5.0	11

*HIPDM = methyl-hydroxy-iodobenzyl propane diamine; HMPAO = d,l-hexamethyl-propyleneamine oxime; IMP = isopropyl-iodo-amphetamine; DDC = diethyldithiocarbonate.

radiation in the head reduces image contrast, and with ^{127}Xe, penetration of the high-energy photons through the collimator causes the same effect (see Table 4–3). Xenon 127 is more costly than ^{133}Xe, but has much more favorable dosimetry (see Table 4–4) because of the higher incidence of photon emission and the absence of electron emission.

Thallium 201 has not been used recently for SPECT studies of the brain because the only useful tracer labeled with ^{201}Tl, diethyl-dithio-carbamate (DDC), gives images of CBF distribution, and this can be measured more effectively with ^{99m}Tc-labeled tracers. Recently, ^{201}Tl has been used to image brain tumors, since it has negligible uptake in normal brain but good extraction into tumors.

SPECT IMAGING OF CEREBRAL BLOOD FLOW

Xenon 133

The tracers available for measurement of CBF by SPECT are all strongly lipophilic and can thus diffuse freely from blood into brain tissue. There are two different types of such tracers, the chemically inert ones, which are not retained in the brain, and the chemically active ones, which are retained.

Xenon 133 is the most widely used of the chemically inert tracers. Others in this category include ^{127}Xe, ^{99m}Tc-propyleneamine-oxime (PnAO), and ^{123}I-iodo-antipyrine, a tracer not yet studied with SPECT. Xenon 133 is usually administered by inhalation over 60–90 seconds. Intravenous injection can be used. The arrival and subsequent cerebral washout of the tracer is followed dynamically for 4–5 minutes with a series of four tomographic images per slice of brain tissue. Regional CBF is calculated in absolute units of mL/100 g per minute from the variation of the count rate of the region in four images and from the arterial input function.[7] This calculation is based on the autoradiographic principle for determining local blood flow with inert tracers.[23]

Arterial sampling is not required for CBF studies with ^{133}Xe. Instead, the count rate over the lung is monitored, and it is assumed that the arterial input function is proportional to the lung curve except for a time delay. The method is quantitative and yet completely atraumatic. Lasting only 4½ minutes, it is well accepted even by children. Repeat studies can readily be carried out. Since ^{133}Xe is rapidly cleared by the expired air, the measurement may be repeated after just 20 minutes.

The limitations of this method are:

- The necessity of using a specialized *dynamic* brain SPECT system that rotates rapidly.
- The fairly poor spatial resolution (1.5–2.0 cm) (see Table 4–2) in only three to five planes per study.
- The artifacts due to tracer in the sinuses and nasopharynx and to scattered radiation.
- The unreliability of taking the lung curve to represent the input in patients with severe pulmonary insufficiency. In such cases the absolute level of the flow may be inaccurate.

NORMAL VALUES

In normal adults, CBF measured in the resting state averages about 55 ml/100 g per minute.[44] With the usual positioning of the head and recording, three 2-cm-thick slices are taken simultaneously with an interslice distance of 4 cm. The lower slice shows the cerebellum and the temporal lobes; the middle slice shows the high flows in the cortex and basal ganglia, and the upper slice depicts the upper parts of the hemispheres (Fig. 4–8). The images are almost symmetrical, often with a 1%–2% higher mean CBF value on the *right* side. A side-to-side asymmetry of a region exceeding 10% is abnormal. The observed gray-white matter flow ratio is 2:1.

Intellectual activity or anxiety increases CBF in all regions by about 10%

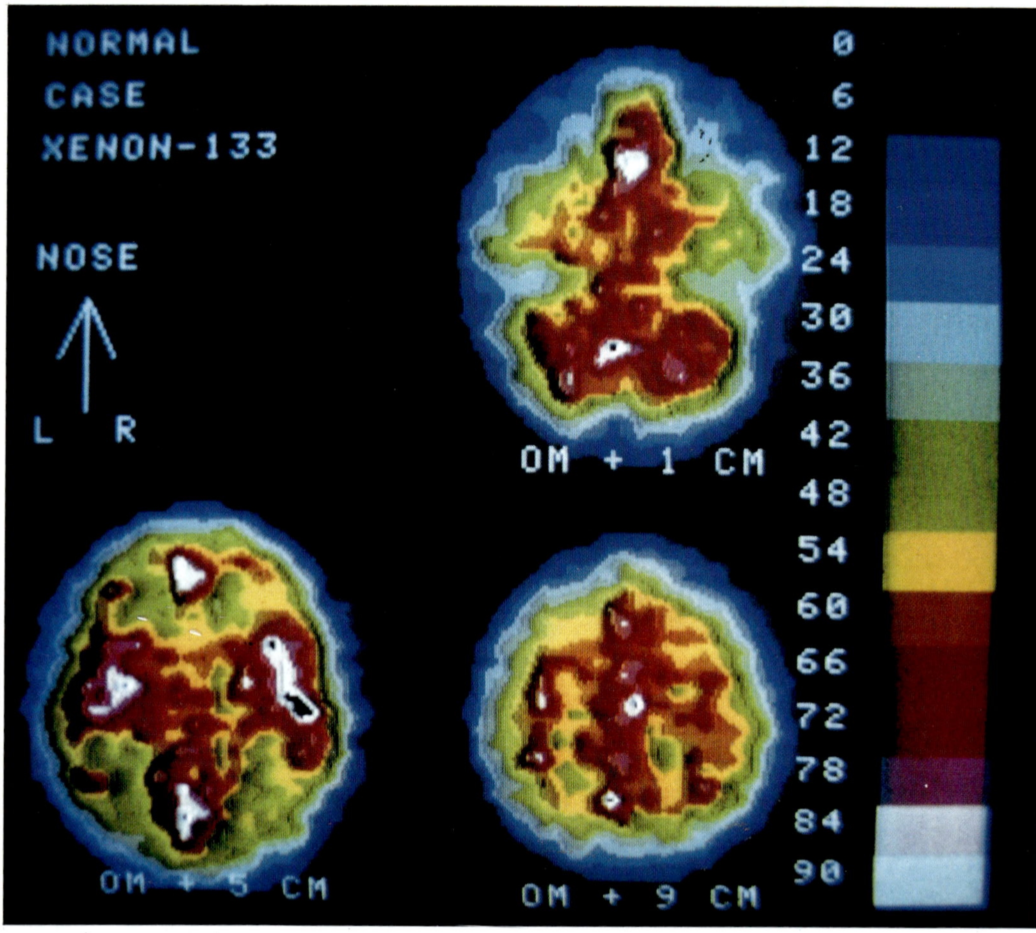

Figure 4–8. Xenon 133 CBF in a normal subject. Spatial resolution is 1.5 to 1.7 cm in the x-y plane, and 2.0 cm in the z-direction (Tomomatic-64).

above the value of the resting state. This increase results from enhancement of the oxidative metabolism of the brain ("metabolic regulation"). Focal changes are also seen. Most easy to record is the augmentation of 20%–30% in the visual cortex when the eyes are kept open. CBF increases with a rise in arterial PCO_2 and decreases with a drop in arterial PCO_2.

ACUTE STROKE

In ischemic stroke, xenon 133 CBF can reveal the evolution of hemodynamic changes.[53] When a major artery occludes, flow decreases immediately, long before changes develop in x-ray CT or MRI. The acute phase of dense focal ischemia lasts a few days (Fig. 4–9*A*). The subacute phase, which lasts some weeks, is characterized by a moderate increase of flow or sometimes by a marked hyperemia ("luxury perfusion," Fig. 4–9*B*). In the chronic phase, after some weeks, local flow of the fully developed infarct is again reduced to very low levels, just as in the acute phase (Fig. 4–9*C*).

Typically, the low-flow area is considerably larger than the structural lesion imaged by x-ray CT or MRI and larger than the area that would be expected from the limitation in resolution. This may be due to borderline ischemia ("ischemic penumbra"), diffuse cell loss, or disconnection between areas of the CNS. With major lesions involving one cerebral hemisphere, CBF also decreases in the opposite cerebellum ("crossed cerebellar diaschisis").[34]

Because it shows the full extent of the functional impact of the stroke, SPECT can be valuable in assessing prognosis. With attempts to treat stroke with acute thrombolytic techniques, ^{133}Xe tomography performed repeatedly may be important, since serial angiographic studies cannot be performed readily.

CAROTID OCCLUSION

Measurements of CBF with ^{133}Xe are useful in chronic internal carotid artery occlusion or high-grade stenosis. When studied in the normal, resting state with the patient lying horizontally, CBF may either be normal and symmetric or show a reduced flow corresponding to the territory of supply of the ICA occlusion. In many cases, however, the reduced flow may be the result of a previous stroke caused by the occlusion. Consequently, if the CBF image is normal or if it shows an asymmetry, the blood supply by way of collaterals may be adequate for maintaining a normal local arterial blood pressure. Patients with this finding have no hemodynamic impediment, and to reveal a hemodynamic insufficiency that results from poor collaterals, it is necessary to perform a "stress test" with a cerebral vasodilator such as carbon dioxide or acetazolamide (Diamox).[51,52] With this test, patients with adequate collaterals will show an increase in CBF on both sides; that is, flow even increases on the side of the carotid occlusion (regardless of the absence or presence of an asymmetry in the control state before the test), although the percentage increase usually is somewhat less on the affected side. Patients with inadequate collaterals and consequently with a much reduced distal blood pressure on the affected side show a marked enhancement of side-to-side asymmetry. In the patients with the lowest distal pressure, flow remains constant or even decreases on the side of the occlusion during the vasodilator stimulus. This paradoxical response is called the "intracerebral-steal" phenomenon. About 10% of all ICA occlusion cases have inadequate collaterals and they often manifest transient ischemic attacks of hemodynamic (orthostatic) type. Such patients are candidates for vascular surgery to bypass the carotid obstruction (Fig. 4–10).

SUBARACHNOID HEMORRHAGE

Patients with spontaneously ruptured arterial aneurysms often develop severe arterial vasospasm some days after the hemorrhage. Serial ^{133}Xe CBF measurements can reveal this complication[37] even before symptoms become clinically evident, because spasms introduce an asymptomatic moderate decrease of regional flow hours before a severe flow decrease develops and causes focal impairment of tissue function.

MIGRAINE

During the visual or sensorimotor prodromes of classic migraine, CBF is reduced in the area corresponding to the focal neurologic symptoms.[32] The low flow is confined to the cortex over the convexity of the brain, sparing the subcortical nuclei. If unilateral, the headache is located on the side of the low flow. The low flow gradually normalizes over some hours as the pain subsides; in many cases a phase of moderate hyperemia of the initial low-flow cortical regions can be found several hours after the attack.[2] Between the attacks, CBF is normal except in cases in which tissue lesions have developed.

In common migraine, which is defined by the absence of focal neurologic prodromes, CBF remains normal during and after the attack. In cluster headache, defined as periods ("clusters") of

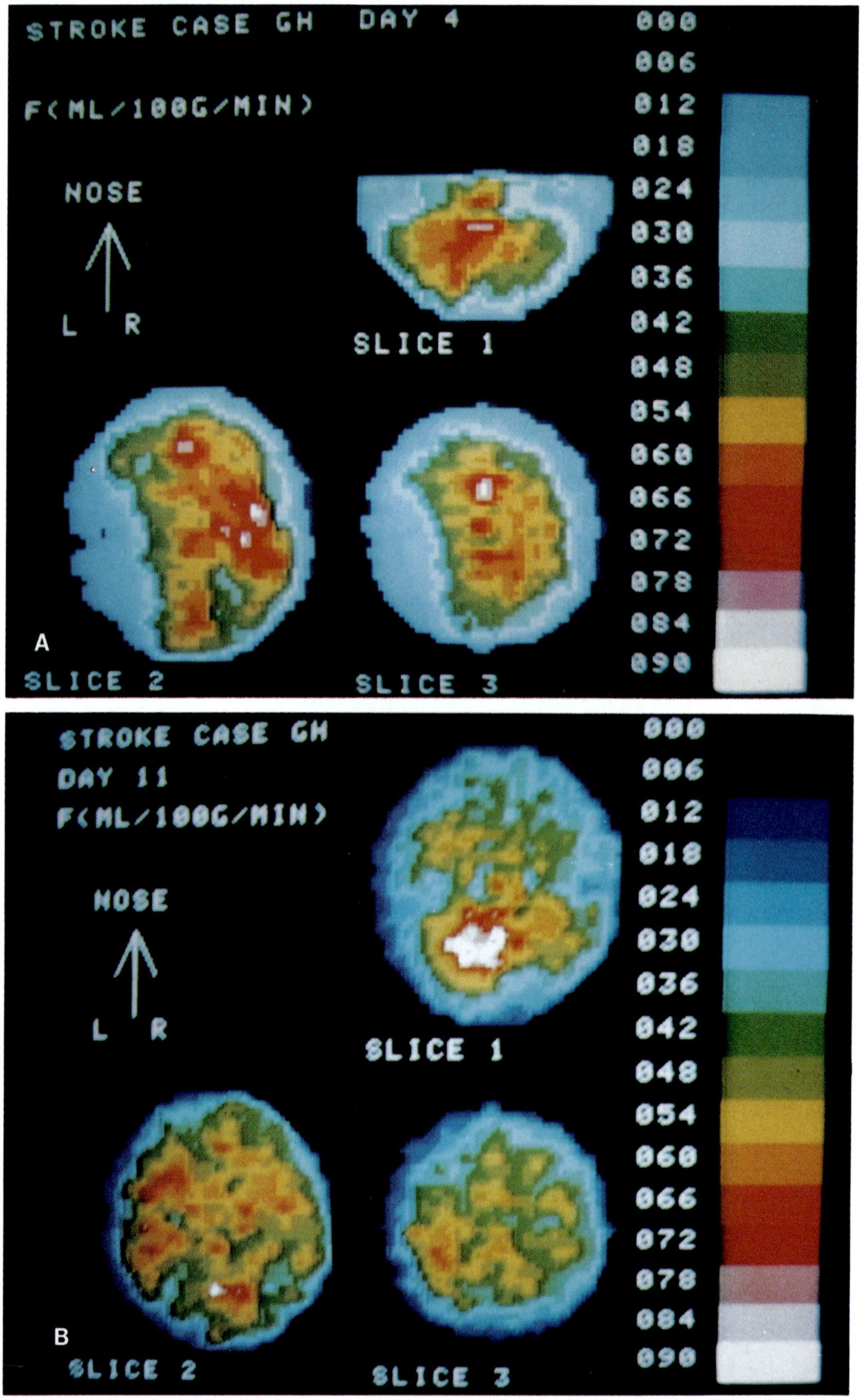

Figure 4–9. CBF by ^{133}Xe studied after (*A*) 4 days, (*B*) 11 days and (*C*). 2 months in a patient with right-sided hemiparesis due to occlusion of the left middle cerebral artery and a large infarction on x-ray CT. This case shows evidence of spontaneous reperfusion with "luxury" perfusion (day 11). The chronic phase looks practically the same as it did initially.

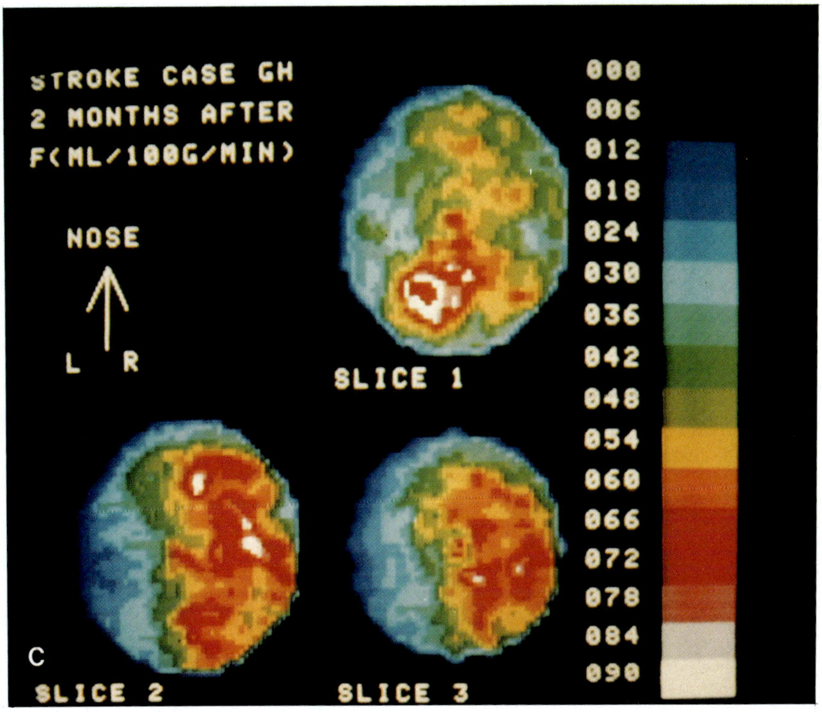

Figure 4–9. *Continued*

some weeks with daily attacks of severe pain in the retro-orbital region, CBF is also normal both during and after the attack.

DEMENTIA AND EPILEPSY

In dementia and epilepsy, ^{133}Xe gives essentially the same results as HMPAO, as discussed in the next section. Because of the better spatial resolution obtainable with HMPAO, this tracer is particularly valuable in such cases.

Technetium 99m-HMPAO

The distribution of CBF can be mapped tomographically with "chemical microspheres." These are chemically active molecules that behave like microspheres, which are trapped locally in the brain in proportion to blood flow. Iodine 123-labeled iso-propyl-iodo-amphetamine (IMP)[24,57] and ^{201}Tl-labeled diethyl-dithio-carbonate (DDC)[6,54] have been used. These tracers are now being rendered obsolete, however, with the advent of ^{99m}Tc-labeled molecules that have prolonged brain retention, such as HMPAO[40,41] and ethyl cysteinate dimer (ECD).[33,55] These two molecules are very similar with respect to the basic mechanism of retention.

As with all chemical microspheres, HMPAO is lipophilic, freely crossing capillary walls. Inside the brain the molecule is rapidly converted to a hydrophilic form which cannot leave the brain. The rate constant (k) of this trapping process is about 0.80 minute^{-1} and appears to be relatively constant at this level, both in normal and in pathologic brain tissue.[29,30] The rapid and yet not instantaneous trapping implies that a certain fraction (about one half) of ^{99m}Tc-HMPAO molecules entering the brain diffuse back into the blood stream

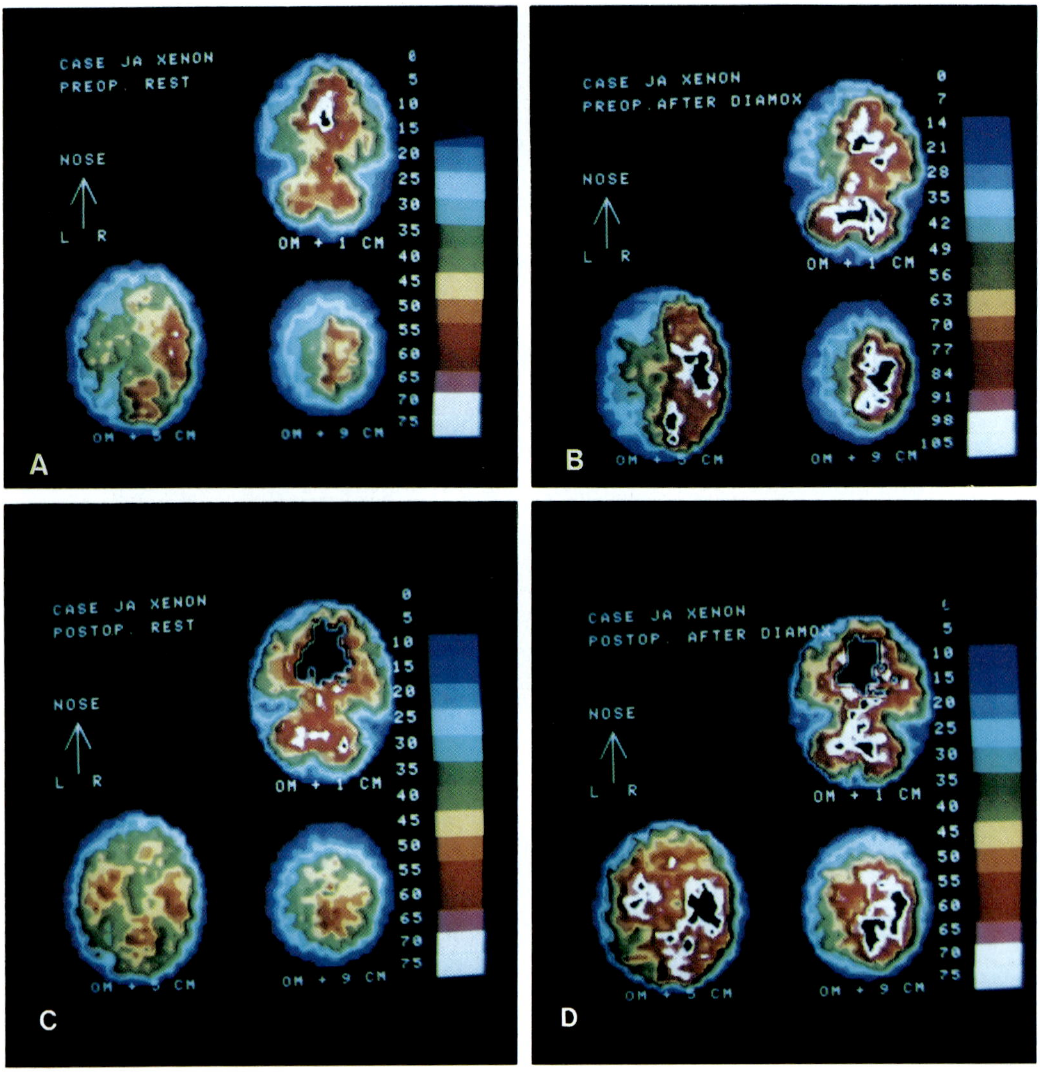

Figure 4–10. Xenon 133 CBF in a case of left internal carotid artery occlusion with multiple TIAs from the same hemisphere and treated by EC-IC bypass surgery. (*A*) Rest preoperatively shows moderate CBF asymmetry. (*B*) Acetazolamide (Diamox) preoperatively enhances CBF asymmetry. (*C*) Rest postoperatively shows almost normal CBF pattern. (*D*) Acetazolamide postoperatively also shows a practically normal pattern. The preoperative diagnosis was TIA of the hemodynamic type and was a key element in the decision for vascular surgery. The operation resulted in cessation of the TIAs and near normalization of the hemodynamic state.

and are cleared by the cerebral venous blood. The faster the blood flow, the greater the fraction cleared by this back-diffusion process. This explains why the contrast in tracer concentration between high-flow and low-flow regions decreases slightly over the first few minutes.[1]

The uptake and trapping of HMPAO is complete after about 10 minutes. Thereafter HMPAO remains fixed in the brain, with a loss of only 0.4% per hour. The steady-state pattern of retention seen in the tomograms also remains stable. Thus there is ample time for prolonged data acquisition over 20 minutes or more by a rotating gamma or multidetector system.

Calculation of CBF in absolute flow units can be performed. Since rapid conversion of HMPAO to the hydrophilic form also takes place in the blood stream, arterial blood must be sampled and analyzed immediately for the lipophilic, primary form of HMPAO to obtain the true input function. One can avoid this traumatic and cumbersome step by calculating CBF only in relative units—that is, percent of flow of a reference region.

The HMPAO technique is technically simple and atraumatic. With a sensitive detector system and conventional doses of radioactivity, a low-resolution SPECT image can be recorded in 1 minute or less. Thus, practically all patients can be studied regardless of age and condition.

The limitations of the technique are:

- It yields quantification of CBF only in terms of relative flow units.
- Repeat studies within a few hours can only be performed by using image subtraction with resulting loss of precision.
- In rare cases with marked local hyperemia, the slow leak of trapped HMPAO is more marked; in such cases scanning must be carried out within about 1 hour of tracer injection.[21,47]

NORMAL VALUES

In normal adults, with linearization using the cerebellum as the reference region,[18a,29,58] the average hemispheric CBF value is slightly above 100%. With a spatial resolution of 0.9–1.0 cm, the CBF of the gray matter–dominated visual area is about 140% and that of the white matter of the centrum semiovale, 70% that of the reference region.

Normal images outline the gray matter areas as high-blood-flow regions (see Fig. 4–11 and healthy side on Fig. 4–12). The images are practically symmetrical. Just as for xenon 133 CBF, however, the right side often has 1%–2% higher values. In young normal subjects the ventricular system and the cortical sulci are too narrow to be visible in the images. In elderly, normal subjects, who on x-ray CT have moderate degrees of enlarged CSF spaces, cortical CBF is slightly reduced. This is probably in part due to the CSF spaces, which cannot be seen distinctly as no-flow regions because of the limited spatial resolution.

CEREBROVASCULAR DISEASE (CVD)

As with the other tomographic CBF techniques, in cerebrovascular disease the low-flow areas seen with ^{99m}Tc-HMPAO typically extend beyond the infarct seen on x-ray CT or MRI scans.[13] The peri-infarct low-flow areas may be due to zones of ischemia ("penumbra") around the core of dense ischemia that causes necrosis. In many cases, however, the low-flow area extends into other vascular territories (Fig. 4–12), suggesting that reduced flow due to deafferentation ("diaschisis") also is involved.

In patients with occlusions of the internal carotid artery, ^{99m}Tc-HMPAO can show collateral flow. Xenon 133 is better suited for this type of study, however, in that a repeat study involving a vasodilator stimulus should be performed as described earlier.

ALZHEIMER'S DISEASE AND OTHER DEGENERATIVE DISEASES

Preliminary studies suggest the clinical utility of applying ^{99m}Tc-HMPAO to the differential diagnosis of Alzheimer's disease (AD) and multi-infarct dementia (MID).[19a,43] Usually AD shows a characteristic pattern of decreased flow in the parietal and temporal regions (Fig. 4–13). Often the changes are somewhat asymmetrical and in severe cases the frontal cortex may also be involved. MID shows more irregular patterns of reduced cortical flow. In both diseases, subcortical areas of reduced flow commonly correspond to subcortical atrophy, a somewhat dilated ven-

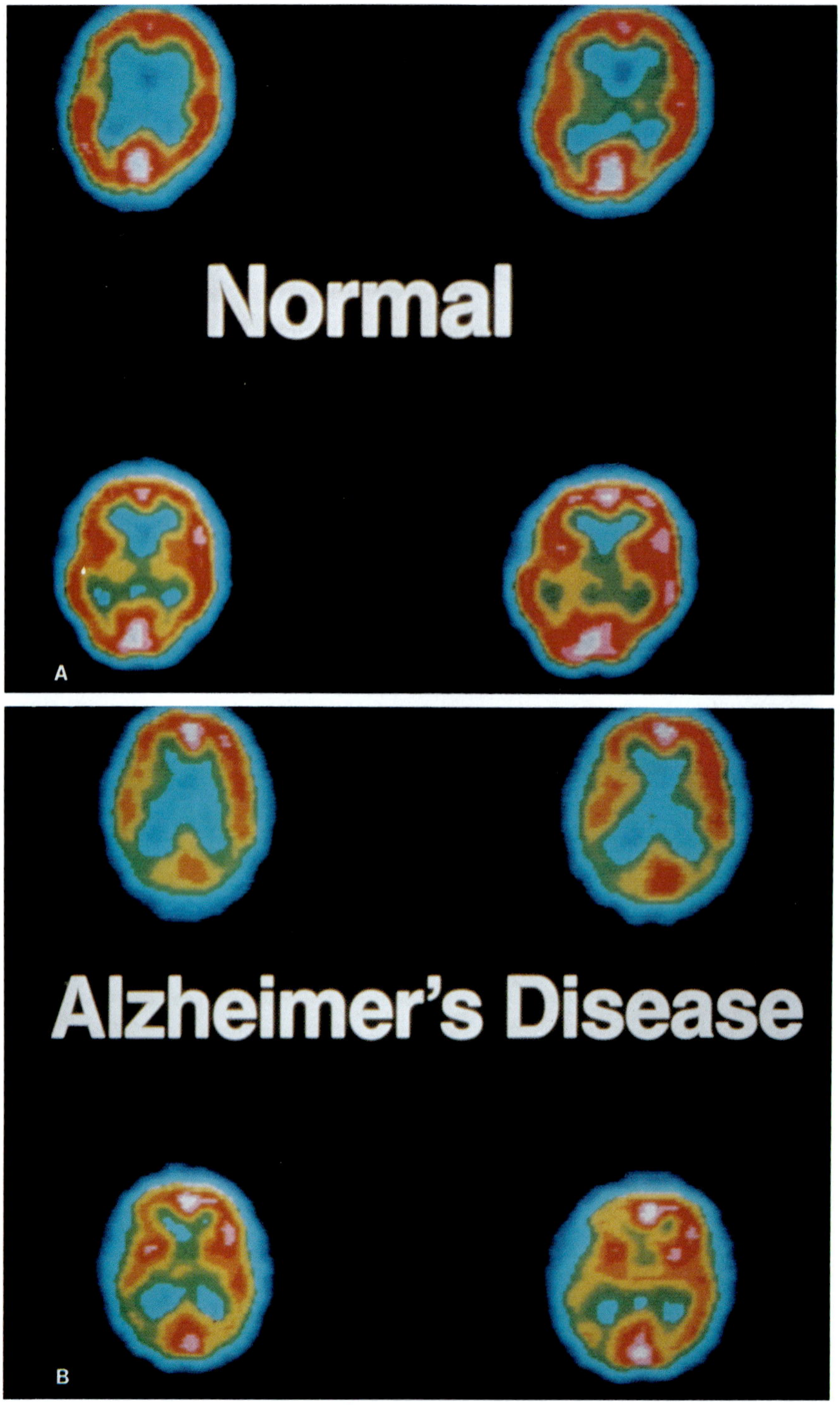

Figure 4–11. SPECT images using the GE-400 system (rotating single-head gamma camera with cut-off camera head) and ^{99m}Tc-HMPAO. (*A*) Normal; (*B*) Alzheimer's disease. (Courtesy of FW Smith, Aberdeen, Scotland.)

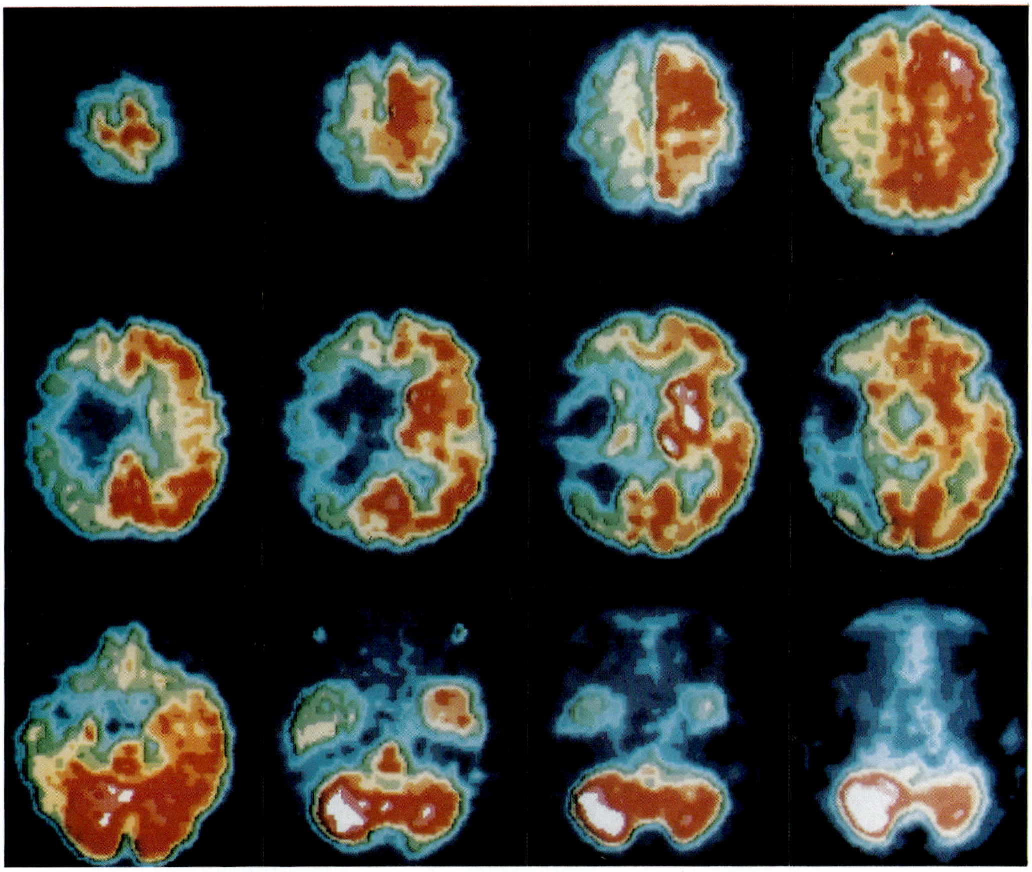

Figure 4–12. Brain-dedicated SPECT using ^{99m}Tc-HMPAO with a stroke patient. Twelve transverse slices parallel to the orbitomeatal plane are shown. Spatial resolution is 0.9 to 1.0 cm with approximately 3×10^6 counts per slice (Tomomatic-64).

tricular system, or both. In Binswanger's subcortical arteriosclerotic encephalopathy, the fairly moderate and diffuse cortical effects caused by the deeper lesions can sometimes be visualized.[10] Technetium 99m-HMPAO may also be valuable in recognizing dementia of frontal lobe type (such as Pick's disease) as a clinical entity separate from AD.[39]

Patients with degenerative disease of the basal ganglia cannot be adequately studied by ^{133}Xe tomography because of its low resolution, but ^{99m}Tc-HMPAO can be used in these patients. In a preliminary study of Huntington's disease,[46] seven of eight such patients showed low blood flow in the caudate nucleus.

TEMPORAL LOBE EPILEPSY

In many patients with this disorder, structural imaging by x-ray CT or MRI does not disclose any abnormality in the temporal lobe. Electroencephalography is usually the definitive diagnostic test, but occasionally equivocal EEG results are obtained. In most cases, functional imaging with PET and SPECT can demonstrate the side of the focus, sometimes even in patients without abnormal EEGs. Functional imaging has become an important diagnostic test since it has been shown that many patients can be treated effectively by surgical removal of part of the involved temporal lobe.

PET studies with ^{18}F-labeled de-

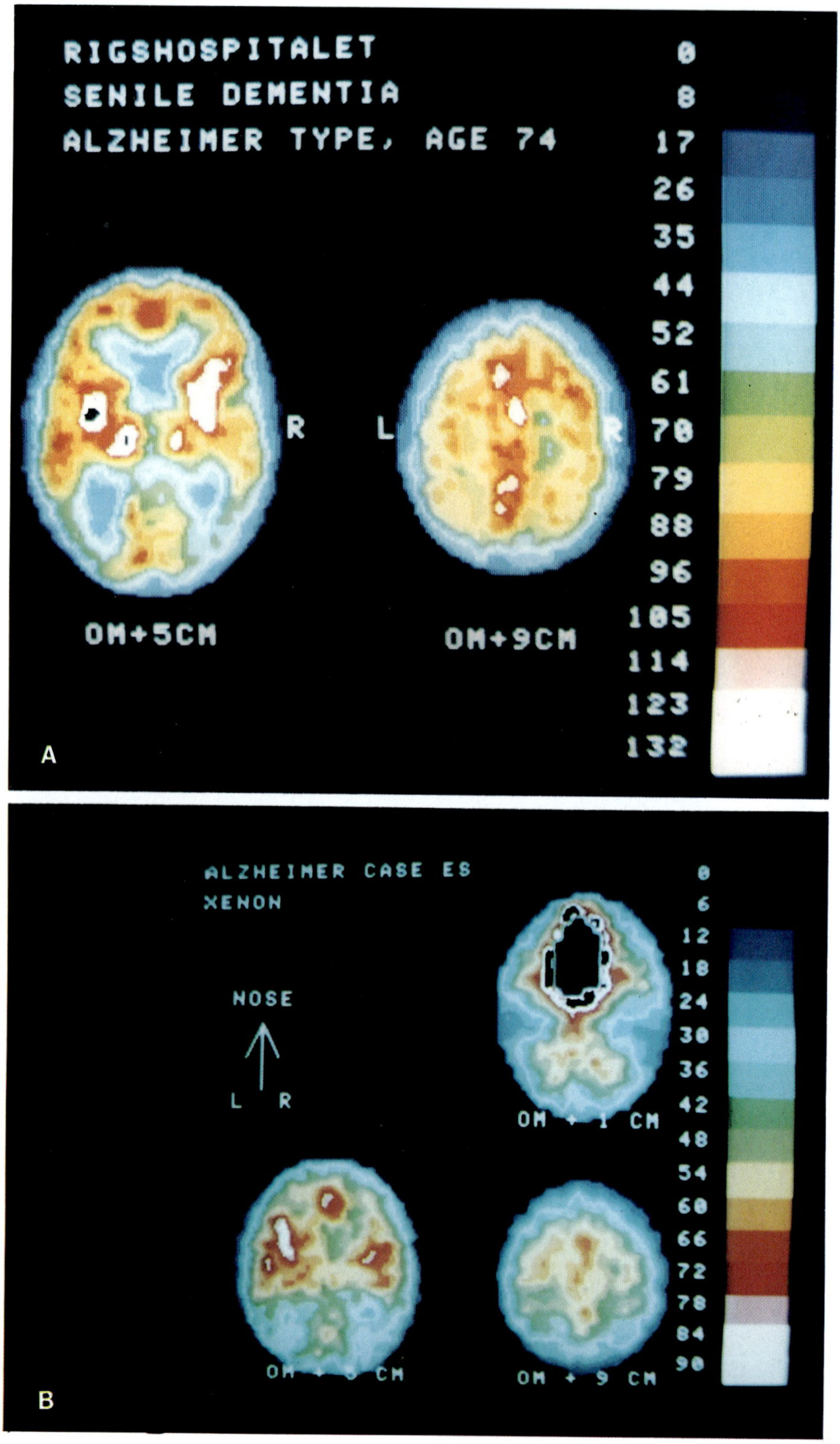
RIGSHOSPITALET
SENILE DEMENTIA
ALZHEIMER TYPE, AGE 74
0
8
17
26
35
44
52
61
70
79
88
96
105
114
123
132
R
L
OM+5CM
OM+9CM
A
ALZHEIMER CASE ES
XENON
NOSE
L R
OM + 1 CM
0
6
12
18
24
30
36
42
48
54
60
66
72
78
84
90
OM + 9 CM
B

oxyglucose demonstrated interictally a widespread *decrease* of the metabolism of the affected temporal lobe, even in some patients without abnormal EEGs.[15–17] This finding was proven to be correct by histologic confirmation and good surgical outcome. With ^{99m}Tc-HMPAO/SPECT, the preliminary results are similar.[3,19b,42] They show an excellent correlation between the side with the lowest CBF in the temporal lobe and the side of the EEG abnormalities. Even cases without a unilateral EEG focus sometimes show an obvious CBF asymmetry, allowing identification of the side primarily involved (Fig. 4–14).

RECEPTOR LIGANDS LABELED WITH IODINE 123

The success of positron-emitting receptor ligands for PET imaging has spurred the search for ligands labeled with single-photon emitters suitable for SPECT. Technetium 99m is difficult to incorporate into organic molecules, and ^{99m}Tc-labeled receptor ligands have not yet been developed. Halogens (F, Cl, Br, and I) are easier to incorporate. Among all the gamma-emitting halogen isotopes, only ^{123}I can be considered well-suited for SPECT. Thus, since other possible gamma tracers (not belonging to the halogen group) are much less flexible for organic chemistry, current efforts are concentrated on developing ^{123}I-labeled ligands.

Certain ^{123}I-labeled amines are well retained in the brain and are used for CBF imaging. Their retention probably results from binding to receptor sites of varying affinity and specificity. Yet, because the total binding capacity is high in all brain areas, the distribution image is flow-dominated. To image the distribution of a receptor in a meaningful way, the tracer must have a very low nonspecific binding. This can be achieved if the amount of tracer is so small that only a small fraction of the specific receptor is occupied. In other words, a very high specific activity must be used, as is well known from PET studies.

Dopaminergic receptor ligands have been studied. In humans, dopaminergic receptors are located in the striatum and, to a lesser degree, in the frontal cortex. Early attempts to label these receptors involved the labeling of spiperone with bromine 77, a gamma emitter with too high energy for high-quality SPECT images. This tracer was used for uptake studies in the basal ganglia of schizophrenic patients.[9]

The dopamine receptor ligand ^{123}I-labeled 4-iodo-spiperone has been synthesized with an exceptionally high specific activity of 100,000 Ci/mmol,[35,36] corresponding to a labeling efficiency of 40%. This means that picomol concentrations can be visualized—that is, such small amounts that specific receptor binding dominates the image. In vitro studies show that 2′-iodo-spiperone has a higher dopaminergic selectivity than 4-iodo-spiperone and therefore 2′-position labeling is proposed for in vivo use.[35] The work on iodinated spiperone compounds (D_2 receptor ligands) has not yet yielded a clinically applicable method for D_2 imaging. This decisive step, however, has been achieved with respect to D_1 receptor imaging, using an iodinated benzazepine IBZM.[5a,25a,26,27,38]

The compounds currently under study include ligands binding within serotonergic systems, benzodiazepine

Figure 4–13. (*A*) Senile dementia of the Alzheimer type (SDAT) in a 74-year-old woman with visual perception difficulties. Initially these difficulties were diagnosed to be of a psychogenic nature. X-ray CT showed slight atrophy. The characteristic symmetrical temporoparietal CBF reduction is diagnostic of SDAT. Images were taken by a Tomomatic brain-dedicated SPECT using ^{99m}Tc-HMPAO at image resolution 0.9 to 1.0 cm. They were linearized and scaled in relative units of CBF in percent of the blood flow of the cerebellum. (*B*) Xenon 133 CBF in the same patient. The same flow abnormalities are seen.

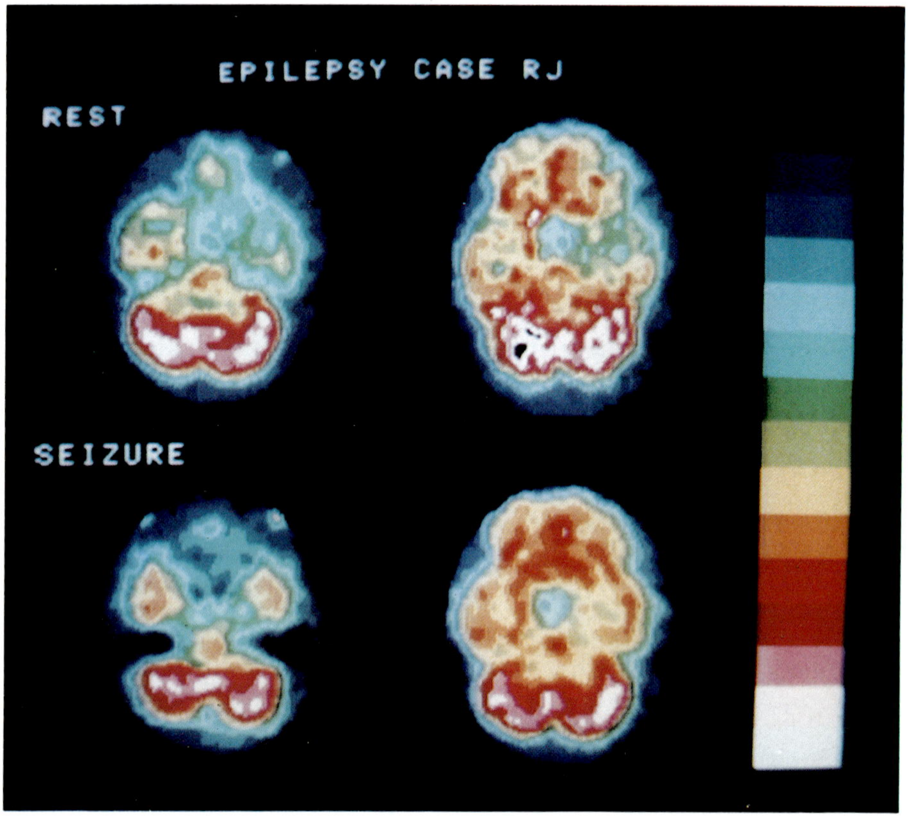

Figure 4–14. Temporal lobe epilepsy. Since infancy, this 20-year-old woman had seizures that, at the age of 5 months, had been noted to be associated with increased tone of the left arm. A feeling of heaviness of the left arm was associated with current attacks. Frequent seizures could not be controlled by drugs, making her a potential candidate for temporal lobectomy. X-ray CT and MRI were normal, and EEG was equivocal as to side localization. To image CBF, ^{99m}Tc-HMPAO was used with a Tomomatic-64 SPECT system. Studies were performed in the interictal phase (rest), and on another day during a seizure. The images show low flow on the right side interictally, and a flow increase in this region alone during a typical psychomotor seizure. Considering favorable results obtained in a series of similar cases, these findings favor surgical intervention on the right side.

receptors, gamma aminobutyric acid (GABA) receptors, and muscarinic cholinergic receptors.[12] With the current massive efforts in this area, rapid progress will be made within the next few years. An important impetus to this research is the prospect that specific receptor ligands for SPECT may allow the study of competing nonradioactive drugs in humans at moderate costs. Thus, SPECT has the potential to become a practical tool in clinical neurochemistry.

REFERENCES

1. Andersen, AR, Friberg, H. Schmidt, J., and Hasselbalch, SG: Quantitative measurements of CBF using SPECT and Tc-99m-d,l-HMPAO compared to

xenon-133. J Cereb Blood Flow Metab 8(Suppl):S69–S81, 1988.

2. Andersen, AR, Friberg, L. Olsen, TS, and Olesen, J: Delayed hyperemia following hypoperfusion in classic migraine. Arch Neurol 45(2):154–159, 1988.
3. Andersen, AR, Gram, L, Kjaer, L, Fuglsang-Frederiksen, A, Herning, M, Lassen, NA, and Dam, M: SPECT in partial epilepsy: Identifying side of the focus. Acta Neurol Scand, suppl. 117, 78:90–95, 1988.
4. Atkins, HL, Robertson, JS, Croft BY, Tsui, B, Susskind, H, Ellis, KJ, Loken, MK, and Treves, S: Estimate of radiation absorbed doses from radioxenons in lung imaging. (MIRD dose estimate report no. 9) J Nucl Med 21:459–465, 1980.
5. Axelson, B, Msaki, P, and Israelsson, A: Subtraction of Compton-scattered photons in single-photon emission computerized tomography. J Nucl Med 25:490–494, 1984.
5a. Beer, H-F, Bläuenstein, PA, Hasler, PH, Delaloye, B, Riccabona, G, Bangerl, I, Hunkler, W, Bonetti, EP, Pieri, L, Richards, JG, and Schubiger, PA. In vitro and in vivo evaluation of iodine-123-R_o 16-0154: A new imaging agent for SPECT investigations of benzodiazepine receptors. J Nucl Med 31:1007–1014, 1990.
6. Bruine J, van Royen E, Vyth A, de Jong, JMBV, and van der Schoot, JB: Thallium-201 diethyldithio-carbamate: An alternative to iodine-123 n-isopropyl-p-iodoamphetamine. J Nucl Med 26:925–929, 1985.
7. Celsis, P, Goldman, T, Henriksen, L, and Lassen, NA: A method for calculating regional cerebral blood flow from emission computed tomography of inert gas concentrations. J Comput Assist Tomogr 5:641–645, 1981.
8. Chang, LT: A method for attenuation correction in radionuclide computed tomography. IEEE. Trans Nucl Sci NS-25:638–639, 1978.
9. Crawley, JCW, Crow, TJ, Johnstone, EC, Oldland, SRD, Owen, F, Owens, DGC, Smith, T, Veall, N, and Zanelli, GD: Uptake of ^{77}Br-spiperone in the striata of schizophrenic patients and controls. Nucl Med Comm 7:599–607, 1986.
10. De Chiara, S, Lassen, NA, Andersen, AR, Gade, A, Lester, J, Thomsen, C, and Henriksen, O: High-resolution nuclear magnetic resonance imaging and single-photon emission computerized tomography: Cerebral blood flow in a case of pure sensory stroke and mild dementia owing to subcortical arteriosclerotic encephalopathy (Binswanger's disease). Amer J Physiol Imaging 2:192–195, 1987.
11. Dige-Petersen, H (Ed): Nuclearmedicin, Munksgaard Pub, Copenhagen, 1986, p 178.
12. Eckelman, WC, Reba, RC, Rzeszotarski, WJ, Gibson, RE, Hill, T, Holman, BL, Budinger, T, Conklin, JJ, Eng, R, and Grissom, MP: External imaging of cerebral muscarinic acetylcholine receptors. Science 223:291–293, 1984.
13. Ell, PJ, Cullum, ID, Costa, DC, Jarritt, PH, Hocknell, JML, Lui, D, Jewkes, RF, Steiner, TJ, Nowotnik, DP, Pickett, RD, and Neirinckx, RD: A new regional cerebral blood flow mapping with Tc-99m-labelled compound. The Lancet ii:50–51, 1985.
14. Ell, P, Costa, DC, Cullum, ID, Jamitt, PH, Lui, D. The clinical application of rCBF imaging by SPET. Amersham International, Little Chalfont, UK, 1987.
15. Engel, J Jr, Brown, WJ, Kuhl, DE, Phelps, ME, Mazziotta, JC, and Crandall, PH: Pathological findings underlying focal temporal lobe hypometabolism in partial epilepsy. Ann Neurol 12:518–528, 1982a.
16. Engel, J Jr, Kuhl, DE, Phelps, ME, and Crandall, PH: Comparative localization of epileptic foci in partial epilepsy by PCT and EEG. Ann Neurol 12:529–537, 1982.
17. Engel, J Jr, Kuhl, DE, Phelps, ME, and Mazziotta, JC: Inter-ictal cerebral glucose metabolism in partial epilepsy and its relation to EEG changes. Ann Neurol 12:510–517, 1982.
18. Floyd, CE, Jaszczak, RJ, and Coleman, RE: A unified reconstruction algorithm

for SPECT. IEEE, Trans Nucl Sci NS-32:779–785, 1985.

18a. Gemmell, HG, Evans, NTS, Besson, JAO, Roeda, D, Davidson, J, Dodd, MG, Sharp, PF, Smith, FW, Crawford, JR, Newton, RH, Kulkarni, V, Mallard, JR: Regional cerebral blood flow imaging: A quantitative comparison of technetium-99m-HMPAO SPECT with $C^{15}O_2$ PET. J Nucl Med 31:1595–1600, 1990.

19. Genna, S, and Smith, AP: The development of ASPECT, an annular single crystal brain camera for high efficiency SPECT. IEEE, Trans Nucle Sci NS-35:654–658, 1988.

19a. Habert, MO, Spampinato, U, Mas, JL, Piketty, ML, Bourdel, MC, deRecondo, J, Rondot, P, and Askienazy, S: Eur J Nucl Med 18:341, 1991.

19b. Grünwald, F, Durwen, HF, Bockisch, A, Hotze, A, Kersjes, W, Elger, CE, and Biersack, HJ: Technetium-99m-HMPAO brain SPECT in medically intractable temporal lobe epilepsy: A postoperative evaluation. J Nucl Med 32(3):388–394, 1991.

20. Holm, S, Andersen, AR, Vorstrup, S, Lassen, NA, Paulson, OB, and Holmes, RA: Dynamic SPECT of the brain using a lipophilic technetium-99m complex, PnAO. J Nucl Med 26:1129–1134, 1985.

20a. Holman, BL, Carvalho, PA, Zimmerman, RE, Johnson, KA, Tumeh, SS, Smith, AP, and Genna, S: Brain perfusion SPECT using an annular single crystal camera: Initial clinical experience. J Nucl Med 31, 9:1456–1561, 1990.

21. Holmes, RA, Gini, A, and Logan, KW: Demonstration of cerebral infarct hyperemia with Tc-99m-HM-PAO. J Nucl Med 28, 4:633, A320, 1987.

22. Kanno, I, Uemura, K, Miura, S, and Miura, Y: HEADTOME: A hybrid emission tomograph for single photon and positron imaging of the brain. J Comput Assist Tomogr 5:216–226, 1981.

23. Kety, SS: The theory and applications of the exchange of inert gas at the lungs and tissues. Pharm Rev 3:1–41, 1951.

24. Kuhl, DE, Barrio, JR, Huang, SC, Selin, C, Ackermann, RF, Lear, JL, Wu, JL, Lin, TH, and Phelps, ME: Quantifying local cerebral blood flow by N-isopropyl-p-I-123 Iodo amphetamine (IMP) tomography. J Nucl Med 23:196–203, 1982.

25. Kuhl, DE, Edwards, RO, Ricci, AR, Yacob, RJ, Mich, TJ, and Alavi, A: The Mark IV system for radionuclide computed tomography of the brain. Radiology 121:405–413, 1976.

25a. Kung, HF, Alavi, A, Chang, W, Kung, M-P, Keyes, JW, Jr, Velchik, MG, Billings, J, Pan, S, Noto, R, Rausch, A, and Reilly, J. In vivo SPECT imaging of CNS D-2 dopamine receptors: Initial studies with iodine-123-IBZM in humans. J Nucl Med 31:573–579, 1990.

26. Kung, HF, Alavi, A, Billings, J, Kung, MP, Pan, S, and Reilley, J: (^{123}I)IBZP: A potential CNS D-1 dopamine receptor imaging agent: In vivo biodistribution in a monkey. J Nucl Med 29(5): 758, A74,1988.

27. Kung, HF, Alavi, A, Kung, MP, Pan, S, Billings, J, Kasliwal, R, and Reilley, J: In vivo and in vitro biodistribution of (^{123})IBZM: A potential CNS D-2 dopamine receptor imaging agent. J Nucl Med 29(5):759,A75,1988.

28. Larsson, SA: Gamma camera emission tomography. Acta Radiol (Suppl) 363, 1980.

29. Lassen, NA, Andersen, AR, Friberg, L, and Paulson, OB: The retention of Tc-99m-d,l-HMPAO in the human brain after intra-carotid bolus injection: A kinetic analysis. J Cereb Blood Flow Metab 8(Suppl):S13–S22, 1988.

30. Lassen, NA, Andersen, AR, Neirinckx, RD, Ell, PJ, and Costa, DC: Validation of Ceretec. In Ell, PJ, Costa, DC, Cullum, ED, Jarritt, PH, and Lui, D (eds): The Clinical Application of rCBF Imaging by SPET. Amersham International, Little Chalfont, UK.

31. Lassen, NA, Sveinsdottir, E, Kanno, I, Stokely, EM, and Rommer, P: A fast moving, single photon emission tomograph for regional cerebral blood flow studies in man (Abstr.) J Comput Assist Tomogr 2:661–662, 1978.

32. Lauritzen, M and Olesen, J: Regional cerebral blood flow during migraine attacks by Xenon-133 inhalation and emission tomography. Brain 107:447–461, 1984.

33. Léveillé, J, Demonceau, G, De Roo, M, Rigo, P, Taillefer, R, Morgan, RA, Kupranick, D, and Walovitch, RC: Characterization of technetium-99m-L,L-ECD for brain perfusion imaging, Part 2: Biodistribution and brain imaging in humans. J Nucl Med 30:1902–1910, 1989.
34. Meneghetti, G, Vorstrup, S, Mickey, B, Lindewald, H, and Lassen, NA: Crossed cerebellar diaschisis in ischemic stroke: A study of regional cerebral blood flow by ^{133}Xe inhalation and single photon emission computerized tomography. J Cereb Blood Flow Metab 4:235–240, 1984.
35. Mertens, J, Terriere, D, Leysen, J, and Ingels, M: N.C.A. 4-I-123(125)-spiperone, new high yield labeling couples to in vitro and SPECT animal studies. J Nucl Med 28:570–571, 1987.
36. Mertens, J, Terriere, D, Vanryckegjem, W, and Gyscmans, M: New method for high yield preparation of carrier free ^{123}I-spiperone applied for in-vitro binding and animal studies. Nucl Med 25:A54, 1986.
37. Mickey, B, Vorstrup, S, Voldby, B, Lindewald, H, Harmsen, A, and Lassen NA: Serial measurement of regional cerebral blood flow in patients with SAH using 133-Xe inhalation and emission computerized tomography. J Neurosurg 60:916–922, 1984.
38. Nakatsuka, I, Saji, H, Shiba, K, Shimizu, H, Okuno, M, Yoshitake, A, and Yokoyama, A: In vitro evaluation of radioiodinated butyrophenones as radiotracer for dopamine receptor study. Life Sciences 41:1989–1997, 1987.
39. Neary, D, Snowden, JS, Northen, B, and Goulding, P: Dementia of frontal lobe type. J Neurol Neurosurg Psychiatry 51:353–361, 1988.
40. Neirinckx, RD, Canning, LR, Piper, IM, Nowotnik, DP, Pickett, RD, Holmes, RA, Volkert, WA, Forster, AM, Weisner, PS, Marriott, JA, and Chaplin, SB: Tc-99m d,l-HMPAO: A new radiopharmaceutical for SPECT imaging of regional cerebral blood perfusion. J Nucl Med 28: 191–202, 1987.
41. Nowotnik, DP, Canning, LR, Cumming, SA, Harrison, RC, Higley, B, Nechvatal, G, Pickett, RD, Piper, IM, Bayne, VJ, Forster, AM, Weisner, PS, and Neirinckx, RD: Development of a Tc-99m-labeled radiopharmaceutical for cerebral blood flow imaging. Nucl Med Commun 6:499–506, 1985.
42. Ryding, E, Rosén, I, Elmqvist, D, and Ingvar, DH: SPECT measurements with 99m-Tc-HMPAO in focal epilepsy. J Cereb Blood Flow Metab 8(suppl): S95–S100, 1988.
43. Sharp, PF, Smith, FW, Gemmell, HG, Lyall, D, Evans, NTS, Gvozdanovic, D, Davidson, J, Tyrell, DA, Pickett, RD, and Neirinckx, RD: Technetium 99m-Tc-HMPAO stereoisomers as potential agents for imaging regional cerebral blood flow: Human volunteer studies. J Nucl Med 27:171–177, 1986.
44. Shirahata, N, Henriksen, L, Vorstrup, S, Holm, S, Lauritzen, M, Paulson, OB, and Lassen, NA: Regional cerebral blood flow assessed by 133-Xe inhalation and emission tomography: Normal values. J Comput Assist Tomogr 9(5): 861–866, 1985.
45. Singh, M and Doria, D: Single photon imaging with electronic collimation. IEEE Trans Nucl Sci NS-32:843-847, 1985.
46. Smith, FW, Besson, JAO, Gemmell, HG, and Sharp, PF: The use of technetium-99m-HMPAO in the assessment of patients with dementia and other neuropsychiatric conditions. J Cereb Blood Flow Metab 8(Suppl):S116–S122, 1988.
47. Hayashida, K, Nishimura, T, Imakita, S, and Vehara, T: Filling out phenomenon with technetium-99m HM-PAO brain SPECT at the site of mild-cerebral ischemia. J Nucl Med 30:591–598, 1989.
48. Stoddart, HF and Stoddart, HA: A new development in single gamma transaxial tomography: Union Carbide focused collimator scanner. IEEE Trans Nucl Sci NS-26:2710–2712, 1979.
49. Stokely, EM, Sveinsdottir, E, Lassen, NA, and Rommer, P: A single photon dynamic computer-assisted tomograph (DCAT) for imaging brain function in multiple cross-sections. J Comput Assist Tomogr 4:230–240, 1980.

50. Tanaka, M, Hirose, Y, Koga, K, and Hattori, H: Engineering aspects of a hybrid emission computed tomograph. IEEE. Trans Nucl Sci NS-28:137–141, 1981.
51. Vorstrup, S, Boysen, G, Brun, B, and Engell, HC: Evaluation of the regional cerebral vasodilatory capacity before carotid endarterectomy by the acetazolamide test. Neurol Research 98:10–18, 1987.
52. Vorstrup, S, Brun, B, and Lassen, NA: Evaluation of the cerebral vasodilatory capacity by the acetazolamide test before EC-IC bypass. Stroke 17:1291–1298, 1986.
53. Vorstrup, S, Paulson, OB, and Lassen, NA: Cerebral blood flow in acute and chronic ischemic stroke using xenon-133 inhalation tomography. Acta Neurol Scand 74:439–451, 1986.
54. Vyth, A, Fennema, P, van der Shoot, J: Tl-201-diethyl-dithiocarbamate: A possible radiopharmaceutical for brain imaging. Pharm Weekbl(Sci)5:213–216, 1983.
55. Walovitch, RC, Hill, TC, Garrity, ST, Cheesman, EH, Burgess, BA, O'Leary, DH, Watson, AD, Ganey, MV, Morgan, RA, and Williams, SJ: Characterization of technetium-99m-L,L-ECD for brain perfusion imaging, Part 1: Pharmacology of technetium-99m ECD in nonhuman primates. J Nucl Med 30: 1892–1901, 1989.
56. Wicks, R, Billings, J, Kung, HF, Steinbach, JJ, Ackerhalt, R and Blau, M: Biodistribution in humans and radiation dose calculations for the brain perfusion agent I-123 HIPDM. J Nucl Med 24: 95, 1983.
57. Winchell, HS, Horst, WD, Braun, L, Oldendorf, WH, Hattner, R, and Parker, HN: N-Isopropyl(^{123}I)p-iodoamphetamine: Single-pass brain uptake and washout; binding to brain synaptosomes; and localization in dog and monkey brain. J Nucl Med 21:947–952, 1980.
58. Yonekura, Y, Nishizawa, S, Mukai, T, Fujita, T, Fukuyama, H, Ishikawa, M, Kikuchi, H, Konishi, J, Lassen, NA, and Andersen, AR: SPECT with Tc-99m-(d,l)-hexamethyl-propyleneamine oxime (HM-PAO) compared with regional cerebral blood flow measured by PET: Effects of linearization. J Cereb Blood Flow Metab 8(Suppl):S82–S89, 1988.

Part II

NEUROIMAGING IN CLINICAL EVALUATION AND MANAGEMENT

Chapter 5

EPILEPSY

William H. Theodore, M.D.

AN APPROACH TO THE PATIENT
PARTIAL SEIZURES ("LOCALIZATION-RELATED EPILEPSY")
GENERALIZED SEIZURES
NUCLEAR MAGNETIC RESONANCE SPECTROSCOPY
PET AND THE NEUROPHARMACOLOGY OF EPILEPSY
A STRATEGY FOR IMAGING EVALUATION OF PATIENTS WITH EPILEPSY

AN APPROACH TO THE PATIENT

The evaluation of a patient suspected of having epilepsy requires confirming the diagnosis, establishing the type of epilepsy (both the seizure type and epilepsy classification) and the presence of a specific cause, and developing a plan of treatment. The history is the most important part of the evaluation, both for differential diagnosis and classification. Electroencephalograms (EEGs), to help distinguish between partial and generalized epilepsy, also are required before deciding on an imaging strategy. Clinical or electrographic features suggestive of focal onset, such as focal slowing or spikes, the presence of an aura, unilateral motor or sensory phenomena, or a postictal hemiparesis, may influence the plan of an imaging evaluation. The high sensitivity of MRI in particular can lead to detection of "lesions" of uncertain significance, which cannot be interpreted without clinical and EEG data.

Experience with x-ray CT also suggests that imaging studies in epilepsy may be difficult to interpret. Correlation between x-ray CT and EEG often is imprecise.[55,67,93] Early reports of x-ray CT duplicated experience with pneumoencephalography and plain skull x-rays, showing a high incidence of nonspecific abnormalities in some series, heavily influenced by patient selection and referral patterns.[12,18,39,94,102] Even in patients evaluated for surgery, the value of routine x-ray CT scanning was not always apparent.

Should an initial scan be unrevealing, or show an abnormality that does not seem related to the seizure disorder, it may be important to reevaluate clinical and electrophysiologic findings and perform additional EEGs. Simultaneous video-EEG monitoring of seizures should be used before positron emission tomography (PET) or single photon emission computed tomography (SPECT), since the pathophysiologic findings of these tests can only be interpreted when accurate ictal localization is available.

Cerebral angiography, demonstrating the intracranial blood vessels by injecting contrast agents, is less commonly used since the development of modern tomographic scanning, especially because it carries a complication risk of about 2%. Nevertheless, arteriography remains important when seizures are related to vascular disease, and it may be used preoperatively to define the vascular supply of regions chosen for focal resection. An intracarotid sodium amytal (Wada) test is a standard procedure to help localize memory and language before temporal lobectomy.

PARTIAL SEIZURES ("LOCALIZATION-RELATED EPILEPSY")

The epileptic discharges accompanying partial seizures begin locally, usually in one temporal lobe, and, by definition, do not involve the entire brain, although spread to additional regions often occurs. A patient may have a single epileptic focus or multiple foci. Neuroimaging studies are most important for partial seizures, which are frequently associated with intracranial lesions. Moreover, patients with partial seizures not controlled by medication may be surgical candidates. Some "localization-related" epilepsies such as benign rolandic epilepsy of childhood, however, are unlikely to be associated with brain lesions, so that a patient with this diagnosis may not benefit from an x-ray CT or MRI scan. The extent of imaging evaluation must be guided by the possibility of therapeutic intervention based on the test results; in some cases imaging tests will have a low yield.

X-Ray CT and MR Imaging

X-ray CT brain imaging has now been available for almost 20 years. Experience over this time, as well as advances in technology, have led to increasingly reliable interpretations of x-ray CT images with and without contrast agents, as well as to the development of standard technical settings for the instrument (Figs. 5–1*A*, 5–2). Many of the technical variables of MRI also have become standardized, and increasing numbers of postmortem or biopsy studies have identified the neuropathology of abnormalities revealed by MRI. Obtaining maximal discrimination with MRI, however, depends upon employing more complex physical variables than are necessary with x-ray CT. Some of these adjustments have been found to be particularly important in studying patients with seizures.

Illustrating the need for special attention to technical factors in MRI, most studies have suggested that heavily weighted T_2 sequences are most sensitive to detecting the types of pathologic changes seen in patients with seizures, such as focal gliosis, low-grade tumors, and small hamartomas or arteriovenous malformations (Figs. 5–1, 5–3).[64,98,107] Abnormal regions of signal intensity appearing at TE 70 may not be detected at TE 35.[93] Taking thin sections of 5-mm as opposed to 10-mm thickness also increases sensitivity.[117] Obtaining images in both coronal and sagittal planes (Fig. 5–3*C*) helps to exclude pulsation artifacts from flowing blood and CSF, since artifacts will change their apparent "location" as slice orientation is varied. Coronal images are particularly valuable for precise anatomic localization of regions of mesial temporal increased signal intensity.[64,98,107,117] But caution is needed, since artifacts due to CSF flow become more prominent at high field strengths and in heavily T_2-weighted images. These may cause confusion with regions of focal gliosis (Fig. 5–4). To minimize error, such CSF flow areas should show the same signal characteristics as ventricular CSF, rather than those of gliosis or a mass lesion, and they should be correlated with identification of the temporal horns on CT or T_1-weighted sequences.

Population studies defining the incidence of image-identified anatomic abnormalities in patients with epilepsy as yet have not been reported with MRI. X-ray CT surveys, however, indicate that in the presence of a normal neurologic examination, abnormal CT scans are unlikely to be found among patients younger than age 30.[8,46,84,87,122] Discrete abnormalities consistent with infarction are more common on x-ray CT scans of patients with seizures begin-

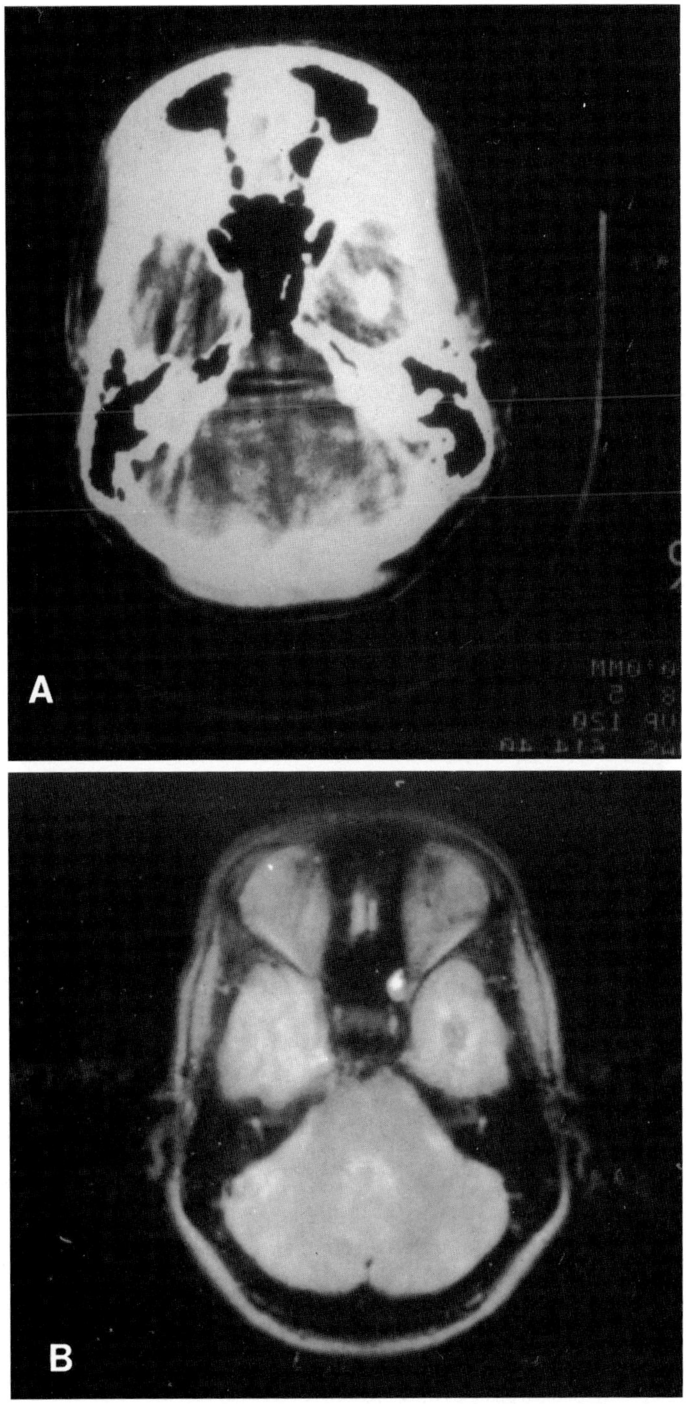

Figure 5–1. (*A*) X-ray CT scan shows temporal calcification in a patient with complex partial seizures (CPS). (*B*) MRI scan of the same patient: TR 2500, TE 80. Pathologic examination showed focal gliosis with features suggestive, but not diagnostic, of an oligodendroglioma. The PET scan showed bitemporal hypometabolism.

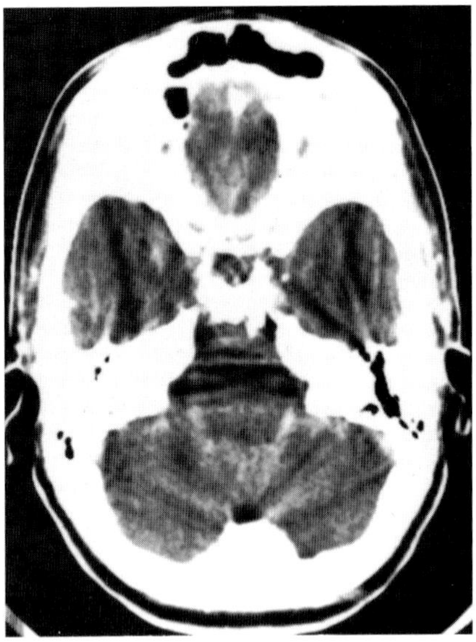

Figure 5–2. X-ray CT scan shows beam hardening artifact, impairing evaluation of temporal lobe.

ning after the age of 50 than for earlier ages.[96] Nonspecific abnormalities such as mild cortical atrophy have no influence on treatment. One study demonstrated that only 2% of x-ray CT scans provided helpful therapeutic information in children with uncontrolled seizures, both focal and generalized.[6]

If x-ray CT is used to evaluate seizures, both pre- and postcontrast films usually should be employed. The presence and degree of contrast enhancement adds an important dimension in identifying small tumors, arteriovenous malformations (AVMs), or the presence of calcium. Five to 10 mg of diazepam given just before the procedure reduces the risk of contrast agent–precipitated seizures in patients with tumor.[79] To emphasize this point, fatal status epilepticus has been reported as an initial presentation of a seizure disorder in three unmedicated patients with metastatic brain tumors given a water-soluble contrast agent for x-ray CT.[4]

Several investigators have used quantitative approaches to x-ray CT to identify temporal lobe abnormalities.[13,50,74,118] Metrizamide infusion and thin (3-mm) sections may help to detect low-grade gliomas, as well as temporal gliosis, by increasing definition of the anatomy of mesial temporal structures and detecting minimal degrees of uncal herniation.[13,24,50,118]

All evidence indicates that MRI is superior to x-ray CT in identifying morphologic abnormalities in patients with epilepsy. MRI is superior to x-ray CT in almost every aspect, especially in the diagnosis of treatable lesions such as small areas of gliosis or AVMs that may be overlooked by CT. An exception to the rule may hold in emergency cases, where the speed of imaging and accessibility of the instrument lend an advantage to CT in evaluating acute central nervous system disorders or trauma. Posttraumatic intracerebral hemorrhages predict a fourfold increase in the risk of posttraumatic seizures and a 15-fold increase in risk if a satellite extracerebral intracranial hematoma coexists.[20] Other x-ray CT abnormalities following trauma have not been associated with an increase of posttraumatic seizures.[20]

Many studies illustrate the superiority of MR images in detecting the incidence and nature of structural lesions in epilepsy. Comparative studies have shown that from 20%–100% of patients with epilepsy had normal x-ray CT scans but abnormal MR images.* Schoerner and colleagues,[93] for example, reported that in 50 patients, x-ray CT detected a focal lesion in 12 but MRI in 16; if regions of discrete attenuation or signal abnormality were included, x-ray CT-detected abnormalities rose to 13 but those detected on MRI increased to 20. Only one small calcification observed on x-ray CT escaped MRI detection, whereas the latter was superior in detecting decreased temporal lobe size. Similarly, Triulzi and coworkers[117] found that among 31 patients with medication-controlled temporal lobe epilepsy and normal x-ray CT findings,

*References 55, 64, 67, 71, 73, 98, 107, 112, 117.

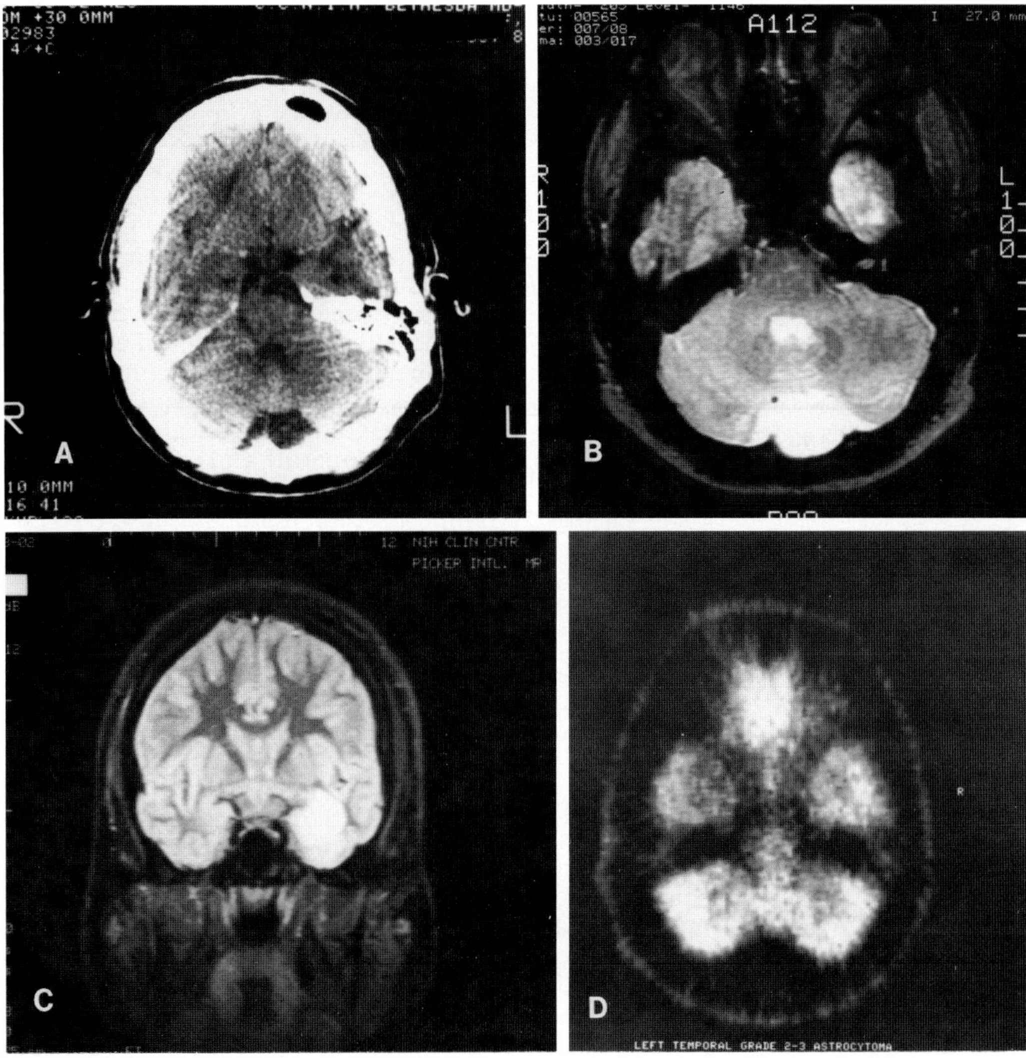

Figure 5–3. (*A*) X-ray CT scan in a patient with CPS. An irregular lucency is present in the inferior temporal region. A large cisterna magna and fourth ventricle are seen as well. There was no contrast enhancement. At surgery, grade 2–3 astrocytoma was found in the anterior temporal lobe. The patient had had seizures for 20 years. (*B*) T_2-weighted MRI scan of the same patient, showing increased signal in the temporal region. (*C*) Coronal MRI scan. There is a large region of increased temporal signal intensity, with probable encroachment on the basal ganglia and displacement of the left middle cerebral artery. Angiography showed straightening of the left middle cerebral artery but no blush or early draining veins. (*D*) PET scan showing temporal hypometabolism.

MR images in 11 showed increased signal intensity on 5-mm T_2-weighted slices through basal or medial temporal regions. Five more patients showed similar alterations in frontoparietal white matter. Axial views imaged the lesions in only 9 patients and short TE sequences in 10.

Pathologic studies generally confirm the superiority of MRI over x-ray CT images. Kuznietsky and colleagues evaluated 48 patients who had temporal lobectomies.[64] Thirty-one (65%) showed abnormal MRI signal intensity, including all those with tumors or vascular malformations, whereas x-ray CT

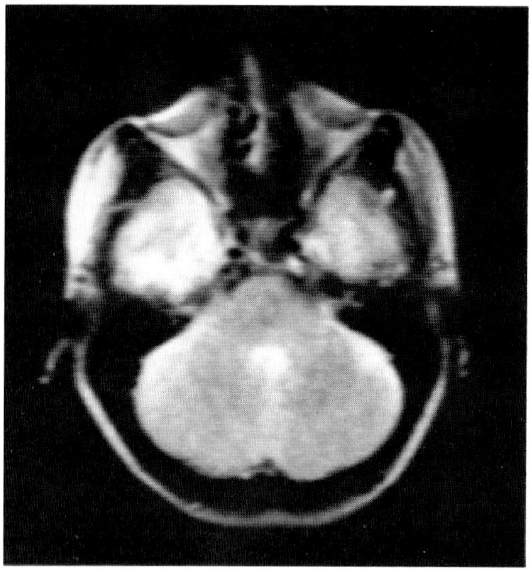

Figure 5–4. MRI scan in a patient with CPS and a unilateral temporal EEG focus. The temporal lobe is normal. Probable "shading" artifact (note difference in signal intensity in temporal soft-tissue structures and globe, as well as inferior temporal lobe) due to inhomogeneity in orienting static magnetic field gradient.

was abnormal in only eight patients (17%). "Mild focal gliosis" was less likely to induce increased signal intensity on MRI.[64] Although early reports suggested that patients with mesial temporal sclerosis, a common pathologic finding in patients with uncontrolled complex partial seizures, had normal MRI scans, more recent studies have shown increased signal intensity in these regions.[64,93,98] One difficulty in interpreting MR-pathologic correlations lies in the quantitative definition of histologic diagnoses: hippocampal cell loss in patients described as having "mesial temporal sclerosis" can vary from 30%–90%, and there may be a correlation between increased signal intensity and degree of cell loss.[98]

Varying pulse sequences sometimes can bring out pathologic regions on MR images. Using pulse sequences of TR 1500 and TE 168, Grant and associates[45] measured T_1 and T_2 values in patients with mesial temporal sclerosis. T_1 was 13% and T_2 was 14% higher in the affected temporal lobe compared with the contralateral one. They detected no abnormalities when they employed pulse sequences of TR 2200 and TE 80. Measures of T_1 and T_2 have not generally proved helpful, however, in detecting pathology in epileptic foci.

In patients with partial seizures, MRI sometimes demonstrates a smaller temporal lobe without increased signal intensity on the side of the lesion.[125] Such asymmetries in the normal population, however, make it difficult to determine the clinical significance of such changes. Although left hemisphere regions related to speech (including planum temporale and parietal operculum) are larger in right-handers, right temporal lobe total volume may be greater than left.[42,57] Recently, Jack and colleagues[58] have reported that MRI volumetric measurements correctly identify epileptogenic temporal lobe in 75% of patients with partial seizures.

Although the determination of a normal x-ray CT, MRI, or both reduces the likelihood that a patient with focal epilepsy has a tumor,[64,98] the procedures are not infallible, especially when the neoplasm is relatively small. MRI is more likely than x-ray CT to detect tumors but can be nonspecific. Abnormal signal intensity without mass effect or distortion of architecture does not distinguish between tumor and gliosis.[64,78] Ormson and coworkers, using a TR 2000, TE 60 pulse sequence, found that eight of nine low-grade gliomas were detected on MRI but only four on x-ray CT.[78] X-ray CT may detect tumors in some patients only after seizures have been present for more than 10 years.[46,56,97] Repeat scans should be performed at appropriate intervals, especially when a change in neurologic examination is detected. Patients with uncontrolled simple partial seizures and with rapid progression of symptoms are more likely to have tumors.[3,46,97] Increased use and understanding of MRI[2,11,85] undoubtedly will reduce the incidence (10%–20%) of normal imaging studies in patients found to have tumors at surgery.

Tumors, however, are by no means

the only reason for change in epileptic patients. Fluctuations in seizure frequency or clinical manifestations, such as progression of simple partial seizures to complex partial seizures, or complex partial seizures to generalized tonic-clonic seizures, occur often in patients with uncontrolled partial seizures. Among other possible causes, these changes can result from fluctuations in antiepileptic drug plasma levels.

False Localization

Even when a tumor or other space-occupying lesion exists, its location may not coincide with that of the electrophysiologically defined seizure focus (Fig. 5–5).[67,97,107] False localization of seizure onset by surface EEG recording to the hemisphere contralateral to a structural lesion has been reported, perhaps due to low electrical amplitude on the side of the lesion. Depth electrode

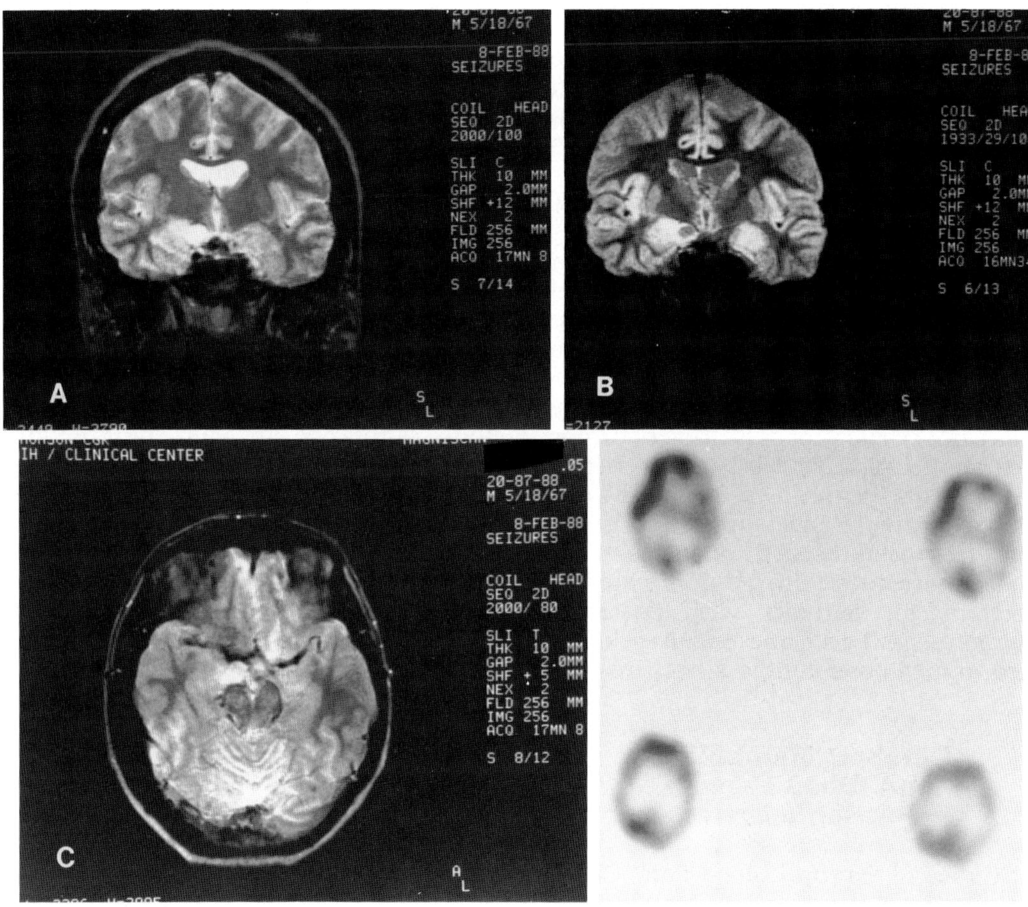

Figure 5–5. (*A*) Complex partial seizures (CPS). Increased right mesial temporal signal intensity on spin echo MRI sequence (TR 2000, TE 80). Possible mesial extension of the increased signal is present. Angiography showed elevation of the right anterior choroid and posterior cerebral arteries, but no evidence of a vascular blush. At surgery, the right temporal lobe evaginated into the prepeduncular space. A low-grade astrocytoma was found. (*B*) Inversion recovery sequence; abnormality still apparent. (*C*) Axial SE image in the same patient. FDG-PET scan showed no hypometabolism. (*D*) ^{123}IMP SPECT scan during a complex partial seizure. Increased blood flow in right frontotemporal region. (Courtesy of Jabbari and Van Nostrand, Walter Reed Army Medical Center.)

studies have been more reliable; a few patients who showed seizure origin in mesial temporal lobe ipsilateral to the radiographic findings became seizure-free after surgery.[90] These considerations indicate that in patients with tumors, additional localizing data are needed for planning resections if seizure control is to be obtained surgically. Moreover, some investigators have suggested that a nonprogressive mass lesion need not always be resected in patients undergoing surgery for uncontrolled seizures.[120] EEG localization of seizure onset is the criterion used by most epilepsy centers to identify tissue for surgical resection. Nevertheless, the advent of MRI and PET has led some centers to place depth electrodes in fewer patients, using imaging tests to confirm the results of surface EEG recording.

X-ray CT has been used to guide stereotactic biopsies of low-density lesions in patients with seizures.[119] In these studies, 34 of 35 patients had tumors; the group was selected for the procedure from among patients whose scans were suggestive of neoplastic disease. With this technique, a craniotomy was unnecessary for definition of tumor extent, decision on surgery or radiotherapy, and planning of ports for radiation therapy.[119] In a similar approach, MRI has been used for computer-assisted stereotactic amygdalohippocampectomy for patients with posterior temporal EEG foci and seizures localized to mediobasolimbic structures.[60]

Cerebral Metabolism and Blood Flow in Partial Seizures

Studies of cerebral blood flow (CBF), metabolism, and neurotransmitter activity hold greater promise than structural imaging to reveal underlying pathophysiology in epilepsy. A pitfall, however, is that underlying cerebral damage, of which seizures may be only one manifestation, may have effects on brain function that go well beyond changes induced by the seizures themselves. Moreover, most patients under study are taking antiepileptic drugs. Although no evidence indicates that such medication can cause focal dysfunction, anticonvulsants can induce global alterations in metabolic rate (Table 5–1).

In 1934 Gibbs and colleagues showed that seizures are accompanied by increased cerebral blood flow.[43] The greatest flow increase was seen in generalized tonic-clonic seizures, but increases also occurred in focal motor and absence attacks.[43] These findings contradicted the older theory that seizures were caused by "cerebral anemia" due to vasospasm in the immediate preictal period. Subsequently, Penfield[81] observed areas of cortical hyperemia during intraoperative stimulation of focal brain regions. No evidence of interictal abnormalities was found. In later studies, the Kety-Schmidt technique was used to examine cerebral blood flow. CBF was calculated by the Fick principle after nitrous oxide was inhaled to equilibrium, and femoral artery and internal jugular vein cannulation was used to measure the cerebral arteriovenous difference in gas content. Increased blood flow and oxygen consumption during seizures and postictal decreases were reported in both monkeys and humans.[61,66] Interictal flow and metabolism were normal.[61,66] Similar results were found with indicator dye dilution methods involving injection of Evans blue into the internal carotid artery and sampling from the internal jugular vein.[66]

Table 5–1 PERCENT REDUCTION OF CEREBRAL GLUCOSE METABOLISM BY ANTIEPILEPTIC DRUGS*

Phenobarbital[137]	37 ± 3†
Phenytoin[135]	13.2 ± 4†
Carbamazepine[142]	10.7 ± 3†
Control	5.2 ± 1.8‡

*Mean ± S.E.M. over all regions of interest.
†(off-drug scan – on-drug scan)/(off-drug scan).
‡Two scans without changes in drug treatment (first scan – second scan)/(first scan).

Seizures due to hypoglycemia were associated with decreased oxygen and glucose consumption when the Kety-Schmidt technique was used.[62] When methods for determining regional cerebral cortical blood flow with ^{133}Xe became available, focal interictal hypoperfusion was detected.[54,68,89] Some patients were reported to have increased interictal flow, but EEG was not monitored during all the studies, and some "interictal" scans may have been ictal or postictal. Selection of patients with tumors or continuous EEG spike discharges and the use of activating procedures such as intermittent light stimulation also may have accounted for some of the findings of increased "interictal" flow.[54,68,89]

Xenon-133–enhanced CT has also been used to detect decreased blood flow in epileptic foci in patients with complex partial seizures.[33] Flow reduction was greater in lateral than in medial temporal regions, but distortion induced by movement artifact impaired resolution of mesial temporal structures. Regions of interest were based on changes in routine x-ray CT images.

Positron Emission Tomography: Interictal Studies

Positron emission tomography (PET) has proved to be of great scientific interest and clinical utility for evaluating patients with partial seizures (see Chapter 3). Most studies have demonstrated interictal hypometabolism or reduced blood flow in 70%–80% of patients with complex partial seizures (Figs. 5–6 to 5–12).[1,28,35,76,88,112,114] Engel and colleagues studied 50 patients, of whom 35 showed hypometabolic regions.[28] Eighteen were unilateral temporal, six temporofrontal, three occipital, two frontal, and two involved an entire hemisphere. Four patients had bilateral temporal hypometabolism.[28] Only eight of these

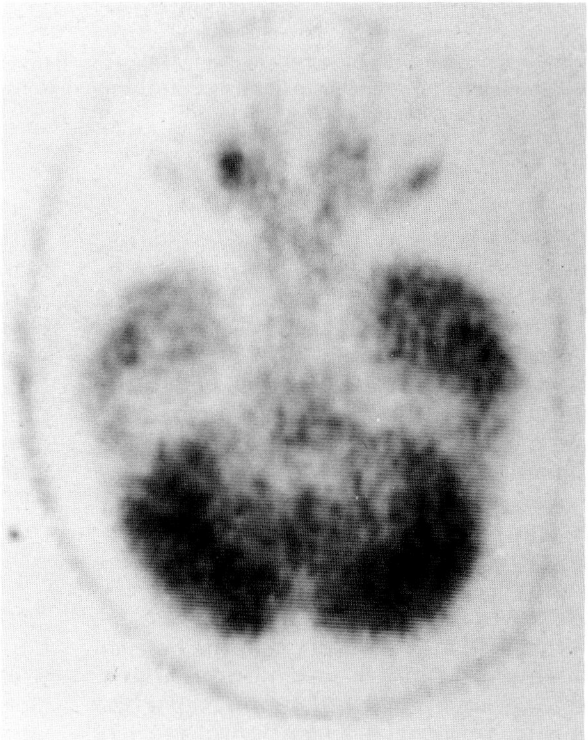

Figure 5–6. Interictal FDG-PET showing unilateral temporal glucose hypometabolism in a patient with CPS. Seizure included an aura of fear, unformed vocalizations, blinking, lip smacking, picking with the left hand, and head and eye deviation away from the affected side. MRI and x-ray CT were normal. Minimal neuronal loss and focal gliosis were found at surgery.

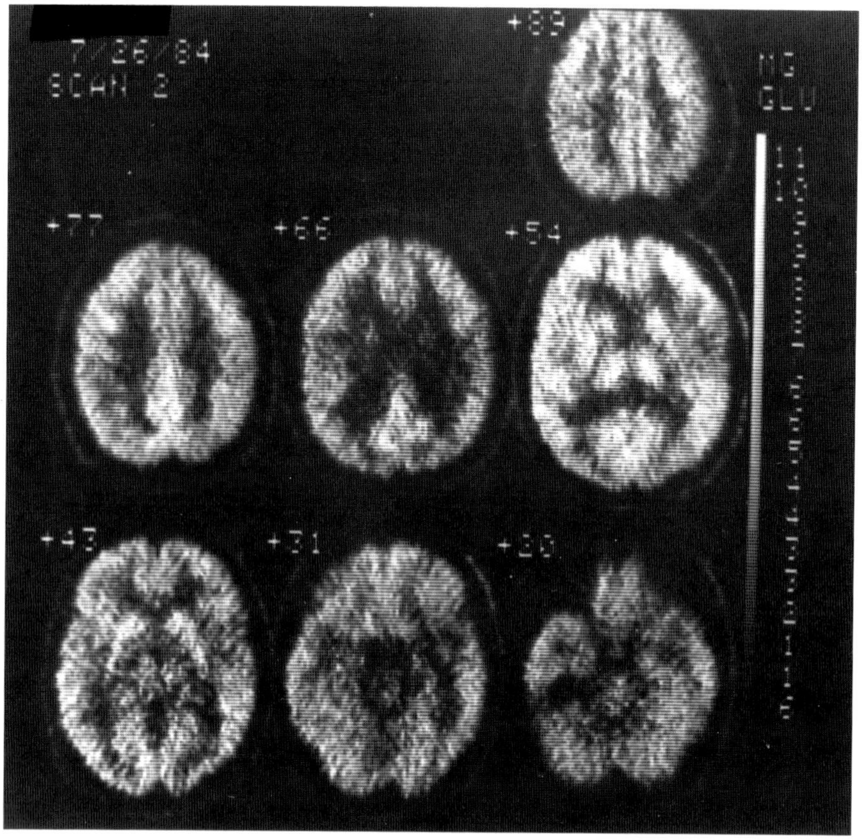

Figure 5–7. Interictal FDG-PET of glucose metabolism in a patient with CPS characterized by severe left shoulder pain radiating to the hand; stare; and twitching of the left side of the mouth. Right parieto-temporal hypometabolism is present on scans marked "+20" to "+66" mm above the canthomeatal scanning baseline.

patients had abnormal x-ray CT scans. Surgical excision was performed on 25; 19 of 22 with PET hypometabolism had a focal lesion. The three patients with normal PET scans had focal EEG changes but no neuropathologic abnormalities.[27] Although the degree of PET hypometabolism was related to the severity of neuronal loss, hypometabolic regions were larger than the area of pathologic abnormality.[27] Subsequently, Abou-Khalil and colleagues found 17 patients with qualitatively identified temporal hypometabolism, as well as 5 with frontotemporal, 3 with bitemporal, and 5 with normal scans among 31 patients with complex partial seizures.[1] Ten of 28 patients studied with MRI had abnormal scans in the region of PET hypometabolism. Patients with well-defined EEG foci had unilateral PET hypometabolism, but scans were often "normal" (nonfocal) when bilateral or diffuse discharges were present.[1] Gur and colleagues[47] found only ipsilateral temporal hypometabolism in 14 patients with left temporal EEG foci; ipsilateral parietal metabolic rates were minimally, though significantly, lower than control.

Bilateral or generalized hypoperfusion and decreased cerebral metabolic rate for oxygen ($CMRO_2$) may be present in patients with partial seizures (see Fig. 5–9). Bernardi and associates[9] compared 10 patients to 10 normal con-

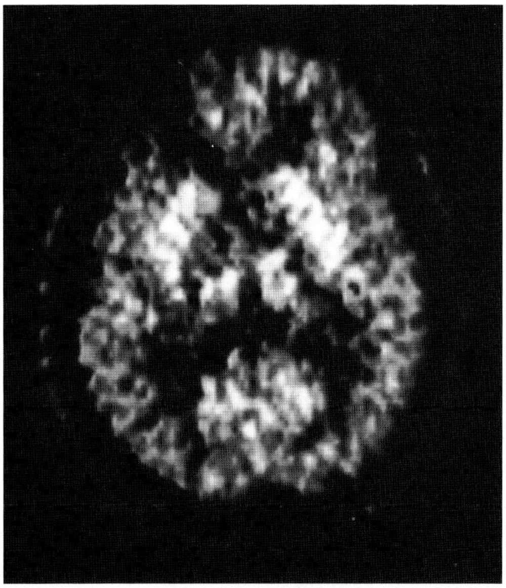

Figure 5–8. FDG-PET of glucose metabolism showing unilateral frontal hypometabolism in a patient with CPS. No specific clinical features suggestive of frontal onset were present, and the EEG showed diffuse discharges.

trols using oxygen-15 inhalation. Reduced $CMRO_2$ in the patient population was found ipsilateral to the EEG focus in temporal and frontal lobes, basal ganglia, and cerebellum. Reduced CBF was found in temporal lobes, basal ganglia, and cerebellum ipsilateral to the EEG focus. Contralateral temporal and cerebellar CBF and $CMRO_2$ were depressed as well. Comparing the two hemispheres in the patients, CBF but not $CMRO_2$ was significantly lower ipsilateral to the epileptic focus. The oxygen extraction fraction (OEF), the percentage of arterial oxygen concentration extracted by brain tissue, which normally averages 35%–45%, however, was significantly higher than controls only in temporal cortex ipsilateral to the EEG focus. Some of these changes may have been due to the effect of antiepileptic drugs or partial-volume effects of x-ray CT-demonstrated structural abnormalities. Other workers found lower OEF in epileptic psychotic patients compared with epileptic nonpsychotic patients in frontal, temporal, and basal ganglia regions, but differences between patients and controls were found only in temporal-lobe and basal ganglia.[38] The prevalence of bitemporal hypometabolism in the latter report could not be assessed because patients with right and left temporal EEG foci were grouped together.

In studies of overall patterns of cerebral metabolism and blood flow, the exclusion of patients with structural lesions is important; even focal lesions can produce widespread metabolic deficits not necessarily predictable by their radiographic features.[110] Extension of hypometabolism to structures beyond the temporal lobe may depend on the degree and extent of epileptiform discharges, the underlying cerebral pathology, and other factors such as the effects of antiepileptic drugs. For example, Sadzot and coworkers[88] found that reduced local cerebral metabolic rate for glucose (LCMRGlc) extended to frontal and thalamic regions ipsilateral to the EEG focus, but not to contralateral cortex. They used large (3.77 cm^2) regions of interest (ROIs) and did not exclude patients with tumors or abnormal x-ray CTs, factors that may have contributed to their identification of extensive hypometabolic zones.[88]

Several groups have calculated "asymmetry indices" (AI) to compare side-to-side variation in patients and normal controls.[1,28,47,109] Because the normal variability in LCMRGlc is wide, regions identified as relatively hypometabolic or asymmetric often have absolute LCMRGlc within the normal range. It is uncertain whether qualitative or quantitative analysis of PET studies should be used to localize epileptic foci for surgical resections. The accuracy of quantitative analysis depends on the size and variability of the control population, as well as on the analytical method, such as the size and shape of the ROIs within which metabolic rates are measured. A standard template may be used, or ROIs may be placed at the nadir of a visually identified hypometabolic zone, thereby accentuating side-to-side asymmetries. Occasion-

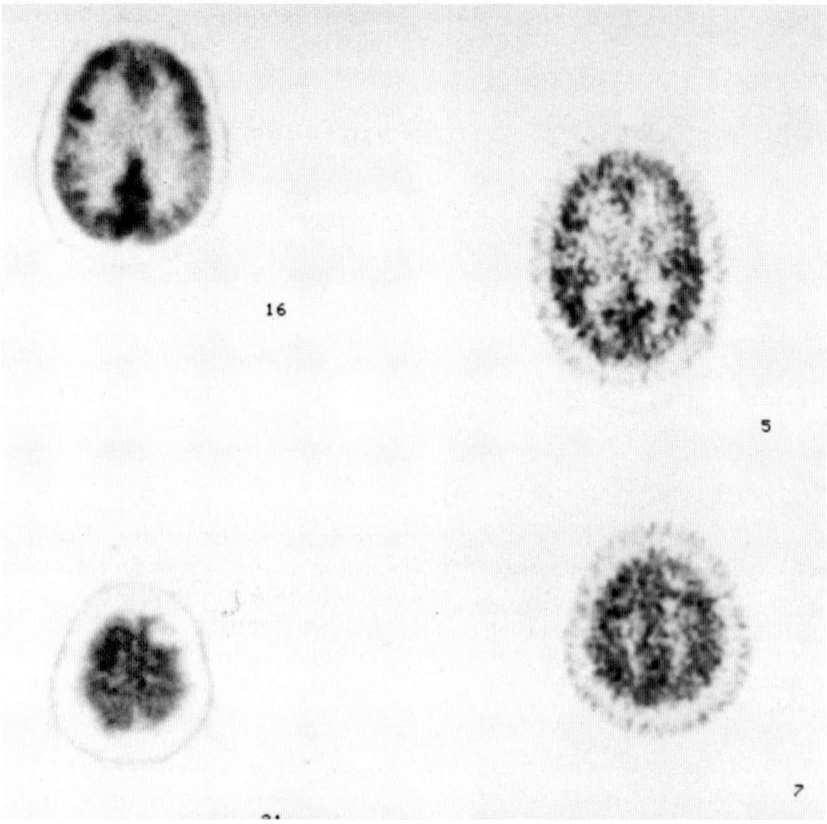

Figure 5–9. Comparison of interictal FDG-PET (*left*) and H_2-^{15}O blood flow (*right*) scans in a patient with CPS. Decreased LCMRGlc at frontal pole is present but much less dramatic on CBF image, which has lower resolution due to higher energy of ^{15}O (see Chap. 3).

ally, AIs may fail to show a significant difference from control in qualitatively identified hypometabolic regions, because of the normal range of side-to-side asymmetry (mean +2 standard deviations = 15% in the National Institutes of Health [NIH] control population).[109] Unless adequate controls are available, it may be impossible to identify bilateral temporal or diffuse hypometabolism. Purely qualitative analysis will never allow this to be done.

The resolution of PET is lower than that of MRI, making identification of small structures and precise anatomic localization more difficult. Several groups of investigators are working on techniques to match MR and PET images, thus improving the anatomic accuracy of the latter.

Positron Emission Tomography: Ictal Studies

During seizures, blood flow and metabolism increase in epileptic areas that show interictal hypometabolism.[21,29,30,114] Metabolic activation during the seizure may spread beyond the region of the interictal abnormality, presumably reflecting propagation of the seizure. Nevertheless, ictal images do depict the metabolic anatomy of sites in the brain activated by seizure activity. Since these sites are larger than the interictal epileptogenic zones, however, ictal PET studies must be used with caution to guide surgical therapy planning.

Clinical as well as theoretical issues affect accurate measurement of

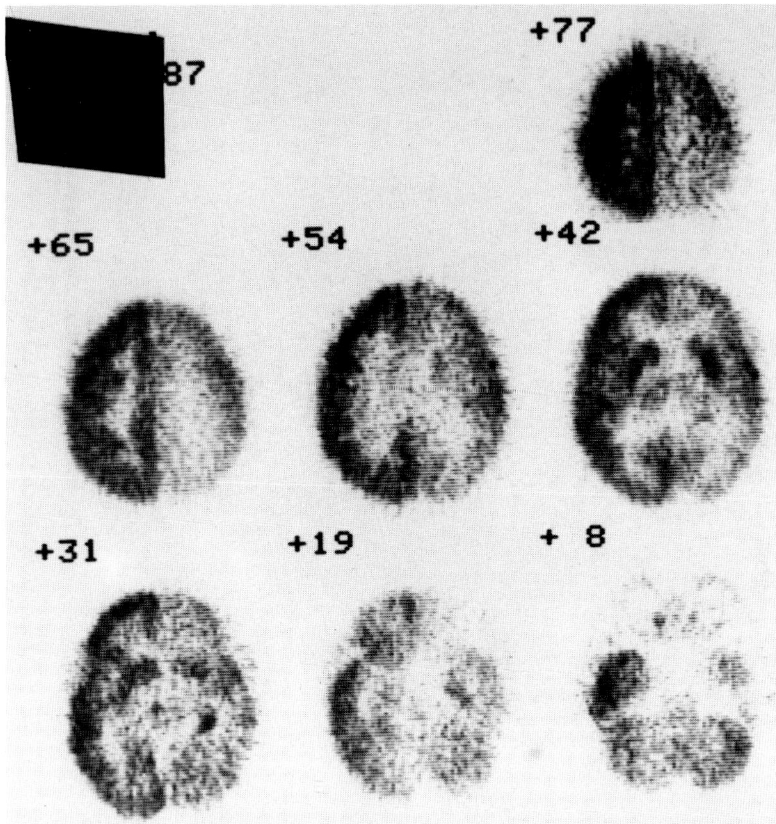

Figure 5–10. Frequent simple partial seizures (SPS); hemiparesis. Marked hypometabolism confined to opposite hemisphere. Subcortical gray structures, including putamen and caudate nucleus, show normal metabolic rates. Possible focus of increased activity in parahippocampal region. Seizure-free posthemispherectomy. Pathology consistent with Rasmussen's encephalitis.

LCMRGlc during fluorodeoxyglucose (FDG) scans. A seizure is usually a short event, compared to the total FDG uptake period of 30–45 minutes, so that "ictal" scans actually include interictal, ictal, and postictal data. The final integrated calculation may reflect combinations of hypometabolic and hypermetabolic regions due to the influence of postictal depression as well as ictal activation.[29,114] Also, because events occurring soon after injection of the isotope have a much greater influence on the final measured metabolic rate than those occurring later, postictal tracer administration may even show hypometabolism compared to the patient's interictal scans. The 2-deoxyglucose model assumes that cerebral glucose metabolism is in a steady state for the uptake period. This condition is violated during a seizure and accurate metabolic rate measurements cannot be made. In addition, the "lumped constant" (see Chapter 3) may change under abnormal circumstances, altering unpredictably the relationship between deoxyglucose and glucose utilization.

Although the time course of resolution of ictal metabolic alterations usually is rapid, elevated CBF and $CMRO_2$ have been reported to persist for up to 1 week after a seizure.[21] The qualitative data derived from comparisons of ictal and interictal scans may be very valuable if interpreted carefully. The limited data available suggest that perfusion

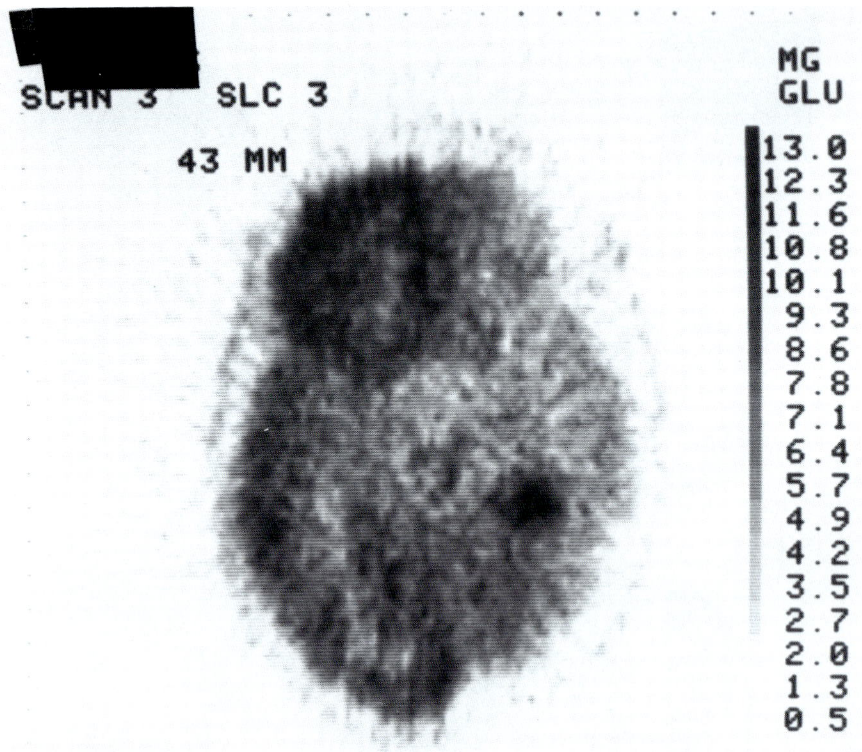

Figure 5–11. Complex partial seizures (CPS). Clinically interictal scan, but EEG showed frequent right temporal epileptiform discharges, in runs of up to 15 seconds. Extensive right frontotemporal hypometabolism; right posterior temporal hypermetabolic region is present as well.

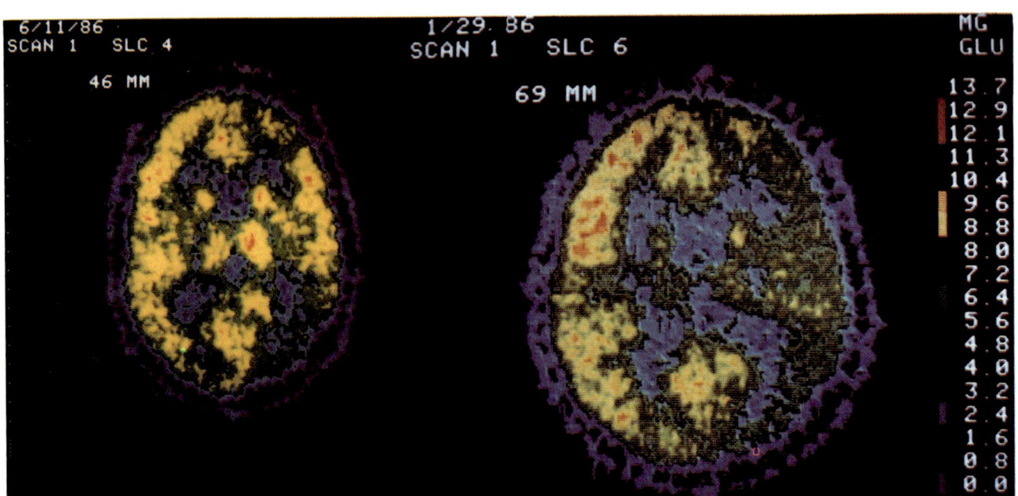

Figure 5–12. FDG-PET of glucose metabolism in SPS. (*Right*) Interictally, right frontotemporal hypometabolism was present. (*Left*) During simple partial seizure (twitching of left face and arm), increased LCMRGlc was present in right frontotemporal region, right thalamus. Increased LCMRGlc was present in right parietal cortex and right cerebellum (not shown) as well.

and metabolism increase equally during short partial seizures in humans.[35]

Single Photon Emission Computerized Tomography

Single photon emission computerized tomography (SPECT) (see Chapter 4) has been used to evaluate patients with complex partial seizures (Fig. 5–5*d*). Some of the practical advantages of this technique, such as reduced expense and the use of commercially available isotopes with longer half-lives, may be counterbalanced by inferior spatial resolution and quantitation. Nevertheless, reduced interictal blood flow has been documented with a number of tracers, including ^{123}IMP, ^{123}I-HIPM, ^{133}Xe, and ^{99m}Tc-HMPAO.[14,53,69,83,89,99] Although specific neuropsychologic deficits have been correlated with lateralized CBF abnormalities in some studies, bitemporal hypoperfusion has been reported frequently, making accurate localization of abnormal regions impossible.[14,53]

Despite the technique's shortcomings, SPECT does appear to be useful in certain settings. In one study, for example, patients were injected with ^{99m}Tc-HMPAO between 2 and 30 (mean = 8) minutes after seizure onset. SPECT detected hyperperfusion in the same temporal lobe as the EEG focus in 15 of 18 patients.[86] Usually, however, ictal flow increases detected by SPECT are more widespread than the region of interictal hypoperfusion. Moreover, the flow increases may be bilateral or even contralateral to the EEG focus.[70,86] Comparison of ictal and interictal SPECT studies, however, has been reported to localize epileptic foci accurately in 70%–90% of patients.[86,95] A preliminary report has suggested that ictal SPECT scans may provide localizing data even when the surface EEG is inconclusive.[70] Many of the same clinical difficulties discussed in regard to ictal PET scanning apply to ictal SPECT as well.

A few studies have directly compared PET and SPECT. Stefan and colleagues[99] performed FDG-PET and ^{99m}Tc-HMPAO SPECT in ten patients. All had focal PET abnormalities, eight had an abnormal MR, five an abnormal SPECT, and three abnormal x-ray CT images. One patient had decreased blood flow on SPECT in a region contralateral to abnormalities detected by x-ray CT, MRI, PET, and EEG. SPECT localization was inferior to MRI and PET, but patients may have been selected for positive PET scans. Another study of 12 patients with complex partial seizures[113] found PET hypometabolism in 8, and SPECT hypoperfusion in 2. Two others had increased CBF during ictal SPECT scans; one of these had a normal interictal PET.[113] Technical advances in SPECT are occurring rapidly, and the distinctions from PET in terms of clinical utility may become less marked.

Functional Images in the Localization of Epileptic Sites

Conversion of interictal hypoperfusion or hypometabolism to ictal hyperperfusion or hypermetabolism can be a convincing demonstration of epileptic activity, especially if EEG and PET localization agree. The wider the region of interictal hypometabolism, the less useful these findings become for surgical localization. CBF or LCMRGlc may be elevated because of projection of discharges from a distant epileptogenic region, especially if secondary generalization of a partial seizure occurs. Data derived from ictal-interictal scan pairs must be evaluated to ensure that the activation observed is not associated with a behavior that is an epiphenomenon of the seizure itself. An example of such an epiphenomenon is increased occipital metabolism due to eye opening and the consequent increase of visual input. Simultaneous EEG recording is crucial to ictal PET studies to confirm seizure occurrence and timing.

Because of the time needed for tracer

incorporation, FDG-PET is less suitable than ^{15}O PET or SPECT for visualization of seizures, but seizures concurring exactly with administration of any isotope are usually fortuitous. Hyperventilation has been used to induce generalized absence seizures.[31,105] The use of drugs such as pentylenetetrazole to provoke partial seizures during PET scans presents a number of problems, including rapid secondary generalization and the possibility that the induced seizures may differ from the spontaneous ictal events. Another approach to localization of epileptic foci is to perform PET during a neuropsychologic activation task. Significant LCMRGlc increases have been reported only contralateral to the stimulated side in some studies, but bilaterally in others.[63,72] Patterns of activation and involvement of extratemporal regions such as frontal and parietal cortex depend on the stimulus presentation paradigm and type of material used, such as understandable or incomprehensible (for example, foreign language) speech (see Chapter 3).

Spontaneous speech by the subject during PET has been reported to lead to widespread metabolic activation, and in epileptics, to increased definition of temporal lobe foci.[49] The demonstration of localized cerebral dysfunction in a patient with seizures, however, does not identify the area as necessarily epileptogenic, since epileptic patients can have structural lesions producing neuropsychologic impairment but not the seizures themselves.

Pathophysiology of Decreased Metabolism and Blood Flow in Epileptic Foci

Although resected temporal lobe specimens from patients with complex partial seizures and focal hypometabolism may be normal to standard light microscopy, pathologic findings usually include "mesial temporal sclerosis," focal gliosis, or small gliomas, hamartomas, or arteriovenous malformations.[27] Hypometabolism usually extends to involve a much wider region than these structural abnormalities. It is uncertain whether the widespread hypometabolism that occurs in these patients represents equally widespread epileptogenic tissue, whether it is caused by the "primary" seizure-inducing lesions, or whether it is secondary to the seizures themselves. Neuropathologic study of resected temporal lobes indicates that the degree of hypometabolism on PET scans is unrelated to the percentage loss of mesial temporal neurons.[51] An alternative explanation is that hypometabolism detected with PET could be due to reduced synaptic activity in projection areas of nonfunctioning inhibitory neurons.[25]

The Role of PET and SPECT in the Evaluation of Patients for Surgery

The presence of hypometabolism in PET scans or an abnormality on MRI may predict good surgical results, but this point remains debated (Table 5–2).

Table 5–2 RELATION OF PET SCAN FINDINGS TO SURGICAL RESULTS AT THREE CENTERS

	NIH Surgical Result[116]		UCLA Surgical Result[26]		Univ. Michigan Surgical Result		Total Surgical Results	
	Good	*Poor*	*Good*	*Poor*	*Good*	*Poor*	*Good*	*Poor*
PET								
Focal	19	2	32	9	12	0	63	11
Nonfocal	3	5	14	3	3	1	20	9

From Engel et al,[26] Theodore et al,[116] and JC Sackellares: personal communication.

Engel and associates[26] found that patients with and without focal hypometabolism were equally likely to improve after temporal lobectomy, and failure to detect a specific mesial temporal lesion on routine pathologic examination of temporal lobe tissue specimens was not necessarily associated with an unfavorable outcome. Engel suggested that degrees of cell loss too mild to be detected by routine pathologic or neuroimaging techniques could still be epileptogenic.[26] In contrast, Falconer and colleagues[32] reported that patients with specific lesions on pathologic examination were likely to be improved by surgery, and other investigators[116] have found the presence of well-localized PET hypometabolism to be predictive of good surgical outcome (see Table 5–2).

GENERALIZED SEIZURES

Imaging Changes in Primary Generalized Seizures

Within the broad category of primary generalized absence epilepsy, a number of syndromes have been identified, based primarily on age of onset. The clinical features of these syndromes are similar and the imaging characteristics are identical. Absence attacks are short, lasting a mean of 10 seconds and rarely longer than 45 seconds. Clonic activity such as eyelid blinking may accompany them; automatisms may occur in longer seizures but are usually restricted to face and hands. In complex partial seizures, automatic behavior often includes the legs and trunk. There is no aura and no postictal confusion associated with absence attacks. About half the patients develop generalized tonic-clonic seizures.

Nonspecific x-ray CT abnormalities, including ventricular and sulcal enlargement, are rare in patients with absence seizures alone, but have been reported in up to 24% of those who had generalized tonic-clonic seizures as well.[40,91] X-ray CT findings may be more frequent in patients with "complex absences," but these too are usually nonspecific.[40] Lagenstein and coworkers[65] reported that 41% of patients had atrophic changes, but included patients with atonic seizures. Patients with abnormal neurologic examinations are more likely to have nonspecific x-ray CT (and probably MRI) findings than patients with normal examinations. Focal pathology, including midline or frontal lobe tumors, has been reported rarely, especially when associated syndromes such as precocious puberty are present.[100,101] In most cases, the discovery of nonlocalizing x-ray CT or MRI abnormalities has little influence on treatment.[91,121] Routine imaging evaluation of patients with pure absence seizures is unnecessary.

CEREBRAL BLOOD FLOW AND METABOLISM

Studies with intracarotid ^{133}Xe showed a diffuse increase in CBF and $CMRO_2$ during electroconvulsive-therapy–induced seizures, which lasted 2–3 minutes; and possible postictal $CMRO_2$ depression.[15] Vasodilatation and impaired autoregulation leading to an increase in CBF was observed despite only a slight change in blood pressure. Diffuse flow elevations also were detected with ^{133}Xe inhalation in four patients with petit mal seizures during 3/second spike wave discharges.[89] Flow during generalized tonic-clonic seizures was increased in the brainstem and cerebellum as well as the cerebral hemispheres.[54]

Interictal PET-FDG studies of patients with absence seizures[31,54] have shown no abnormalities, but during attacks, generalized metabolic rate increased by a factor of three times interictal values.[31] (Fig. 5–13). Hyperventilation without EEG discharges did not change the pattern or magnitude of LCMRGlc.[31,75] Ochs and associates[75] reported no consistent increases in LCMRGlc during spike wave discharges, but the amount of spike wave activity was considerably less than described in other studies, and baseline FDG metabolism was reduced compared with that of normal controls.

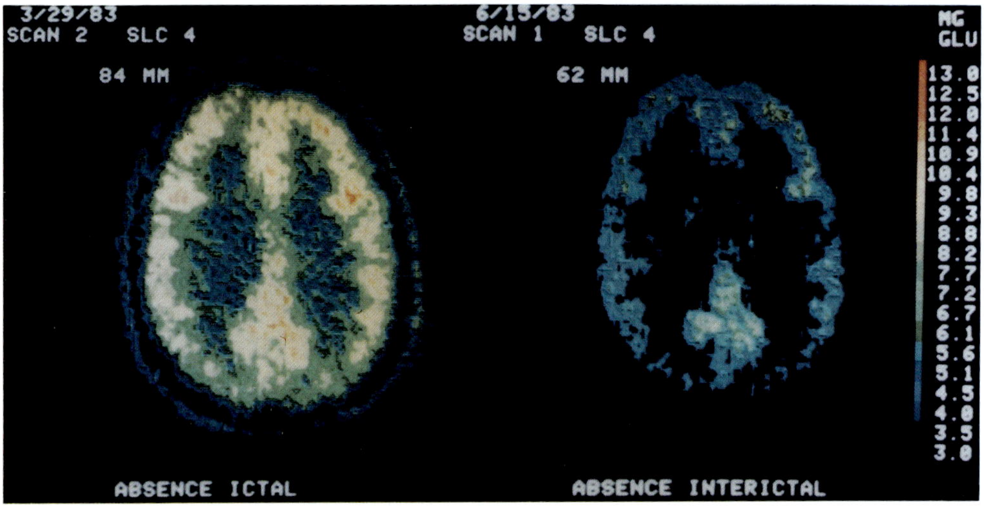

Figure 5–13. Comparison of ictal and interictal FDG-PET scans of glucose metabolism in a patient with absence seizures. (*Right*) Interictal image has LCMRGlc within normal range (color scale changed to range of ictal scan). (*Left*) Diffuse hypermetabolism during seizures, increased by a factor of two.

Some of the patients in this study had cerebral atrophy, ventricular asymmetry, or evidence of lateralized neuropsychologic dysfunction. Moreover, possible medication effects were not controlled, making the results difficult to compare with earlier reports.[31,75,105]

Podreka and colleagues[83] reported that seven of nine patients with "generalized seizures" had focal SPECT abnormalities, but two of the patients had abnormal x-ray CT scans, and four had focal EEG discharges, suggesting that secondarily generalized partial seizures were involved. The lack of a postictal contribution may account for the much higher ictal increases measured in petit mal than in partial seizures, where the 30 minutes required for accurately measuring cerebral uptake and phosphorylation of FDG includes ictal, postictal, and interictal periods.

Imaging Changes in Secondary Generalized Epilepsy: Infantile Spasms and the Lennox-Gastaut Syndrome

X-ray CT abnormalities, including agenesis of the corpus callosum, infarctions, and arachnoid and porencephalic cysts, have been reported in 80%–90% of patients with infantile spasms (see Chapter 12). Diffuse atrophy and ventricular enlargement are the most common findings. Patients with normal x-ray CT scans are likely to have normal neurologic examinations and to be seizure-free at follow-up.[19,41] Decreased cortical volume may appear after ACTH therapy in patients with a normal pretreatment x-ray CT.[44] MRI scans, which may miss small intracranial calcifications, may be less sensitive than x-ray CT in detecting evidence of tuberous sclerosis.[52] PET hypometabolism in tuberous sclerosis is reportedly more extensive than the lesions detected by x-ray CT or MRI.[107]

The Lennox-Gastaut Syndrome (LGS) is a severe childhood epileptic encephalopathy of diverse etiology, including metabolic encephalopathy, phakomatoses, infections, and perinatal compromise. The cause is unknown in 30%–70% of cases. The types of seizures include atonic episodes, prolonged absence with clonic components, and "astatic-myoclonic" seizures (a jerk precedes a fall). Sixty percent have generalized tonic-clonic, tonic, or clonic seizures, and these may be the initial episodes in older children.

Neuropsychologic evidence of static encephalopathy, and generalized 1.5–2.5/second spike wave discharges on EEG ("slow spike wave") are usually found. Cerebral atrophy occurs in up to 70% of patients with LGS, but focal changes are found in only one third.[41] The presence of a variety of radiologic findings, including tuberous sclerosis, agenesis of the corpus callosum, infarctions, arachnoid and porencephalic cysts in patients with the stereotyped EEG and clinical features of LGS, suggest that the lesions seen on x-ray CT may not be directly responsible for the clinical problems. The incidence of scans showing cerebral atrophy increases with age. Atrophy might be a consequence rather than a cause of the seizures.[41]

The interictal FDG metabolic patterns in LGS include unilateral focal, bilateral multifocal, and diffuse hypometabolism.[17] The hypometabolic regions in some of these patients are related to structural abnormalities. Frontal and diffuse hypometabolism have also been found in patients without abnormalities on x-ray CT.[115] Gur and associates[48] reported profound unilateral temporal hypometabolism in two patients with LGS. Following corpus callosum section, the hypometabolism resolved in one case, but persisted after clinically unsuccessful section in the other. In four other cases of LGS, metabolic rates increased with increased EEG discharges in one, but the others had lower metabolic rates during EEG-recorded epileptiform discharges.[115] The patients were taking barbiturates, however, which may explain the decrease in LCMRGlc.

MAGNETIC RESONANCE SPECTROSCOPY

MR spectroscopy (MRS) can rapidly and serially measure metabolites of glucose and ATP during induction and resolution of seizures. Presently, spatial resolution is inferior to other metabolic imaging techniques. Petroff and coworkers[82] showed by NMRS a fall in phosphocreatine and intracellular pH during bicuculline-induced seizures in rats. Lactate remained modestly elevated up to 2 hours after seizures stopped, even though pH and the EEG returned to near baseline levels. In neonatal dogs, brain lactate levels rose markedly during seizures despite insulin-induced hypoglycemia, suggesting that a low blood glucose level might not protect against lactic-acid–induced brain damage.[123] In eight children with neonatal seizures, the phosphocreatine: inorganic phosphate ratio was decreased, suggesting compromise of cerebral energy supply. This was correlated with the severity of neurologic sequelae. When seizures were stopped by antiepileptic drugs during MRS data acquisition, the ratio of phosphocreatine to inorganic phosphate returned to normal.[124] These and other studies suggest that neonates and young children may be particularly susceptible to seizure-related brain damage.[5,22,23]

PET AND THE NEUROPHARMACOLOGY OF EPILEPSY

The effects of antiepileptic drugs on cerebral glucose metabolism can be studied by PET. In contrast to earlier global metabolic measurements obtained with the Kety-Schmidt method, PET analyses show that phenobarbital decreases LCMRGlc significantly, with less dramatic effects associated with phenytoin and carbamazepine (see Table 5–1).[103,106,111] Phenytoin had only a weak effect on cerebellar metabolism, which is reduced in patients with complex partial but not primary generalized seizures, whether or not they are taking the drug.[108] Baron and associates used PET to study the distribution of ^{11}C-phenytoin in patients with complex partial seizures. Uniform ^{11}C activity was found and there was no increased accumulation in the epileptic focus.[7]

Different effects among pharmacologic agents on LCMRGlc may be related to the mechanisms of action, since the antiepileptic actions of barbiturates may be mediated through the GABA-benzodiazepine receptor complex, which is linked to the chloride channel, whereas phenytoin and carbamazepine directly alter conductance at active sodium channels in neuronal membranes.[77] In rats, intravenous injection of GABA agonists leads to widespread reduction of LCMRGlc.[59,80] Intravenous diazepam also depresses global glucose metabolism.[34] The reduction in LCMRGlc due to barbiturates may be related to their interactions with GABA receptors.

Barbiturate anesthesia in patients with brain tumors led to greater reductions of LCMRGlc in normal cortex and enhancement of tumor visualization.[10] Unfortunately, the effect of barbiturates in patients with seizures is generalized, and the epileptic focus is affected as much as the contralateral cortex.[98]

Initial studies in patients with complex partial seizures[37] suggested increased μ-opiate receptor binding in temporal neocortex, but not in hippocampus or amygdala, ipsilateral to FDG hypometabolic foci. The anticonvulsant effect of opiates may be mediated by μ- and the convulsant effect by δ-receptors.[36] Enkephalin seizures increase LCMRGlc primarily in limbic structures, while high-dose naloxone activates pyramidal and extrapyramidal motor areas.[16] The increased μ-opiate receptor binding in association with epileptic foci may represent an autochthonous anticonvulsant response.[37] Using a ligand that may have mixed μ- and κ-opiate receptor binding, another group found no difference between epileptic foci and contralateral temporal lobe.[104]

Several ligands under development will permit study of dopamine, benzodiazepine, and other receptors using PET. Recently, for example, Savic and colleagues[92] reported that in patients with partial seizures, benzodiazepine receptor binding measured with [^{11}C]R015-1788 was significantly lower in epileptic foci than in contralateral neocortex. This suggests that GABAergic inhibitory mechanisms might be disturbed in these patients.[92]

A STRATEGY FOR IMAGING EVALUATION OF PATIENTS WITH EPILEPSY

The first step in the evaluation of patients with seizures is proper clinical and EEG classification of the seizure type (Figs. 5–14, 5–15). Children with primary generalized absence seizures do not need any imaging tests on initial presentation. Failure to respond to antiepileptic drugs should lead to re-evaluation of these patients, and an MRI scan is appropriate at that point. Focal lesions are rare; PET or SPECT are unlikely to provide additional information of clinical value. The same considerations apply to the less common generalized syndromes such as benign juvenile myoclonus or occipital epilepsy. In these patients, progressive lesions are unusual, and follow-up scans are rarely indicated. Decisions about the use of imaging procedures in children presenting with generalized tonic-clonic seizures will depend on EEG and clinical analysis in each case, since the seizures may be of either "primary" or "secondary" origin, and imaging studies are more likely to be abnormal in the latter. Children in the broad category of the Lennox-Gastaut syndrome often have abnormal imaging studies, but the results are still unlikely to change their treatment unless surgery is contemplated. Tumors are unusual in these patients.

The evaluation of patients presenting with new-onset partial seizures (Fig. 5–15) is more complex than of those with primary generalized epilepsy. The peculiar appeal of complex technology leads most patients to expect imaging procedures even when the history, examination, and EEG do not suggest a specific intracranial lesion. In any event, obtaining both x-ray CT and MRI is redundant and unnecessary (Table 5–3). MRI is the procedure of choice be-

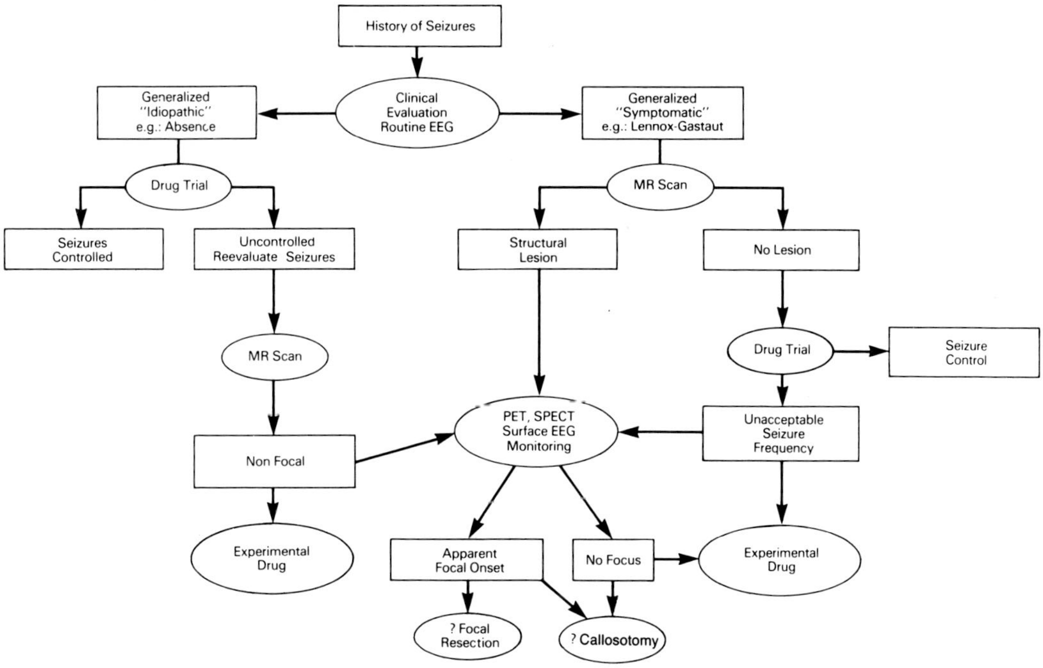

Figure 5–14. Suggested outline for evaluation of patients with generalized seizures.

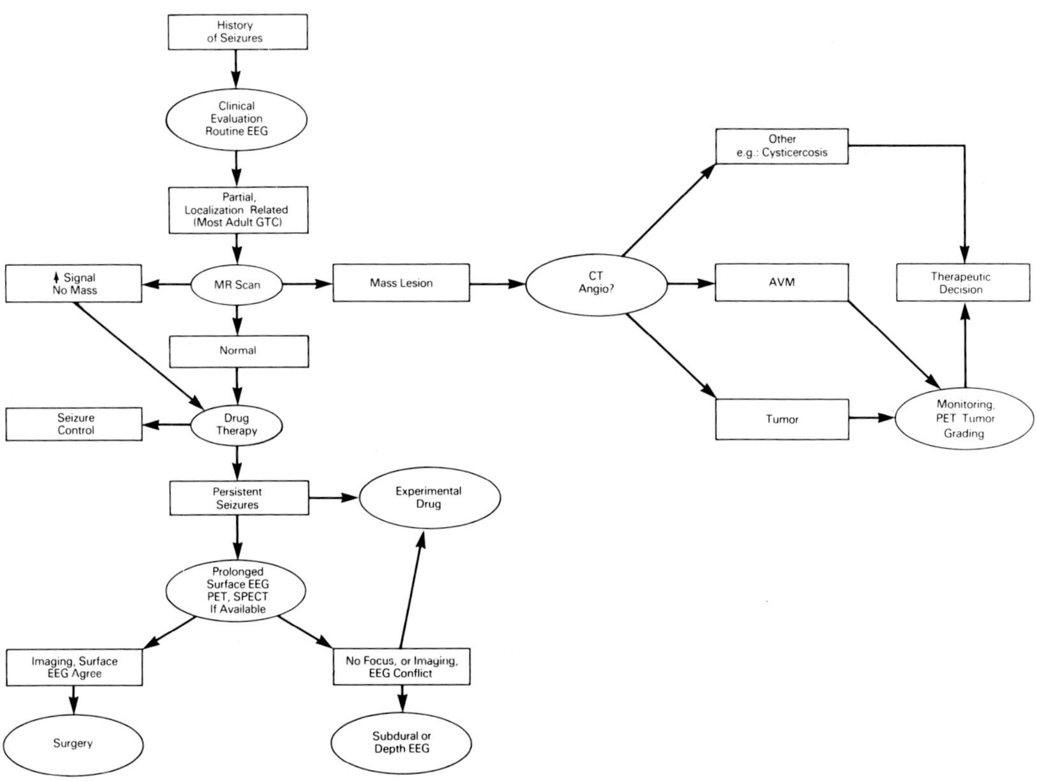

Figure 5–15. Suggested outline for evaluation of patients with partial seizures.

Table 5–3. ADVANTAGES AND DISADVANTAGES OF IMAGING TECHNIQUES FOR THE EVALUATION OF PATIENTS WITH SEIZURES

	Advantages	Disadvantages
CT	Rapid scans Detects calcification Vascular anatomy may be imaged with contrast Detects acute bleeding	Low sensitivity to focal gliosis (mesial temporal sclerosis) Bone artifact at temporal levels Radiation exposure IV contrast Detection of structural lesion may not co-localize with epileptic focus
MRI	Sensitive to gliosis and low-grade tumors Excellent display of temporal lobe anatomy No radiation	Long procedure; children may need sedation More expensive than CT Misses occasional calcification Detects "abnormalities" of uncertain significance Functional imaging not proven
PET	Versatile: can measure metabolic rate, blood flow, neurotransmitter activity, and others Often abnormal when CT, MRI normal Decreased CBF / LCMRGlc / $CMRO_2$ may correlate with neuropsychologic dysfunction as well as with epileptic focus Identifies abnormal function that may be characteristic of epilepsy Clinical role in surgical planning	Need cyclotron Radiation exposure Expensive, long (1 hr) procedure Spatial resolution inferior to x-ray CT, MRI
SPECT	Uses commercially available longer-lived isotopes Can use standard nuclear medicine cameras Easily integrated into routine procedures Ictal studies easier than with PET	Low resolution Only blood flow measurable at present Quantitation uncertain Clinical application less defined than for PET High cost

cause of higher yield of evidence of neuropathology and lack of exposure to radiation and contrast agents. Because of the design of the camera, x-ray CT is preferable when patients need continuous physiologic monitoring, intravenous fluids, or assisted ventilation during the scan.

Mass lesions are less likely to be found in children than in adults unless clinical suspicion of a progressive lesion is high, as when findings on the neurologic examination change. Accordingly, follow-up scans may be delayed for at least several years. It is important to recognize special syndromes such as benign rolandic epilepsy of childhood, which, even though "localization-related," behaves like primary generalized epilepsy in prognosis and etiology. Adults presenting with generalized tonic-clonic seizures who do not have a history of childhood absence seizures are likely to have secondarily generalized partial seizures.

Even if a tumor or arteriovenous malformation is detected, a full seizure evaluation should be performed before surgery, including prolonged EEG monitoring. Because the site of origin of the seizures may not coincide with the anatomy of the mass lesion, surgery must provide both tumor removal and seizure control. Discovery of multifocal epileptiform discharges may also affect decisions about whether to pursue surgical therapy for seizure control.

The decision to refer a patient for a PET or SPECT scan should be made in the context of consideration of surgery for intractable seizures. It is more important for a patient with uncontrolled seizures to have a comprehensive evaluation in an epilepsy center than a particular test. Individual tests may be uninterpretable unless they are put in the context of the appropriate clinical and laboratory information.

REFERENCES

1. Abou-Khalil, BW, Siegel, GJ, Sackellares, JC, Gilman, S, Hichwa, RD, Marshall, R: Positron emission tomography studies of cerebral glucose metabolism in chronic partial epilepsy. Ann Neurol 22:480–486, 1987.
2. Adams, CBT, Anslow, P, Molyneux, A, and Oxbury, J: Radiological detection of surgically treatable pathology. In Engel, J Jr (ed): Surgical Treatment of the Epilepsies. Raven Press, New York, 1987, pp 213–233.
3. Angeleri, F, Provinciali, L, and Salvolini, U: Computerized tomography in partial epilepsy. In Canger, R, Angeleri, F, and Penry, JK (eds): Advances in Epileptology: 11th Epilepsy International Symposium. Raven Press, New York, 1980, pp 53–64.
4. Avrahami, E, Weiss-Peretz, J, and Cohn, DF: Focal epileptic activity following intravenous contrast material injection in patients with metastatic brain disease. J Neurol Neurosurg Psychiatr 50:221–223, 1987.
5. Babb, TL and Brown, WJ: Pathological findings in epilepsy. In Engel JP (ed): Surgical Treatment of the Epilepsies. Raven Press, New York, 1987, pp 511–540.
6. Bachman, DS, Hodges, FJ, and Freeman, JM: Computerized axial tomography in chronic seizure disorders of childhood. Pediatrics 58:828–831, 1976.
7. Baron, JC, Roeda, D, Munari, C, et al: Brain regional pharmacokinetics of 11-C labeled diphenylhydantoin: Positron emission tomography in humans. Neurology 33:580–585, 1983.
8. Bauer, G, Mayr, U, and Pallua, A: Computerized axial tomography in chronic partial epilepsies. Epilepsia 21:227–233, 1980.
9. Bernardi, S, Trimble, MR, Frackowiak RSJ, Wise, RJS, and Jones, T: An interictal study of partial epilepsy using positron emission tomography and the oxygen-15 inhalation technique. J Neurol Neurosurg Psychiatr 46:473–477, 1983.
10. Blacklock, JB, Oldfield, EH, Di Chiro, G, Tran, D, Theodore, WH, Wright, DC, and Larson, SM: Selective suppression of glucose utilization in normal brain versus gliomas: Positron emission tomography during barbiturate coma in humans. J Neurosurg 67:71–75, 1987.
11. Blom, RJ, Vinuela, F, Fox, AJ, et al: Computed tomography in temporal lobe epilepsy. J Comput Assist Tomogr 8:401–405, 1984.
12. Bogdanoff, BM, Stafford, CR, Green, L, et al: Computerized transaxial tomography in the evaluation of patients with focal epilepsy. Neurology 25: 1013–1017, 1975.
13. Bolender, NF and Wyler, AR: CT measurements of mesial temporal herniation. Epilepsia 23:409–416, 1982.
14. Bonte FJ, Devous MD Sr, Stokely, EM, et al: Single photon tomographic determination of regional cerebral blood flow in epilepsy. AJNR 4:544–546, 1983
15. Broderson, P, Paulson, OB, Bolwig, TG, et al: Cerebral hyperemia in electrically induced seizures. Arch Neurol 28:334–338, 1973.
16. Chugani, HT, Ackermann, RF, Chugani, DC, and Engel J Jr: Opioid-induced epileptogenic phenomena: Anatomical, behavioral, and electrographic features. Ann Neurol 15:361–368, 1984.
17. Chugani, HT, Engel, J Jr, Mazziotta, JC, and Phelps ME: The Lennox-Gastaut syndrome: Metabolic subtypes determined by 2-deoxy-2-[18F]-fluoro-D-glucose positron emission tomography. Ann Neurol 21:4–13, 1987.
18. Collard, M, Dupont, H, and Noel, G: Computerized transverse axial tomography in epilepsy. Epilepsia 17:339–342, 1975.
19. Curatolo, P, Pelliccia, A, and Cotroneo, E: Prognostic significance of CT finding in West syndrome. In Akimoto, H, Kazamatsuri, H, Seino, M, Ward, AA Jr (eds): Advances in Epileptology; 13th Epilepsy International Symposium. Raven Press, New York 1982, pp 191–194.
20. D'Alessandro, R, Ferrara, R, Benassi,

G, Lenzi, PL, and Sabattini, L: Computed tomographic scans in post-traumatic epilepsy. Arch Neurol 45:42–44, 1988.
21. Depresseux, JC, Frank, G, and Sadzot, B: Regional cerebral blood flow and oxygen uptake in human focal epilepsy. In Baldy-Moulinier, M, Ingvar, DG, and Meldrum, BS (eds): Cerebral Blood Flow, Metabolism and Epilepsy. John Libby, London, 1983, pp 76–81.
22. Doose, H, Volzke, E: Petit mal status in early childhood and dementia. Neuropediatrie 10:10, 1979.
23. Dwyer, BE, Wasterlain, CG, Fujikawa, DG, and Yamada, L: Brain protein metabolism in epilepsy. In Delgado-Escueta, AV, Ward, AA Jr, Woodbury, DM, Porter, RJ (eds): Basic Mechanisms of the Epilepsies: Molecular and Cellular Approaches. Raven Press, New York, 1986, pp 903–918.
24. El Gammal, T, Adams, RJ, King, DW, So, E, and Gallagher, BB: Modified CT techniques in the evaluation of temporal lobe epilepsy prior to lobectomy. AJNR 8:131–134, 1987.
25. Engel, J Jr: Metabolic patterns of human epilepsy: Clinical observations and possible animal correlates. In Baldy-Moulinier, M, Ingvar, DH, and Meldrum BS (eds): Cerebral Blood Flow, Metabolism and Epilepsy. John Libby, London, 1983, pp 6–18.
26. Engel, J, Babb, TL, and Phelps, ME: Contribution of positron emission tomography to understanding mechanisms of epilepsy. In Engel, J Jr, Ojemann, GA, Lüders, HO, and Williamson, PD (eds): Fundamental Mechanisms of Human Brain Function. Raven Press, New York, 1987, pp 209–218.
27. Engel, J Jr, Brown, WJ, Kuhl, DE, Phelps, ME, Mazziotta, JC, and Crandall, PH: Pathological findings underlying focal temporal lobe hypometabolism in partial epilepsy. Ann Neurol 12:518–529, 1982.
28. Engel, J Jr, Kuhl, DE, Phelps, ME, and Mazziotta, JC: Interictal cerebral glucose metabolism in partial epilepsy and its relation to EEG changes. Ann Neurol 12:510–517, 1982.
29. Engel, J Jr, Kuhl, DE, Phelps, ME: Patterns of human local cerebral glucose metabolism during epileptic seizures. Science 218:64–66, 1982.
30. Engel, J Jr, Kuhl, DE, Phelps, ME, Rausch, R, and Nuwer, M: Local cerebral metabolism during partial seizures. Neurology 33:400–413, 1983.
31. Engel J Jr, Lubens, P, Kuhl, DE, and Phelps, ME: Local cerebral metabolic rate for glucose during petit mal absences. Ann Neurol 17:121–128, 1985.
32. Falconer, MA, Serefetinides, EA, and Corsellis, JAN: Aetiology and pathogenesis of temporal lobe epilepsy. Arch Neurol 19:233–240, 1964.
33. Fish, DR, Lewis, TT, Brooks, DJ, Zilka, E, Wise, RJS, and Kendall, BE: Regional cerebral blood flow of patients with focal epilepsy studied using xenon-enhanced CT brain scanning. J Neurol Neurosurg Psychiatr 50:1584–1588, 1987.
34. Foster, NL, VanDerSpek, AFL, Aldrich, MS, Berent, S, Hichwa, RH, Sackellares, JC, Gilman, S, and Agranoff, BW: The effect of diazepam sedation on cerebral glucose metabolism in Alzheimer's disease as measured using positron emission tomography. J Cereb Blood Flow Metab 7:415–420, 1987.
35. Franck, G, Sadzot, B, Salmon, E, Depresseux, JC, Grisar, T, Peters, JM, Guillaume, M, Quaglia, L, Delfiore, G, and Lamotte, D: Regional cerebral blood flow and metabolic rates in human focal epilepsy and status epilepticus. In Delgado-Escueta, AV, Ward, AA Jr, Woodbury, DM, Porter, RJ (eds): Basic Mechanisms of the Epilepsies: Molecular and Cellular Approaches. Raven Press, New York, 1986, pp 935–948.
36. Frenk, H: Pro- and anticonvulsant actions of morphine and the endogenous opioids: Involvement and interactions of multiple opiate and non-opiate systems. Brain Res Rev 6:197–210, 1983.
37. Frost, JJ, Mayberg, HS, Fisher, RS, Douglass, KH, Dannals, RF, Links, JM, Wilson, AA, Ravert, HT, Rosenbaum, AE, Snyder, SH, and Wagner, HN: Mu-opiate receptors measured by positron emission tomography are increased in

temporal lobe epilepsy. Ann Neurol 23:231–237, 1988.

38. Gallhofer, B, Trimble, MR, Frackowiack, RSJ, Gibbs, J, and Jones, T: A study of cerebral blood flow and metabolism in epileptic psychosis using positron emission tomography and oxygen. J Neurol Neurosurg Psychiatr 48:201–206, 1985.
39. Gastaut, H and Gastaut, JL: Computerized transverse axial tomography in epilepsy. Epilepsia 17:325–336, 1976.
40. Gastaut, H and Gastaut, JL: Computerized axial tomography in epilepsy. In Penry, JK (ed): Epilepsy: The 8th International Symposium. Raven Press, New York, 1977, pp 5–15.
41. Gastaut, H, Pinsard, N, and Genton, P: Electroclinical correlations of CT scans in secondary generalized epilepsies. In Canger, R, Angeleri, F, and Penry, JK (eds): Advances In Epileptology: 11th Epilepsy International Symposium. Raven Press, New York, 1980, pp 45–52.
42. Geschwind, N and Levitsky, W: Human brain: Left-right asymmetries in temporal speech region. Science 161:186–187, 1968.
43. Gibbs, F, Lennox, WG, and Gibbs, EL: Cerebral blood flow preceding and accompanying epileptic seizures in man. Arch Neurol Psychiatr 32:257–272, 1934.
44. Glaze, DG, Hrachovy, RV, Frost, JD Jr, Zion, TE, and Bryan, RN: Computed tomography in infantile spasms: Effects of hormonal therapy. Pediatr Neurol 2:23–27, 1986.
45. Grant, R, Hadley, DM, Condon, E, Doyle, D, Patterson, J, Bone, I, Galbraith, SL, and Teasdale, GM: Magnetic resonance imaging in the management of resistant focal epilepsy: Pathological case report and experience of 12 cases. J Neurol Neurosurg Psychiatr 50: 1529–1532, 1987.
46. Guberman, A: The role of computed cranial tomography in epilepsy. Can J Neurol Sci 10:16–21, 1983.
47. Gur, RC, Sussman, NM, Gur, RE, et al: Regional hypometabolism in focal epilepsy: A positron emission tomographic study. Neurology 37(Suppl 1), 1987.
48. Gur, RE, Sussman, NM, Alavi, A, Gur, RC, Rosen, AD, O'Connor, M, Goldberg, HI, Greenberg, JH, and Reivich, M: Positron emission tomography in two cases of childhood epileptic encephalopathy (Lennox-Gastaut syndrome). Neurology 32:1191–1194, 1982.
49. Heiss, W-D, Pawlik, G, Hebold, I, Herholtz, K, Wagner, R, and Wienhard, K: Metabolic pattern of speech activation in healthy volunteers, aphasics, and focal epileptics. J Cereb Blood Flow Metab 7(Suppl 1), 1987.
50. Hekster, REM, Zapletal, BJ, and Marticali, B: Comparison of CT and conventional neuroradiological procedures in lesions in the proximity of the tentorial hiatus. Neuroradiology 6:510–511, 1978.
51. Henry, TR, Engel, J Jr, Babbs, TE, and Phelps, ME: Correlation of neuronal cell loss with degree of interictal focal temporal hypometabolism in complex partial epilepsy. Neurology 38(Suppl 1): 156, 1988.
52. Holland, BA, Kucharcyzk, WA, Brant-Zawadzki, M, Norman, D, and Hass, DK: MR imaging of calcified intracranial lesions. Radiology 157:353–356, 1985.
53. Homan, RW, Paulman, RG, Devous, MD, et al: Neuropsychological function and regional cerebral blood flow in epilepsy. In Porter, RJ, Mattson, RJ, Ward, AA, et al (eds.): Advances in Epileptology: 15th International Symposium. Raven Press, New York, 1984, pp 115–120.
54. Hougaard, K, Oikawa, T, Sveinsdottir, E, et al: Regional cerebral blood flow in focal cortical epilepsy. Arch Neurol 33:527–535, 1976.
55. Jabbari, B, Gundersen, CH, Wippold, F, Citrin, C, Sherman, JK, Bartoszek, D, Daigh, JD, and Mitchell, MH: Magnetic resonance imaging in partial complex epilepsy. Arch Neurol 43:869–872, 1986.
56. Jabbari, B, Huott, AD, Di Chiro, G, et al: Surgically correctable lesions detected by CT in 143 patients with partial epilepsy. Surg Neurol 10:319–322, 1978.
57. Jack, CR, Gehring, DG, Sharbrough, FW, Felmlee, JP, Forbes, G, Hench, VS,

and Zinsmeister, AR: Temporal lobe volume measurement from MR images: Accuracy and left-right asymmetry in normal persons. J Comput Assist Tomogr 12:21–29, 1988.

58. Jack, CJ, Sharbrough, FW, Twomey, CK, et al: Temporal lobe seizures: Lateralization with MR volume measurements of the hippocampal formation. Radiology 175:40:423–429, 1990.
59. Kelly, PAT and McCulloch, J: Effects of the putative GABAergic agonists, muscimol and THIP, upon local cerebral glucose utilization. J Neurochem 39:613–624, 1982.
60. Kelly, PJ, Sharbrough, FW, Kall, BA, and Goerss, SJ: Magnetic resonance imaging–based computer-assisted stereotactic resection of the hippocampus and amygdala in patients with temporal lobe epilepsy. Mayo Clin Proc 62:103–108, 1987.
61. Kety, S, and Schmidt, CF. The nitrous oxide method for the quantitative determination of cerebral blood flow in man: Theory, procedure, and normal values. J Clin Invest 27:476–483, 1947.
62. Kety, SS, Woodford, RB, Hormel, MH, et al: Cerebral blood flow and metabolism in schizophrenia: The effect of barbiturate seminarcosis, insulin coma, and electroshock. Am J Psychiatr 104:765–770, 1948.
63. Kushner, MJ, Schwartz, R, Alavi, A, Dann, R, Rosen, M, Silver, F, and Reivich, M: Cerebral glucose consumption following verbal auditory stimulation. Brain Research 409:79–87, 1987.
64. Kuzniecky, R, de la Sayette, V, Ethier, R, Melanson, D, Andermann, F, Berkovic, S, Robitaille, Y, Olivier, A, Peters, T, and Feindel, W: Magnetic resonance imaging in temporal lobe epilepsy: Pathological correlations. Ann Neurol 22:341–347, 1987.
65. Lagenstein, I, Kuhne, D, Sternowsky, HJ, et al: Computerized transverse axial tomography (CTAT) in 145 patients with primary and secondary generalized epilepsies, West syndrome, myoclonic-astatic petit mal, absence epilepsy. Neuropaediatrie 10:15–28, 1979.
66. Lassen, NA: Cerebral blood flow and oxygen consumption in man. Physiol Rev 39:183, 1959.
67. Latack, JT, Abou-Khalil, BW, Siegel, GJ, Sackellares, JC, Gabrielsen, TO, and Aisen, AM: Patients with partial seizures: Evaluation by MR, CT, and PET imaging. Radiology 159:159–163, 1986.
68. Lavy, S, Melamed, E, Portnoy, Z, et al: Interictal regional cerebral blood flow in patients with partial seizures. Neurology 26:418–422, 1976.
69. Lee, BI, Markand, ON, Siddiqui, AR, Park, HM, Mock, B, Wellman, HH, Worth, RM, and Edwards, MK: Single photon emission computed tomography (SPECT) brain imaging using N,N,N′-trimethyl-N′-(2 hydroxy-3-methyl-5-123I-iodobenzyl)-1,3-propanediamine 2 HCl (HIPDM): Intractable complex partial seizures. Neurology 36:1471–1477, 1986.
70. Lee, BI, Markand, ON, Wellman, HN, Siddiqui, AR, Park, HM, Mock, B, Worth, RM, Edwards, MK, and Krepshaw, J: HIPDM-SPECT in patients with medically intractable complex partial seizures: Ictal study. Arch Neurol 45:397–402, 1988.
71. Lesser, RP, Modic, MT, Weinstein, MW, Duchesneau, PM, Luders, H, Dinner, D, Morris, HH III, Estes, M, Chou, S, and Hahn, J: Magnetic resonance imaging (1.5 Tesla) in patients with intractable focal seizures. Arch Neurol 43: 367–371, 1986.
72. Mazziotta, JC, Phelps, ME, Carson, RE, and Kuhl, DE: Tomographic mapping of human cerebral metabolism: Auditory stimulation. Neurology 31: 503–516, 1981.
73. Mclachon, RS, Nicholson, RL, Black, S, et al: Nuclear magnetic resonance, a new approach to the investigation of refractory temporal lobe epilepsy. Epilepsia 26:555–562, 1985.
74. Oakley, J, Ojemann, GA, Ojemann, LM, and Cromwell, L: Identifying epileptic foci on contrast enhanced computerized tomographic scans. Arch Neurol 36:669–671, 1979.
75. Ochs, RF, Gloor, P, Tyler, JF, Wolfson, T, Worsley, T, Andermann, F, Diksic, M, Meyer, E, and Evans, A: Ef-

fect of generalized spike-and-wave discharge on glucose metabolism measured by positron emission tomography. Ann Neurol 21:458–464, 1987.

76. Ochs, RF, Yamamoto, Y, Gloor, P, et al: Correlation between the positron emission tomography measurement of glucose metabolism and oxygen utilization with focal epilepsy. Neurology 34(Suppl 1):125, 1984.

77. Olsen, RW: Drug interactions and the GABA receptor ionophor complex. Ann Rev Pharmacol Toxicol 22:245–277, 1982.

78. Ormson, MJ, Kispert, DB, Sharbrough, FW, Houser, OW, Earnest, F, Scheithauer, BW, and Laws, ER: Cryptic structural lesions in refractory partial epilepsy: MR imaging and CT studies. Radiology 160:215–219, 1986.

79. Pagani, JJ, Hayman, LA, Bigelow, RHJ, et al: Prophylactic diazepam in prevention of contrast media associated seizures in glioma patients undergoing cerebral computed tomography. Cancer 54:2200–2204, 1984.

80. Palacios, JM, Kuhar, MJ, Rapoport, SI, and London, ED: Effects of G-aminobutyric acid agonist and antagonist drugs on local cerebral glucose utilization. J Neurosci 2:853–860, 1983.

81. Penfield, W and Jasper, H: Epilepsy and the Functional Anatomy of the Human Brain. Little, Brown & Co, Boston, 1954, pp 251–263.

82. Petroff, OAC, Prichard, JW, Ogino, T, Avison, M, Alger, JR, and Shulman, RG: Combined 1H and 31P nuclear magnetic resonance spectroscopy studies of bicuculline-induced seizures in vitro. Ann Neurol 20:185–193, 1986.

83. Podreka, I, Suess, E, Goldenberg, G, Steiner, M, Brucke, T, Muller, CH, Lang, W, Neirinckx, RD, and Deecke, L: Initial experience with technetium 99-M HMPAO brain SPECT. J Nucl Med 28: 1657–1666, 1987.

84. Ramirez-Lassepas, M, Cipolle, RJ, Morillo, LR, and Gumnit, RJ: Value of computed tomographic scan in the evaluation of adult patients after their first seizure. Ann Neurol 15:536–543, 1984.

85. Rasmussen, TB: Surgical treatment of complex partial seizures: Results, lessons, and problems. Epilepsia 24 (Suppl):65–76, 1983.

86. Rowe, CC, Berkovic, SF, Sia, B, Austin, M, Bladin, PF, and McKay, WJ: Localization of epileptic foci by postictal single photon computed tomography (SPECT) and 99m TC-HMPAO: Comparison with ictal EEG in 22 patients. Annals of Neurology 26:660–668, 1989.

87. Russo, LS and Goldstein, KH: The diagnostic assessment of single seizures: Is cranial computed tomography necessary? Arch Neurol 40:744–746, 1983.

88. Sadzot, B, Salmon, E, Maquet, P, et al: Assessment of the interest of PET and MRI in complex partial seizures. J Cereb Blood Flow Metab 7(Suppl 1):432, 1987.

89. Sakai, F, Meyer, JS, Naritomi, H, et al: Regional cerebral blood flow and EEG in patients with epilepsy. Arch Neurol 35:648–657, 1978.

90. Sammaritano, M, de Lotbiniere, A, Andermann, F, Olivier, A, Gloor, P, and Quesney, LF: False lateralization by surface EEG of seizure onset in patients with temporal lobe epilepsy and gross focal cerebral lesions. Ann Neurol 21:361–369, 1987.

91. Sato, S, Dreifuss, FE, Penry, JK, et al: Long-term follow-up study of absence seizures. In Akimoto, H, Kazamatsuri, H, Seino, M, Ward, AA (eds): Advances in Epileptology; 13th International Symposium. Raven Press, New York, 1982, pp 41–42.

92. Savic, I, Roland, P, Sedvall, G, Persson, A, Pauli, S, and Widen, L: In-vivo demonstration of reduced benzodiazepine receptor binding in human epileptic foci. Lancet 863–866; October 15, 1988.

93. Schorner, W, Meencke, HJ, and Felix, R: Temporal lobe epilepsy: Comparison of CT and MR imaging. AJR 149:1231–1239, 1987.

94. Scollo-Lavizzari, G, Eichorn, H, and Wuthrich, R: Computerized transaxial tomography in the diagnosis of epilepsy. Eur Neurol 15:5–8, 1977.

95. Shen, W, Lee, BI, Park, HM, et al:

HIPDM-SPECT brain imaging in evaluation of intractable epilepsy for temporal lobectomy. Neurology 39(Suppl 1):132, 1989.

96. Shorvon, SD, Gilliatt, RW, Cox, TC, et al: Evidence of vascular disease from CT scanning in late-onset epilepsy. J Neurol Neurosurg Psychiatr 47:225–230, 1984.
97. Spencer, DD, Spencer, SS, Mattson, RH, and Williamson, PD: Intracerebral masses in patients with intractable partial epilepsy. Neurology 34:432–436, 1984.
98. Sperling, MR, Wilson, G, Engel, J Jr, Babb, TW, Phelps, M, and Bradley, W: Magnetic resonance imaging in intractable partial epilepsy: Correlative studies. Ann Neurol 20:57–62, 1986.
99. Stefan, H, Pawlik, G, Bocher-Schwarz, HG, Biersack, HJ, Burr, W, Penin, H, and Heiss, W-D. Functional and morphological abnormalities in temporal lobe epilepsy: A comparison of interictal and ictal EEG, CT, MRI, SPECT, and PET. J Neurol 234:377–384, 1987.
100. Stevens, JR. Focal abnormality in petit mal epilepsy. Neurology 20:1069–1075, 1970.
101. Stewart, LF and Dreifuss, FE. "Centrencephalic" seizure discharges in focal hemisphere lesions. Arch Neurol 17:60–68, 1967.
102. Theodore, WH: Neuroimaging. In Porter, RJ and Theodore, WH (eds): Epilepsy. Neurologic Clin North Am 4:645–668, 1986.
103. Theodore, WH, Bairamian, D, Newmark, ME, Di Chiro, G, Porter, RJ, Larson, S, and Fishbein, D: The effect of phenytoin on human cerebral glucose metabolism. J Cereb Blood Flow Metab 6:315–320, 1986.
104. Theodore, WH, Blasberg, R, Leiderman, D, et al: PET imaging of opiate receptor binding in human epilepsy using ^{18}F-cyclofoxy. Neurology 40 (Suppl 1):257, 1990.
105. Theodore, WH, Brooks, R, Margolin, R, and Patronas, N, Sato, S, Porter, RJ, Mansi, L, Bairamian, D, and Di Chiro, G: Positron emission tomography in generalized seizures. Neurology 35: 684–690, 1985.
106. Theodore, WH, Di Chiro G, Margolin R, Fishbein, D, Porter, RJ, and Brooks, RA: Barbiturates reduce human cerebral glucose metabolism. Neurology 36:60–64, 1986.
107. Theodore, WH, Dorwart, R, Holmes, M, Porter, RJ, and Di Chiro, G: Neuroimaging in refractory partial seizures: Comparison of PET, CT, and MRI. Neurology 36:750–759, 1986.
108. Theodore, WH, Fishbein, D, Deitz, M, and Baldwin, P: Complex partial seizures: Cerebellar metabolism. Epilepsia 28:319–323, 1987.
109. Theodore, WH, Fishbein, D, and Dubinsky, R: Patterns of cerebral glucose metabolism in patients with partial seizures. Neurology 38:1201–1206, 1988.
110. Theodore, WH, Holmes, MD, Dorwart, RH, Porter, RJ, Di Chiro, G, Sato, S, and Rose, D: Complex partial seizures: Cerebral structure and cerebral function. Epilepsia 27:576–582, 1986.
111. Theodore, WH, Ito, B, Devinsky, O, Porter, RJ, Jacobs, G: Carbamazepine and cerebral glucose metabolism. Neurology 37(Suppl 1):104, 1987.
112. Theodore, WH, Jabbari, B, Leiderman, DB, McBurney, J, and Van Nostrand, DV: Positron emission tomography and single photon emission tomography in epilepsy. Ann Neurol 28:262–263, 1990.
113. Theodore, WH, Katz, D, Kufta, C, Sato, S, Patronas, N, Smothers, P, and Bromfield, E: Pathology of temporal lobe foci: Correlation with CT, MRI, and PET. Neurology 40:797–803, 1990.
114. Theodore, WH, Newmark, ME, Sato, S, De La Paz, R, Di Chiro, G, Brooks, R, Patronas, N, Kessler, RM, Manning, R, Margolin, R, Channing, M, and Porter, RJ: ^{18}F-fluorodeoxyglucose positron emission tomography in refractory complex partial seizures. Ann Neurol 14:429–437, 1983.
115. Theodore, WH, Rose, D, Patronas, N, Sato, S, Holmes, M, Bairamian, D, Porter, RJ, Di Chiro, G, Larson, S, and Fishbein, D: Cerebral glucose metabolism in the Lennox-Gastaut syndrome. Ann Neurol 21:14–21, 1987.
116. Theodore, WH, Sato, S, Kufta, C, Bare,

M, Porter, RJ, Ito, B, Rose, D, and Devinsky, O: Strategy for surgical selection of patients with partial seizures: The role of positron emission tomography. Ann Neurol 22:133, 1987.

117. Triulzi, F, Franceschi, M, Fazio, F, Del Maschio, A: Nonrefractory temporal lobe epilepsy: 1.5T MR imaging. Radiology 166:181–185, 1988.

118. Turner DA, Wyler AR: Temporal lobectomy for epilepsy: Mesial temporal herniation as an operative and prognostic finding. Epilepsia 22:623–629, 1981.

119. Wilden, JN and Kelly, PJ: Computerized stereotactic biopsy for low density CT lesions presenting with epilepsy. J Neurol Neurosurg Psychiatr 50: 1302–1305, 1987.

120. Wyllie, E, Lüders, H, Morris, HH III, Lesser, RP, Dinner, DS, Hahn, J, Estes, ML, Rothner, AD, Erenberg, G, Cruse, R, and Friedman, D: Clinical outcome after complete or partial cortical resection for intractable epilepsy. Neurology 37:1634–1641, 1987.

121. Yang, PJ, Berger, PE, Cohen, ME, and Duffner, PK: Computed tomography in childhood seizure disorders. Neurology 29:1084–1088, 1979.

122. Young, AC, Mohr, PD, Constanzi, JB, et al: Is routine computerized axial tomography in epilepsy worthwhile? Lancet 2:1146–1147, 1982.

123. Young, RSK, Cowen, BE, Petroff, OAC, Novotny, E, Dunham, SL, and Briggs, RW: In vivo 31P and in vitro 1H nuclear magnetic resonance study of hypoglycemia during neonatal seizure. Ann Neurol 22:622–628, 1987.

124. Younkin, DP, Delivoria-Papadopoulos, M, Maris, J, Donlon, E, Clancy, R, and Chance, B: Cerebral metabolic effects of neonatal seizures measured with in vivo 31P NMR spectroscopy. Ann Neurol 20:513–519, 1986.

125. Zimmerman, RA, Sperling, M, Bilaniuk, LA, O'Connor, M, Hackney, DB, Grossman, RI, Goldberg, HI, and Gonatas, N: MR imaging findings in patients with mesial temporal sclerosis. Radiology 165(Suppl):249, 1987.

Chapter 6

NEOPLASTIC DISORDERS

Jane L. Tyler, M.D. and
Thomas N. Byrne, M.D.

NEUROIMAGING MODALITIES IN THE EVALUATION OF INTRACRANIAL NEOPLASMS
SPECIFIC NEOPLASTIC DISORDERS
REMOTE EFFECTS OF INTRACEREBRAL TUMORS
RESPONSE OF TUMORS TO TREATMENT
THE DIFFERENTIATION OF RADIATION NECROSIS FROM RECURRENT TUMOR

Patients with intracranial neoplasms constitute a substantial population in the clinical practice of medicine. Up to 20% of patients dying of cancer have evidence of intracerebral metastases at the time of their death. Primary intracerebral tumors comprise approximately 2% of all neoplasms.

Classification of tumors based on their degree of malignancy or aggressiveness requires an understanding of their pathophysiology.[216] In 1838 Johannes Müller proposed a method of classifying tumors based on their "chemical nature, microscopic structure, mode of development, and embryological origin."[139] Virchow provided the first useful classification based on his work on glial cells, describing the similarities between cells from brain tumors and the basic structure of glia.[197,198] The first classification of intracranial tumors based on histologic criteria derived from the study of normal cells was proposed by Borst in 1902.[17] The more detailed classification in current use was proposed by Pick and Bielschowsky in 1911, based on their study of ganglion cell tumors,[159] and by Ribburt in 1918 from his work on gliomas,[167] and is dependent on the "degree of maturation" of the neoplastic cells. This system was refined and enlarged by Bailey and Cushing in 1926,[7] and it remains the basis of the present system of classification.

The types of primary intracranial tumors reported in previous series[42,149,215] are shown in Table 6–1, comprising data on approximately 15,000 patients. Patient age is closely related to tumor type, with medulloblastomas seen primarily before the age of 20 years. Heredity is a factor in retinoblastomas, neurofibromas, and hemangioblastomas.

For the clinician caring for patients with intracranial neoplasms, an understanding of the pathophysiology of these lesions is essential as diagnostic and therapeutic decisions are being made. Factors such as tumor location, rate of tumor growth, tumor vascularity, the amount of peritumoral edema, and the degree of disruption of the blood-brain barrier (BBB) in and around the tumor must all be evaluated.

The symptoms caused by tumor growth are attributable to increased pressure in the limited intracranial

Table 6–1 TYPES OF INTRACRANIAL TUMORS SEEN IN THE COMBINED SERIES OF ZÜLICH, CUSHING AND OLIVECRONA*

Tumor	*Percentage of Total*
Gliomas†	
Glioblastoma multiforme	20
Astrocytoma	10
Ependymoma	6
Meduloblastoma	4
Oligodendrocytoma	5
Meningioma	15
Pituitary adenoma	7
Neurinoma (schwannoma)	7
Metastatic carcinoma	6
Craniopharyngioma, dermoid, epidermoid, teratoma	4
Angioma	4
Sarcoma	4
Unclassified	5
Miscellaneous (pinealoma, chordoma, granuloma)	3
TOTAL	100

*Expressed in percentage of total (approximately 15,000 cases).

†In children, the proportions differ: astrocytoma 48%, medulloblastoma 44%, ependymoma 8%.

From Adams and Victor[1] p. 475, with permission.

space and to the direct impingement on or damage to neuronal tissue caused by the tumor. Many patients present with focal deficits and seizures. Others present with less specific symptoms such as irritability, emotional lability, decreased spontaneity, drowsiness and forgetfulness because of general impairment of cognitive function and mentation. These latter symptoms are usually not attributable to a site-specific brain lesion, but rather to increased intracranial pressure (ICP) due to the tumor mass and peritumoral edema. The signs of brain tumors are related to their location in the nervous system; site-specific effects will be totally dependent on the location. For example, lesions in the occipital lobes will produce visual field deficits, whereas tumors interrupting motor pathways will cause weakness and increased tone. General increases in intracranial pressure are usually associated with the global symptoms described above, plus papilledema and sixth cranial nerve abnormalities.

The tight endothelial junctions comprising the BBB of the normal brain are defective in brain tumors,[93] allowing electrolytes and proteins to pass from tumor capillaries into the extracellular space, thereby contributing to local edema and raising the protein content of the cerebrospinal fluid. Further damage to capillaries from the release of toxins and the local accumulation of lactic acid also contributes to the edema associated with cerebral tumors. This type of edema, termed "vasogenic",[111] is largely confined to white matter. The increased capillary permeability that occurs with plasma entering the extracellular space may be due both to breakdown of endothelial-cell tight junctions and to increased vesicular transport across those cells.[1] The accumulation of the extracellular fluid with increased protein content may itself alter the ionic balance of nerve fibers in the white matter, thereby altering neuronal function. Vasogenic edema, seen with intracranial tumors as well as with localized toxic injuries to blood vessels (e.g., lead encephalopathy), contrasts with "cytotoxic" edema seen with hypoxic injury, in which all cellular elements take up fluid and swell.[1]

Information on the degree of BBB breakdown and the extent of peritumoral edema are extremely important in the initial diagnosis and characterization of intracranial neoplasms. In addition, treatment of these tumors with chemotherapeutic agents often depends upon BBB disruption for delivery of drugs selectively to tumor tissue, either through BBB breakdown within and around the tumor, or through the action of osmotic agents such as mannitol.[143]

The tumor mass itself is comprised of a mixture of actively growing cells, areas of necrosis, and tumor blood vessels. Assessing the rate of growth of this heterogeneous mass obviously is important in the grading of the lesion and in the selection of therapeutic interventions. The ability to detect changes in the rate of growth is useful in monitoring the response to treatment. Measurements of tumor vascularity and intratumor blood volume may indicate the degree of tumor aggressiveness and may also be helpful in assessing the effects of treatment.

NEUROIMAGING MODALITIES IN THE EVALUATION OF INTRACRANIAL NEOPLASMS

A variety of neuroimaging techniques are now available to aid in the assessment of the patient with a brain tumor. Despite rapid advances in magnetic resonance angiography (MRA), conventional angiography must remain the standard of care in that it provides the precise size and location of arteries supplying the tumor, the extent of tumor vascularity, the degree of arteriovenous shunting of blood, and the size and location of draining veins. This information is often important diagnostically. For example, meningiomas are typically dura-based, highly vascular, and have calcifications. On conventional angiography this high vascularity is easily identified and provides a high degree of confidence about the ultimate histologic diagnosis. Similarly, angiographic data also are important to the neurosurgeon planning biopsy, debulking, or resection of a tumor. With the advent of intraarterial administration of chemotherapy, determination of tumor vascular anatomy becomes even more important. The invasive nature of angiography and its inherent risk, however, have prompted the search for other, less hazardous vascular imaging techniques that can provide information on tumor vascularity, such as magnetic resonance angiography (see Chapters 2 and 13).

In the last 15 years, x-ray computed tomography (CT) (see Chapter 1) has transformed the diagnosis and management of cerebral lesions. With its speed, accuracy, and low radiation dose, x-ray CT has replaced previous radiologic procedures such as pneumoencephalography and cisternography, which were both uncomfortable and hazardous for the tumor patient. The role of high-resolution, contrast-enhanced CT in the diagnosis of intracranial tumors is now well established.[2,84,188,200] X-ray CT is also widely used in following the response of these neoplasms to treatment. In addition, considerable work has been done to evaluate the correlation of tumor appearance on CT scan with histologic grade and prognosis.[2,21,84]

Magnetic resonance imaging (MRI), with its high contrast resolution, has proven to be more sensitive than x-ray CT in the detection of small intracranial tumors.[21] For example, although CT scans capably demonstrate acoustic neuromas that have extended into the cerebellopontine angle, injection of air into this subarachnoid space may be necessary for the CT diagnosis of small intracanalicular neuromas.[183] These small lesions are usually seen noninvasively with MRI, which has become the diagnostic study of choice for evaluating patients suspected of harboring acoustic neuromas. Furthermore, gadolinium-DTPA–enhanced MRI has been found to be more sensitive than unenhanced MRI in detecting cerebellopontine angle masses and intracanalicular tumors. Whether MRI is as sensitive as air-contrast CT remains to be determined. Likewise, MRI is more sensitive than x-ray CT in the detection of pituitary and pineal neoplasms. MRI is often more useful than x-ray CT in the evaluation of posterior fossa disease, regardless of the size of the lesion (see Chapters 2 and 11), because of the limitations of CT scans owing to artifacts caused by bony structures (Figure 6–1).[153]

Despite its high sensitivity in detecting intracranial tumors, MRI may, in certain cases, be less specific than x-ray CT. Characteristic appearances on CT scans of some tumors, such as in

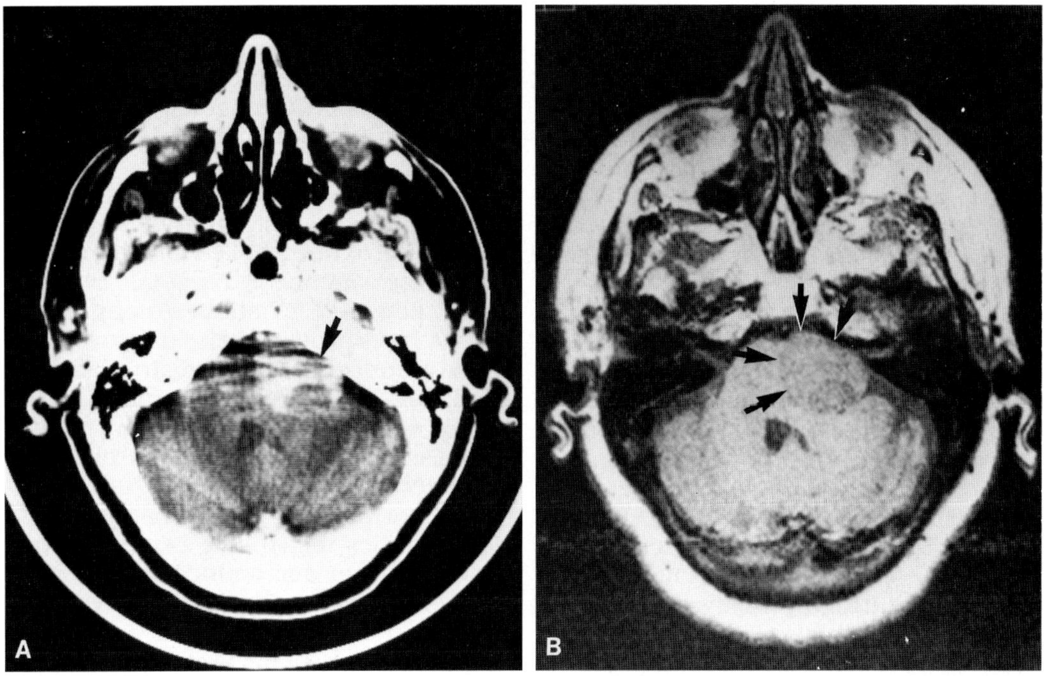

Figure 6–1. (*A*) The x-ray CT scan of a patient with a right cerebellar tumor contains considerable beam hardening artifact (*arrow*) (see Chapter 1). (*B*) An MRI scan demonstrates the extent of the lesion (*arrows*) and its distortion of the fourth ventricle. On this and all further illustrations, the right side of the scan is to the right in the figure.

oligodendrogliomas or the nodular pattern seen in meningiomas, may lead to a more specific diagnosis with x-ray CT, whereas MRI merely detects the presence of the lesions.[20]

Because of the considerable past experience with x-ray CT scanning, the histologic type of many tumors such as meningiomas and glioblastomas[188] can be estimated from the intracranial location of the tumor, presence or absence of calcifications, and pattern and intensity of contrast enhancement. The considerable anatomic information provided by angiography and x-ray CT scanning is surpassed by the data supplied by MRI, which can provide even better resolution for the detection of small lesions, and allows assessment of tumoral and peritumoral water content. Although both x-ray CT and MRI provide data that are "anatomic" in nature, neither has been able to distinguish tumor types reliably based on their characteristics.

Past studies attempting to characterize cerebral neoplasms in terms of clinical behavior and response to therapy have been fraught with a number of methodologic and practical problems. For example, the use of x-ray CT with iodinated contrast material delivered intravenously depicts alterations in the BBB but does not necessarily identify viable tumor or areas of cerebral necrosis.[83,144,171] It is also known that the tumor may extend beyond the boundaries of CT enhancement or hypodensity.* In fact, it has been estimated that the boundary of x-ray CT enhancement may only show half of the actual tumor volume.[104]

Similar ambiguities occur in the examination of cerebral neoplasms with T_2-weighted MR images.[105,106] As with CT, gadolinium-ethylenediaminete-

*References 26–27, 45, 46, 104, 106, 128, 137, 203.

traacetic acid (Gd-EDTA)–enhanced MR images typically depict BBB alterations and not viable tumor.[173] Although it is generally accepted that MRI information exceeds that of CT in terms of image quality,[22,33,67,108] neither technique provides biochemically based estimates of active tumor growth, three-dimensional tumor extent, or malignancy grade.[36,46,97]

Standard imaging techniques can sometimes produce ambiguous information about differential diagnosis when one is trying to distinguish neoplastic lesions from infectious disorders. For example, ring enhancement with contrast CT or signal characteristics with MRI may produce confusion between bacterial cerebral abscesses or cysticercosis lesions and neoplastic disease, resulting in misdiagnosis.

The attempt to develop "functional" imaging of brain tumors was the impetus that led to the birth of the field of nuclear medicine. Initial radionuclide studies of brain tumors between the 1950s and 1970s, with inhaled krypton gas or injected technetium-labeled compounds, gave only crude estimates of blood flow and BBB integrity. Recently, CT image reconstructions developed for x-ray CT scanning have been combined with radionuclide imaging to produce single photon emission tomography (SPECT) (see Chapter 4) and positron emission tomography (PET) (see Chapter 3). Both of these modalities provide important diagnostic information to the clinician, but both present limitations as well. In the past, SPECT studies have been hampered, to some extent, by lower image resolution than that available with PET, and with a difficulty in labeling appropriate radiopharmaceuticals. PET in turn has been limited by its higher costs and the requirement for an onsite cyclotron.

The reconstruction process used in SPECT removes the contributions of activities in tissues lying above or below the plane of interest, thereby improving lesion contrast (see Chapter 4). In two large studies,[34,91] sensitivity in lesion detection was increased significantly without loss of specificity with the use of tomography, compared with planar nuclear medicine imaging. The application of radiopharmaceuticals for SPECT imaging such as iodine-123 iodoamphetamine, xenon-133 gas, and technetium-labeled hexamethylene-propyleneamine oxime (^{99m}Tc-HMPAO) allows the assessment of regional cerebral blood flow. SPECT studies using ^{99m}Tc-DTPA have proven useful in the evaluation of cerebrospinal fluid circulation,[11] and SPECT has also been used in the detection of areas of BBB abnormality. Good correlations have been obtained between results from ^{99m}Tc-HMPAO and continuous-inhalation oxygen-15 PET studies measuring cerebral blood flow.[120] Other compounds labeled with ^{99m}Tc are currently under investigation.[60]

Thallium-201 was first used for myocardial imaging and was noted, incidentally, to show uptake in lung carcinoma.[193] Subsequent studies demonstrated that there was a substantial retention of this radioisotope in primary and metastatic cerebral tumors.[3,193] Actual retention is related to a combination of factors, including regional blood flow, BBB permeability, and cellular retention.[4] Increased BBB permeability alone does not necessarily increase thallium retention, since nonneoplastic lesions that cause BBB breakdown, such as areas of radiation necrosis or resolving hematomas, have little or no thallium retention.[15] Experimental evidence suggests that ionic movement of thallium and potassium are related to active transport by way of a cell-membrane ATP pump and that thallium retention is related to cellular growth rates.[44,61] Because thallium uptake does not simply rely on BBB abnormalities, whereas iodinated contrast agents in x-ray CT and Gd-EDTA in MRI do, it is not surprising that thallium imaging has been found superior to x-ray CT in a series of 198 imaging studies on patients with recurrent tumors.[103] More recently, thallium-SPECT imaging has been used to differentiate high- and low-grade gliomas in a series of 25 patients.[110]

Truly functional or metabolic evaluations of brain tumors, however, have remained in the realm of positron emission tomography. The introduction of radioactive oxygen, carbon, nitrogen or fluorine into a wide variety of substances, including naturally occurring water, O_2 and CO_2 gases and amino acids, as well as into glucose analogs and drugs, only minimally alters their physiologic charactcristics and allows for their in vivo autoradiographic imaging in the living human brain (see Chapter 3). As new radiopharmaceuticals are developed and tested, an even wider number of physiologic functions can be measured.

An increased understanding of tumor pathophysiology is needed to design better treatment plans. Noninvasive metabolic and hemodynamic evaluations possible with SPECT and PET may provide the means to an improved understanding of tumor growth and behavior. For example, it is still extremely difficult to determine the size, position, and residual volume of viable tumor cells before or after surgery. In addition, it is difficult using only clinical signs or symptoms, or structural imaging to differentiate recurrent tumor from radiation injury to the brain. Biochemical measurements with PET have provided advances in these areas.

SPECIFIC NEOPLASTIC DISORDERS

Intracerebral Gliomas

Gliomas comprise approximately 45% of primary intracerebral tumors. Approximately half of these are highly malignant (see Table 6–1). Because of the frequency with which gliomas are seen and their often devastating consequences, most of the work in the neuroimaging of cerebral neoplasms has been concentrated on this type of tumor.

These lesions are graded, in terms of growth rate and malignancy, from I to IV. Low-grade lesions (I, II) have minimal growth rates, minimal disruption of BBB and the best prognosis. High-grade lesions (III, IV) are typically heterogeneous, with areas of tissue necrosis and hemorrhage, are rapidly growing, and have a poor prognosis. Gliomas typically recur after therapy and frequently transform from lower to higher grades with recurrence.

There is little doubt that gliomas are highly lethal. In patients with moderate to high-grade gliomas, median survival is 35 weeks for patients having symptoms of less than 16 weeks' duration.[210] For patients in whom symptoms have lasted more than 16 weeks, the average survival is 88 weeks.[210] Thus, despite optimal surgery, radiation therapy (RT), and medical therapy, survival of these patients is extremely limited. Any insights into the fundamental nature of tumor development and growth should provide new tools and avenues for intervention aimed at prolonging both the duration and quality of patients' lives.

High-grade (IV) gliomas are estimated to account for 2500–5000 deaths per year. Despite intense and extensive study of these lesions for the past 50 years, there is still a wide range of unanswered questions about the fundamental basis of these tumors and their response to therapy. One recent review[142] demonstrated that in the past 50 years of surgical management of patients with supratentorial gliomas, the literature substantiates the value of neurosurgical approaches to the treatment of gliomas with regard to tissue diagnosis and decompression, but provides little definitive information about the role of cytoreductive surgery on survival, recurrence, or ultimate prognosis.[75,172,175,186,201,203]

Significant factors affecting the prognosis of patients with cerebral gliomas include a number of well-described variables such as patient age, preopera-

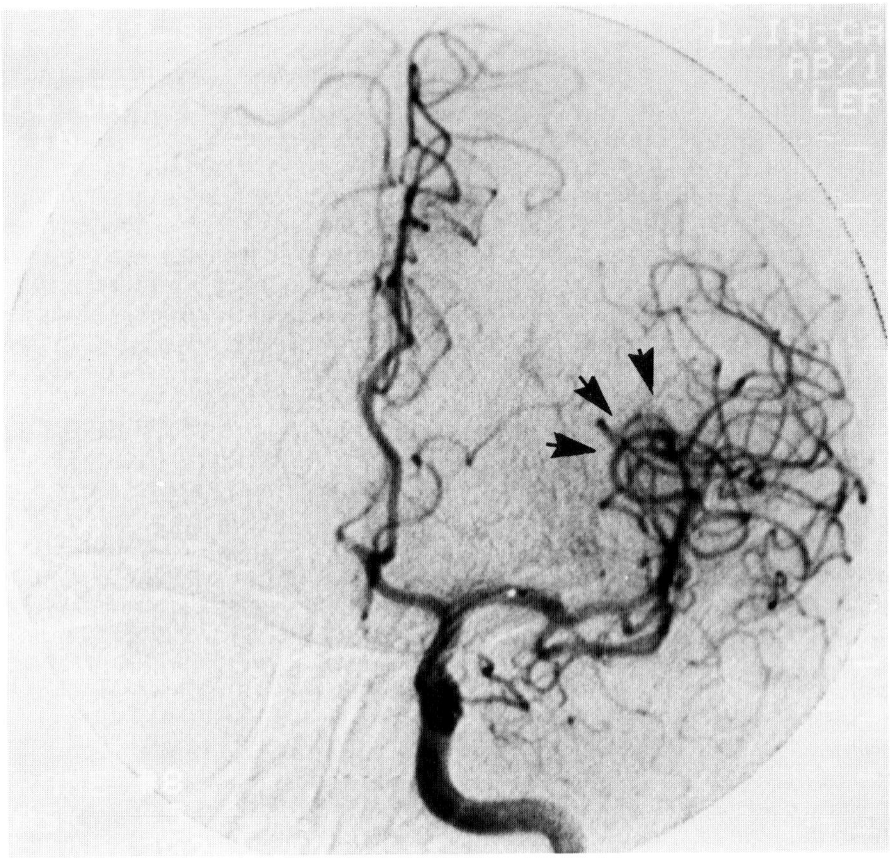

Figure 6–2. This left carotid angiogram demonstrates markedly increased vasculature in the region of an occipital glioblastoma multiforme (*arrows*).

tive functional status, tumor site, adequacy of resection, duration of symptoms, and tumor type. Clinical studies designed to evaluate new medical or surgical therapies are confounded by all of these issues.[142] It is possible that the combination of modern structural and functional imaging information will provide the necessary anatomic and biochemical foundation for a data base for the examination of patients, and an objective means of monitoring clinical trials of medical or surgical interventions for the treatment of patients with gliomas.

ANGIOGRAPHY

On angiography, gliomas are typically highly vascular, with a network of abnormal vessels within the tumor (Fig. 6–2), and displacement of surrounding vessels by the tumor mass. The degree of vascularity correlates somewhat with tumor grade, and the angioarchitecture of the glioma can be very helpful in the differential diagnosis.

X-RAY CT

Typically, an untreated intracerebral glioma appears on CT as an area of variable, though usually low, attenuation.[144a] Following the infusion of iodinated contrast material, ringlike patterns of enhancement may be seen that can be homogeneous or heterogeneous (Fig. 6–3).[30,125,188] Edematous brain tissue on the unenhanced x-ray CT has a slightly lower mean attenua-

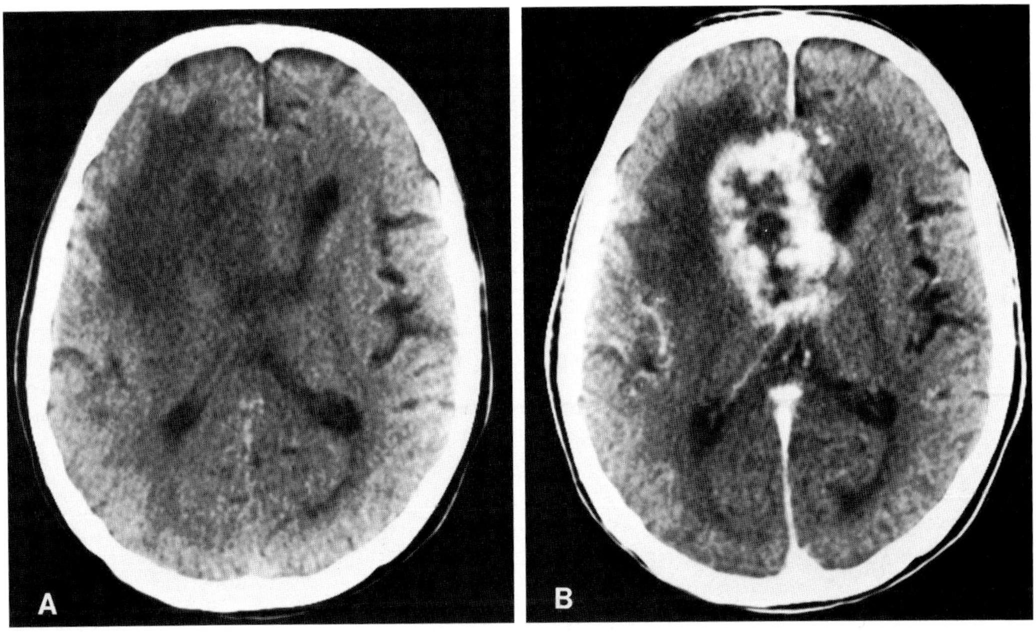

Figure 6–3. (*A*) This unenhanced x-ray CT scan demonstrates a large low-density area in the left frontoparietal region. (*B*) In the same patient, following contrast enhancement, the full extent of the blood-brain barrier (BBB) disruption in the medially located lesion is seen. Biopsy later proved this to be a glioblastoma multiforme.

tion than normal brain. The contrast enhancement that occurs in tumors is due to accumulation of iodinated contrast material in the extracellular space, which is blocked in normal brain by the intact BBB. There is also some contribution from iodine in the increased vascular space of the tumor blood vessels. Steroids seem to reestablish the BBB partially,[122] thereby decreasing the permeability of brain tissue to contrast material.[41] Tumor blood volume may not be appreciably diminished by steroids,[115] and thus the decreased enhancement seen is likely due to their effect on the BBB.

After early studies[36,107,187] suggested that x-ray CT could provide an accuracy approaching 90% in the diagnosis of glioma, it was suggested that contrast enhancement of gliomas correlated with the degree of anaplastic change. In one study,[30] contrast enhancement was found in 100% of grade III and IV astrocytomas (Fig. 6–4) but in only 3 (15%) of 20 grade I and II astrocytomas. Another study[123] found enhancement in 48% of grade I and II astrocytomas and 96% of grade III and IV gliomas. The observation that contrast enhancement predicted degree of malignancy could be explained by the electron microscopic observation that the defects in the endothelial cells and tight junctions that correlate with malignancy were the defects through which iodine extravasated into the extravascular space, resulting in enhancement.

More recent studies, however, have shown that some malignant gliomas may not enhance. In a study of 229 consecutive patients with supratentorial malignant gliomas,[36] no enhancement was seen in 4% of 93 patients with glioblastoma multiforme, 10% of 10 with gemistocytic astrocytoma, 31% of 74 with highly anaplastic astrocytoma, and 54% of 52 with moderately anaplastic astrocytoma. Since the histologic findings did not correlate with contrast enhancement, the authors concluded that it is important to obtain

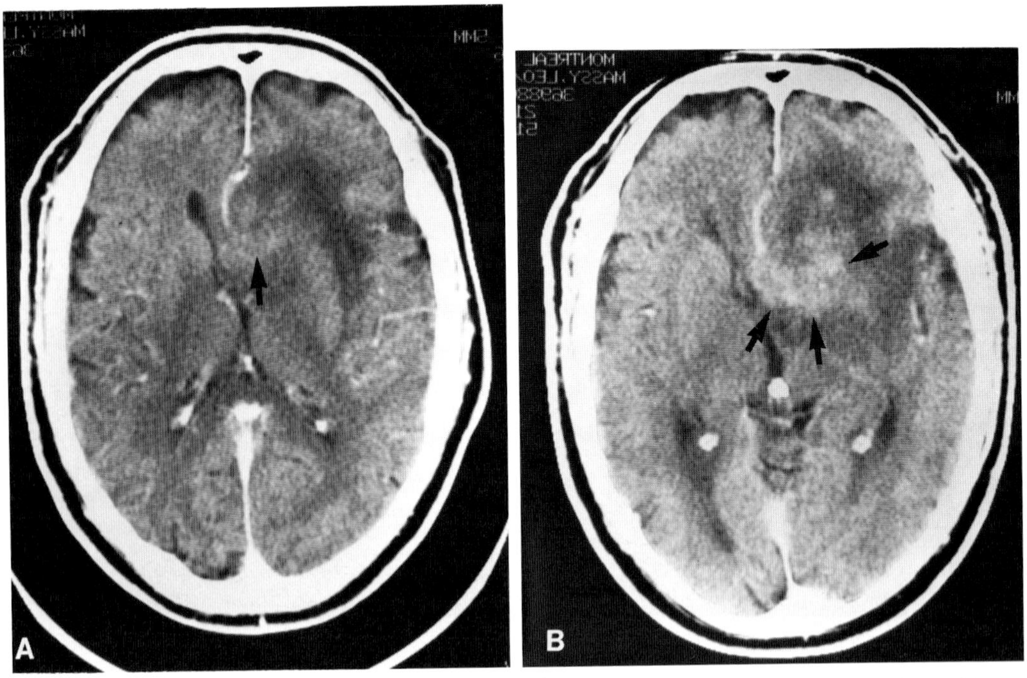

Figure 6–4. This x-ray CT scan with contrast demonstrates no enhancement in a right frontal lesion (*arrow*). Biopsy revealed a grade II astrocytoma. (*B*) Six months later, the enhanced CT scan was repeated because of clinical deterioration in the patient. Enhancement was then seen in the lesion (*arrows*); repeat biopsy was consistent with a grade III/IV tumor.

histologic confirmation of supratentorial gliomas regardless of the presence or absence of enhancement. Piepmeier[160] has reported that 20% of low-grade astrocytomas show contrast enhancement; the prognosis among those patients with enhancing tumors was worse (mean survival, 3.9 years) than that in tumors without enhancement (mean survival, 7.9 years). A study of the x-ray CT appearance of pediatric brain tumors[156] found that the degree of contrast enhancement only weakly correlated with the degree of malignancy.

A major question being investigated is whether the area of contrast enhancement or surrounding low attenuation identifies the topographic anatomy of a glioma. An early retrospective autopsy study of 16 untreated and 19 treated glioblastomas[94] demonstrated that tumor cells are typically confined to within 2 cm peripheral to the region of contrast enhancement on x-ray CT. A more recent autopsy study of untreated glioblastomas[27] showed that tumor could be identified beyond 2 cm of the area of contrast enhancement in 3 of 15 patients. Furthermore, in a study of image-based stereotaxic biopsies in untreated glial tumors, Kelly and colleagues[105] found the following:

1. Low-grade glial tumors were usually hypodense but could be isodense with contrast injection;
2. Contrast enhancement correlated with the degree of neovascularity;
3. Central low-density regions in glioblastoma multiforme revealed necrosis;
4. Areas of contrast enhancement usually corresponded to tumor tissue without intervening brain parenchyma;
5. Adjacent to contrast-enhancing regions, nonenhancing hypodense areas could represent brain paren-

chyma with infiltrating tumor cells in high-grade gliomas, or tumor tissue in low-grade gliomas, or edema alone; and

6. Isolated tumor cells could be found in isodense regions of brain beyond the area of low attenuation.

These findings indicate that tumor may extend well beyond the area of enhancement, and thus have a profound impact on our understanding of glial neoplasms and the planning of regional forms of therapy such as surgery, external beam RT, interstitial radiation, and chemotherapy.

Oligodendrogliomas, comprising approximately 5%–7% of intracranial gliomas, are most commonly located in the frontal lobes (40%–70%). They are often deep in the white matter, with little or no surrounding edema, and are often calcified.[1] They typically grow slowly and are similar to low-grade astrocytomas in their x-ray CT appearance (Fig. 6–5). Ependymomas, constituting about 5% of intracranial gliomas in adults (about 8% in children) are usually identified by their location and their growth into ventricles and adjacent brain. Three fourths of ependymomas occur in the posterior fossa. The remainder are supratentorial; they are frequently isodense on the precontrast CT scan, and have patchy enhancement more commonly than a homogeneous pattern following contrast infusion. Fifty percent are calcified.

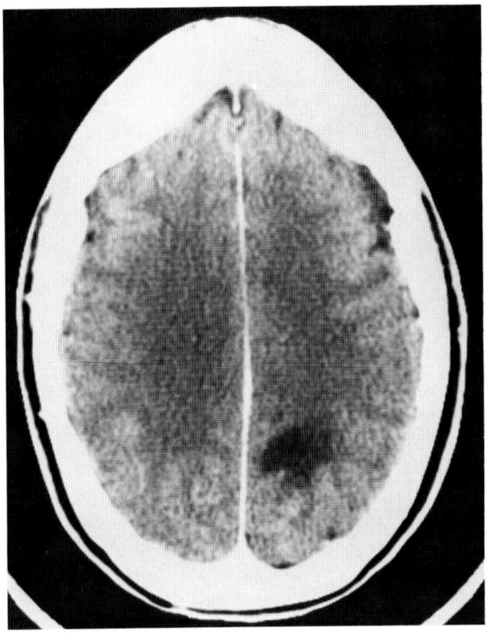

Figure 6–5. X-ray CT scan with contrast shows no enhancement in a right posterior parietal oligodendroglioma.

The predictive value of x-ray CT in glioma patients, with regard to prognosis or response to treatment, has been investigated in a number of studies.* As noted earlier, variables that are important in prognosis include patient age, preoperative functional status, site, adequacy of resection, duration of symptoms, and tumor cell type. Variables that consistently have demonstrated a more favorable prognosis include younger age at onset and the location of the tumor in the optic tract, spinal cord, or cerebellum.[77,124,132]

Commonly, serial x-ray CT scans are compared in order to assess response to treatment. There are pitfalls, however, in determining whether regions of enhancement and edema are due to specific treatments such as surgery, radiation therapy, or chemotherapy. For example, Cairncross and associates[31] have emphasized that changes on consecutive CT scans that appear to show tumor "response" or "progression" may be due to changes in corticosteroid dosage alone.

Contrast enhancement may occur secondary to surgical trauma and may be difficult to differentiate from residual or progressive tumor. Cairncross' group[32] studied the evolution of postsurgical changes in patients undergoing resection of gliomas, and found that enhancement due to surgical trauma typically occurred as early as the fifth postoperative day, became maximum at 2 weeks, and persisted for several months. Alternatively, contrast enhancement before the fifth postoperative day identified residual tumor. Since postsurgical artifacts were prominent

*References 66,77,124,131,132,165,177,179.

during the first 2 postoperative days, however, the authors recommend postoperative CT scans on days 3 or 4 in order to assess enhancing residual tumor.

MRI

Although significant anatomic information can be obtained with MRI, it is not completely interchangeable with x-ray CT as a tumor-imaging technique. Whereas CT values reflect the mean electron densities and atomic numbers of the tissue, proton MRI values are related to the concentration and chemical environment of hydrogen nuclei. Since biochemical differences between structures can serve as a basis of contrast resolution in MRI, and since abnormal chemical and physiologic changes probably precede pathologic changes in gross tissue structure, MRI has proved to have wider diagnostic applications than x-ray CT in tumor evaluations.

When magnetic resonance imaging of gliomas became available, it was evident that much larger regions of abnormality were identified than were seen on x-ray CT. In a comparative study of CT and MR imaging of untreated gliomas,[105] Kelly and colleagues performed stereotaxic biopsies to identify the histologic correlate of abnormalities seen on imaging. They found that the region of prolonged T_2 was generally much larger than the CT region of abnormal low attenuation surrounding contrast enhancement (Fig. 6–6). Stereotaxic biopsies revealed that infiltrating tumor cells are present in regions of prolonged T_2, areas that may be isodense on CT scanning. These authors concluded that in the majority of high-grade and low-grade glial tumors, tumor infiltration occurred in the re-

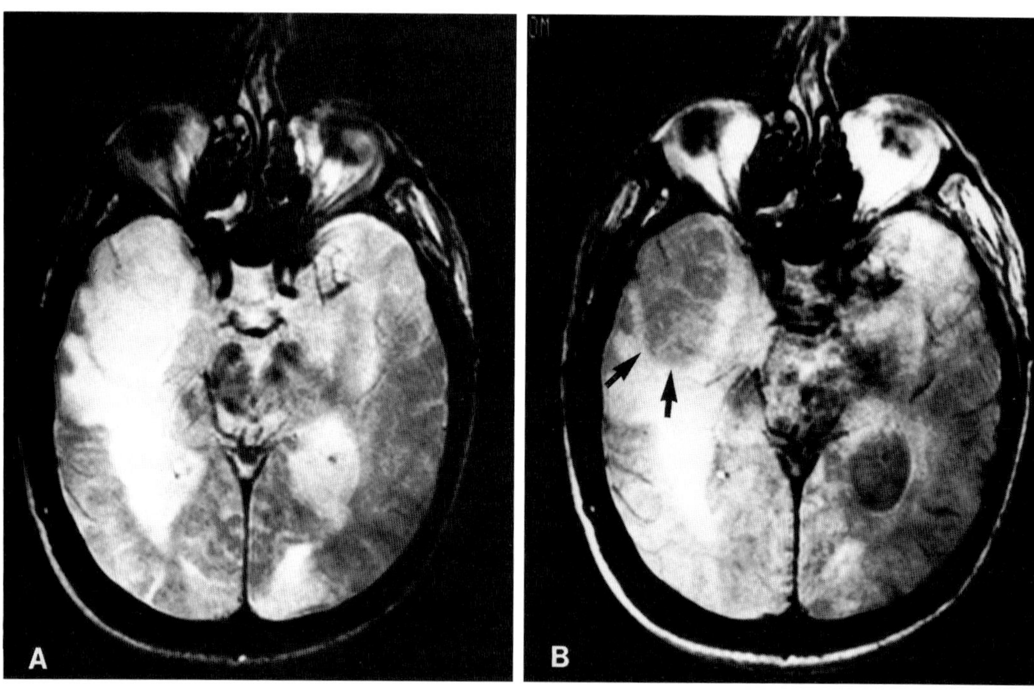

Figure 6–6. (*A*) A T_2-weighted MRI (TR 2100, TE 30) demonstrates an area of increased signal in the left temporal region, reflecting an increased water content in this glioma and in surrounding edematous brain. (*B*) A proton density (intermediate-echo) MRI scan (TR 2100, TE 60) in the same patient shows the margins of the tumor itself more clearly (*arrows*).

gion of T_2 prolongation. Furthermore, 50% of biopsies of brain adjacent to that with T_2 prolongation revealed infiltrating tumor cells. Thus, tumor infiltration could occur beyond the limits of abnormalities seen on MRI. These findings have dramatic implications for the planning of regional therapy.

A similar histopathologic correlation study using stereotaxic biopsies of contrast-enhanced regions on MRI[59] demonstrated that gadolinium-labeled diethylenetriamine penta-acetic acid enhancement on T_1-weighted MR images was equal to or greater than that seen on contrast-enhanced x-ray CT in four of six gliomas. As in CT studies, Gd-DTPA enhancement corresponded histopathologically to regions of neovascularity and endothelial proliferation. Central zones of decreased intensity corresponded to necrosis pathologically. Tumor boundaries could not be defined by contrast enhancement on T_1- or T_2-weighted MR imaging. This study concluded that x-ray CT and MRI were insensitive in identifying tumor boundaries and that histologic assessment was required.

Preliminary studies[39] suggest that Gd-DTPA–enhanced MRI may be useful in differentiating postoperative scar from recurrent or residual tumor, but further studies are necessary to confirm this. Gd-DTPA–enhanced studies also have proved sensitive in the diagnosis of leptomeningeal metastases.[189] Because the T_1 and T_2 relaxation times are similar for tumor nodules and proteinaceous CSF, unenhanced MRI has been insensitive in the diagnosis of these metastases.

It has been postulated that T_1 and/or T_2 images could be used in determining tumor cell type,[43] but the results thus far have not validated this hypothesis. The use of calculated T_2 values for lesion identification has been studied.[43] Infarcts, gliomas, and multiple sclerosis plaques all display a wide range of overlapping values. Although MRI is more sensitive than x-ray CT in the detection of small tumors, CT may be more specific, as in the CT demonstration of subtle calcifications in oligodendrogliomas.[19]

Recently, MRI has been used to evaluate blood flow.* This work is based on the principle that the motion of magnetic nuclei within a field relative to an external field gradient will alter the precession frequency and phase angle of nuclei in the field. Although this measurement demonstrates blood flow effects and does not directly quantify flow or perfusion, the development of this technique holds promise for the future and may be able to provide an estimate of tumor blood flow (see Chapter 13). Regional MR spectroscopy promises to provide additional valuable information. Evaluations of the metabolic state of tissues have already been carried out with ^{31}P spectra to quantitate adenosine triphosphate (ATP), phosphocreatine and inorganic phosphate. Studies of implanted neuroectodermal tumors derived from primary brain tumors have shown low phosphocreatine and high phosphomonoester levels compared with those in the normal brain.[140] Sequential ^{31}P MR spectroscopy may provide important metabolic information on tumor growth and response to treatment. As more expertise and information are accumulated, spectroscopy may be used in the future to evaluate a variety of biologic processes in tumors and surrounding tissues.

SPECT

Functional imaging studies with PET and SPECT complement anatomic images derived from x-ray CT or MRI. The physiologic information available from these techniques, however, can and should be correlated with structural information available with CT and MRI. Most SPECT agents have been used to estimate cerebral blood flow (CBF) or perfusion in neoplasms. To date, however, except for large, highly vascular tumors such as meningiomas

*References 19,58,76,89,112,141,180,181.

or glioblastomas, CBF studies have had limited ability to detect tumors, determine their type, or predict their behavior.

An exception to this rule has been the use of thallium-SPECT imaging to differentiate between high- and low-grade gliomas. In a series of 25 such patients,[110] thallium-201 retention indices were able to differentiate the spectrum of malignancies in the glioma series with a mean thallium index of 1.27 ± 0.40 in 14 patients with low-grade gliomas, as compared to a mean index of $2.40 + 0.61$ in 11 patients with high-grade gliomas. Classification errors using this technique were found to be related to partial-volume effects due to the limited spatial resolution of SPECT instrumentation. This work also demonstrated that the use of routine attenuation correction for SPECT improved the sensitivity of the technique (Fig. 6–7).

IMAGING BBB DEFECTS

As mentioned previously, the tight junctions of the capillary endothelial cells in normal brain are disrupted in brain tumors. A defect in the BBB can be seen on electron microscopy as fenestrated endothelium, gaps between endothelial cells, and increased pinocytosis, allowing the passage of charged ions and macromolecules from the vascular space into the brain parenchyma.[129] Abnormal BBB permeability has been used with contrast-enhanced CT, Gd-EDTA MRI and ^{99m}Tc-pertechnetate imaging[70] to visualize intracranial tumors such as gliomas. Gallium-67 citrate, a single-photon–emitting isotope, rapidly accumulates in brain tumors and has proved useful in the diagnosis of intracerebral gliomas using conventional radionuclide brain scanning.[102,121,207]

Potassium transport across the BBB

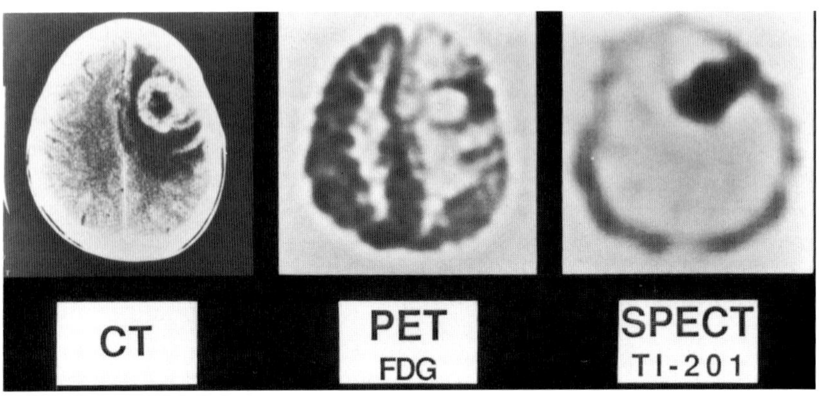

Figure 6–7. Frontal lobe glioblastoma imaged with x-ray CT, PET, and SPECT. The CT image (*left*), performed after iodinated contrast material was administered intravenously, demonstrates a ring-shaped zone of increased attenuation surrounding a central zone of reduced attenuation consistent with a necrotic central core. Edema surrounding the lesion is manifest as low attenuation throughout the frontal lobe and extending posteriorly into the anterior parietal lobe. The PET study (*center*), performed after the administration of FDG to measure glucose metabolism, demonstrates the necrotic tumor core as an ametabolic zone surrounded by a region of hypermetabolism, indicative of a high-grade glioma. Hypometabolism of the frontal cortex surrounding the tumor reflects its dysfunction secondary to mass effect, edema, and neuronal disconnection. The SPECT study, performed after administration of ^{201}Tl, shows uptake in the scalp and the tumor as well as its central core. Normally ^{201}Tl is excluded from the brain parenchyma by the BBB. Studies are underway to determine if the degree of thallium uptake correlates with the degree of malignancy in the tumor. (Courtesy of B Guze and JC Mazziotta, UCLA School of Medicine.)

is thought to be regulated by endothelial ATPases, and the normal brain is relatively impermeable to potassium cations. Rubidium-82 (^{82}Rb), a positron-emitting cation (half-life = 75 seconds) that acts in a manner analogous to potassium ions, has been employed with PET to evaluate the BBB. The extraction of ^{82}Rb is significantly increased in tumors relative to normal brain; this increase is directly proportional to the degree of contrast enhancement seen on x-ray CT imaging.[18] There is, however, no correlation between ^{82}Rb extraction and glioma grade. Rubidium-82 extraction is normal in areas of peritumoral edema, consistent with the normal potassium level seen in regions of vasogenic (as opposed to cytotoxic) edema.[95] Another compound used with PET for evaluation of the BBB is gallium-68-EDTA, a nondiffusible, biologically inert tracer. Both ^{82}Rb and ^{68}Ga are available through generator systems (^{82}Sr/^{82}Rb and ^{68}Ge/^{68}Ga generators respectively; see Chapter 3). PET ^{68}Ga-EDTA scans are somewhat more sensitive in the detection of BBB abnormalities than x-ray CT imaging.[136,148] There is a relationship between ^{68}Ga-EDTA uptake and tumor type, with malignant gliomas demonstrating the highest uptake and low-grade gliomas showing the least uptake[98] (Fig. 6–8).

PET EVALUATIONS OF GLIOMA METABOLISM, BLOOD FLOW, pH AND AMINO ACID UPTAKE

Metabolism. Since the original observations of Warburg on the rate of aerobic glycolysis of tumor slices in vitro,[205] it has been apparent that the metabolism of tumors differs in many ways from that of normal tissue. Accelerated glycolysis is probably one of the most widely accepted biochemical signatures of the malignant state.[204,208] It is accompanied by accelerated activity for the key rate-controlling enzymes of glycolysis, including hexokinase, phosphofructokinase, and pyruvate dehydrogenase.[204] The neoplastic transformation of certain cell lines has been shown to be associated with a functional increase in the cell membrane's ability to transport glucose, and cancer cells have been demonstrated to have an enzyme composition that favors this increased glycolysis. Investigators[72,184] have demonstrated that ^{18}F-fluorodeoxyglucose (FDG), a fluorinated glucose analog, is rapidly taken up by tumor cells with sufficiently high tumor-to-normal-tissue and tumor-to-blood ratios for tumor localization. Absolute quantification of the local cerebral metabolic rate of glucose utilization (LCMRGlc) in rats with intracranial tumors by compartmental kinetic modeling with ^{14}C-labeled deoxyglucose and autoradiography was developed by Sokoloff[182] (see Chapter 3).

The application of PET to the study of cerebral gliomas is not new. Pioneered by the work of Di Chiro and colleagues,[50,51,53,54,152] it has been determined that glucose metabolism is correlated with histologic grade of gliomas. Higher-grade lesions typically have metabolism that equals or exceeds that of normal gray matter, whereas low-grade lesions have metabolic rates that are less than or equal to that of white matter.[51] Increased FDG uptake has also been demonstrated in other tumors, including sarcomas,[109] head and neck cancers,[135] and lymphomas.[154] The use of FDG to evaluate cerebral gliomas is becoming a clinical practice, as has the application of this technique to the differential diagnosis of recurrent tumor versus radiation-induced brain necrosis.[54]

More recently, it has been determined that other intracerebral lesions such as abscesses[174] can have the qualitative appearance of cerebral gliomas on PET and also have high metabolic rates, presumably because of the high utilization of glucose by macrophages and other white blood cells in the wall of the abscess cavity.

In the original report by Di Chiro and associates,[51] 28 studies were performed

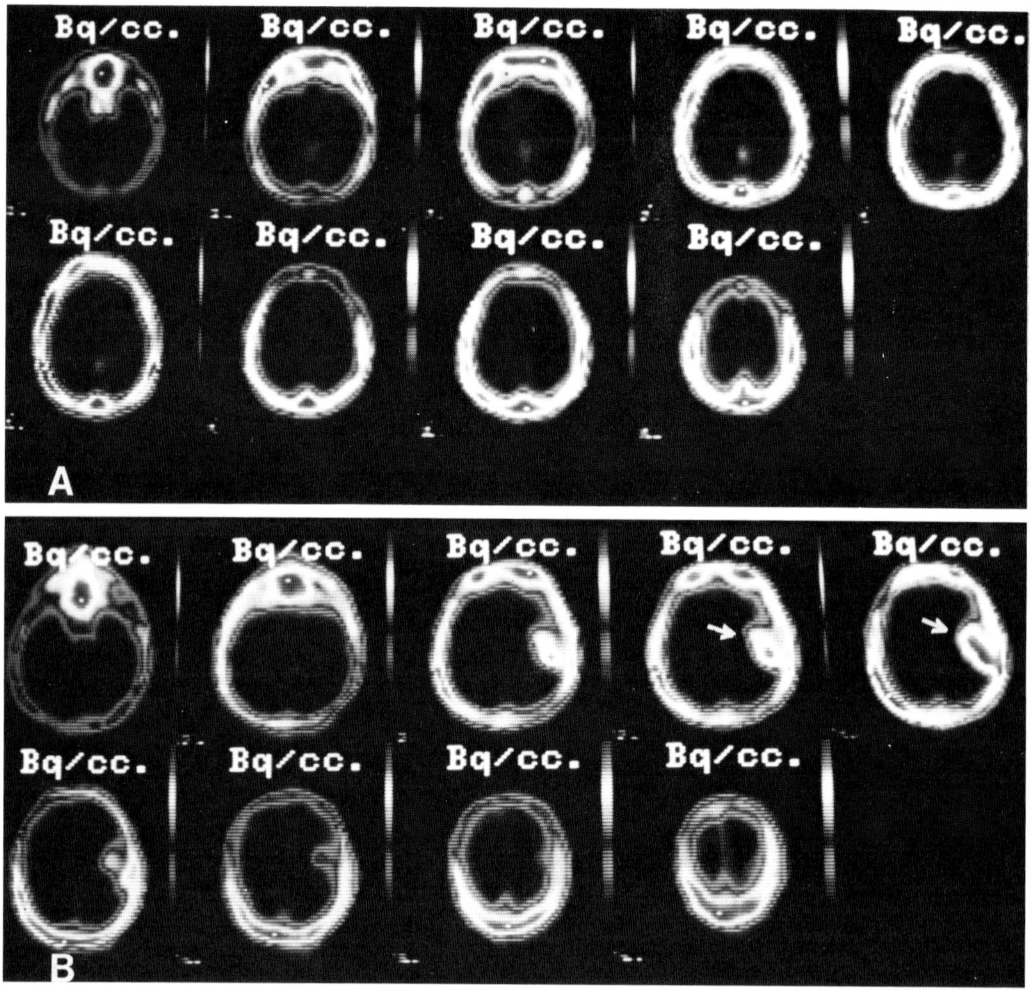

Figure 6–8. (*A*) ^{68}Ga-EDTA tomographic images in a patient with a grade I astrocytoma. Tomographic cuts were obtained at 9-mm intervals, starting at the inferior orbitomeatal (OM) line (*upper left-hand scan*). No disruption of the BBB is seen. (*B*) In similar tomographic images of a patient with a grade IV astrocytoma, ^{68}Ga-EDTA clearly demonstrates an area of BBB breakdown (*arrows*) around the tumor.

in 23 patients. A positive correlation was found between tumor grade and tumor glucose metabolism. In this group, 14 patients were scanned before surgery, chemotherapy, or radiation therapy. Of these cases, half had histologic confirmation of the grade of the tumor. While there was overlap between low-grade and high-grade lesions, in general, the groups were separable.

A different group of investigators[166] studied seven patients, five before treatment, in whom tumor regional glucose consumption did not differ significantly from that of the contralateral cortex. A study of 16 patients with cerebral gliomas scanned before any treatment demonstrated variable metabolism of the gliomas (Fig. 6–9, Table 6–2).[194] The findings of variable rates of glucose metabolism in gliomas indicate that this parameter, taken alone, may not be absolutely reliable as a predictor of tumor grade in untreated gliomas, and that there may be significant differences in glioma metabolism before and after therapy. The variabil-

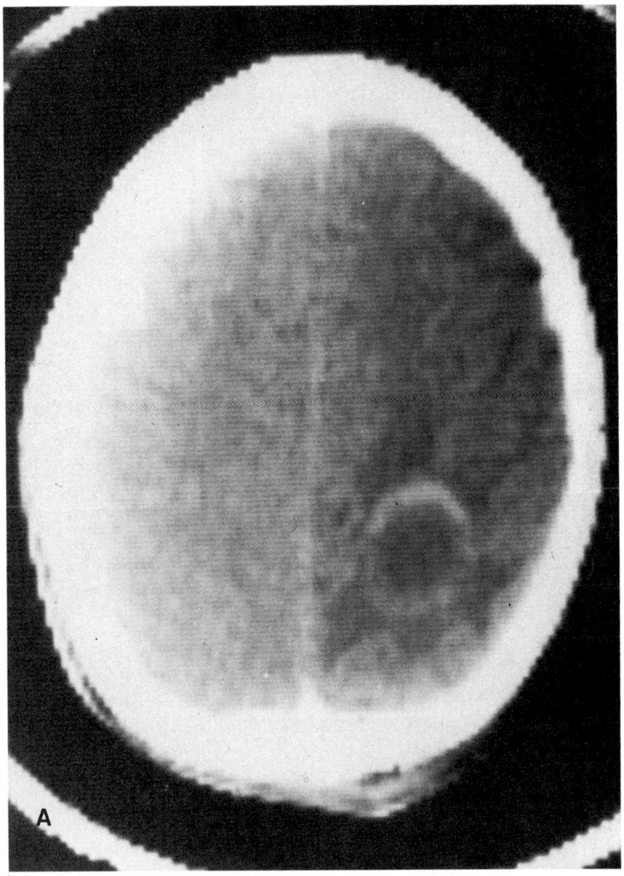

Figure 6–9. (*A*) An x-ray CT scan shows a grade IV glioma in the right parietal region. PET scans of the same area show

ity in the findings of different investigators studying tumor glucose metabolism may be related to several factors. The duration of the patient's illness, the amount of tumor necrosis, the criteria for determining tumor grade, partial-volume effects, and data acquisition and analysis techniques can all affect the results. For example, a better correlation exists between tumor grade and glucose metabolism when peak values are used within the tumor mass for assignment of metabolic rates, as opposed to the use of average values for the entire tumor. This is logical because these tumors tend to be heterogeneous and prognosis is based on the areas having the highest growth rates and, therefore, highest malignancy potential. Another critical factor may be prior treatment of the tumor, and most of the reports in the literature have concerned a combination of treated and untreated patients. There may be differences in the metabolism of malignant cells before and after exposure to radiation and chemotherapy, so that despite the cells' similar pathologic appearances, variable metabolic results may be found. Alternatively, attempts at tumor cell killing with radiation and chemotherapy may select for the most malignant cell types, which have more aggressive metabolic characteristics and higher rates of glucose metabolism.

PET studies of tumor glucose and oxygen metabolism are in agreement with many in vitro studies, which have demonstrated alterations in glycolytic metabolism,[73,205] decreased numbers of mitochondria[157] and depressed activity of the electron transport system.[126]

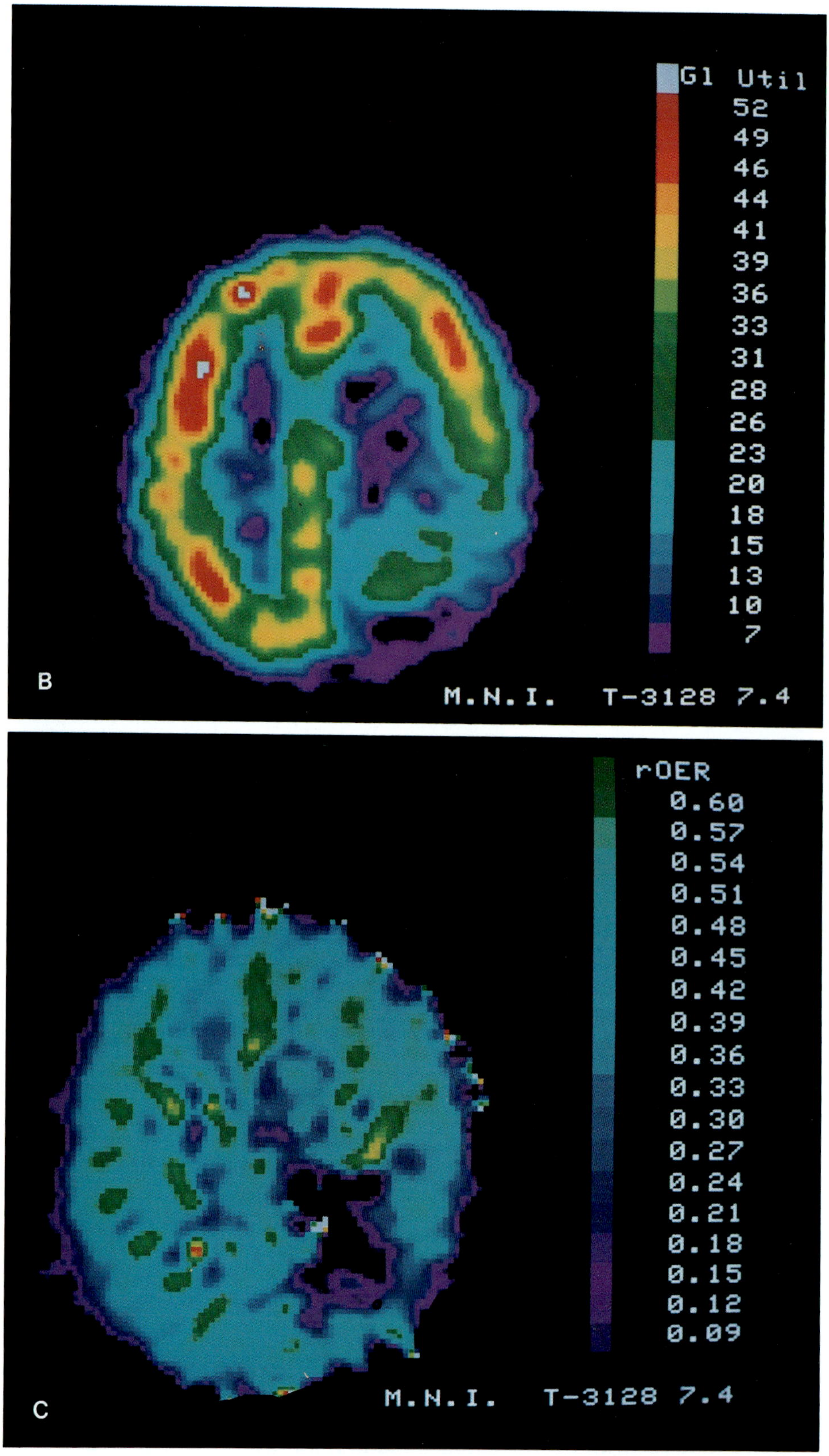

Figure 6–9. *Continued.* (*B*) low glucose metabolism (measured in μmol per 100 g tissue per minute); (*C*) low oxygen extraction (measured as a fraction of 1.00, with normal being 0.45);

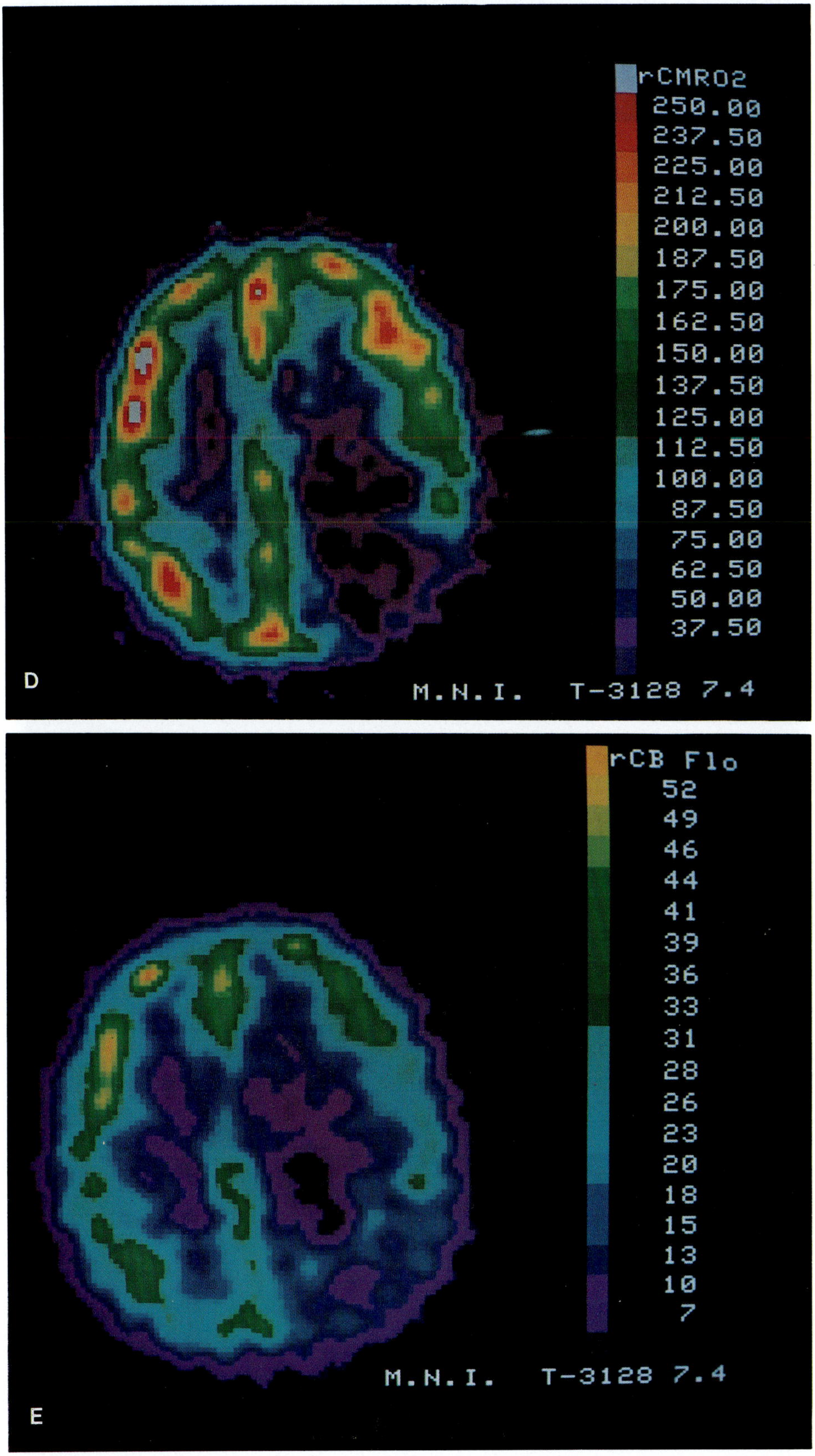

Figure 6–9. *Continued.* (*D*) low oxygen utilization (in μmol per 100 g per minute); (*E*) low blood flow (in ml per 100 g per minute);

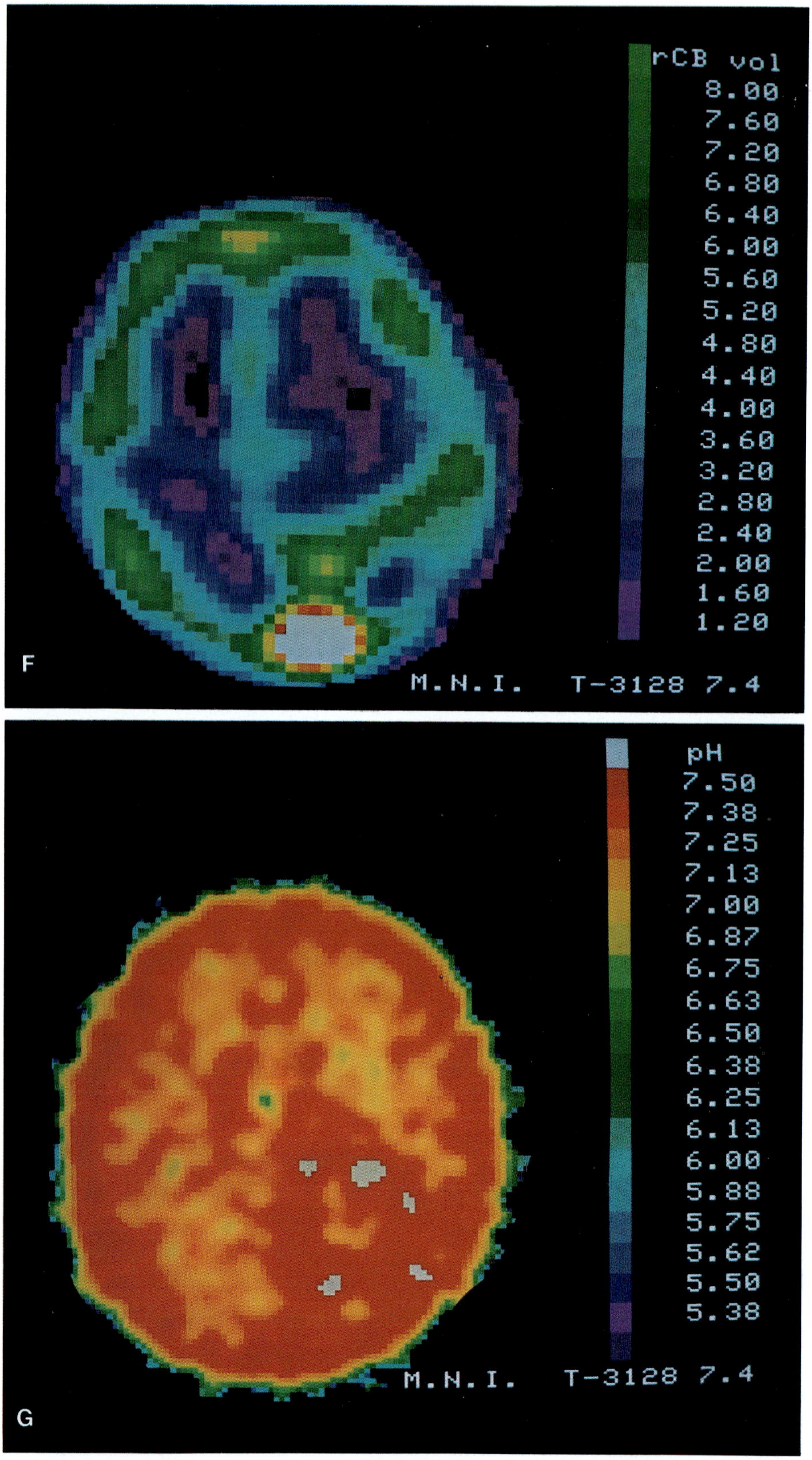

Figure 6–9. *Continued.* (*F*) increased blood volume (as a percentage of brain volume); and (*G*) alkalotic pH relative to contralateral cortex. Scans are located approximately 79 mm above the orbitomeatal line. (From Tyler et al,[194] p. 1127, with permission.)

Table 6–2 METABOLIC AND HEMODYNAMIC RESULTS IN 16 PATIENTS WITH PET GLIOMAS

Patient No.	Tumor Grade	LCMRGlc* Mean	LCMRGlc* Range	CBF†	CBV‡	OER§	$CMRO_2$¶	MR** = $CMRO_2$/LCMRGlc	pH
4	II	22	(17–31)	43	4.3	0.41	132	6.00	—
7	II	25	(20–34)	46	5.9	0.29	112	4.48	—
Mean ±SD		23.5 ±2.1		45 ±2	4.8 ±0.6	0.35 ±0.08	122 ±14	5.24 ±1.07	
10	III	25	(10–38)	14	3.6	0.46	66	2.64	7.34
2	III	28	(12–31)	63	5.4	0.15	106	3.79	—
1	IV	19	(8–35)	31	7.3	0.27	80	4.21	—
3	IV	35	(32–37)	45	5.1	0.18	69	1.97	—
5	IV	32	(25–53)	62	8.2	0.13	102	3.19	7.35
6	IV	39	(20–65)	30	6.0	0.25	62	1.59	—
8	IV	24	(15–35)	24	3.8	0.21	42	1.75	—
9	IV	42	(24–56)	25	10.0	0.12	25	0.60	—
11	IV	25	(20–39)	20	4.2	0.40	77	3.08	—
12	IV	27	(19–42)	42	5.7	0.21	90	3.33	6.99
13	IV	25	(19–33)	23	6.4	0.42	88	3.52	6.81
14	IV	16	(10–22)	13	3.7	0.44	65	7.06	7.06
15	IV	18	(10–25)	19	6.3	0.27	46	2.56	7.43
16	IV	23	(18–26)	20	5.9	0.40	109	4.74	7.18
Mean ±SD		27 ±7.7		31 ±16	5.8 ±1.8	0.28 ±0.12	73 ±25	2.93 ±1.15	
Normal Values (±SD)	—	45.5 2.9	(39–51)	39.8 7.8	3.2 0.7	0.48 0.05	171 32	3.77 0.75	7.00

*LCMRGlc (local cerebral metabolic rate for glucose) in μmol/100 g tissue per min.
†CBF (cerebral blood flow) in ml/100 g per min.
‡CBV (cerebral blood volume) as a fraction of 100%.
§OER (oxygen extraction ratio) as a percentage of 1.00.
¶$CMRO_2$ (cerebral metabolic rate for oxygen) in μmol/100 g tissue per min.
**MR (metabolic rate) as the ratio of oxygen to glucose utilization.
Adapted from Tyler et al,[194] p. 1125.

This is evidenced by decreased metabolic ratio (MR = $CMRO_2$/LCMRGlc) as seen on combined FDG and ^{15}O PET study of metabolism.[166,194] The derangement of metabolic ratio may be due to a primary depression in oxygen metabolism or a release of glucose utilization from its normal control.[16]

Blood Flow. Because cancer cells grown in vitro have abnormal rates of glycolysis and impaired respiratory capacity,[205] there has been considerable interest in the application of PET techniques to study tumor oxygen metabolism and hemodynamics in vivo. Cerebral blood flow and the cerebral metabolic rate for oxygen ($CMRO_2$) have been evaluated with steady-state inhalation of ^{15}O PET[100] (see Fig. 6–9). Although early studies were limited by small, mixed-patient groups, the findings demonstrated a relative uncoupling of tumor blood flow and oxygen consumption. Low levels of oxygen extraction (OER) were seen in these tumors, with normal OER values in edematous tissue, and increased OER in nontumor cerebral tissue (Table 6–3). Other studies of tumor oxidative metabolism[100,117,166,194] also have reported that both oxygen extraction and consumption are decreased (Figs. 6–9 and 6–10, Table 6–2).

Tumor blood flow in gliomas is variable but is generally lower than that of normal cortex[117,166,192,194] (see Fig. 6–9, Tables 6–2 and 6–3). Blood volume in gliomas is also variable,[117] but is typically higher[194] (see Table 6–2) in gliomas than in normal cortex (see Figs. 6–9 and 6–10). It is now known that quantitation of tumor blood volume is necessary not only for the information it provides about the tumor itself, but also for correct quantification of $CMRO_2$ and OER[118] (Chapter 3). Without CBV correction, both OER and $CMRO_2$ tend to be overestimated, due to the signal from intravascular ^{15}O. The correction is especially important in the situation of low regional OER and high CBV, as occurs in intracerebral gliomas.

Glioma pH. Because most enzymes are acutely sensitive to fluctuations in pH,[28,40] pathologic alterations in tissue pH would be expected to alter tissue metabolism. Changes in pH also may affect the distribution and action of drugs such as chemotherapeutic agents[143] and affect the response of tumors to radiotherapy.[170]

Because of the important role that pH plays in the behavior of cells, attempts have been made to use PET to evaluate glioma pH in vivo. Measurements using CO_2[162] and the weak acid dimethyloxazolidinedione (DMO)[169] labeled with ^{11}C have shown that primary intracranial tumor tissue pH (both extracellular and intracellular) is more alkalotic than that of normal gray matter (see Figs. 6–9 and 6–10).[25,169,194] Although DMO measurement of pH is not without error,[25,169] the consistency of the findings suggests that this information about relative regional tissue pH may complement other metabolic information obtained form glucose and oxygen metabolism studies, and may prove to

Table 6–3 PET MEASUREMENTS OF BLOOD FLOW AND OXYGEN UTILIZATION OF TUMORS AND CEREBRAL TISSUES*

	CBF (mL/100g per min)	*OER*	*$LCMRO_2$ (μmol/100g per min)*
Tumors	19 (10)	0.34 (0.03)	58 (31)
Edema	13 (4)	0.49 (0.09)	54 (22)
Contralateral gray	32 (7)	0.57 (0.06)	156 (31)
Normals	46 (9)	0.52 (0.10)	183 (36)

*Mean values (±SD)
From Ito, et al.,[100] p. 68, with permission.

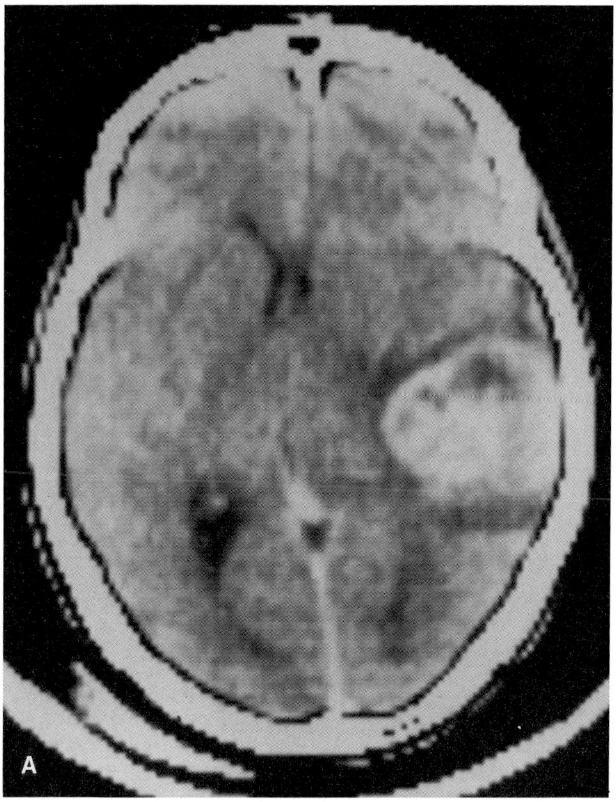

Figure 6–10. (*A*) An x-ray CT scan shows a grade IV right parietal glioma. PET scans demonstrate

have therapeutic implications for the design of radiotherapy and chemotherapy protocols.

Amino Acid Uptake. PET imaging also has been used with radiolabeled amino acids to evaluate amino acid uptake and protein synthesis. The establishment of a biological model for amino acid utilization is difficult, since labeled amino acids may be incorporated into carbohydrates, neurotransmitters, and neuropeptides, as well as protein. A variety of amino acids has been found to accumulate preferentially in tumors: D,L-tryptophan[96]; D,L-valine[96]; L-methionine[13,29,63,127]; L-leucine[87]; and L-tyrosine.[88] This accumulation does not appear to be due solely to a disruption in the BBB.[63,127] In fact, low-grade tumors may be better delineated on amino acid PET imaging than on x-ray CT scans or ^{68}Ga-EDTA or FDG-PET studies (Fig. 6–11).[63,127] Of the amino acids, ^{11}C-methionine has been studied most extensively. It is well suited for PET scanning because it functions as an essential amino acid that is not synthesized or recycled in the brain, and because of its relatively slow rate of transmethylation.[29] Carbon 11-labeled methionine has been found to accumulate readily in gliomas, and there are indications that this degree of uptake gives an approximation of the rate of protein synthesis and correlates with tumor grade.[29]

The concept of tumor detection with amino acids is based on achieving significant metabolic differences in the incorporation of labeled amino acids into neoplastic versus nonneoplastic tissue. Labeled amino acid concentrations may be greater in tumor cells as a consequence of cell membrane changes that permit increased amino acid transport. Both natural amino acids and their analogs have been labeled with ^{11}C, as noted above, and studied in both labora-

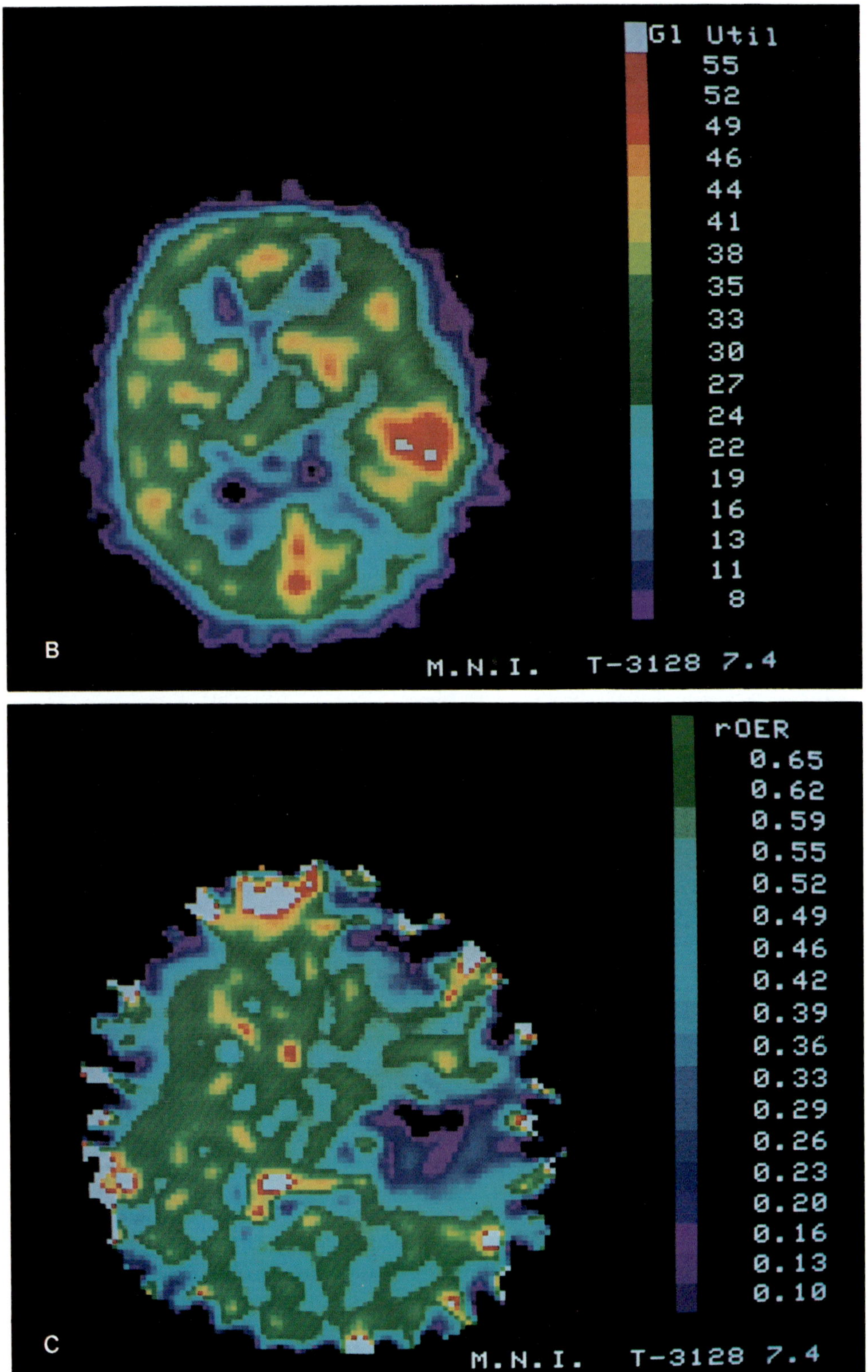

Figure 6–10. *Continued.* (*B*) increased glucose metabolism, (*C*) low oxygen extraction,

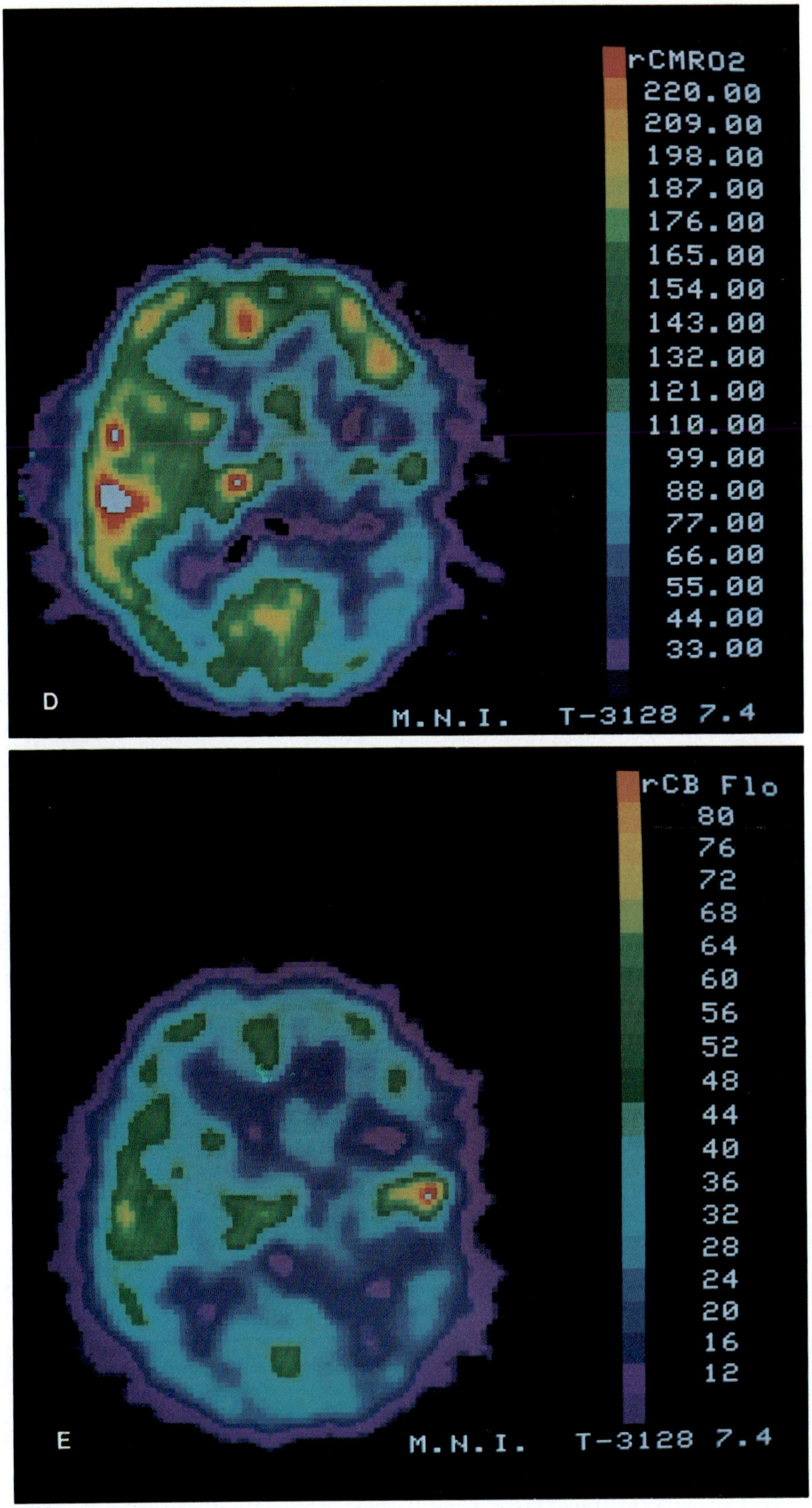

Figure 6–10. *Continued.* (*D*) low oxygen consumption, (*E*) high blood flow,

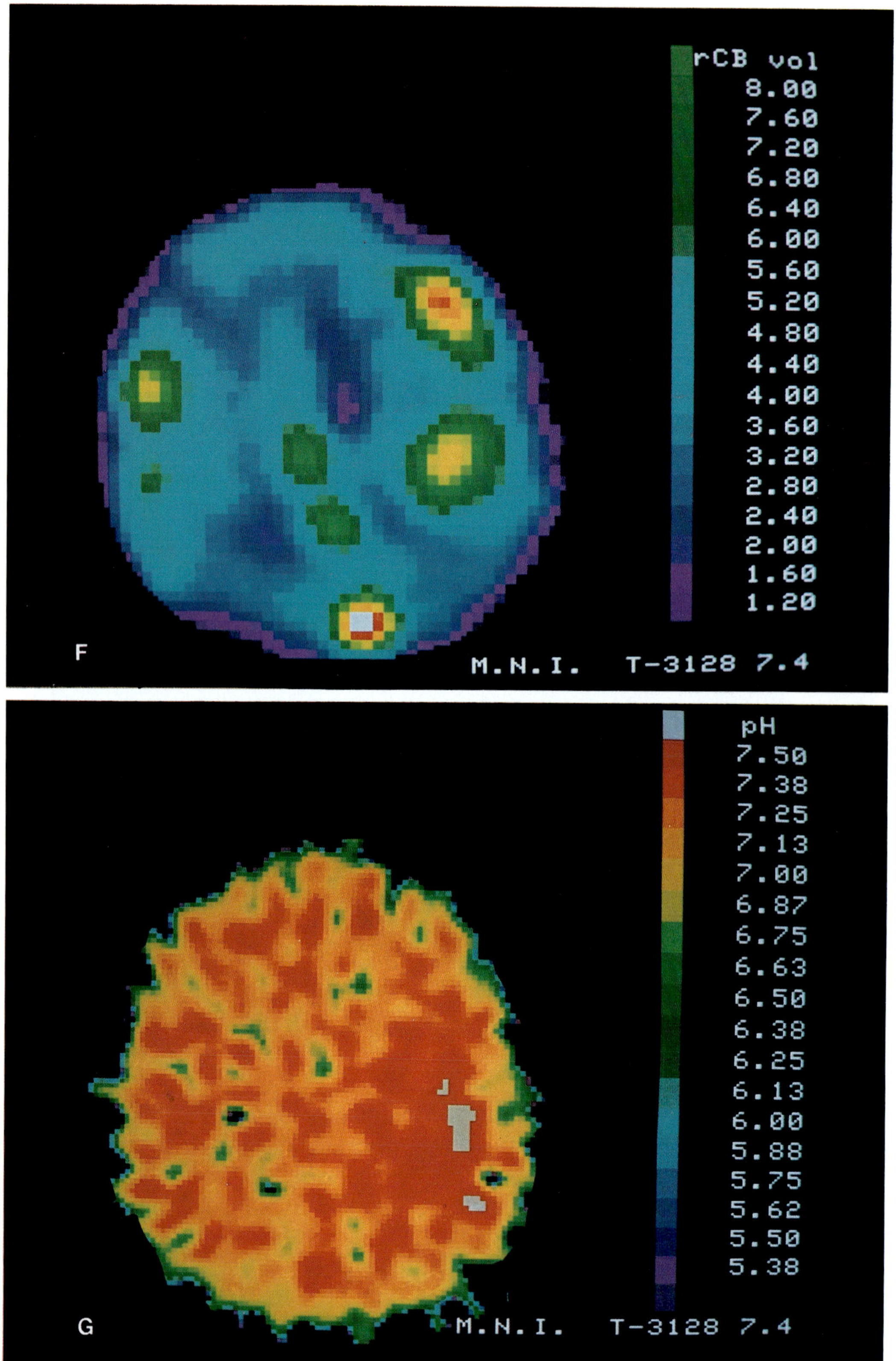

Figure 6–10. *Continued.* (*F*) high blood volume, and (*G*) alkalotic pH. Note that while glucose metabolism was within the normal range in the tumor, it was suppressed in other areas of the right hemisphere; a similar right-sided remote suppression of oxygen metabolism was seen. (Metabolic units are the same as those detailed in Fig. 6–9.) These scans are located approximately 50 mm above the OM line. (From Tyler et al.,[194] p 1128, with permission.)

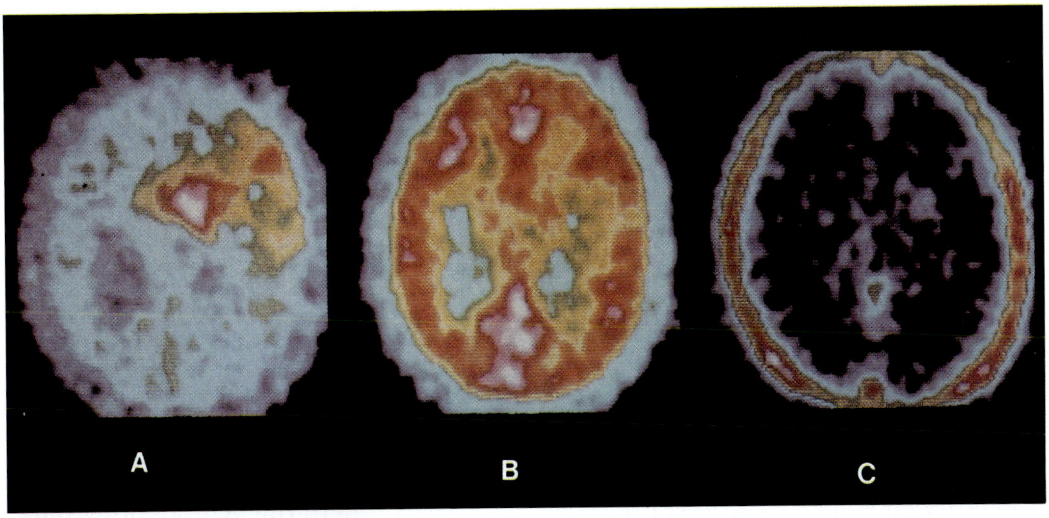

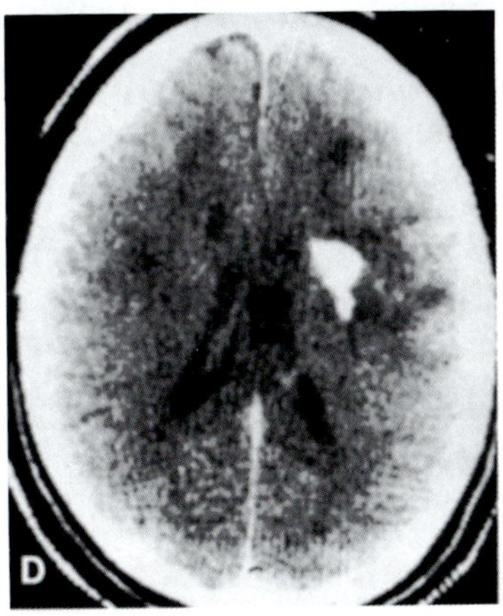

Figure 6–11. (*A*) An ^{11}C-methionine study in a patient with an oligoastrocytoma demonstrates intense accumulation in a large area extending across the midline. (*B*) An FDG study in the same patient demonstrates decreased glucose uptake, and (*C*) the ^{68}Ga-EDTA study shows no evidence of BBB disruption. (*D*) An x-ray CT scan reveals an expanding lesion with irregular hypodense areas and a central calcification, without contrast enhancement. (From Ericson et al.,[63] p. 685, with permission)

tory animals and in humans.[114,206] Several studies have compared the uptake of these compounds in different human tumors, including astrocytomas, pancreatic cancers, and bronchogenic carcinomas.* A study of children with brain tumors using ^{11}C-labeled L-methionine and PET[150] demonstrated that, in patients with high-grade astrocytomas, medulloblastomas or ependymomas, tumor-to-brain uptake ratios were 1.5 ± 0.57. Retention was lower in lower-grade lesions.

*References 12–14,29,63,64,88,99,206.

Other Areas of PET Investigation. Recent investigations using PET to identify various biochemical aspects of cerebral gliomas have included the application of positron-emitting analogs of nucleosides such as deoxyuridine.[193a] This compound, labeled with ^{18}F, has been effectively localized in rodent models of gliomas with a tumor-to-background ratio of 12 : 1. Additionally, ^{11}C-labeled thymidine has been synthesized[178] as a PET-measurable indicator of DNA synthesis in neoplasms. The application of this approach to the study of cerebral gliomas seems inevitable. Another area of recent PET investigation has been in the labeling of neurotransmitter receptors in the diagnosis and evaluation of brain tumors. Human glioma cell lines grown in nude mice and rats have shown selective binding of two peripheral benzodiazepine receptors, flunitrazepam and PK 11195.[10,38,130] Binding sites appear to be located in cell nuclei and/or mitochondria, and the binding of labeled compounds is blocked by the pre-administration of unlabeled PK 11195. Studies of such receptor binding may prove more accurate than currently used metabolic studies, such as glucose metabolism, in defining areas of viable tumor and in assessing responses to treatment. It is not yet fully determined, however, how specific these markers will be for gliomas; early indications are that they may label numerous alterations in glial tissues and macrophages, such as those that can be induced by infarction or inflammation.

Meningiomas

These typically benign tumors comprise approximately 15% of all primary intracerebral neoplasms. They are more common in women than men (2 : 1) and have their peak incidence in the seventh decade of life. As noted above, they frequently are found along the dural surfaces, particularly at the base of the brain, along the falx cerebri, and at the tentorium. Malignant forms are more rarely found. Prognosis and outcome frequently depend on the initial size at the time of diagnosis and on their location, which dictates surgical accessibility.

ANGIOGRAPHY

The highly vascular nature of meningiomas becomes apparent by their characteristic appearance on angiography. Meningiomas are most commonly located in the Sylvian region, superior parasagittal surface of the frontal and parietal lobes, olfactory grooves, lesser wings of the sphenoid bones, tuberculum sellae, superior surface of the cerebellum, cerebellopontine angle, and spinal canal. They may show a direct meningeal blood supply and they typically demonstrate a marked vascular "blush" on angiography (Fig. 6–12).[8]

X-RAY CT

Because of their extra-axial location, dural attachments, and vascularity, meningiomas have a characteristic appearance on enhanced x-ray CT images (Figure 6–12*B*).[38] Approximately 97% of meningiomas have a nodular appearance on CT and 59% are surrounded by edema.[188] The diagnostic accuracy of CT scanning in the evaluation of meningiomas approaches 100% in a technically optimal study.[145]

Using an early-generation CT x-ray scanner, Vassilouthis and Ambrose[196] identified CT characteristics that correlated with histologic subtypes of meningiomas. The x-ray CT appearances of 102 meningiomas confirmed at operation formed the basis of their study. These authors found that calcium aggregates suggested a diagnosis of transitional or fibroblastic meningioma. The tumor attenuation seen on precontrast studies did not correlate with histologic subtypes, but homogeneous enhancement was most commonly seen in transitional types. Angioblastic and syncytial types commonly demonstrated nonenhancing "cystic" areas surrounded by irregular, poorly defined tumor margins. Transitional, fibroblastic, or mixed fibroblastic and transitional variants were typically characterized by well-defined shapes. The x-ray CT characteristics that typically predicted an aggressive or invasive meningioma of the angioblastic or syncytial subtypes included absence of calcium aggregates and marked peritumoral edema, nonhomogeneous contrast enhancement with a nonenhancing "cystic" portion, and poorly defined, irregular margins.

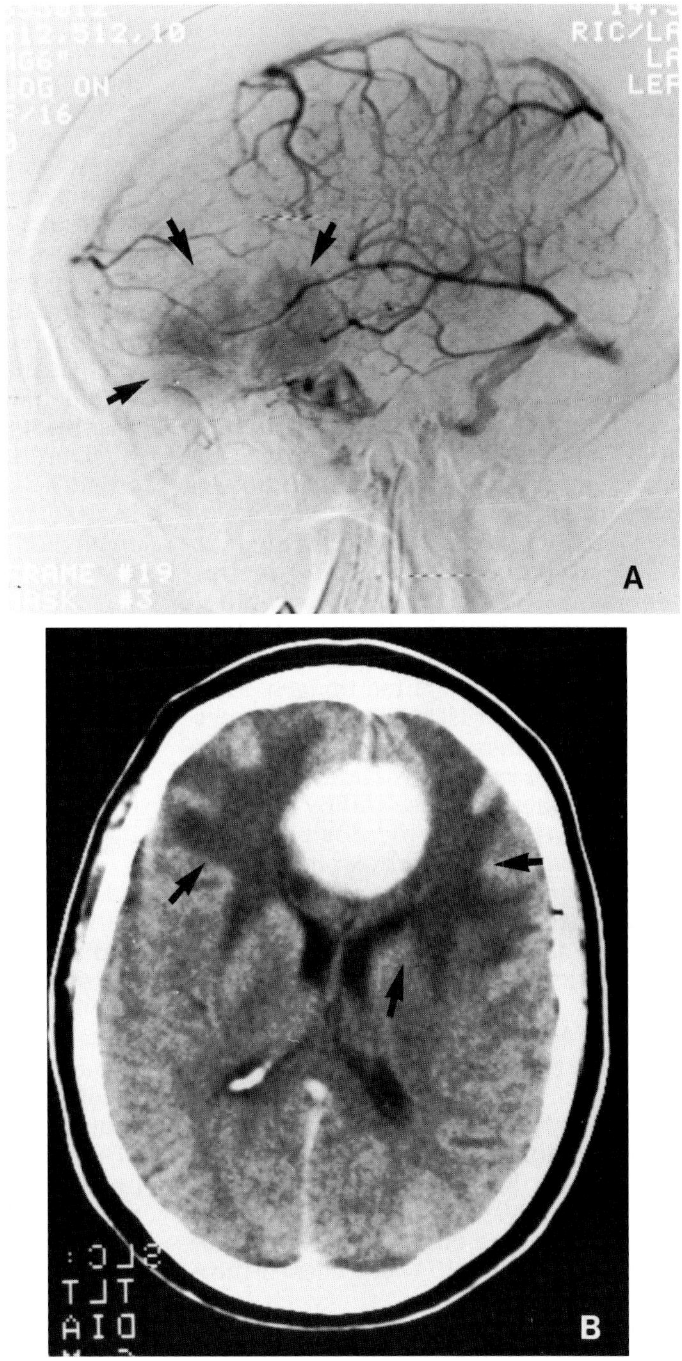

Figure 6–12. (*A*) The left-lateral-view angiogram demonstrates the markedly increased vascularity in a large midline meningioma (*arrows*). (*B*) The well-demarcated, intense enhancement in the lesion on CT scan is typical of these tumors. Note marked peritumoral edema (*arrows*).

MRI

MRI has a predictive accuracy of 86% in the diagnosis and evaluation of meningiomas.[133] Meningiomas demonstrate relatively short T_1 and T_2 values compared with other tumors.[115] Despite its superiority in detecting small lesions, MRI is not able to demonstrate subtle calcifications that can be seen readily on x-ray CT, and for this reason, CT may be more specific than MRI in the diagnosis of meningioma in certain patients.

In one study of 25 patients with meningiomas,[185] the lesions showed low signal intensity on T_1-weighted images and increased signal intensity on T_2-weighted images, relative to white matter.[185] Relative to the cortex, meningiomas were reportedly low or equal in signal intensity on T_1-weighted images, and showed equal or increased signal intensity on T_2-weighted images. Meningiomas were distinguished by a heterogeneous signal pattern probably resulting from vascular structures, cystic foci and calcifications, and by an interface between the meningioma and brain composed of cerebrospinal fluid, a vascular rim, or a dural margin. MRI was judged to be superior to x-ray CT in defining location, vascularity, arterial encasement, and venous-sinus invasion.[185]

There have been recent attempts to correlate the MRI appearance of meningiomas with the histologic pattern. One study[62] reported that whereas T_1-weighted images were not useful in discriminating between histologic types, signal intensity and features on T_2-weighted images correlated with histologic findings in 75% of cases. Fibroblastic or transitional subtypes were typically hypointense to cortex on T_2-weighted images. Alternatively, syncytial or angioblastic subtypes were generally hyperintense. Other features such as calcification, cyst formation, and edema helped to predict histopathologic subtypes further.

Gadolinium-DTPA–enhanced MRI has been useful in aiding in the diagnosis of meningiomas.[86] There may still be difficulty, however, in differentiating meningiomas from other extra-axial lesions such as nerve sheath tumors in the cerebellopontine angle. Atypical meningiomas with cyst formation or hemorrhage may also be difficult to diagnose even with the use of Gd-DTPA–enhanced MRI. Goldsher and colleagues,[81] however, found a linear enhancing "tail" extending from the tumor mass along the dural surface in 60% of meningiomas, which differentiated meningiomas from other extra-axial lesions. This "tail" was not demonstrated on the x-ray CT scans of these tumors. Pathologic material demonstrated meningothelial tumor nodules in regions that corresponded to the "tail."

SPECT

The SPECT techniques described in the foregoing section on cerebral gliomas are all applicable to the study of meningiomas.

BBB IMAGING

Meningiomas cause significant abnormalities of the BBB and readily accumulate agents such as ^{99m}Tc-pertechnetate and ^{68}Ga-EDTA. The intensity of uptake of this latter compound, as judged by the ratio of tumor-to-sagittal-sinus activity (TSR), is intermediate (mean TSR = 0.52) between that of malignant gliomas (mean TSR = 0.63) and metastatic tumors (mean TSR = 0.39).[98] Although, as previously discussed, enhancement on x-ray CT imaging reflects BBB integrity, PET using ^{68}Ga-EDTA seems to be somewhat superior to CT in detecting BBB disruption.[136]

PET

Extensive metabolic evaluations of meningiomas have not yet been reported. The rate of glucose utilization in meningiomas has been proposed as being at least as reliable as histologic classification and other currently proposed criteria for predicting the behavior and recurrence of meningiomas.[49] In this work, tumors showing no recurrence in a 3–5 year follow-up had significantly lower glucose metabolic rates (10.6 ± 5.6 mmol/100 g per minute) compared with tumors that recurred (25.0 ± 10.6 mmol/100 g per minute). Other researchers[126] have studied meningioma glucose metabolism in vivo with PET, followed by in vitro evaluation of biopsy specimens of these tumors. They found depressed electron transport in vitro and elevated glucose metabolism in vivo, and concluded that decreases in oxidative metabolism and corresponding increases in glycolytic rate are not correlated with "malignancy." In another study comparing ^{68}Ga-EDTA, ^{11}C-glucose, and ^{11}C-methionine uptake in tumors,[63] meningiomas showed increased glucose utilization, with similar tumor volume estimates made from glucose and methionine images. More recent work has indicated that meningioma uptake of L-methionine is extremely high and helps contribute to the differential diagnosis of these lesions.

As would be expected, meningiomas have very high cerebral blood flow.[211] Similar to other intracerebral tumors, meningioma tissue is alkalotic relative to normal brain.[169]

Pituitary Adenomas

Pituitary adenomas comprise approximately 7% of intracranial tumors. Anatomically, they may be classified as microadenomas, adenomas with sellar enlargement (Fig. 6–13*A*), locally invasive adenomas, and diffusely invasive adenomas.[119] Alternatively, pituitary adenomas may be classified by their cell type and, hence, the compounds that they secrete (e.g., prolactinomas, growth hormone–secreting tumors).

Pituitary adenomas usually present with endocrine dysfunction caused by compression of normal pituitary tissue, and/or visual field deficits, since the most common site for injury outside of the sellae is directly superior at the level of the optic chiasm. Mass effect at the level of the optic chiasm produces bitemporal visual field deficits. Patients with pituitary adenomas are frequently treated surgically and, if the size of the tumor is sufficiently small, a transphenoidal-sinus surgical approach obviates the need for a craniotomy. Patients who have adenomas with dopamine D_2 receptors on their cell surface can be treated with dopamine agonists, which result in shrinkage of the tumor. This approach may be used to manage exceedingly large tumors before surgery or to minimize tumor volume at any point in their course.

ANGIOGRAPHY

Tumors located at the base of the skull, such as pituitary adenomas, usually do not show abnormal tumor vascularity on routine angiography. A relatively large pituitary adenoma may cause displacement of the first segment of the anterior cerebral artery (Fig. 6–13*B*) and elevation and straightening of the supraclinoid portion of the internal carotid artery. In rare instances, a malignant pituitary adenoma with extrasellar extension may have demonstrable vascular supply from meningeal branches of the internal carotid artery.[113] Recent experience with magnification and subtraction angiography, however, has revealed the highly vascular nature of many chromophobe adenomas.[146]

X-RAY CT

In patients with pituitary adenomas, x-ray CT images may show focal bulging, atrophy, or sloping of the floor of the sella, or the dorsum sellae may be thin. Other findings may include a focal area of low attenuation in the tumor, displacement of the pituitary stalk, focal convexity at the top of the gland, or focal "erosion" of the floor of the pituitary fossa. X-ray CT changes are commonly identified when the tumors are greater

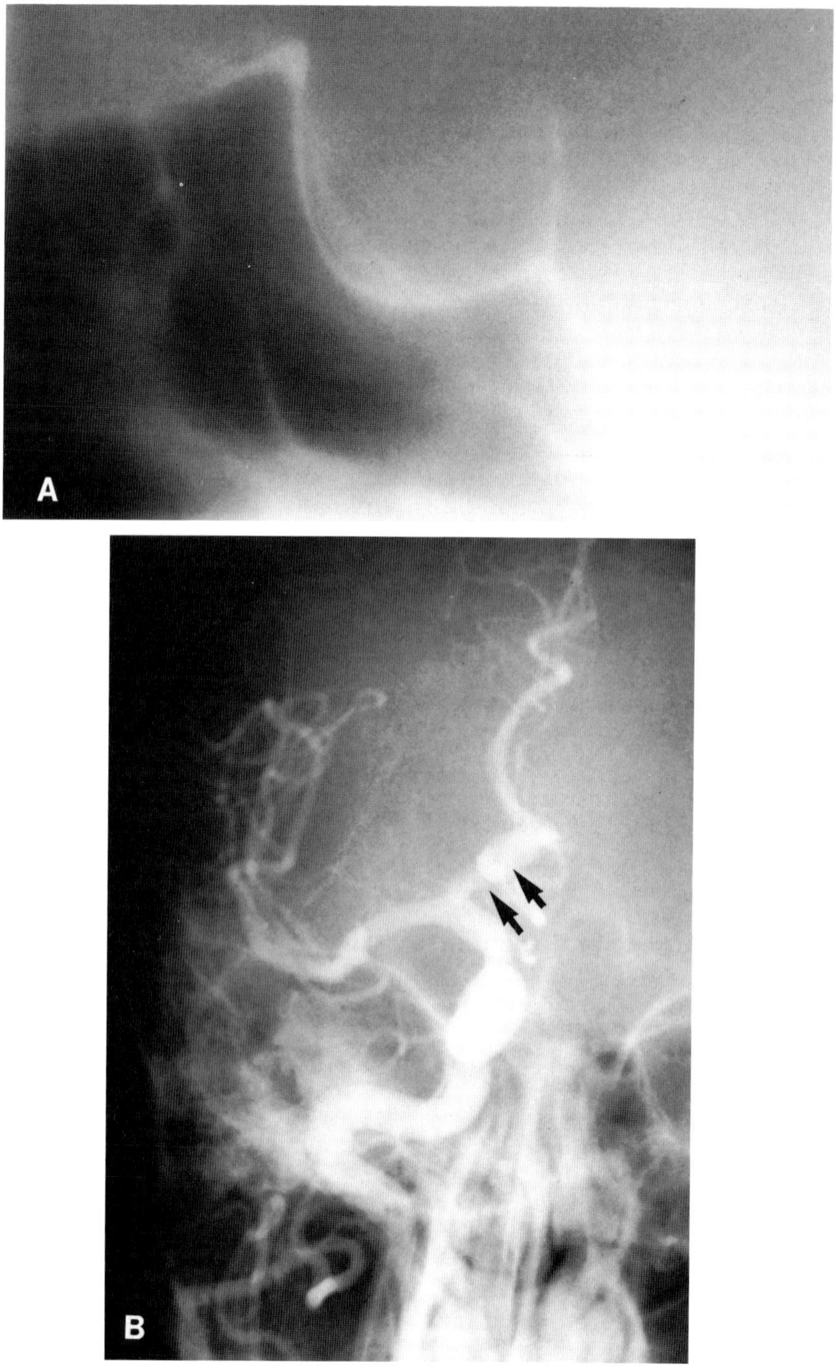

Figure 6–13. (*A*) The lateral skull x-ray in this patient with a large pituitary adenoma shows the increased size of the sella turcica. (*B*) The angiogram shows upward displacement of the anterior cerebral artery (*arrows*).

than 10 mm in size; adenomas smaller than 3 mm will go undetected. With progressive increase in the size of these tumors, the dorsum sellae becomes lengthened and thinned, and there may be erosion of the posterior clinoid processes.[113] High-dose intravenous contrast enhancement can improve the diagnosis of suprasellar and lateral extension of chromophobe adenomas, since most of these tumors are sufficiently vascular to make such contrast-enhanced scans worthwhile.[146] In fact, there is evidence that the intense enhancement seen in some pituitary adenomas is due to extravascular diffusion of contrast medium into the tumors. Differential diagnosis of pituitary adenoma, suprasellar meningioma, hypothalamic glioma, or granuloma is often difficult on x-ray CT scans alone, however. Thin-slice imaging through the optic chiasm and sella with CT are ways by which to optimize the examination.

MRI

The improved contrast resolution that can be obtained with MRI makes this modality superior to x-ray CT in the evaluation of pituitary tumors.[47] Direct sagittal and coronal images can demonstrate irregularities in the floor of the sella caused by small adenomas and show any suprasellar extension present.[19] Although x-ray CT may be more sensitive than MRI in detecting focal lesions and invasion of the sellar floor, MRI is superior in identifying infundibular abnormalities, focal abnormalities of the diaphragma sellae, cavernous sinus invasion, and optic chiasm compression.[47] Overall, MRI imaging is the diagnostic procedure of choice for defining the structure of these lesions.

When visualized, microadenomas usually appear as round areas of lower signal on T_1-weighted images and higher signal on T_2-weighted images. Although macroadenomas are often partially cystic and/or hemorrhagic, they may have signal characteristics similar to the normal gland. Subacute hemorrhage in adenomas may be difficult to differentiate from proteinaceous material in craniopharyngiomas.[35]

SPECT

In the past, the small size of most pituitary adenomas has put them outside the realm of practical imaging with SPECT. With improving spatial resolution from newer instruments, evaluation of pituitary adenomas with SPECT may become more realistic.

PET

Relatively few published articles exist evaluating the use of PET imaging for pituitary adenoma diagnosis. One study of tumor glucose metabolism[126] included two cases of pituitary chromophobe adenomas; these two tumors showed disparate rates of glucose metabolism of 21.2 and 87.9 mmol/100 g per minute. The lower rate of metabolism was seen in a tumor with larger areas of necrosis, but the accuracy of these values must be judged in light of the relatively poor spatial resolution of the imaging system used (1.95 cm), resulting in a mixture of tumor and nontumor tissues within the field of view.

Recently, pituitary adenomas have been studied with PET and ^{11}C-labeled L-methionine. These studies demonstrated that prolactinomas have high methionine uptake.

One of the most exciting areas of current PET research involves the study of receptor binding. Many pituitary adenomas contain dopamine receptors on their cell surfaces,[23,163,176] resulting in high uptake of dopamine-D_2-receptor ligands labeled with positron-emitting isotopes. These receptors can be imaged with ^{11}C-labeled raclopride or N-methylspiperone[138] and other ligands (see Chapter 3). Receptor quantification may provide valuable information about the pathophysiology, pharmacology, and response of pituitary adenomas to treatment with such dopamine agonists as bromocriptine.[138] Preliminary data indicate that with dopamine agonist therapy, pituitary adenomas decrease in size and demonstrate reductions in the uptake of such positron-labeled radiopharmaceuticals.

Intracerebral Metastases

A large percentage of patients with melanoma and carcinoma of the lung and colon have multiple intracerebral metastases at the time of initial diagnosis.[74] Single intracerebral metastases are common in patients with breast, renal, and ovarian carcinomas and osteogenic sarcomas.

ANGIOGRAPHY

Angiography is an important preoperative procedure, providing information about the vascular supply of metastatic lesions and the presence of shifted surrounding vessels. Angiography is, however, less useful than x-ray CT scanning in the demonstration of metastases. The angiographic picture is nonspecific, giving no information on the type of primary tumor.[113]

X-RAY CT

Traditionally, x-ray CT scanning has been used as the primary diagnostic modality when intracerebral metastases are suspected. A contrast-enhanced scan alone is usually performed because many metastases (especially those of melanomas and carcinomas of the colon or stomach) are isodense with brain on plain CT.[74] Although modern high-resolution x-ray CT imaging devices and the use of contrast enhancement have improved detection rates, many lesions of 5 mm or less still are not seen.[164] In addition, lesions located in the posterior fossa, at the base of the brain, and high on the cerebral convexities may go undetected. The use of higher doses of contrast material and delayed imaging increases the sensitivity of x-ray CT in these situations.

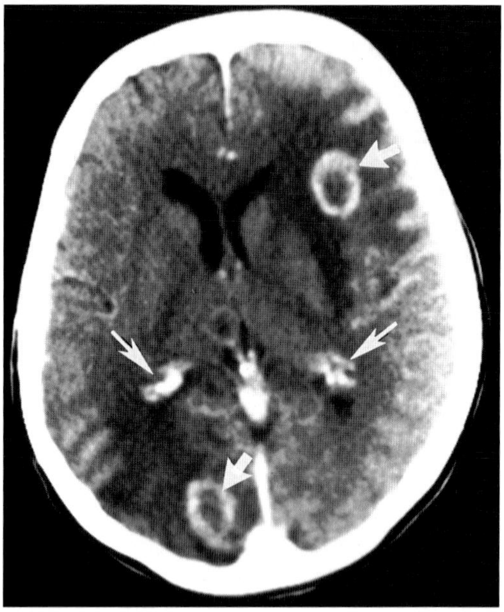

Figure 6–14. An x-ray CT scan demonstrating multiple metastatic lesions, with both irregular (*arrows*) and ring-shaped enhancement, in a patient with a known lung carcinoma.

On CT scans, metastases are most often seen as enhancing ring-shaped lesions (33%), as enhancing nodular masses (42%), or as a mixture of the two (16%).[84] Intracranial metastases are often multiple (Fig. 6–14), and individual lesions may closely resemble the appearance of glioblastomas.

MRI

Although MRI is recognized for providing unequalled contrast resolution and anatomic definition, in a recent study comparing noncontrast MRI and contrast-enhanced x-ray CT in the detection of brain metastases, neither was consistently superior.[191] In this study, contrast-enhanced CT tended to miss punctate hemorrhagic metastases and posterior fossa lesions, whereas MRI, at times, could not identify some metastases in regions surrounded by edema of adjacent metastases, and occasionally metastases were isointense with normal surrounding brain.

In a more recent study[190] contrast-enhanced MRI was compared to unenhanced MRI and contrast-enhanced x-ray CT in the detection of brain metastases. Among 50 consecutive patients, postcontrast MRI scans proved to be superior to both of the other imaging techniques. In the evaluation of suspected intraparenchymal metastases, these authors recommended a single long-TR postcontrast scan followed by a single short-TR postcontrast scan. They emphasized that precontrast MRI may be helpful if bone lesions or hemorrhagic metastases are present.

MRI may be especially useful in the evaluation of hemorrhagic metastases[5] and metastases from malignant melanoma.[6] Although early enhancement, multiple hemorrhagic sites, and atypical locations on x-ray CT may often help diagnose a hemorrhagic neoplasm, CT patterns of intratumor hemorrhage are variable, and it is sometimes impossible on CT to differentiate tumor hemorrhage from other causes of intracranial hemorrhage (see Chapter 7). MRI signal intensity patterns produced by hemorrhagic tumors differ significantly, however, from the patterns that result from nonneoplastic intracerebral hemorrhage.[5] Hemorrhagic neoplasms are characterized by an overall heterogeneity of signal intensity, which is more complex than that typically seen in nonneoplastic intracerebral hematomas. In addition, hemorrhagic neoplasms contain focal areas of abnormal tissue that are hypointense or isointense compared with the cortex on short-TR/short-TE images, and hyperintense compared with cortex on long-TR/long-TE images. Presumably, this effect corresponds to areas of tumor tissue (see Chapter 2). So, too, the x-ray CT appearance of intracerebral metastases from melanoma is varied and unspecific, whereas definite MRI signal-intensity patterns have been reported.[6]

SPECT

Radionuclide studies have been used in the past when metastatic intracerebral lesions were suspected and x-ray CT scanning was inconclusive. Occasionally, a radionuclide scan has demonstrated a lesion not seen with CT,[69] but the low false-negative rate of high-resolution CT and MRI scans have made radionuclide studies virtually obsolete, despite the improved detection from SPECT imaging devices. As noted above, ^{201}Tl can be used for the detection of intracerebral neoplasms, including metastatic lesions.[110]

BBB IMAGING

BBB disruption usually accompanies intracerebral metastases, as evidenced by ^{99m}Tc-pertechnetate uptake on radionuclide scans and contrast enhancement on x-ray CT. ^{68}Ga-EDTA studies have shown uptake in metastases, with intensity of uptake close to that of low-grade gliomas.[98] Uptake of ^{82}Rb in metastases occurs in lesions that demonstrate enhancement on x-ray CT.[24]

PET

Metastatic tumors have been studied with PET less extensively than cerebral gliomas, but the reported cases show similar decreases in CBF, OER, and $CMRO_2$.[100,117] As in the case of reported glucose metabolic rates in gliomas, investigators studying metastatic lesions have found both increased and decreased glucose metabolism.[90,101] Also, as in gliomas, metastatic lesions have been shown to be more alkalotic than contralateral normal cortex.[25,169] Variable rates of cell growth have been reported for intracerebral metastatic lesions, as reflected by the uptake of [1-^{11}C]putrescine.[90] This polyamine passes through the disrupted BBB in tumors and is retained by metabolic trapping, which reflects polyamine synthesis. Since putrescine is not taken up by normal brain with intact BBB, ^{11}C-labeled putrescine provides a higher tumor-to-normal-brain contrast than do images of glucose metabolism; this is especially important in the detection of small, hypometabolic tumors.

Other CNS Tumors

It is beyond the scope of this chapter to describe fully the neuroimaging features of all types of intracerebral neoplastic processes. Volumes have been devoted to the angiographic, x-ray CT, and MRI characteristics of various other tumors, and experience with PET is rapidly accumulating. In preliminary studies of CNS lymphoma, for example, PET has shown depressed oxygen metabolism[161] and increased glucose metabolism[116,154] relative to gray matter, with blood flow in the normal range.[161]

REMOTE EFFECTS OF INTRACEREBRAL TUMORS

The remote depression of cerebral function by circumscribed brain lesions was first described by von Monakow[199]; the full extent of this effect from brain tumors is now being appreciated with functional imaging. The local effects of peritumoral edema have long been visualized on x-ray CT scans, and the extent of this edema can now be better delineated with MRI. A combination of tumor volume and edema volume within the fixed intracranial space may cause midline shifts with compression of contralateral structures (Figs. 6–4, 6–10*G*, 6–15), and eventually may result in herniation.

In addition to these gross morphologic changes due to tumors, far more subtle metabolic and hemodynamic effects of tumor growth on surrounding and re-

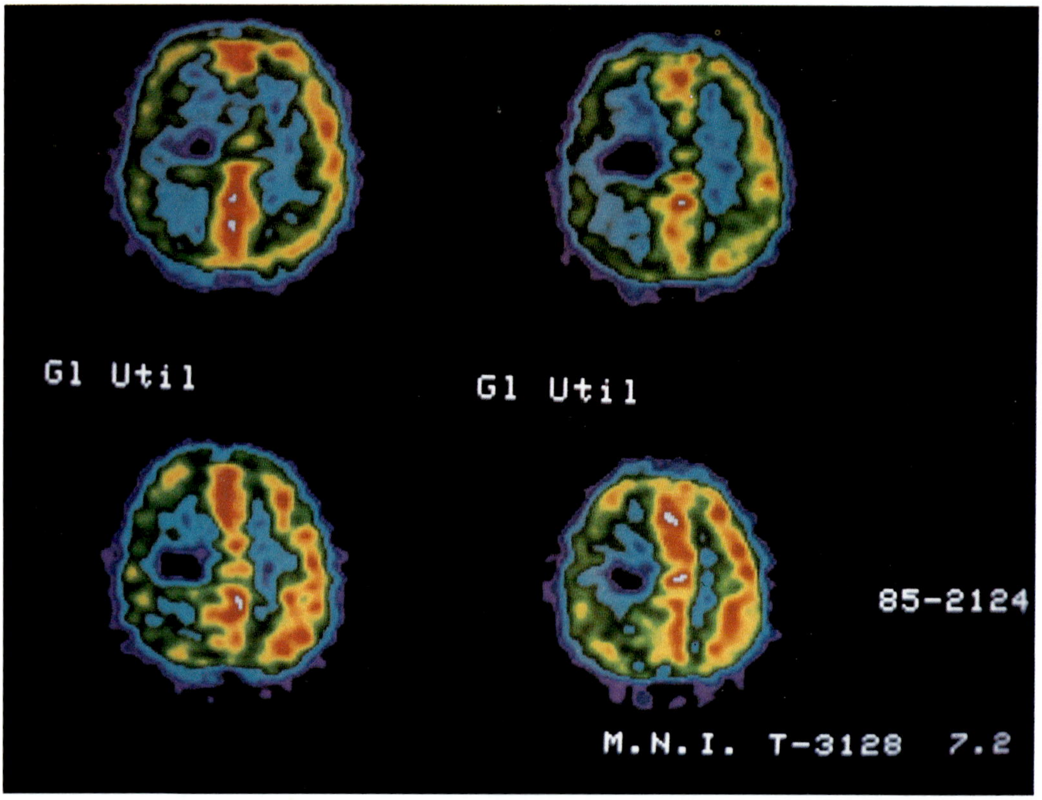

Figure 6–15. Depressed glucose metabolism is evident in the entire left hemisphere at multiple levels in this patient with a centrally located, cystic grade IV astrocytoma.

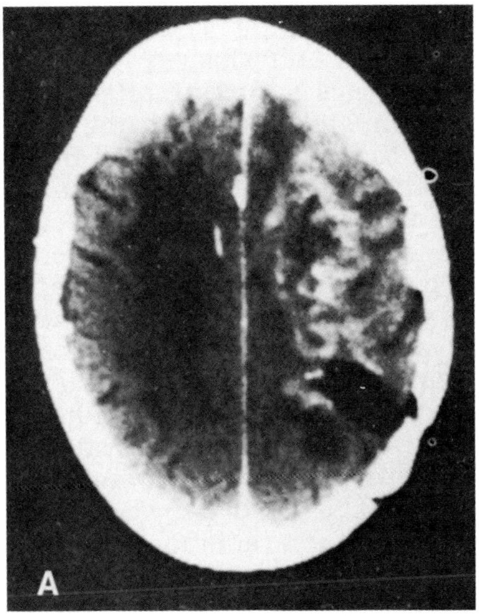

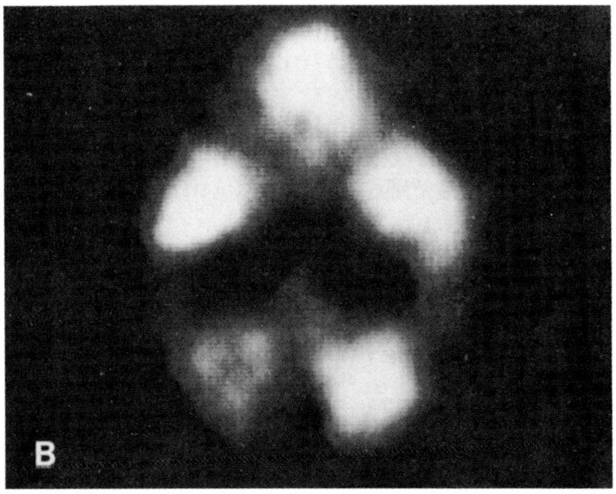

Figure 6–16. (*A*) An x-ray CT scan shows an irregular enhancing mass in the right frontoparietal region in a patient who had undergone radiation for a tumor. (*B*) An FDG–PET image demonstrates marked hypometabolism in the contralateral cerebellar hemisphere. (From Patronas et al.,[153] p. 98, with permission.)

mote brain are now being discovered with PET. Studies of tumor metabolism have shown that glucose utilization is often decreased in cortical regions adjacent to or neuronally connected with tumor sites (Figs. 6–10, 6–16).[48,52,194] Blood flow and oxygen utilization have also been found to be depressed in cortex remote from brain tumors (see Fig. 6–10).[9,117,194] Decreased $CMRO_2$ is thought to be a primary effect rather than a by-product of depressed CBF, since no increase in OER has been seen to suggest ischemia. This depression of oxygen utilization can be partially reversed with surgical decompression.[9]

Functional interconnections of the cerebral and cerebellar cortices can be visualized with PET in patients who have tumors (see Fig. 6–16).[122] Numerous studies have demonstrated bilateral and/or contralateral suppression of cerebellar cortical glucose metabolism from intracerebral tumors.[47,48,153] This metabolic suppression is hypothesized to be due to interruptions of the functional connections between the cerebellar cortex and the cerebral cortex; the location of the tumor is a crucial factor in producing this remote effect. Tumors and their resultant edema in the motor cortex, anterior corona radiata, and the thalamus, areas all neuronally connected to the cerebellum, produced the most marked suppression of contralateral cerebellar cortical metabolism.[153] Metabolic suppression does not seem to depend on single characteristics of the tumors such as size or type, or on the duration of symptoms, but may be related to rapid growth with prominent edema, as seen with higher-grade lesions.[153] These cerebellar effects spare the dentate nuclei and other deep structures and appear to affect primarily the cerebellar cortex.[71]

RESPONSE OF TUMORS TO TREATMENT

The currently accepted treatment of intracranial gliomas is maximum possible surgical resection followed by radiation therapy and chemotherapy. Morphologically, a variety of changes are known to occur following radiation and chemotherapy. In addition to necrosis and vascular response, nonspecific changes are seen, including formation of multinucleated giant cells and irregular hyperchromatic nuclei, and inhibition of cell division.[78] Currently, the most frequently used chemotherapeutic agent for intracerebral tumors is 1,3-bis(2-chloroethyl)-1-nitrosourea (BCNU). A combination of this drug with radiation produces more hypocellular areas and more bizarre giant cells than does radiation alone,[209] suggesting that BCNU plus radiation therapy inhibits cell division, and that the number of giant and monstrous cells subsequently increases. In clinical trials,[82,202] the combination of radiotherapy and chemotherapy seems to provide longer survival times than does either therapy alone. Understanding and measuring posttreatment changes in vivo would greatly benefit the evaluation of response to therapy and might lead to better design of treatment programs.

Both x-ray CT and MRI have thus far provided mainly morphologic information on posttreatment changes (Fig. 6–17). It was hoped that planar or SPECT radionuclide imaging could provide complementary physiologic information on changes occurring after therapy. Radionuclide brain scans have been used to monitor changes of brain tumors after surgery.[68,85] Technetium-99m–pertechnetate tends to concentrate in areas of edema, however,[92] making it difficult to differentiate viable residual tumor from posttreatment edema. In addition, radionuclide scanning is limited in postoperative patients because of the accumulation of radioactivity in the surgical calvarial defects.[158] Although x-ray CT and MRI overall have slightly better sensitivity and specificity than radionuclide scans in the long-term follow-up of persistent or recurrent neoplasms,[134] the radiologic and nuclear medicine studies are complementary modalities.

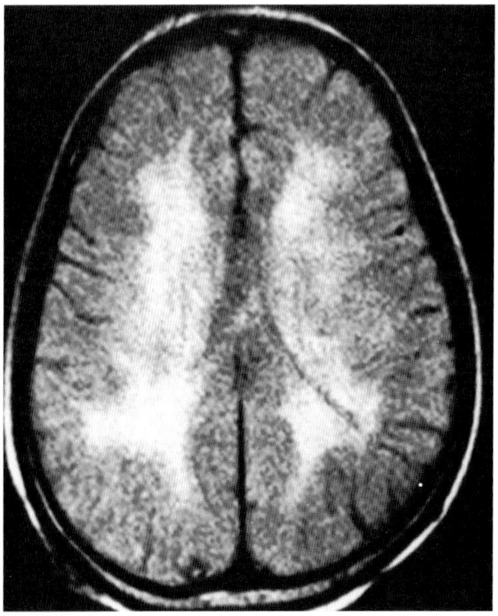

Figure 6–17. This MRI scan at 0.5 T was performed after surgery for a medulloblastoma of the fourth ventricle, and 60-Gy radiation therapy. The diffuse hyperintensity of the white matter is typical of postirradiation changes.

PET, with its capacity to study multiple metabolic and hemodynamic parameters in vivo, is the most promising single modality for the evaluation of response to treatment. Because glucose metabolism is relatively unaltered by surgery or use of corticosteroids,[80] PET can be used to study the kinetics of tracer amounts of radiolabeled chemotherapeutic drugs administered intravenously (Fig. 6–18) and intra-arterially,[79,195] and this information may potentially be helpful in designing individual treatment schedules.[168] PET results can also be used in the performance of stereotaxic biopsies of tumors that appear inhomogeneous metabolically, to obtain separate histologic specimens from areas of tumor that may be functionally different.[213] PET imaging can be combined in several evaluations with techniques such as digital subtraction angiography[212] and stereotaxic x-ray CT and MRI to obtain even more accurate anatomic-functional information. Attempts have been made to predict posttreatment outcome with PET. In one series,[152] tumor glucose utilization was inversely proportional to survival time. As noted above, PET determinations of dopamine-D_2-receptor binding and methionine uptake have also been used to monitor pituitary ade-

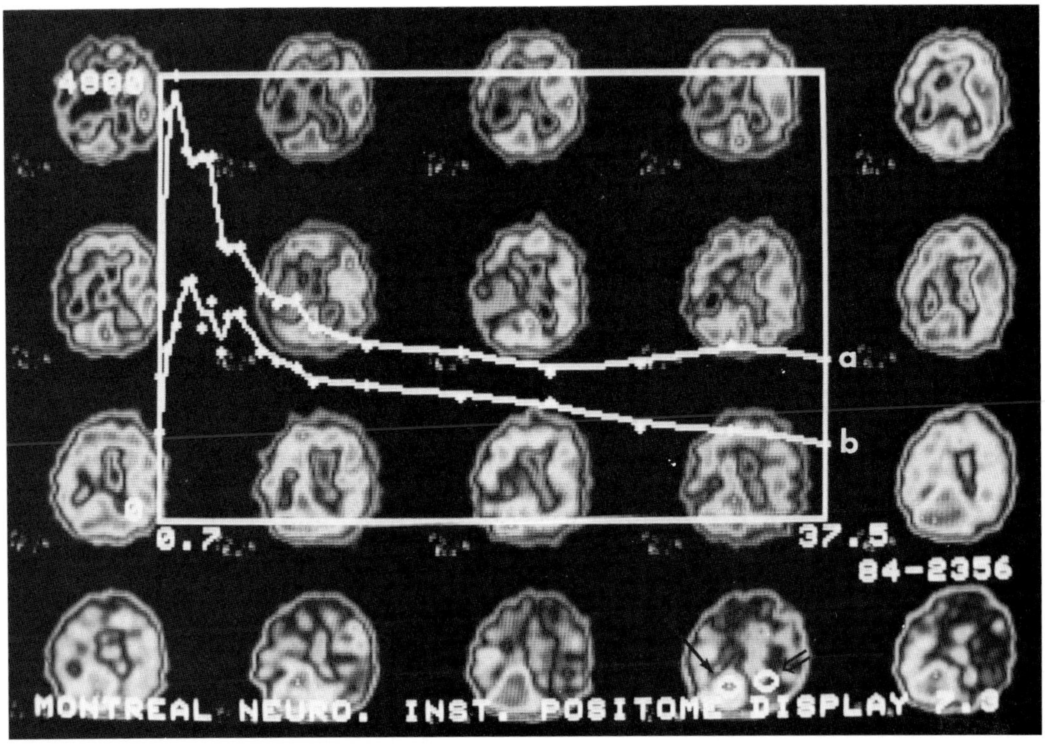

Figure 6–18. Time-activity curves are seen here superimposed over PET scans that were obtained sequentially over 40 minutes after the intravenous injection of ^{11}C-BCNU. ^{11}C activity in Bq per ml is plotted on the y axis, and time in minutes along the x axis. Curve "a" is derived from a region of interest (see image on bottom row, second from right) placed over a left occipital glioblastoma (*closed arrow*). Curve "b" represents a comparable contralateral region (*open arrow*). Significantly more activity accumulates in the region of the left occipital tumor, showing the concentration of the active breakdown product of BCNU in the glioma.

nomas. The differentiation of radiation necrosis from tumor recurrence, another critical issue for which PET provides specific information, is discussed in the next section.

PET studies done serially after treatment not only can assess metabolic changes in the tumor due to therapy, but also can be used to monitor the effects of radiation or chemotherapy on the surrounding brain. Because of the heterogeneous nature of brain tumors, and because of the significant and varied effects of treatment on tumor metabolism, posttreatment evaluation is often difficult. It is believed that a combination of these imaging modalities may provide objective means by which to follow patients, monitor therapy, and select patients for subsequent treatment approaches.

THE DIFFERENTIATION OF RADIATION NECROSIS FROM RECURRENT TUMOR

The differentiation of postradiation necrosis from tumor recurrence has been clinically impossible without biopsy. A typical situation is one in which a patient returns approximately 4 to 6 months after surgery and radiation therapy for a cerebral glioma. On return, the patient complains of symptoms and has signs referable to the site of the initial lesion. Contrast-enhanced x-ray CT, or MRI with Gd-EDTA, demonstrates mass effect and alteration in the BBB with surrounding edema. These findings, as well as the physical examination and history, do not help to differentiate between radiation necrosis and tumor recurrence.[65,147]

PET metabolic evaluation seems ideal for differentiating between these two entities. The finding of increased glucose metabolism on PET imaging is virtually diagnostic for recurrence (Figs. 6–19 and 6–20).[151] This finding is in agreement with the study[52] showing high glucose metabolism in high-grade tumors after surgery, radiation, and chemotherapy. In contrast, glucose metabolism is severely reduced in areas of the brain affected by radiation necrosis. A combination of glucose utilization and ^{82}Rb studies of BBB disruption may offer even more specificity in differentiating tumor recurrence from changes caused by radiation damage alone.[57] The use of PET in the differential diagnosis of radiation necrosis versus recurrent brain tumor has now become an accepted clinical modality.[80]

SUMMARY

Many imaging modalities are available to a clinician managing a patient with an intracerebral tumor. Noninvasive techniques such as MRI are providing increasing anatomic information without discomfort or risk to the patient and have replaced more invasive radiologic procedures. Anatomic information obtained from angiography, x-ray CT, or MRI is complemented by functional data provided by PET, SPECT, and, perhaps in the future, MR spectroscopy. The integration and correlation of these modalities promises to provide not only greater sensitivity and specificity in the identification of intracerebral tumors, but also insights into the biology and behavior of these lesions. With this information, more efficacious treatments can be devised and response to therapy more closely followed.

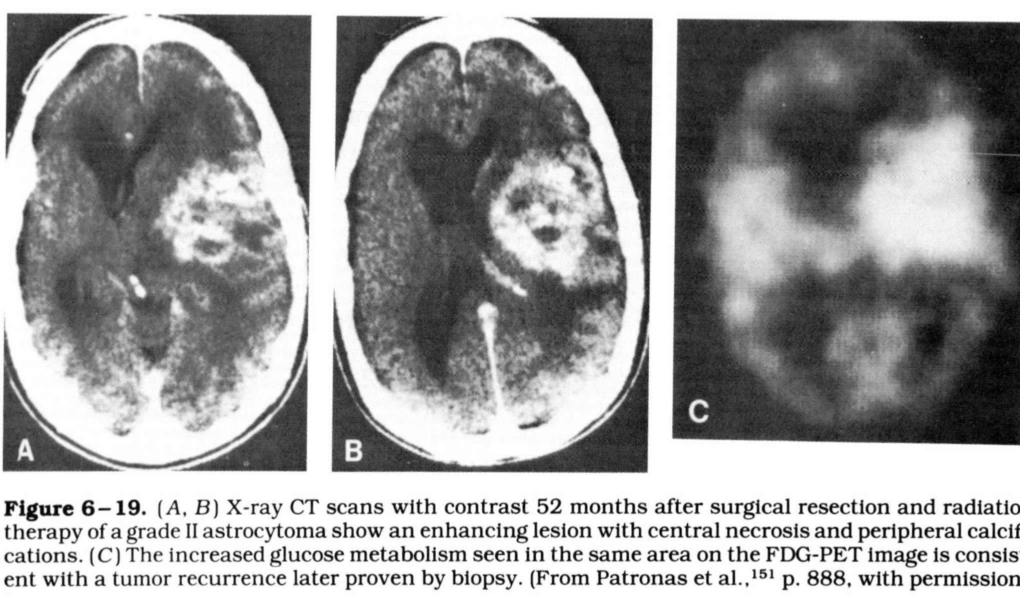

Figure 6–19. (*A, B*) X-ray CT scans with contrast 52 months after surgical resection and radiation therapy of a grade II astrocytoma show an enhancing lesion with central necrosis and peripheral calcifications. (*C*) The increased glucose metabolism seen in the same area on the FDG-PET image is consistent with a tumor recurrence later proven by biopsy. (From Patronas et al.,[151] p. 888, with permission.)

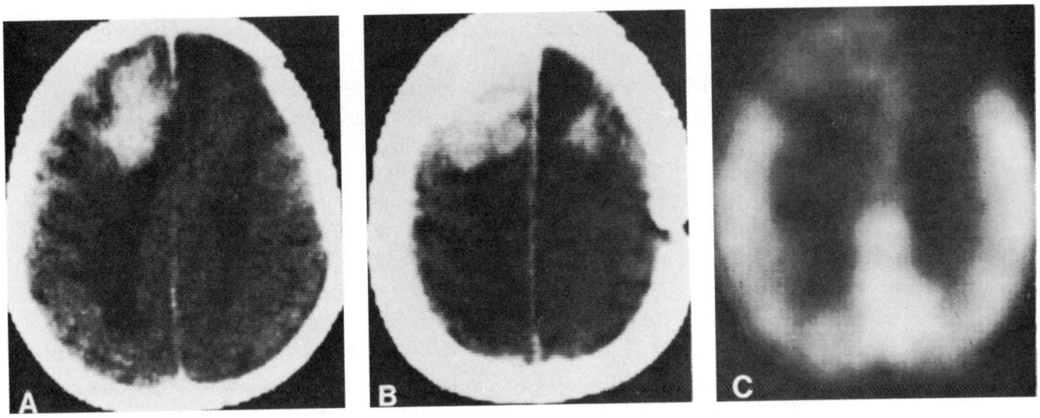

Figure 6–20. (*A*, *B*) Contrast-enhanced x-ray CT scans 28 months after surgery and radiation therapy for a grade II astrocytoma show a small, enhancing lesion in the right frontal lobe and a larger, enhancing lesion in the left frontal area. (*C*) The FDG-PET scan shows decreased metabolism in both frontal regions, consistent with postradiation changes later confirmed on biopsy. (From Patronas et al.,[151] p. 886, with permission.)

ACKNOWLEDGMENT

The authors thank Dr. Denis Melançon of the Montreal Neurological Institute for providing many of the radiologic images for this chapter, and Ms. Carolyn Elliot for her secretarial assistance.

REFERENCES

1. Adams, RD and Victor, M: Principles of Neurology, ed 3. McGraw-Hill. New York, 1985, p 474.
2. Ambrose, J, Gooding, MR, and Richardson, AE: An assessment of the accuracy of computerized transverse axial scanning (EMI scanner) in the diagnosis of intracranial tumor. A review of 366 patients. Brain 98:569–582, 1975.
3. Ancri, D and Bassett, JY: Diagnosis of cerebral metastases by thallium-201. Br J Radiol 53:443–445, 1980.
4. Atkins, HL, et al: Thallium-201 for medical use. J Nucl Med 18:133–140, 1977.
5. Atlas, SW, Grossman, RI, Gomori, JM, Hackney, DB, Goldberg, HI, Zimmerman, RA, and Bilaniuk, LT: Hemorrhagic intracranial malignant neoplasms: Spin-echo MR imaging. Radiology 164:71–77, 1987.
6. Atlas, SW, Grossman, RI, Gomori, JM, Guerry, D, Hackney, DB, Goldberg, HI, Zimmerman, RA, and Bilaniuk, LT: MR imaging of intracranial metastatic melanoma. J Comput Assist Tomogr 11:577–582, 1987.
7. Bailey, P and Cushing, H: A Classification of Tumors of the Glioma Group on a Histogenetic Basis with a Correlated Study of Prognosis. JB Lippincott, Philadelphia, 1926.
8. Banna, M and Appleby, A: Some observations on the angiography of supratentorial meningiomas. Clin Radiol 20:375–386, 1969.
9. Beaney, RP, Brooks, DJ, Leenders, KL, Thomas, D, Jones, T, and Halnan, K: Blood flow and oxygen utilization in the contralateral cerebral cortex of patients with untreated intracranial tumours as studied by positron emission tomography, with observations on the effect of decompressive surgery. J Neurol Neurosurg Psych 48:310–319, 1985.
10. Benavides, J, Quarteronet, D, Imbault, F, Malgouris, C, Uzan, A, Renault, C, Dubroeucq, MC, Gueremy, C, and Le Fur, G: Labelling of "peripheral type" benzodiazepine binding sites in

the rat brain by using [^{3}H]PK 11195 and isoquinoline carboxamide derivative: Kinetic studies and autoradiographic localization. J Neurochem 41:1744–1750, 1983.

11. Bergstrand, G, Larsson, S, Berström, M, Eriksson L, and Edner, G: Cerebrospinal fluid circulation: Evaluation by single-photon and positron emission tomography. AJNR 4:557–559, 1983.
12. Bergström, M, Collins, VP, Ehrin, E, Ericson, K, Eriksson, L, Greitz, T, Halldin, C, von Holst, H, Långström, B, Lilja, A, Lundquist, H, and Någren, K: Discrepancies in brain tumor extent as shown by CT and PET using [^{68}Ga]EDTA, [^{11}C]glucose, and [^{11}C]methionine. J Comput Assist Tomogr 7:1062–1066, 1983.
13. Bergström, M, Ericson, K, Hagenfeldt, L, Mosskin, M, von Holst, H, Norén, G, Eriksson, L, Ehrin, E, and Johnström, P: PET study of methionine accumulation in glioma and normal brain tissue: Competition with branched chain amino acids. J Comput Assist Tomogr 11:208–213, 1987.
14. Bergström, M, Muhr, C, Lundberg, PO, Bergström, K, Gee, AD, Fasth, K-J, and Långström, B: Rapid decrease in amino acid metabolism in prolactin-secreting pituitary adenomas after bromocriptine treatment: A PET study. J Comput Assist Tomogr 11:815–819, 1987.
15. Black, KL, Hawkins, RA, Kim, KT, Becker, DP, Lerner, C, and Marciano, D: Thallium-201 (SPECT): A quantitative technique to distinguish low-grade from malignant brain tumors. J Neurosurg 71:342–346, 1989.
16. Blacklock, JB, Oldfield, EH, Di Chiro G, Tran, D, Theodore, W, Wright, DC, and Larson, SM: Effect of barbiturate coma on glucose utilization in normal brain versus gliomas: Positron emission tomography studies. J Neurosurg 67:71–75, 1987.
17. Borst, M: Die Lehre von den Geschwülsten. Bergmann, Wiesbaden, 1902.
18. Bradbury, MWB and Davson, H: The transport of potassium between blood, cerebrospinal fluid and brain. J Physiol(Lond) 181:151–174, 1965.
19. Bradley, WG: Magnetic resonance imaging of the central nervous system. Neurol Res 6:91–106, 1984.
20. Bradley, WG, Jr, Waluch, V, Yadley, RA, and Wycoff, RR: Comparison of CT and MR in 400 patients with suspected disease of the brain and cervical spinal cord. Radiology 152:695–702, 1984.
21. Brant-Zawadzki, M, Davis, PL, Crooks, LE, Mills, CM, Norman, D, Newton, TH, Sheldon, P, and Kaufman, L: NMR demonstration of cerebral abnormalities: Comparison with CT. AJR 140:857–864, 1983.
22. Brant-Zawadzki, M, Berry, I, Osaki, L, Brasch, R, Murovic, J, and Norman, D: Gd-DTPA in clinical MR of the brain. AJR 147:1223–1230, 1986.
23. Bression, D, Brandi, AM, Martes, MP, Nousbaum, A, Cesselin, F, Racadot, J, and Peillon, F: Dopaminergic receptors in human prolactin-secreting adenomas: A quantitative study. J Clin Endocrinol Metab 51:1037–1043, 1980.
24. Brooks, DJ, Beaney, RP, Lammertsma, AA, Leenders, KL, Horlock, PL, Kensett, MJ, Marshall, J, Thomas, DG, and Jones, T: Quantitative measurement of blood-brain barrier permeability using Rubidium-82 and positron emission tomography. J Cereb Blood Flow Metab 4:535–545, 1984.
25. Brooks, DJ, Beaney, RP, Thomas, DGT, Marshall, J, and Jones, T: Studies on regional cerebral pH in patients with cerebral tumors using continuous inhalation of $^{11}CO_2$ and positron emission tomography. J Cereb Blood Flow Metab 6:529–535, 1986
26. Burger, PC, Dubois, PJ, Schold, SC, Smith, KR, Odom, GL, Crafts, DC, and Giangaspero, F: Computerized Tomographic and pathologic studies of the untreated, quiescent, and recurrent glioblastoma multiforme. J Neurosurg 58:159–169, 1983.
27. Burger, PC, Heinz, ER, Shibata, T, and Kleihues, P: Topographic anatomy and CT correlations in the untreated glioblastoma multiforme. J Neurosurg 68:698–704, 1988.
28. Busa, WB and Nuccitelli, R: Metabolic regulation via intracellular pH. Am J Physiol 246:R409–R438, 1984.

29. Bustany, P, Chatel, M, Derlon, JM, Darcel, F, Sgouropoulos, P, Soussaline, F, and Syrota, A: Brain tumor protein synthesis and histological grades: A study by positron emission tomography (PET) and C-11-L-methionine. J Neuro-Oncol 3:397–404, 1986.
30. Butler, AR, Horii, SC, Kricheff, II, Shannon, MB, and Budzilovich, GN: Computed tomography in astrocytomas. A statistical analysis of the parameters of malignancy and the positive contrast-enhanced CT scan. Radiology 129:433–439, 1978.
31. Cairncross, JG, Macdonald, DR, Pexman, JH, and Ives, FJ: Steroid-induced CT changes in patients with recurrent malignant glioma. Neurology 38:724–726, 1988.
32. Cairncross, JG, Pexman, JHW, Rathbone, MP, and DelMaestro, RF: Postoperative contrast enhancement in patients with brain tumor. Ann Neurol 17:570–572, 1985.
33. Carr, DH, Brown, J, Bydder, GM, Steiner, RE, Weinmann, HJ, Speck, U, Hall, AS, and Young, IR: Gadolinium DTPA as a contrast agent in MRI: Initial clinical experience in 20 patients. AJR 143:215–224, 1984.
34. Carril, JM, MacDonald, AF, Dendy, PP, Keyes, WI, Undrill, PE, and Mallard, JR: Cranial scintigraphy: Value of adding emission computed tomographic sections to conventional pertechnetate images (512 cases). J Nucl Med 20:1117–1123, 1979.
35. Chakares, DW, Curtin, A, and Ford, G: Magnetic resonance imaging of pituitary and parasellar abnormalities. Radiol Clin North Am 27:265–281, 1989.
36. Chamberlain, MC, Murovic, JA, and Levin, VA: Absence of contrast enhancement on CT brain scans of patients with supratentorial malignant gliomas. Neurology 38:1371–1374, 1988.
37. Chatterji, DC, Greene, RF, and Gallelli, JF: Mechanism of hydrolysis of halogenated nitrosoureas. J Pharm Sci 67:1527–1532, 1978.
38. Ciliax, BJ, Starosta-Rubinstein, S, McKeever, P, Young, AB, and Penny, JB: In vivo brain tumor imaging using peripheral benzodiazepine ligands. Neurology 37 (Suppl 1):328, 1987.
39. Cohen, BH, Bury, E, Packer, RJ, Sutton, LN, Bilaniuk, LT, and Zimmerman, RA: Gadolinium-DTPA-enhanced magnetic resonance imaging in childhood brain tumors. Neurology 39:1178–1183, 1989.
40. Cohen, RD and Iles, RA: Intracellular pH measurement control, and metabolic interrelationships. Crit Rev Clin Lab Sci 6:101–143, 1975.
41. Crocker, EF, Zimmerman, RA, Phelps, ME, Kuhl, DE: The effects of steroids on the extravascular distribution of radiographic contrast material and technetium pertechnetate in brain tumors as determined by computed tomography. Radiology 119:471–474, 1976.
42. Cushing, H: Intracranial Tumors: Notes upon a Series of 2000 Verified Cases with Surgical-Mortality Percentages Pertaining Thereto. Charles C Thomas, Springfield, Ill, 1932.
43. Darwin, RH, Drayer, BP, Riederer, SJ, Wang, HZ, and MacFall, JR: T_2 estimates in healthy and diseased brain tissue: A comparison using various MR pulse sequences. Radiology 160:375–381, 1986.
44. Dasarov, LB and Friedman, H: Enhanced Na^+-K^+ activated adenosine triphosphatase activity in transformed fibroblasts. Cancer Res 34:1862–1865, 1974.
45. Daumas-Duport, C, Monsaigneon, V, Blond, S, Munari, C, Musolino, A, Chodkiewicz, JP, Missir, O: Serial stereotactic biopsies and CT scan in gliomas: Correlative study in 100 astrocytomas. J Neurooncol 4:317–328, 1987.
46. Daumas-Duport, C, Monsaingeon, V, Szenthe, L, and Szikla, G: Serial stereotactic biopsies. Appl Neurophysiol 45:431–437, 1982.
47. Davis PC, Hoffman JC Jr, Spencer, T, Tindall, GT, and Braun, IF: MR imaging of pituitary adenomas: CT, clinical and surgical correlation. AJR 148:797–802, 1987.
48. De La Paz, RL, Patronas, NJ, Brooks, RA, Smith, BH, Kornblith, PL, Milam, H, and Di Chiro, G: Positron emission to-

mographic study of suppression of gray matter glucose utilization by brain tumors. AJNR 4:826–829, 1983.
49. Di Chiro, F, Hatazawa, J, Katz, DA, Rizzoli, HV, and De Michele, DJ: Glucose utilization by intracranial meningiomas as an index of tumor aggressivity and probability of recurrence: A PET study. Radiology 164:521–526, 1987.
50. Di Chiro, G: Positron emission tomography using [^{18}F]fluorodeoxyglucose in brain tumors. Invest Radiol 22:360–371, 1987.
51. Di Chiro, G, De La Paz, RL, Brooks, RA, Sokoloff, L, Kornblith, PL, Smith, BH, Patronas, NJ, Kufta, CV, Kessler, RM, Johnston, GS, Manning, RG, and Wolf, AP: Glucose utilization of cerebral gliomas measured by ^{18}F-fluorodeoxyglucose and PET. Neurology 32:1323–1329, 1982.
52. Di Chiro, G, Brooks, Ra, Patronas, NJ, Bairamian, D, Kornblith, PL, Smith, BH, Mansi, L, and Barker, J: Issues in the in vivo measurement of glucose metabolism of human central nervous system tumors. Ann Neurol 15(Suppl): S138–S146, 1984.
53. Di Chiro, G and Brooks, RA: PET-FDG of untreated and treated cerebral gliomas. J Nucl Med 29:421–422, 1988.
54. Di Chiro, G, Oldfield, E, Wright, DC, De Michele, P, Katz, DA, Patronas, NJ, Doppman, JL, Larson, SM, Ito, M, and Kufta, CV: Cerebral necrosis after radiotherapy and/or intraarterial chemotherapy for brain tumors: PET and neuropathologic studies. AJR 150: 189–197, 1988.
55. Digenis, GA, Cheng, YC, McQuinn, RL, Freed, BR, and Tilbury, RS: ^{13}N-labeling of a substituted nitrosourea, its carbamate, and nitrosocarbaryl: In vivo and in vitro studies. In Root, JW and Krohn, KA (eds): Short-Lived Radionuclides in Chemistry and Biology, American Chemical Society 1981, pp 351–367.
56. Digenis, GA and Issidorides, CH: Some biochemical aspects of N-nitroso compounds. Bioorg Chem 8:97–137, 1979.
57. Doyle, WK, Budinger, TF, Valk, PE, Levin, VA, and Gutin, PH: Differentiation of cerebral radiation necrosis from tumor recurrence by [^{18}F]FDG and ^{82}Rb positron emission tomography. J Comput Assist Tomogr 11:563–570, 1987.
58. Dumoulin, CL, Hart, HR Jr: Magnetic resonance angiography. Radiology 161:717–720, 1986.
59. Earnest, F IV, Kelly, PJ, Scheithauer, BW, Kall, BA, Cascino, TL, Ehman, RL, Forbes, GS, and Axley, PL: Cerebral astrocytomas: Histopathologic correlation of MR and CT contrast enhancement with stereotaxic biopsy. Radiology 166:823–827, 1988.
60. Efange, SMN, Kung, HF, Billings, J, Guo, Y-Z, and Blau, M: Technetium-99m bis (Aminoethanethiol) complexes with amine side chains: Potential perfusion imaging agents for SPECT. J Nucl Med 28:1012–1019, 1987.
61. Elligsen, JD, Thompson, JE, Frey, HE, and Kruuv, J: Correlation of (Na^+-K^+) ATPase activity with growth of normal and transformed cells. Exp Cell Res 87:233–240, 1974.
62. Elster, AD, Challa, VR, Gilbert, TH, Richardson, DN, and Contento, JC: Meningiomas: MR and histopathological features. Radiology 170:857–862, 1989.
63. Ericson, K, Lilja, A, Bergström, M, Collins, VP, Eriksson, L, Ehrin, E, von Holst, H, Lundqvist, H, Långström, B, and Mosskin, M: Positron emission tomography with ([^{11}C]methyl)-L-methionine, [^{11}C]D-glucose, and [^{68}Ga]EDTA in supratentorial tumors. J Comput Assist Tomogr 9:683–689, 1985.
64. Ericson, K, Lilja, A, and Bergström, M: PET with ^{11}C methionine in brain tumors: Methionine kinetics, tumor delineation, and follow-up studies after therapy. In Heiss, WD, Pawlik, G, Herholz, K, Wienhard, K (eds): Clinical Efficacy of Positron Emission Tomography. Martinus Nijhoff, Dordrecht, 1987, pp 379–390.
65. Eyster, EF, Nielsen, SL, Sheline, GE, and Wilson, CB: Cerebral radiation necrosis simulating a brain tumor. J Neurosurg 40:267–271, 1974.
66. Fazekas, JT: Treatment of grades I

and II brain astrocytomas: The role of radiotherapy. Int J Radiat Oncol Biol Phys 2: 661–666, 1977.
67. Felix, R, et al: Brain tumors: MR imaging with gadolinium-DTPA. Radiology 156:681–688, 1985.
68. Fletcher, JW, George, EA, Henry, RE, Schörner, W, Laniado, M, Niendorf, HP, Claussen, C, Fiegler, W, Speck, U, and Donati, RM: Brain scans, dexamethasone therapy, and brain tumors. JAMA 232:1261–1263, 1975.
69. Fordham, EW: The complementary role of computerized axial transmission tomography and radionuclide imaging of the brain. Semin Nucl Med 7:137–159, 1977.
70. Front, D and Israel, O: Scintigraphy and ultrastructure of the blood-brain and blood-tissue barriers of human brain tumors: Radionuclides as in vivo indicators of tumor permeability. In Magistretti, PH (ed): Functional Radionuclide Imaging of the Brain. Raven Press, New York, 1983, pp 47–59.
71. Fulham, M and Dickens, G: J Cerebral Blood Flow, 1989.
72. Gallagher, BM, Fowler, JS, Gutterson, NI, MacGregor, RR, Wan, C-N, and Wolf, AP: Metabolic trapping as a principle of radiopharmaceutical design. J Nucl Med 19:1154–1161, 1978.
73. Galarraga, J, Loreck, DJ, Graham, JF, De La Paz, RL, Smith, BH, Hallgren, D, and Cummins, CJ: Glucose metabolism in human gliomas: Correspondence of in situ and in vitro metabolic rates and altered energy metabolism. Metab Brain Dis 1:279–291, 1986.
74. Gamache, FW Jr, Posner, JB, and Patterson, RH Jr: Metastatic brain tumors. In Youmans, JR (ed): Neurological Surgery, Vol 5. WB Saunders, Philadelphia, 1982, pp 2872–2898.
75. Garfield, J: Surgery of cerebral gliomas. In Thomas, DGT and Graham, DI (eds): Brain Tumors: Scientific Basis, Clinical Investigation and Current Therapy. Butterworths, London, 1980, pp 301–321.
76. Garroway, AN: Velocity measurements in flowing fluids by NMR. J Physics D (Appl Phys) 7:L159–163, 1974.
77. Gehan, EA and Walker, MD: Prognostic factors for patients with brain tumors. NCI Monogr 46:189–195, 1977.
78. Gerstner, L, Jellinger, K, Heiss, W-D, and Wöber, G: Morphological changes in anaplastic gliomas treated with radiation and chemotherapy. Acta Neurochirugica 36:117–138, 1977.
79. Ginos, JZ, Cooper, AJL, Dhawan, V, Lai, JCK, Strother, SC, Alcock, N, and Rottenberg, DA: [^{13}N]cisplatin PET to assess pharmacokinetics of intra-arterial versus intravenous chemotherapy for malignant brain tumors. J Nucl Med 28:1844–1852, 1987.
80. Glantz, MJ, Hoffman, JM, Coleman, RE, Friedman, AH, Hanson, MW, Burger, PC, Herndon, JE II, Meisler, WJ, and Schold, SC Jr: Identification of early recurrence of primary central nervous system tumors by F-18 FDG-PET. Ann Neurol 29:347–355, 1991.
81. Goldsher, D, Litt, AW, Pinto, RS, and others: Dural "tail" associated with meningiomas on Gd-DTPA-enhanced MR images: Characteristics, differential diagnostic value, and possible implications for treatment. Radiology 176: 447–450, 1990.
82. Green, SB, Byar, DP, Walker, MD, Pistenmaa, DA, Alexander, E Jr, Batzdorf, U, Brooks, WH, Hunt, WE, Mealey, J Jr, Odon, GL, Paoletti, P, Ransohoff, J II, Robertson, JT, Selker, RG, Shapiro, WR, Smith, KR, Wilson, GB, and Strike, TA: Comparisons of carmustine, procarbazine, and high-dose methylprednisolone as additions to surgery and radiotherapy for the treatment of malignant glioma. Cancer Treat Rep 67:121–132, 1983.
83. Greig, NH: Brain tumors and the blood-tumor barrier. In Neuwelt, EA (ed): Implications of the Blood-Brain Barrier and Its Manipulation: Vol 2, Clinical Aspects. Plenum Press, New York, 1989, pp 77–106.
84. Greitz, T: Computer tomography for diagnosis of intracranial tumors compared with other neuroradiologic procedures. Acta Radiol (Suppl)346:14–20, 1975.
85. Handel, SF, Powell, MR, Wilson, CB, Enot, KJ: Scinti-photographic evalua-

tion of response of brain neoplasms to systemic chemotherapy. J Nucl Med 12:292–296, 1971.
86. Haughton, VM, Rimm, AA, and Cverionke, LF: Sensitivity of Gd-DTPA-enhanced MR imaging of benign extraaxial tumors. Radiology 166:829–833, 1988.
87. Hawkins, RA, Huang, S-C, Barrio, JR, Keen, RE, Feng, D, Mazziotta, JC, and Phelps, ME: Estimation of local cerebral protein synthesis rates with L-[1-^{11}C]leucine and PET: Methods, model and results in animals and humans. J Cereb Blood Flow Metab 9:446–460, 1989.
88. Heiss, WD, Coenen, HH, Wienhard, K, Herholz, K, Rudolf, J, Kling, P, and Stoecklin, G: L-[2-^{18}F]fluorotyrosine uptake in gliomas studied with dynamic PET. J Nucl Med 31(5):799, 1990.
89. Hemminga, MA, DeJager, PA, and Sonneveld, A: The study of flow by pulsed nuclear magnetic resonance: Measurement of flow rates in the presence of stationary phase using a different method. J Magn Reson 27:359–370, 1977.
90. Hiesiger, E, Fowler, JS, Wolf, AP, Logan, J, Brodie, JD, McPherson, D, MacGregor, RR, Christman, DR, Volkow, ND, and Flamm, E: Serial PET studies of human cerebral malignancy with [1-^{11}C]putrescine and [1-^{11}C]2-deoxy-D-glucose. J Nucl Med 28:1251–1261, 1987.
91. Hill, TC, Lovett, RD, and McNeil, BJ: Observations on the clinical value of emission tomography. J Nucl Med 21:613–616, 1980.
92. Hindo, WA, Clasen, RA, Raynda, GVS, and Pandolfi, S: Technetium in cryogenic cerebral injury and edema. Arch Neurol 27:526–534, 1972.
93. Hirano, A and Matsui, T: Vascular structures in brain tumors. Hum Path 6:611–621, 1975.
94. Hochberg, FH and Pruitt, A: Assumptions in the radiotherapy of glioblastoma. Neurology 30:907–911, 1980.
95. Hossmann, KA, Wechsler, W, and Wilmes, F: Experimental peritumourous oedema. Morphological and pathophysiological observations. Acta Neuropathol 45:195–203, 1979.
96. Hübner, KF, Purvis, JT, Mahaley, SM, Robertson, JT, Rogers, S, Gibbs, WD, King, P, and Partain, CL: Brain tumor imaging by positron emission computed tomography using ^{11}C-labeled amino acids. J Comput Assist Tomogr 6:544–550, 1982.
97. Hylton, PD and Reichman, OH: Clinical manifestation of glioma before computed tomographic appearance: The dilemma of a negative scan. Neurosurgery 21:27–32, 1987.
98. Ilsen, HW, Sato, M, Pawlik, G, Herholz, K, Wienhard, K, and Heiss, W-D: (^{68}Ga)-EDTA positron emission tomography in the diagnosis of brain tumors. Neuroradiology 26:393–398, 1984.
99. Ishiwata, K, Ido, T, Abe, Y, Matsuzawa, T, and Iwata, R: Tumor uptake studies of S-adenosyl-L-[methyl-^{11}C] methionine and L-[methyl-^{11}C]methionine. Int J Rad Appl Instrum [B] 15:123–126, 1988.
100. Ito, M, Lammertsma, AA, Wise, RSJ, Bernardi, S, Frackowiak, RSJ, Heather, JD, McKenzie, CG, Thomas, DGT, and Jones, T: Measurement of regional cerebral blood flow and oxygen utilization in patients with cerebral tumors using ^{15}O and positron emission tomography: Analytical techniques and preliminary results. Neuroradiology 23:63–74, 1982.
101. Joensuu, H and Ahonen, A: Imaging of metastases of thyroid carcinoma with fluorine-18 fluorodeoxyglucose. J Nucl Med 28:910–914, 1987.
102. Jones, EA, Koslow, M, and Johnston, GS: Scintigraphic detection of intracranial tumors with ^{67}Ga-citrate. J Nucl Med 13:439–440, 1972.
103. Kaplan, WD, Takvorian, T, Morris, JH, Rumbaugh, CL, Connolly, BT, and Atkins, HL: Thallium-201 brain tumor imaging: A comparative study with pathologic correlation. J Nucl Med 28:47–52, 1987.
104. Kelly, PJ: Stereotactic technology in tumor surgery. Clin Neurosurg 35: 215–253, 1987.
105. Kelly, PJ, Daumas-Duport, C, Kispert, DB, Kall, BA, Scheithauer, BW,

and Illig, JJ: Imaging-based stereotaxic serial biopsies in untreated intracranial glial neoplasms. J Neurosurg 66:865–874, 1987.

106. Kelly, PJ, Daumas-Duport, C, Scheithauer, BW, Kall, BA, and Kispert, DB: Stereotactic histologic correlations of CT- and MRI-defined abnormalities in patients with glial neoplasms. Mayo Clin Proc 62:450–459, 1987.

107. Kendall, BE, Jabukowski, J, Pullicino, P, and Symon, L: Difficulties in diagnosis of supratentorial gliomas on CAT scan. J Neurol Neurosurg Psychiat 42:485–492, 1979.

108. Kent, DL and Larson, EB: Magnetic resonance imaging of the brain and spine: Is clinical efficacy established after the first decade? Ann Intern Med 107:402–424, 1988.

109. Kern, KA, Brunetti, A, and Norton, JA, Chang, AE, Malawer, M, Lack, E, Finn, RD, Rosenberg, SA, and Larson, SM: Metabolic imaging of human extremity musculoskeletal tumors by PET. J Nucl Med 29:181–186, 1988.

110. Kim, KT, Black, KL, Marciano, D, Mazziotta, JC, Guze, BH, Grafton, S, Hawkins, RA, and Becker, DP: Thallium-201 SPECT imaging of brain tumors. J Nucl Med 31:965–969, 1990.

111. Klatzo, I: Neuropathologic aspects of brain edema. J Neuropath Exp Neurol 26:1–14, 1967.

112. Kolin, A: Improved apparatus and technique for electromagnetic determination of blood flow. Rev Sci Instrum 23:235–242, 1952.

113. Krayenbühl, HA and Yasargil, MG: Cerebral Angiography. JB Lippincott, Philadelphia, 1968, pp 313–319.

114. Kubota, K, Matsuzawa, T, Ito, M, Ito, K, Fujiwara, T, Abe, Y, Yoshioka, S, Fukuda, H, Hatazawa, J, Iwata, K, Watanuki, S, and Ido, T: Lung tumor imaging by PET using C-11 methionine. J Nucl Med 26:37–42, 1985.

115. Kuhl, DR, Reivich, M, Alavi, H, Nyary, I, and Staum, MM: Local cerebral blood volume determined by three-dimensional reconstruction of radionuclide scan data. Circ Res 36:610–619, 1975.

116. Kuwabara, Y, Ichiya, Y, Otsuka, M, Miyake, Y, Gunasekera, R, Hasuo, K, Masuda, K, Takeshita, I, and Fukui, H: High [^{18}F]FDG uptake in primary cerebral lymphoma: A PET study. J Comput Assist Tomogr 12:47–48, 1988.

117. Lammertsma, AA, Wise, R, Gibbs, J, Thomas, D, and Jones, T: The pathophysiology of human cerebral tumor and surrounding white matter and remote cortex. J Cereb Blood Flow Metab 3:S9–S10, 1983.

118. Lammertsma, AA, Wise, RJS, Heather, JD, Gibbs, JM, Leenders, KL, Frackowiak, RSJ, Rhodes, CG, and Jones, T: Correction for the presence of intravascular oxygen-15 in the steady-state technique for measuring regional oxygen extraction ratio in the brain: 2. Results in normal subjects and brain tumor and stroke patients. J Cereb Blood Flow Metab 3:425–431, 1983.

119. Landolt, AM, Wilson, CB: Tumors of the sella and parasellar area in adults. In Youman, JR (ed): Neurological Surgery, Vol 5. WB Saunders, Philadelphia, 1982, pp 3107–3162.

120. Langen, K-J, Herzog, H, Kuwert, T, Roosen, N, Rota, E, Kiwit, JCW, Bock, WJ, and Feinendegen, LE: Tomographic studies of RCBF with Tc-99m-HM-PAO SPECT in patients with primary brain tumors: Comparison with continuous inhalation of $C^{15}O_2$ and PET. J Nucl Med 28:591, 1987.

121. Langhammer, H, Glaubitt, G, and Grebe, SF: ^{67}Ga for tumor scanning. J Nucl Med 13:196–201, 1972.

122. Larsell, O and Jansen, J: The Comparative Anatomy and Histology of the Cerebellum: The Human Cerebellum, Cerebellar Connections and Cerebellar Cortex. University of Minnesota Press, Minneapolis, 1972, p 268.

123. Leeds, NE, Elkin, CM and Zimmerman, RD: Gliomas of the brain. Semin Roentgenol 19:27–43, 1984.

124. Leibel SA, Sheline GE, Wara, WM, Boldrey, EB, and Nielsen, SL: The role of radiation therapy in the treatment of astrocytomas. Cancer 35:1551–1557, 1975.

125. Lewander, R: Contrast enhancement with time in gliomas: Stereotactic computer tomography following contrast

medium infusion. Acta Radiol (Diagn) 20:689–702, 1979.

126. Lichtor, J and Dohrmann, GJ: Oxidative metabolism and glycolysis in benign brain tumors. J Neurosurg 67: 336–340, 1987.
127. Lilja, A, Bergström, K, Hartvig, P, Spännare, B, Halldin, C, Lundqvist, H, and Långström, B: Dynamic study of supratentorial gliomas with L-(methyl-^{11}C)-methionine and positron emission tomography. AJNR 6:505–514, 1985.
128. Lilja, A, Bergström, K, Spännare, and Olsson, Y: Reliability of computed tomography in assessing histopathological features of malignant supratentorial gliomas. J Comput Assist Tomogr 5:625–636, 1981.
129. Long, DM: Capillary ultrastructure and the blood brain barrier in human malignant brain tumors. J Neurosurg 32:127–144, 1970.
130. Marangos, PJ, Patel, J, Boulenger, J-P, and Clark-Rosenberg, R: Characterization of peripheral-type benzodiazepine binding sites in brain using [^{3}H]RO 5-4864. Molecular Pharm 22:26–32, 1982.
131. Marks, JE and Gado, M: Serial computed tomography of primary brain tumors following surgery, irradiation, and chemotherapy. Radiology 125: 119–125, 1977.
132. Marsa, GW, Goffinet, DR, Rubenstein, LJ, and Bagshaw, MA: Megavoltage irradiation in the treatment of gliomas of the brain and spinal cord. Cancer 36:1681–1689, 1975.
133. Mawhinney, RR, Buckley, JH, Holland, IM, and Worthington, BS: The value of magnetic resonance imaging in the diagnosis of intracranial meningiomas. Clin Radiol 37:429–439, 1986.
134. Miller, JH, Weinblatt, ME, Smith, JC, Fishman, LS, Segall, HD, and Ortega, JA: Combined computed tomographic and radionuclide imaging in the long-term follow-up of children with primary intraaxial intracranial neoplasms. Radiology 146:681–686, 1983.
135. Minn, H, Joensuu, H, Ahonen, A, and Klemi, P: Fluorodeoxyglucose imaging: A method to assess the proliferative activity of human cancer in vivo. Comparison with DNA flow cytometry. Cancer 61:1776–1781, 1988.
136. Mosskin, M, von Holst, H, Ericson, K, and Norén, G: The blood tumour barrier in intracranial tumours studied with x-ray computed tomography and positron emission tomography using 68-Ga-EDTA. Neuroradiology 28:259–263, 1986.
137. Mosskin, M, von Holst, H, Bergström, M, Collins, VP, Eriksson, L, Johnström, P, and Norén, G: PET with ^{11}C-methionine and CT of intracranial tumours compared with histopathologic examination of multiple biopsies. Acta Radiol 28:673–680, 1987.
138. Muhr, C, Bergström, M, Lundberg, PO, Bergström, K, Hartvig, P, Lundqvist, H, Antoni, G, and Långström, B: Dopamine receptors in pituitary adenomas: PET visualization with ^{11}C-N-methylspiperone. J Comput Assist Tomogr 10:175–180, 1986.
139. Müller, JP: Über den feineren Bau und die Formen der Krankhaften Geschwülste. G. Reimer, Berlin, 1838.
140. Naruse, S, Hirakawa, K, Horikawa, J, et al.: Measurements of in vivo ^{31}P nuclear magnetic resonance spectra in neuroectodermal tumors for the evaluation of chemotherapy. Cancer Res 45:2429–2433, 1985.
141. Nayler, GL, Firmin, DN, and Longmor, DB: Blood flow imaging by cine magnetic resonance. J Comput Assist Tomogr 10:715–722, 1986.
142. Nazarro, JM and Neuwelt, EA: The role of surgery in the management of supratentorial intermediate and high-grade astrocytomas in adults. J Neurosurg 73:331–344, 1990.
143. Neuwelt, EA, Rapoport, SI: Modification of the blood-brain barrier in the chemotherapy of malignant brain tumors. Federation Proc 43:214–219, 1984.
144. Neuwelt, EA and Barnett, PA: Blood-brain barrier disruption in the treatment of brain tumors: Animal studies. In Neuwelt, EA (ed): Implications of the Blood-Brain Barrier and Its Manipulation, Vol 2, Clinical Aspects. Plenum Press, New York, 1989, pp 107–194.

144a. New, PFJ and Scott, WR: Gliomas. In Computed Tomography of the Brain and Orbit. Williams & Wilkins, Baltimore, 1975, pp 123–129.

145. New, PFJ and Scott, WR: Meningiomas. In Computed Tomography of the Brain and Orbit. Williams & Wilkins, Baltimore, 1975, pp 160–177.

146. New, PFJ, Scott, WR: Pituitary adenomas and craniopharyngiomas. In Computed Tomography of the Brain and Orbit. Williams & Wilkins, Baltimore, 1975, pp 178–193.

147. Norman, E and Rekonen, A: Interpretation of ^{99m}Tc-pertechnetate scintigraphy after irradiation of brain tumors. Int J Nucl Med Biol 2:25–29, 1975.

148. Nukui, H, Yamamoto, YL, Thompson, CJ, and Feindel, W: Positron emission tomography with Positome II: With special reference to ^{68}Ga-EDTA positron emission tomography in cases with brain tumor. Neurol Med Chir 19:941–954, 1979.

149. Olivecrona, H: The surgical treatment of intracranial tumors. In Handbuch der Neurochirugie, Vol 4. Springer Verlag, Berlin, 1967, pp 1–301.

150. O'Tuama, LA, Phillips, PC, Straus, LC, Carson, BC, Uno, Y, Smith, QR, Dannals, RF, Wilson, AA, Ravert, HT, and Loats, S: Two-phase [^{11}C]L-methionine PET in childhood brain tumors. Pediatr Neurol 6(3):163–170, 1990.

151. Patronas, NJ, DiChiro, G, Brooks, RA, De La Paz, RL, Kornblith, PL, Smith, BH, Rizzoli, HV, Kessler, RM, Manning, RG, Channing, M, Wolf, AP, and O'Connor, CM: Work in progress: [^{18}F]fluorodeoxyglucose and positron emission tomography in the evaluation of radiation necrosis of the brain. Radiology 144:885–889, 1982.

152. Patronas, NJ, DiChiro, G, Kufta, C, Bairamian, D, Kornblith, PL, Simon, R, and Larson, SM: Prediction of survival in glioma patients by means of positron emission tomography. J Neurosurg 62:816–822, 1985.

153. Patronas, NJ, DiChiro, G, Smith, BH, De La Paz, R, Brooks, RA, Milam, HL, Kornblith, PL, Bairamian, D, and Mansi, L: Depressed cerebellar glucose metabolism in supratentorial tumors. Brain Res 291:93–101, 1984.

154. Paul, R and Parviainen, S: Dynamic [^{18}F]-2-fluoro-2-deoxy-D-glucose (FDG) scintigraphy of normal and tumor-bearing rats. Res Exp Med 186:249–258, 1986.

155. Paul, R: Comparison of fluorine-18-2-fluorodeoxyglucose and gallium-67 citrate imaging for detection of lymphoma. J Nucl Med 28:288–292, 1987.

156. Pedersen, H, Gjerris, F, and Klinken, L: Malignancy criteria in computed tomography of primary supratentorial tumors in infancy and childhood. Neuroradiology 31:24–28, 1989.

157. Pederson, PL: Tumor mitochondria and the bioenergetics of cancer cells. Prog Exp Tumor Res 22:190–274, 1978.

158. Pendergrass, HP, McKusick, KA, New, PFJ, and Potsaid, MS: Relative efficacy of radionuclide imaging and computed tomography of the brain. Radiology 116:363–366, 1975.

159. Pick, L, Bielschowsky, M: Über das System der Neurome und Beobachtungen an einem Ganglioneurom des Gehirns nebst Untersuchung über die Genese der Nervenfasern in 'Neurinomen'. Z ges Neurol Psychiatr 6:391–437, 1911.

160. Piepmeier, JM: Observations on the current treatment of low-grade astrocytic tumors of the cerebral hemispheres. J Neurosurg 67:177–181, 1987.

161. Plowman, PN and Wise, RJS: Intracerebral lymphoma deposits: Investigation and treatment. Int J Radiat Oncol Biol Phys 10:843–849, 1984.

162. Raichle, ME, Grubb, RL, and Higgins, CS: Measurement of brain tissue carbon dioxide content in vivo by emission tomography. Brain Res 166:413–417, 1979.

163. Ramsdell, JS, Bethea, CL, Jaffe, RB, Wilson, CB, and Weiner, RJ: Characterization of dopamine and α-adrenergic receptors in human prolactin-secreting adenomas with (^{3}H)-dihydroergocriptine. Neuroendocrinology 40:518–525, 1985.

164. Rao, KCVG and Williams, JP: Intracranial tumors: Metastatic. In Lee, SH

and Rao, KCVG (eds): Cranial Computed Tomography. McGraw-Hill, New York, 1983, pp 345–369.

165. Reeves, GI and Marks, JE: Prognostic significance of lesion size for glioblastoma multiforme. Radiology 132: 469–471, 1979.

166. Rhodes, CG, Wise, RJS, Gibbs, JM, Frackowiak, RSJ, Hatazawa, J, Palmer, AJ, Thomas, DGT, and Jones, T: In vivo disturbance of the oxidative metabolism of glucose in human cerebral gliomas. Ann Neurol 14:614–626, 1983.

167. Ribbert, H: Über das Spongioblastom und das Gliom. Virchows Arch Path Anat 225:195–213, 1918.

168. Rottenberg, DA, Dhawan, V, Cooper, AJL, Strother, SC, Alcock, N, and Ginos, JZ: Assessment of the pharmacologic advantage of intra-arterial versus intravenous chemotherapy using ^{13}N-cisplatin and positron emission tomography. Neurology 37:335, 1987.

169. Rottenberg, DA, Ginos, JZ, Kearfott, KJ, Junck, ScDL, Dhawan, V, and Jarden, JO: In vivo measurement of brain tumor pH using [^{11}C]DMO and positron emission tomography. Ann Neurol 17: 70–79, 1985.

170. Röttinger, EM and Mendouca, BA: Modification of pH induced cellular inactivation by irradiation: Glial cells. Int J Radiat Oncol Biol Phys 6:1659–1662, 1980.

171. Russell, DS and Rubinstein, LJ: Pathology of Tumours of the Nervous System, ed 4. Baltimore, 1977, pp. 95–161.

172. Sachs, E: The History and Development of Neurological Surgery. Cassell, London, 1952.

173. Sage, MR, Turski, PA, and Levin, A: CNS imaging and the brain barriers. In Neuwelt, EA (ed): Implications of the Blood-Brain Barrier and Its Manipulation, Vol 2, Clinical Aspects. Plenum Press, New York, 1989, pp 1–52.

174. Sasaki, M, Ichiya, Y, Kuwabara, Y, Otsuka, M, Tahara, T, Fukumura, T, Gunasekera, R, and Masuda, K: Ringlike uptake of [^{18}F]FDG in brain abscess. J Comput Assist Tomogr 14(3):486–487, 1990.

175. Schoenberg, BS: The epidemiology of central nervous system tumors. In Walker, MD (ed): Oncology of the Nervous System. Martinus Nijhoff, Boston, 1983, pp 1–29.

176. Serri, O, Marchisio, AM, Collu, R, Hardy, J, and Somma, M: Dopaminergic binding sites in human pituitary adenomas other than prolactinomas. Horm Res 19:97–102, 1984.

177. Sheline, GE: Radiation therapy of primary tumors. Semin Oncol 2:29–43, 1975.

178. Shields, AF, Lim, K, Grierson, J, Link, J, and Krohn, KA: Utilization of labeled thymidine in DNA synthesis: Studies for PET. J Nucl Med 31:337–342, 1990

179. Silverman, C, Marks, JE: Prognostic significance of contrast enhancement in low-grade astrocytomas of the adult cerebrum. Radiology 139:211–213, 1981.

180. Singer, JR: Blood-flow rates by NMR measurements. Science 130:1652–1653, 1959.

181. Singer, JR: Blood flow measurements by NMR of the intact body. IEEE Trans Nucl Sci 27:1245–1249, 1980.

182. Sokoloff, L, Reivich, M, Kennedy, C, Des Rosiers, MH, Patlak, CS, Pettigrew, KD, Sakurada, O, and Shinohara, M: The [^{14}C]deoxyglucose method for the measurement of local cerebral glucose utilization: Theory, procedure and normal values in the albino rat. J Neurochem 28:897–916, 1977.

183. Solti-Bohman, LG, Magram, DL, Lo, WM, Wade, CT, Witlen, RM, Shimizu, FH, McMonigle, EM, and Rao, AK: Gas CT cisternography for detection of small acoustic tumors. Radiology 150:403–407, 1984.

184. Som, P, Atkins, HL, Bandopadhyay, D, Fowler, JS, MacGregor, RR, Matsui, K, Oster, ZH, Sacker, DF, Shiue, CY, Turner, H, Wan, C-N, Wolf, AP, and Zabinski, SV: A fluorinated glucose analog, 2-fluoro-2-deoxy-D-glucose (F-18): Nontoxic tracer for rapid tumor detection. J Nucl Med 21:670–675, 1980.

185. Spagnoli, MV, Goldberg, HI, Grossman, RI, Bilaniuk, LT, Gomori, JM, Hackney, DB, and Zimmerman, RA: Intracranial meningiomas: High-field

MR imaging. Radiology 160:369–375, 1986.

186. Staquet, MJ: Preface. In Staquet, MJ (ed): Cancer Therapy, Prognostic Factors and Criteria of Response. Raven Press, New York, 1975, pp v–vi.

187. Steinhoff, H, Grumme, TH, Kazner, E, Lange, S, Lanksch, W, Meese, W, and Wüllenweber, R: Axial transverse computerized tomography in 73 glioblastomas. Acta Neurochir (Wien) 42:45–56, 1978.

188. Steinhoff, H, Lanksch, W, Kazner, E, Grumme, T, Meese, W, Lange, S, Aulich, A, Schindler, E, and Wende, S: Computed tomography in the diagnosis and differential diagnosis of glioblastomas. Neuroradiology 14:193–200, 1977.

189. Sze, G, Abramson, A, Krol, G, Liu, D, Amster, J, Zimmerman, RD, and Deck, MD: Gadolinium-DTPA in the evaluation of intradural extramedullary spinal disease. AJNR 9:153–163, 1988.

190. Sze, G, Milano, E, Johnson, C, and Heier, L: Detection of brain metastases: Comparison of contrast-enhanced MR with unenhanced MR and enhanced CT. AJNR 11:785–791, 1990.

191. Sze, G, Shin, J, Krol, G, Johnson, C, Liu, D, and Deck, MD: Intraparenchymal brain metastases: MR imaging versus contrast-enhanced CT. Radiology 168:187–194, 1988.

192. Thomas, DGT, Beaney, RP, and Brooks, DJ: Positron emission tomography in the study of cerebral tumors. Neurosurg Rev 7:253–258, 1984.

193. Tonami, N and Hisada, K: Clinical experience of tumor imaging with 201-Tl-chloride. Clin Nucl Med 2:75–81, 1977.

193a. Tsurumi, T, Kameyama, M, Ishiwata, K, Katakura, R, Monma, M, Ido, T, and Suzuki, J: ^{18}F-2′-deoxyuridine as a tracer of nucleic acid metabolism in brain tumors. J Neurosurg 72:110–113, 1990.

194. Tyler, JL, Diksic, M, Villemure, J-G, Evans, AC, Meyer, E, Yamamoto, YL, and Feindel, W: Metabolic and hemodynamic evaluation of gliomas using positron emission tomography. J Nucl Med 28:1123–1133, 1987.

195. Tyler, JL, Yamamoto, YL, Diksic, M, Théron, J, Villemure, J-G, Worthington, C, Evans, AC, and Feindel, W: Pharmacokinetics of superselective intra-arterial and intravenous [^{11}C] BCNU evaluated by PET. J Nucl Med 27:775–780, 1986.

196. Vassilouthis, J and Ambrose, J: Computerized tomography scanning appearances of intracranial meningiomas: An attempt to predict histological features. J Neurosurg 50:320–327, 1979.

197. Virchow, R: Zur Entwicklungsgeschichte des Krebses. Virchows Arch Path Anat, Vol 1, Berlin, 1847, p 94.

198. Virchow, R: Die krankhaften Geschwülste. Hirschwald, Berlin, 1863–1865.

199. von Monakow, C: Die lokalisation im Grosshirm und der abbau der funktion durch kortikale Herde. JF Bergman, Wiesbaden, 1914.

200. Vonofakos, D, Marcu, H, and Hacker H: Oligodendrogliomas: CT patterns with emphasis on features indicating malignancy. J Comput Assist Tomogr 3:783–788, 1979.

201. Walker, AE: A History of Neurological Surgery. Williams & Wilkins, Baltimore, 1951.

202. Walker, MD, Green, SB, Byar, DP, Alexander, E Jr, Batzdorf, U, Brooks, WH, Hunt, WE, MacCarty, CS, Mahaley, MS Jr, Mealey, J Jr, Owens, G, Ransohoff, J II, Robertson, JT, Shapiro, WR, Smith, KR Jr, Wilson, CB, and Strike, TA: Randomized comparisons of radiotherapy and nitrosoureas for the treatment of malignant glioma after surgery. N Engl J Med 303:1323–1329, 1980.

203. Walker, RW and Posner, JB: Central nervous system neoplasms. Curr Neurol 5:285–320, 1984.

204. Warburg, O: The Metabolism of Tumors. Richard R. Smith Inc, New York, 1931 pp. 75–199.

205. Warburg, O: On the origin of cancer cells. Science 123:309–314, 1956.

206. Washburn, LC, Sun, TT, Anon, JB, and Hayes, RL: Effect of structure on tumor specificity of alicyclic alpha amino acids. Cancer Res 38: 2271–2273, 1978.

207. Waxman, AD, Lee, G, Wolfstein, R, and Siemsen, JK: Differential diagnosis

of brain lesions by gallium scanning. J Nucl Med 14:903–906, 1973.

208. Weber, G: Enzymology of cancer cells. N Engl J Med 296:486–493, 541, 551, 1977.

209. Willson, N and Duffy, PE: Morphological changes associated with combined BCNU and radiation therapy in glioblastoma multiforme. Neurology Volume #24:465–471, 1974.

210. Winger, MJ, MacDonald, DR, and Cairncross, JG: Supratentorial anaplastic gliomas in adults: The prognostic importance of extent of resection and prior low-grade glioma. J Neurosurg 71:487–493, 1989.

211. Wise, RJS, Thomas, DGT, Lammertsma, AA, and Rhodes, CG: PET scanning of human brain tumors. Prog Exp Tumor Res 27:154–169, 1984.

212. Worthington, C, Peter, TM, Ethier, R, Melanson, D, Théron, J, Villemure, J-G, Olivier, A, Clark, J, and Mawko, G: Stereoscopic digital subtraction angiography in neuroradiologic assessment. AJNR 6:802–808, 1985.

213. Worthington, C, Tyler, JL, and Villemure, J-G: Stereotaxic biopsy and positron emission tomography correlation of cerebral gliomas. Surg Neurol 27:87–92, 1987.

214. Young, IR, Burl, M, Clarke, GJ, Hall, AS, Pasmore, T, Collins, AG, Smith, DT, Orr, JS, Bydder, GM, Doyle, FH, Greenspan, RH, and Steiner, RE: Magnetic resonance properties of hydrogen: Imaging the posterior fossa. AJR 137:895–901, 1981.

215. Zülich KJ: Brain Tumors: Their Biology and Pathology. ed 2. Springer Verlag, New York, 1965.

216. Zülich, KJ, Mennell, HD: The biology of brain tumors. In Vinken, PJ and Bruyn, GW (eds): Handbook of Clinical Neurology, Vol 16. Elsevier, New York, 1974.

Chapter 7

CEREBROVASCULAR DISEASE

D. J. Brooks, M.D., and
R. S. J. Frackowiak, M.D.

THE PATHOPHYSIOLOGY OF ISCHEMIA
THE USE OF STRUCTURAL SCANNING IN THE DIAGNOSIS OF CEREBROVASCULAR DISEASE
THE USE OF FUNCTIONAL IMAGING FOR THE INVESTIGATION OF CEREBROVASCULAR DISEASE
THE ROLE OF NEUROIMAGING IN THE MANAGEMENT OF CEREBROVASCULAR DISEASE

THE PATHOPHYSIOLOGY OF ISCHEMIA

In human adults, about 20% of the total cardiac output is assigned to supplying the metabolic requirements of the brain. In normal brain tissue, under resting conditions, regional cerebral oxygen metabolism ($LCMRO_2$) and blood flow (LCBF) are closely coupled, and are highest in peripheral cortical and central gray matter.[25] As a consequence of this coupling, the fraction of the arterial oxygen supply extracted regionally (LOEF) by brain tissue under resting conditions is uniform throughout the brain. Roughly 40% of the oxygen in the blood reserve is metabolized by both gray and white matter.[44] This means, in practice, that there is a considerable oxygen reserve in the arterial blood supply. Should cerebral perfusion fall because of cardiac failure, or because of occlusions of extracranial and intracranial vessels, then the fraction of the arterial oxygen supply extracted can rise from a normal 40% level up to a theoretical maximum level of 100%.[73] When the LOEF reaches 100%, the level of cerebral oxygen utilization ($LCMRO_2$) becomes blood-flow–dependent. Further falls in blood flow lead to a state of ischemia (Fig. 7–1).

The brain is subject to hemodynamic autoregulation; that is, over a range of mean cerebral perfusion pressure of roughly 70–140 mm Hg, regional cerebral blood flow (LCBF) is maintained constant.[36] In normal brain, LCBF and blood volume (LCBV) are closely coupled, LCBF and LCBV being highest in gray matter.[14] This coupling results in a uniform CBF/CBV ratio throughout the brain, with a value of approximately 10 min^{-1} for both gray and white matter (Fig. 7–2). This ratio represents the transit rate of the cerebral blood supply. When a fall in perfusion pressure occurs, cerebral blood flow is initially maintained by a reactive vasodilatation that reduces vascular resistance. As a consequence, the LCBV rises and the LCBF/LCBV ratio falls. When this ratio drops to a value of about 6 min^{-1}, vasodilatation is maximal. At this point, cerebral blood flow can no longer be maintained by reactive vasodilatation when further falls in cerebral perfusion pressure occur. Thus, there are two ho-

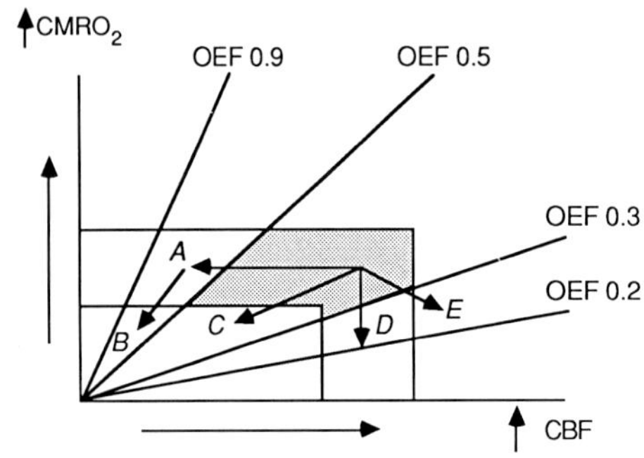

A Compensated Hypoperfusion
B True Ischemia
C Matched Fall of Oxygen Utilization and Perfusion
D Relative] Luxury Perfusion
E Absolute

Indicates Normal Zone

Figure 7–1. The relationship between cerebral oxygen utilization ($CMRO_2$) and blood flow (CBF). The shaded area is the normal zone.

meostatic mechanisms for preserving levels of cerebral oxygen utilization in the presence of falling perfusion pressure: initially the brain exhausts its vascular reserve (with vasodilatation occurring to maintain LCBF), and then it exhausts its oxygen reserve, LOEF increasing from 40% towards 100% once vasodilatation has become maximal and LCBF has started to fall.[26]

When cerebral ischemia occurs as a consequence of focal or generalized interruption of the cerebral circulation, neuronal dysfunction becomes apparent within minutes.[33] The immediate biochemical consequence is a cessation of oxidative phosphorylation; that is, the respiratory chain of enzymes fails to generate ATP and phosphocreatine from the reduction of oxygen.[48] There is a far larger glucose than oxygen reserve in normal brain tissue, only 10% of the arterial glucose supply (as opposed to 40% of the oxygen supply) being extracted under fasting conditions at rest.[67] When it becomes ischemic, brain tissue utilizes the less efficient glycolytic pathway to generate ATP, converting glucose to lactic acid. The result is a fall in levels of ATP and phosphocreatine from preischemic levels within minutes of the onset of ischemia, and a fall in cerebral pH as lactic acid forms.[16] Na^+/K^+ and Mg^{2+}/Ca^{2+} ATPases are reliant on available ATP to maintain the cellular electrolyte homeostasis. As ATP concentrations fall following ischemia, intracellular levels of Na^+, Ca^{2+}, and water rise, while K^+ leaks extracellularly. The result is the formation of cytotoxic edema within minutes of the onset of ischemia.[33]

Initially, the blood-brain barrier

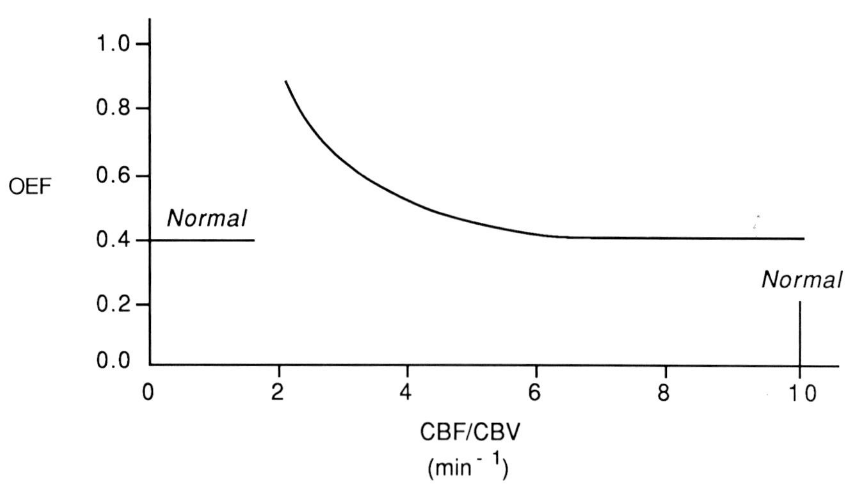

Figure 7–2. The relationship between oxygen extraction by brain tissue (OEF) and cerebral vascular reserves (CBF/CBV).

(BBB) remains intact following ischemia or infarction, but after several hours the tight junctions linking endothelial cells become disrupted and pinocytosis increases.[33] As a consequence, water, electrolytes, and protein can leak from the vascular compartment into the infarcted tissue. The result is formation of vasogenic as well as cytotoxic edema. Resumption of the circulation at this point may result in a secondary hemorrhage owing to the disruption of the tight junctions between endothelial cells.

Once ischemia has become established, failure to restore the circulation within minutes results in irreversible neuronal damage.[7] Over the course of several weeks, the tight junctions comprising the BBB re-form and the edema resulting from infarction subsides. At this stage, neuronal loss with variable degrees of gliosis and cystic necrosis is present. The circulation becomes reestablished and frequently "luxury perfusion" results, the blood supply far exceeding the metabolic requirements of the infarcted tissue[24] (see Fig. 7–1). After some months the infarcted tissue becomes a gliotic scar with a low, but coupled, cerebral oxygen utilization and blood flow.

With functional and structural imaging, the pathophysiology of preischemic and ischemic states can be followed. Single photon emission computerized tomography (SPECT) and positron emission tomography (PET) enable LCBF and LCBV to be estimated, and PET also can be used to measure LOEF, $LCMRO_2$, regional cerebral pH (LpH), and glucose metabolism (LCMRGlc). Magnetic resonance imaging (MRI) detects changes in water proton environment and so is highly sensitive to edema formation. It is also highly sensitive to the presence of paramagnetic agents such as methemoglobin, and to changes in magnetic susceptibility caused by the presence of deoxyhemoglobin and hemosiderin. Thus, MRI is ideally suited for detecting hemorrhagic infarcts and hematomas after 24–48 hours, as paramagnetic breakdown products form within the blood clot. Magnetic resonance spectroscopy (MRS) is able to detect regional changes in levels of phosphorus-31 (^{31}P) metabolites such as ATP, phosphocreatine, and phosphate, plus local formation of lactic acid and alterations in cellular pH. Currently, with surface coils, the effective resolution of MRS is limited to tissue volumes of around 25 ml.[32]

THE USE OF STRUCTURAL SCANNING IN THE DIAGNOSIS OF CEREBROVASCULAR DISEASE

Cerebral Hemorrhages and Hematomas

Following a parenchymal hemorrhage, clot formation takes place over the next 1–2 hours. As the clot develops, hemoconcentration and progressive deoxygenation of the oxyhemoglobin results. X-ray CT scanning is a highly sensitive means of detecting the presence of hemorrhage in the first 24 to 48 hours, the blood clot causing a marked focal attenuation of the x-rays[22] (see Chapter 1). The presence of oxyhemoglobin has little effect on local magnetic fields, or influence on the spin-lattice (T_1) and spin-spin (T_2) relaxation times of bulk water protons.[31] However, a focal prolongation of water T_1 and T_2 relaxation times is found in hematomas in the first few hours following their formation, reflecting their increased water content. T_1-weighted, spin echo MRI sequences show isointense or low signal, and T_2-weighted sequences show increased signal. In the 24–48 hours prior to deoxygenation of the blood, MRI is less sensitive than x-ray CT for detecting hemorrhage unless special phase-sensitive sequences are used to demonstrate these subtle changes in magnetic susceptibility.[20,54]

In the presence of a static magnetic field, paramagnetic substances lead to an increase in local field strength, whereas diamagnetic substances lead to a slight decrease. Both ferrous ions and molecular oxygen are paramagnetic when uncomplexed, having four and two unpaired electrons respectively. In oxyhemoglobin the paramagnetic effects of the ferrous ions and oxygen are largely self-cancelling. Deoxyhemoglobin, by contrast, is strongly paramagnetic.

As the blood in the cerebral hematoma becomes deoxygenated over the first few days, the presence of deoxyhemoglobin results in local changes in magnetic susceptibility. As a consequence, the water protons in the blood continually diffuse through a locally fluctuating magnetic field. This results in a selective decrease of the T_2 values of the water protons, while their T_1 values remain relatively unaffected. The selective shortening of the water proton T_2 values is dependent on the square of the applied field strength.[31] When T_2-weighted spin echo sequences are used, low signal develops in hematomas older than several hours, because of deoxyhemoglobin formation. This low signal is more apparent at higher field strengths (for example, 1.5 T) than at conventional field strengths (0.15–0.6 T).[31] The local changes in magnetic susceptibility caused by deoxyhemoglobin formation in blood clots can, however, easily be visualized at conventional field strengths if partial saturation rather than spin echo sequences are employed[20] (Fig. 7–3*A*). In practice, MRI is a far more sensitive technique than x-ray CT scanning for detecting the presence of blood in cerebral hemorrhages older than 24 hours.[54]

After 1–2 weeks, the center of the blood clot contains methemoglobin as well as deoxyhemoglobin. Methemoglobin contains iron in the form of paramagnetic ferric ions with five unpaired

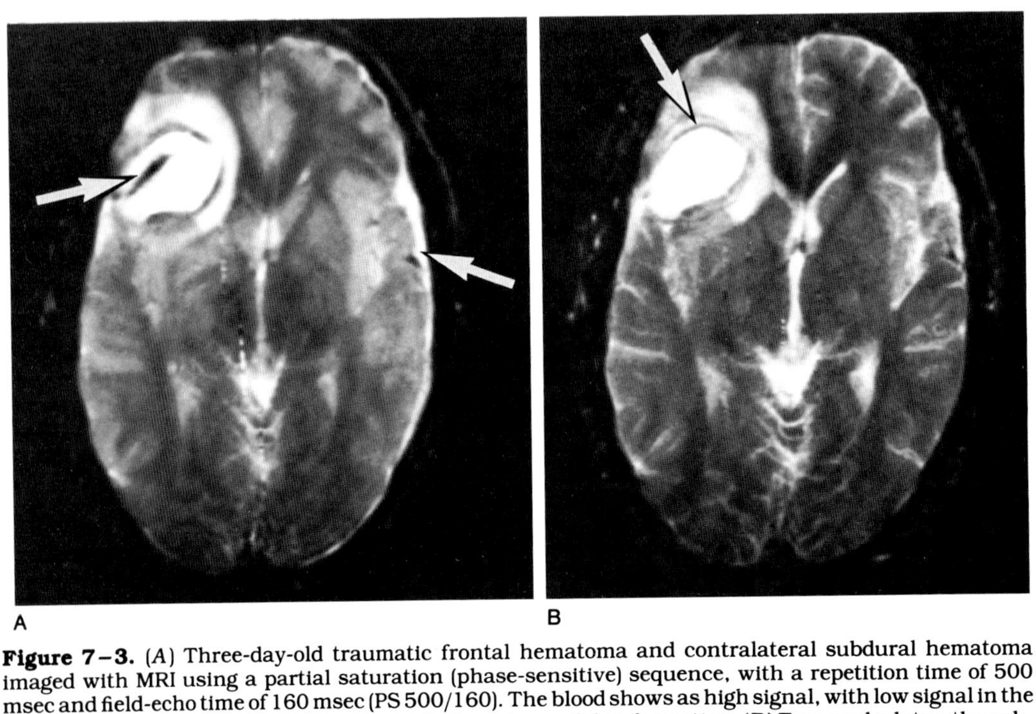

Figure 7–3. (*A*) Three-day-old traumatic frontal hematoma and contralateral subdural hematoma imaged with MRI using a partial saturation (phase-sensitive) sequence, with a repetition time of 500 msec and field-echo time of 160 msec (PS 500/160). The blood shows as high signal, with low signal in the center of the hematoma due to paramagnetic deoxyhemoglobin formation. (*B*) Two weeks later, the subdural hematoma is resolving. A rim of low signal is evident around the hematoma due to hemosiderin deposition.

electrons. Water molecules are able to bind directly to these ferric ions, forming a coordination sphere, and to pass in and out of this water coordination sphere. As a consequence, the bulk water proton T_1 and T_2 values both become shortened by scalar dipole interactions between the water protons and unpaired electrons in the ferric ions in a manner independent of applied field strength. With spin echo sequences, the clot now yields variable signal on T_1-weighted, and low signal on T_2-weighted MRI scans at both conventional and high field strengths.[31]

A rim of low T_2 signal is often evident from the hemosiderin deposited at the boundary of the hematoma[54] (Figs. 7–3*B*, 7–4). Hemosiderin, like deoxyhemoglobin, causes local variations in magnetic susceptibility that in turn lead to a selective decrease in water proton T_2 values.

After some months, cerebral hematomas and hemorrhages resolve, leaving a scar containing hemosiderin. These scars appear as nonspecific, focal low attenuation on x-ray CT scans. They can be shown, however, to have resulted from hemorrhage by the presence of a selectively decreased signal on T_2-weighted spin echo sequences, or by the presence of altered magnetic susceptibility with partial saturation sequences.

Figure 7–5 indicates the appropriate use of structural neuroimaging for investigating cerebral hematomas and hemorrhages. The changes in radiologic appearance of the blood clot as a function of time are detailed in Table 7–1.

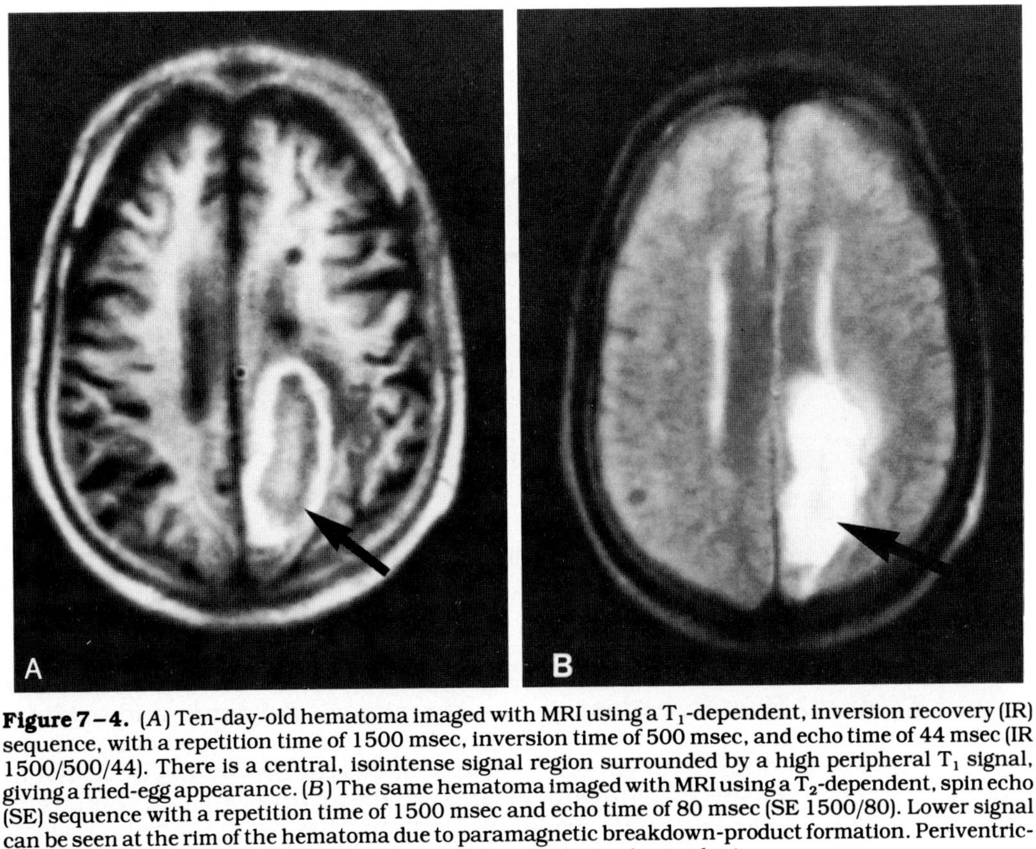

Figure 7–4. (*A*) Ten-day-old hematoma imaged with MRI using a T_1-dependent, inversion recovery (IR) sequence, with a repetition time of 1500 msec, inversion time of 500 msec, and echo time of 44 msec (IR 1500/500/44). There is a central, isointense signal region surrounded by a high peripheral T_1 signal, giving a fried-egg appearance. (*B*) The same hematoma imaged with MRI using a T_2-dependent, spin echo (SE) sequence with a repetition time of 1500 msec and echo time of 80 msec (SE 1500/80). Lower signal can be seen at the rim of the hematoma due to paramagnetic breakdown-product formation. Periventricular high T_2 signal due to ischemic white matter disease is also evident.

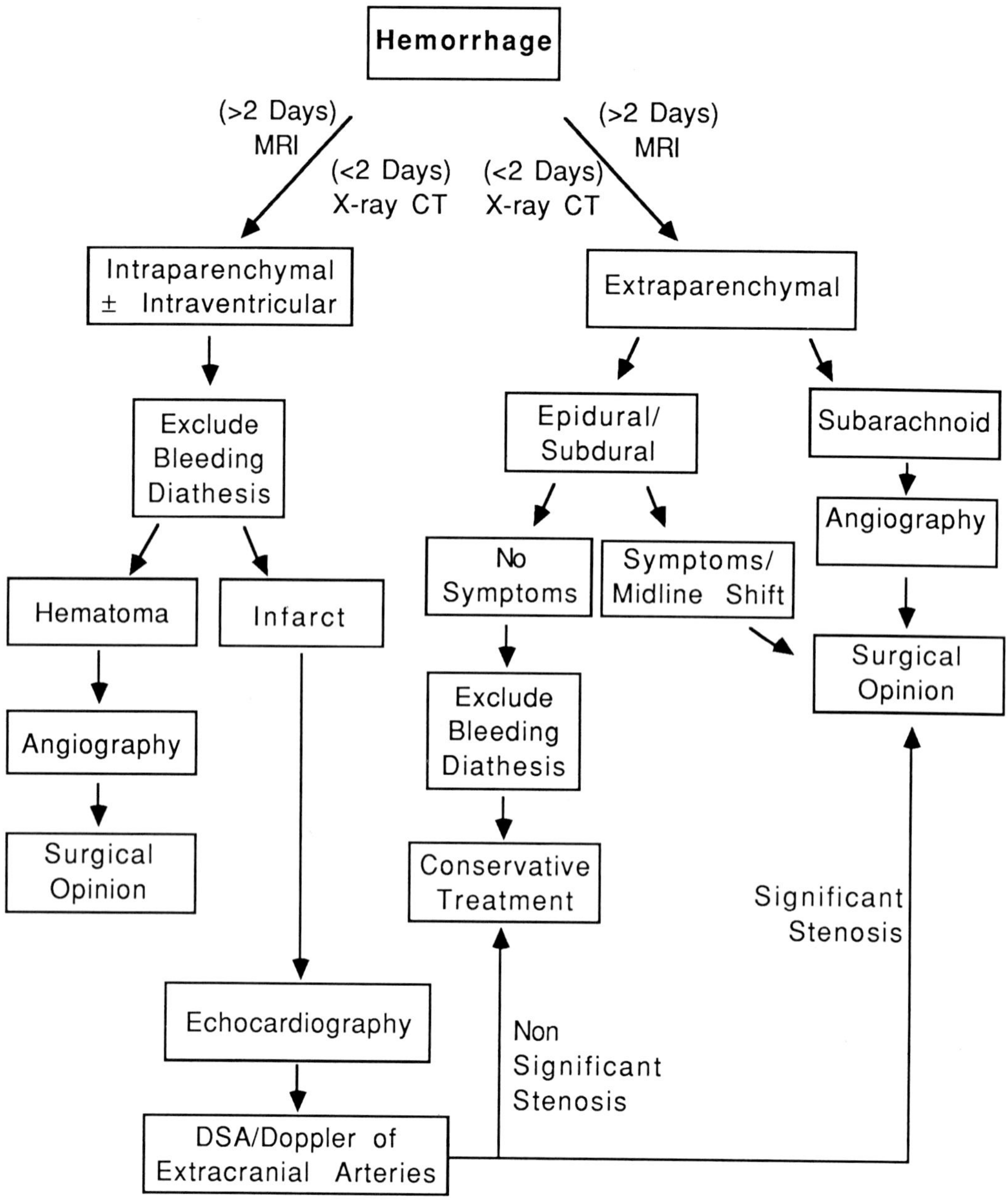

Figure 7–5. Management of cerebral hemorrhage.

Subarachnoid, Subdural, and Epidural Hemorrhages

For the reasons discussed earlier, x-ray CT is more sensitive than MRI (unless special phase-sensitive sequences are employed) when used to image the presence of fresh blood in the subarachnoid, subdural, and epidural spaces. In the first few hours following a hemorrhage, the oxyhemoglobin present shows up as an area of high signal attenuation on the x-ray CT scan. Because oxyhemoglobin is only weakly

Table 7–1 CHEMICAL AND RADIOLOGIC CHANGES IN CEREBRAL HEMORRHAGE

	Day			
	1	*3*	*7*	*50*
Constituents	Oxyhemoglobin	Deoxyhemoglobin	Deoxyhemoglobin Methemoglobin Hemosiderin	Hemosiderin
CT Findings	High attenuation	Resolving high attenuation	Resolving high attenuation	Scar with low attenuation
MRI Findings	Normal T_1, T_2 $\downarrow$susceptibility with phase-sensitive sequence	$T_1\uparrow$ $T_2\downarrow$ $\downarrow$susceptibility	Central $T_1\uparrow$ $T_2\downarrow$ Surrounding T_1 $\uparrow$ $T_2\downarrow$ Peripheral $T_2\downarrow$	Scar with low T_2 and surroundings with high T_1 and T_2
Test of Choice	X-ray CT	MRI	MRI	MRI

paramagnetic, spin echo MRI scans generally show little change in water proton T_1 and T_2 signals at this stage, but phase-sensitive partial saturation sequences may show local susceptibility changes. Once paramagnetic deoxyhemoglobin and methemoglobin have formed within the hemorrhage, MRI scans become more sensitive, showing variable signal changes on T_1- and low signal on T_2-weighted spin echo sequences. After one week, the hematoma generally has high signal on both T_1- and T_2-weighted spin echo sequences. As a consequence, extracerebral collections of altered blood that may be isodense on x-ray CT scans become clearly visible with MRI. MRI is, therefore, the technique of choice for imaging chronic subdural hematomas, and for detecting altered blood in the subarachnoid space.[52] Occasionally, evidence of a previous subarachnoid hemorrhage can be found in the form of superficial streaks of low signal on T_2-weighted spin echo sequences, caused by hemosiderin deposition on the brain surface.

Nonhemorrhagic Cerebral Infarcts

Numerous studies have demonstrated the superior ability of MRI compared to x-ray CT to detect lacunar and early infarcts, particularly when lesions involve the brainstem and cerebellum.[41,62,68] To detect an infarct, x-ray CT scanning requires a change in tissue attenuation of x-rays (Fig. 7–6), or the presence of BBB breakdown. As a consequence, cerebral infarcts may remain isodense for several days after the

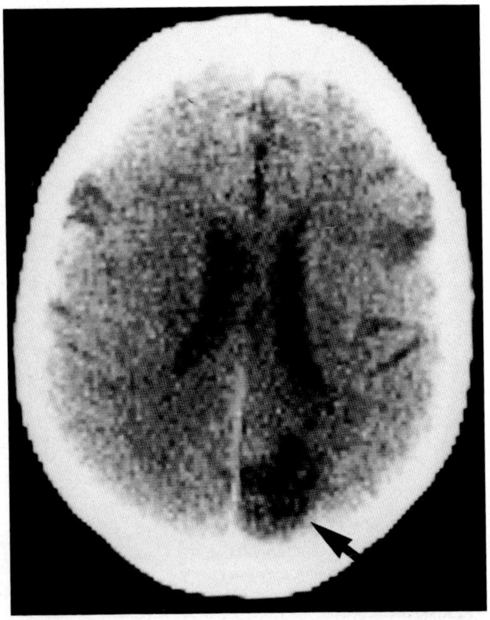

Figure 7–6. An x-ray CT scan of a patient with a left homonymous hemianopia, showing an infarct in right posterior cerebral artery territory.

ictus. By contrast, MRI simply requires a change in the chemical environment of the bulk water protons to produce alterations in signal. Experimental models of ischemia show that significant prolongation of proton T_1 and T_2 values occurs within an hour of infarction, in association with cytotoxic edema formation.[11] Unfortunately, chronic infarcts, where gliosis and cystic necrosis are present, also show prolonged T_1 and T_2 values. Consequently, infarcts of all ages appear as regions of low signal on T_1-weighted and high signal on T_2-weighted spin echo sequences. This appearance is nonspecific, in that any pathology leading to edema formation, gliosis, or demyelination will produce similar MRI appearances. As a result, it can be difficult to distinguish demyelinating disease and encephalitis from multi-infarct disease (Fig. 7–7). Infarcts may also mimic the appearance of low-grade gliomas.

A second problem is the interpretation of the significance of MRI findings in elderly subjects. In 30% of normal subjects over age 65, MRI shows multifocal areas of increased signal in central white matter and periventricular regions, when T_2-weighted spin echo sequences are employed.[8] Autopsy studies suggest that this increased signal results from the presence of silent multiple infarcts in the deep white matter of the elderly.[55] The finding of multiple areas of increased signal in the deep white matter of elderly subjects on T_2-weighted MRI scans must therefore be interpreted with caution, since they may not be related to the clinical problem under investigation.

The presence of BBB breakdown can help to date infarcts. It generally occurs some hours after infarction, and then resolves after a few weeks. BBB breakdown results in focal contrast enhancement on x-ray CT scans, but can be detected with far greater sensitivity with MRI and the paramagnetic contrast agent gadolinium diethylenetriamine penta-acetic acid (Gd-DTPA).[9] This agent produces marked decrease of bulk water proton T_1 values, and lesser

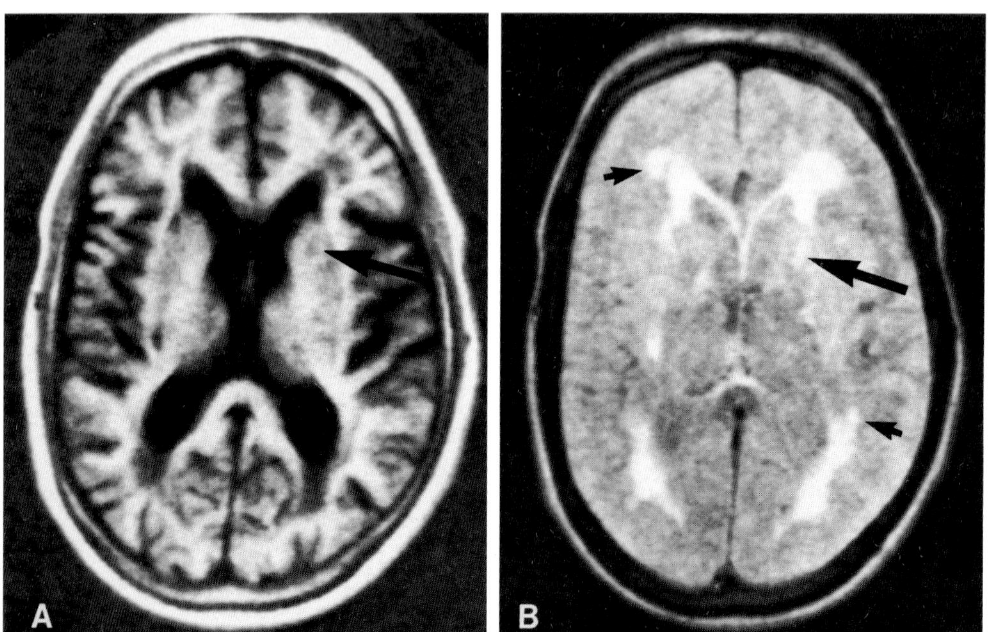

Figure 7–7. (*A*) A T_1-sensitive MRI IR 1500/500/44 sequence showing lacunar infarcts in the left caudate and right lentiform nuclei of a hypertensive patient. (*B*) Imaged with a T_2-sensitive SE 1500/80 sequence, more extensive ischemic basal ganglia and white matter disease is now evident.

decreases of their T_2-weighted spin echo sequences. Unfortunately, focal enhancement with Gd-DTPA is nonspecific. Recently formed plaques of demyelination and some high-grade gliomas can have the same Gd-DTPA appearance as recent infarcts.[51]

Because MRI is highly sensitive to the presence of edema, one might expect this technique to be able to detect focal reversible changes in signal in patients experiencing transient ischemic attacks (TIAs). So far, only fixed MRI lesions have been demonstrated in patients experiencing TIAs.[10] Resolving MRI lesions have been reported, however, in patients with fluctuating neurologic signs in association with systemic lupus erythematosus.[70]

An important question is whether functional imaging can distinguish between the various causes of cerebral infarction—embolus, thrombus, vasculitis, hypotension, and vascular malformation. Embolic infarcts are frequently multiple and occur in different arterial territories. A 60% incidence of secondary hemorrhage after embolic infarction in the first 4 weeks following the ictus has also been reported in one prospective study.[40] Forty percent of thrombotic infarcts, however, also produced some secondary hemorrhage within this time period. The presence of hemorrhage therefore is not specific for embolic infarction.

The presence of infarction in watershed territories (Fig. 7–8) is suggestive either of previous episodes of hypotension or of the presence of extracranial artery occlusion. Watershed infarcts also may result from vascular spasm secondary to subarachnoid hemorrhage. Vasculitides such as systemic lupus erythematosus may lead to lacunar infarcts at gray-white matter interfaces, watershed zones, and the basal ganglia, and may also lead to hemorrhage.[2] Basal ganglia calcification is also occasionally present,[53] although this finding is nonspecific and is seen occasionally in normal subjects and in a variety of other disorders (see Chapter 8).

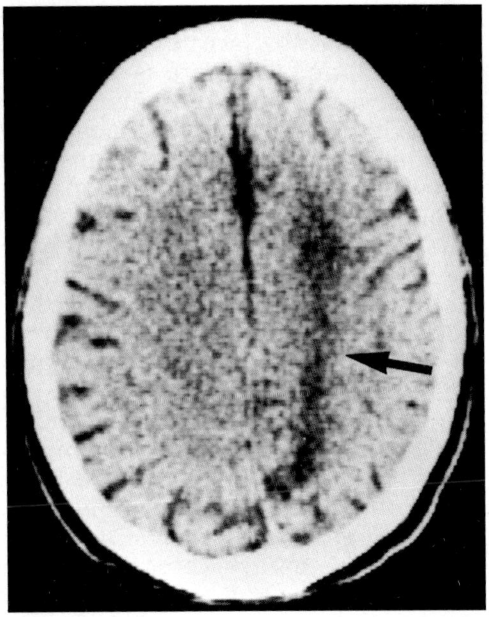

Figure 7–8. An x-ray CT scan of a subject with an occluded right internal carotid artery who developed acute left-sided neglect. The scan shows extensive watershed infarction between right anterior, middle, and posterior artery territories.

Vascular Malformations and Extracranial Artery Disease

Intracranial aneurysms and arteriovenous (AV) malformations are the most important causes of intraparenchymal and subarachnoid hemorrhages, and also may lead to thrombotic infarction. AV malformations can produce a progressive infarction syndrome mimicking space-occupying lesions. Stenosed and occluded carotid and vertebrobasilar arteries can result in both embolic and watershed infarcts, and such infarctions can also be caused by spontaneous and traumatic dissections of extracranial arteries. Other vascular pathologies associated with infarction include fibromuscular dysplasia, Moya Moya disease, congenital redundant arterial loops, and venous sinus thrombosis. Until the advent of MRI, these vascular pathologies were conventionally imaged with angiography with or without digital subtraction techniques. MRI, however, is capable of imaging blood flow (see next section and Chapter 2) and therefore is capable of demonstrating these vascular lesions by providing noninvasive angiography.

The spin echo MRI approach assumes that water protons remain stationary in a volume element (voxel) between the time of the excitatory pulse of radiofrequency electromagnetic radiation and the detection of the spin echo. An excitatory pulse of radiation is used to bring the magnetic moments of the water protons in the voxel into phase. These moments then dephase at a rate dependent on T_1 and T_2, but after a fixed time are flipped through 180° by a second pulse of radiation, experience varying static field strengths, and become dephased relative to stationary water protons. As a consequence, a flowing column of blood appears as a signal void in T_1- and T_2-weighted MRI spin echo sequences[71] (Fig. 7–9).

MRI uses the above phenomenon to image intracranial and extracranial vasculature. In practice, aneurysms and AV malformations give complex signal intensities as the blood flows through them with varying velocity and degrees of turbulence (Fig. 7–10). Calcifications and the presence of hemosiderin and methemoglobin in the thrombus may also reduce the MRI signal. The lamellar appearance of aneurysms and serpiginous appearance of AV malformations, however, makes them easy to identify, and MRI can also be used to reveal calcified cryptic AV malformations, which often appear indistinguishable from gliomas on x-ray CT.[30] Recently, MRI has been used to produce high-resolution angiograms capable of detecting carotid artery stenoses and dissections with accuracy (see Chapter 13).[54]

Venous sinus thrombosis is conventionally demonstrated by examining the delayed phase of an intravenous digital subtraction angiogram, although it may be evident as lack of contrast enhancement of the lateral and sagittal venous sinuses on x-ray CT. After some hours, venous sinus thrombosis appears isointense on T_1-weighted MRI images and as low signal on T_2-weighted images because of the presence of deoxyhemoglobin. After 1–2 weeks, however, high signal is found using both T_1- and T_2-weighted spin echo sequences.[50]

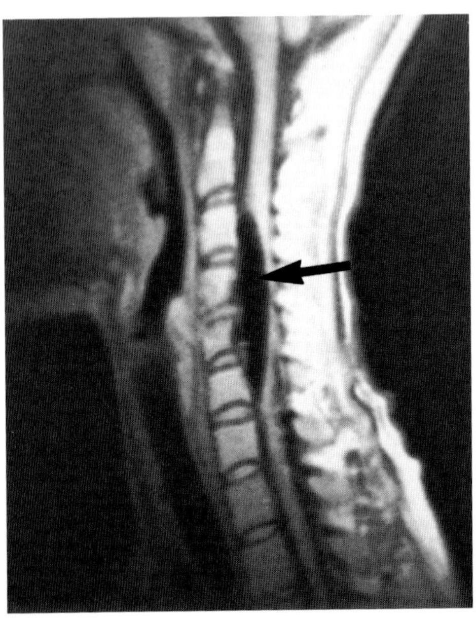

Figure 7–9. A high cervical AV malformation imaged with a T_1-weighted SE 544/44 sequence. The AV malformation shows as signal void because of flow effects.

Conclusions: Applications of Structural Scanning

MRI is more sensitive than x-ray CT scanning for detecting cerebral infarction, although the changes in signal seen are nonspecific, reflecting edema formation and gliosis. It also is the technique of choice for studying the posterior fossa. MRI cannot date infarction unless BBB disruption is present, in which case Gd-DTPA administration will result in a high signal on T_1-weighted spin echo sequences. The etiology of infarctions frequently may be inferred by the radiologic distribution of the lesions. MRI is able to image abnormalities in both intracranial and extracranial vasculature, using the signal void effect caused by flowing blood. In

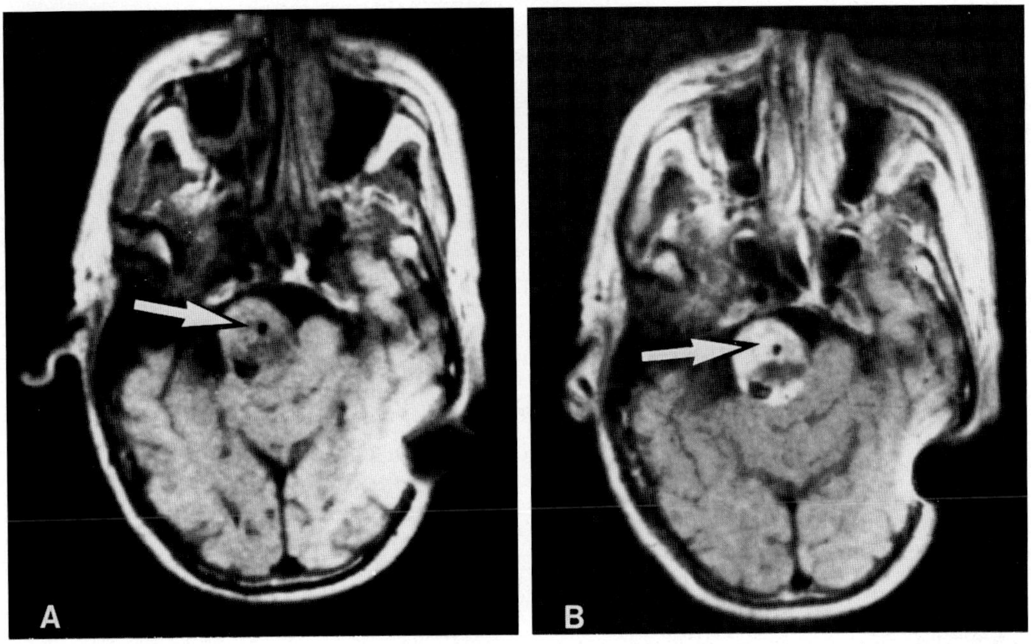

Figure 7–10. (*A*) A giant pontine basilar artery aneurysm imaged with a T_1-sensitive MRI SE 544/44 sequence. Low signal is seen from the mural thrombus because of the dephasing of water proton magnetization in flowing blood. (*B*) The same aneurysm imaged with the same T_1-weighted SE 544/44 sequence and the paramagnetic contrast agent Gd-DTPA. High signal is seen in the lumen of the pontine aneurysm.

this way, aneurysms, AV malformations, and extracranial artery lesions can be detected. X-ray CT scanning is more sensitive than MRI for imaging acute cerebral hemorrhages unless special phase-sensitive sequences are used, but after 24 hours, when altered blood is present, MRI becomes the more sensitive approach for detecting the presence of cerebral hemorrhage.

THE USE OF FUNCTIONAL IMAGING FOR THE INVESTIGATION OF CEREBROVASCULAR DISEASE

Methods of Functional Imaging

The various methods of imaging regional cerebral function are discussed in Chapters 3 and 4. These issues are reviewed briefly here with reference to cerebrovascular disease.

CEREBRAL BLOOD FLOW

Monitoring cerebral ^{133}Xe washout with multiple external detectors enables the estimation of regional cortical blood flow with a resolution of up to 2 cm. If the subject is given acetazolamide, breathes 5% carbon dioxide, or hyperventilates air prior to intravenous ^{133}Xe administration, the reactivity of the cerebral blood flow to changes in CSF pH and PCO_2 also can be determined. A normal subject increases his cerebral blood flow by 4%–5% per mm Hg rise in $PaCO_2$. An impaired vasoreactivity implies either that the microcirculation of the subject is already vasodilated to compensate for a low perfusion pressure or that microvascular disease is present.[15]

Regional cerebral blood flow also can be measured quantitatively by enhancement of x-ray CT scans by way of inhalation of nonradioactive xenon.[37,76] This technique has been used to demonstrate infarcts but has a functional resolution of at best $1.5 \times 1.5 \times 0.8$ cm^3. With SPECT and tracers such as ^{99m}Tc-hexamethyl-propyleneamine oxime (^{99m}Tc-HMPAO) and ^{123}I-isopropyl-iodoamphetamine (^{123}I-AMP), LCBF can be imaged qualitatively with a resolution of about 1 cm.[3,18,23,37] LCBF vasoreactivity following acetazolamide administration can also be assessed with SPECT.

At present, the most accurate method of measuring LCBF is PET. The most commonly employed PET tracer is $H_2{}^{15}O$, which is administered either as an intravenous bolus or by $C^{15}O_2$ inhalation. Comparison of regional cerebral and arterial blood ^{15}O levels under dynamic or steady-state conditions enables LCBF to be determined.[25,63] In practice, with $H_2{}^{15}O$, current PET scanners can achieve a resolution of $7 \times 6 \times 6$ mm^3.

MRI can be adapted to measure intravoxel incoherent motion of water protons, this motion being influenced by capillary blood velocity. With strong static field gradients pulsed between spin echo pulses of radiofrequency magnetic radiation, capillary blood velocity can be determined from the phase and amplitude of the resultant MRI signals.[45,77] The functional resolution of this approach is about $6 \times 6 \times 8$ mm^3 and its application to cerebrovascular disorders is currently being validated.

CEREBRAL BLOOD VOLUME

This can be determined quantitatively with PET and positron-emitting tracers that bind to red cells, such as ^{11}CO or $C^{15}O$, or tracers that remain in the plasma compartment, such as ^{11}C-methyl-albumin, ^{68}Ga-EDTA, and ^{68}Ga-transferrin.[57] Comparison of regional red-cell and plasma volumes of distribution enables the regional microvascular hematocrit, a measure of vessel caliber, to be computed.[43] Regional cerebral blood volume can be imaged qualitatively, and microvascular hematocrit can be imaged quantitatively with SPECT using tracers such as ^{99m}Tc-labeled red cells and albumin.[47]

CEREBRAL OXYGEN AND GLUCOSE UTILIZATION

Regional cerebral oxygen utilization (LCMRO$_2$) and the arterial oxygen extraction fraction (LOEF) can be determined using PET by means of inhalation of $^{15}O_2$.[25] Oxygen-15 binds to hemoglobin, and roughly 40% of the arterial $^{15}O_2$ supply is extracted regionally by normal brain tissue. The extracted $^{15}O_2$ is then metabolized rapidly to $H_2{}^{15}O$. A comparison of regional cerebral and arterial plasma ^{15}O, plus a knowledge of LCBF, enable LCMRO$_2$ and LOEF to be computed.

Regional cerebral glucose utilization (LCMRGlc) can be computed using PET by administration of the positron-emitting D-glucose analog ^{18}F-2-fluoro-2-deoxy-D-glucose (^{18}FDG) intravenously. ^{18}FDG is transported across the BBB by the D-hexose carrier and is then phosphorylated by hexokinase. ^{18}FDG-6-P is not metabolized further and is only slowly hydrolyzed. As a consequence, regional cerebral ^{18}F levels reflect regional cerebral hexokinase activity, which in turn reflects the rate of glycolysis of native D-glucose.[56]

In theory, 6 mol of O_2 should be consumed per mol of glucose converted to carbon dioxide and water. In practice, in normal resting brain, only 5.6 mol of O_2 are consumed, as some glucose is metabolized by way of the pentose phosphate pathway, and some glucose is used in lipid and amino acid synthesis.[67] The normal metabolic molar ratio (that is, LCMRO$_2$: LCMRGlc) is therefore 5.6. In ischemic conditions, measurement of the molar ratio with PET enables the relative contributions of respiration and glycolysis to glucose metabolism to be estimated.

CEREBRAL pH

Cerebral pH can be measured with PET and positron-emitting weak acids such as $^{11}CO_2$ or ^{11}C-dimethyloxazolidinedione (^{11}C-DMO)[12,69] The anions of these weak acids are unable to cross the BBB, and so the partition of ^{11}C activity between plasma and brain reflects the regional pH difference between the two compartments. Phosphorus-31 magnetic resonance spectroscopy (MRS) also enables intracellular pH to be estimated, since the difference in shifts between inorganic phosphate and phosphocreatine peaks is pH-dependent.[16]

BBB INTEGRITY

The integrity of the BBB can be studied quantitatively using positron-emitting tracers such as $^{82}Rb^+$ and ^{68}Ga-EDTA, or qualitatively with Gd-DTPA-enhanced MRI, SPECT tracers such as ^{99m}Tc-albumin and ^{67}Ga-EDTA, and x-ray CT scanning with iodinated contrast agents.

CEREBRAL HIGH-ENERGY PHOSPHATE AND LACTATE LEVELS

As conventionally used, ^{31}P-MRS measures relative, but not absolute, levels of intracellular cerebral phosphocreatine, ATP, hexose phosphates, and inorganic phosphate. In practice, current surface-coil MRS scanners sample signal from hemispheric voxels approximately 15–25 cm^3. With ^{1}H-MRS it is also possible to measure lactate levels and so assess the contribution of glycolysis to glucose metabolism. A comparison of MRS findings with ^{18}FDG and $^{15}O_2$ PET studies enables determination of the efficiency of coupling of respiration to oxidative phosphorylation, and the role of glycolysis in generating ATP and phosphocreatine.

Clinical Applications of Functional Imaging

ASSESSMENT OF PREISCHEMIC CEREBROVASCULAR DISEASE

A 60% or greater stenosis of a carotid artery results in a fall of cerebral perfusion pressure in the affected carotid territory.[61] This in turn leads to a reactive vasodilatation to reduce the vascular resistance and to maintain cerebral blood flow.[34] This vasodilatation can be detected as a reduction in the CO_2 or acetazolamide-induced reactivity of CBF as measured with ^{133}Xe washout, PET, and SPECT,[15] or as a rise in LCBV or fall in the LCBF : LCBV ratio, measured with either SPECT or PET.[26] The degree of reduction of the LCBF : LCBV ratio caused by vasodilatation correlates well with the degree of occlusive disease (Fig. 7–11) and the presence of collateral circulation demonstrated angiographically.[26,61] If the LCBF : LCBV ratio is less than 6 min^{-1}, maximal vasodilatation is present.[26] This is a common situation when both carotid arteries are occluded[26] (Fig. 7–12). The perfusion of the microcirculation is now compromised to the extent that the fractional arterial oxygen extraction (LOEF) becomes elevated above its normal level of 40% in order to maintain the level of oxygen metabolism, and may approach a theoretical maximum of 100%. These various situations are shown in Figures 7–1 and 7–2.

It would appear logical, on hemodynamic grounds, to revascularize patients with occlusive carotid artery disease and exhausted vasodilatory and oxygen reserves. Such patients frequently experience hemodynamic transient ischemic attacks (TIAs), with symptoms induced by changes in posture, exercise, and following ingestion of meals.[26] Several PET and SPECT studies have reported the hemodynamic effects of revascularization in patients with carotid artery stenoses and occlusions (Fig. 7–13). Most subjects experienced relief from their TIAs following extracranial/intracranial bypass (EC-IC), and this was accompanied by a rise in the LCBF : LCBV ratio in the affected carotid territory.[18,28,65] Variable effects of EC-IC bypass on the individual values of LCBF and LCBV in affected carotid territory have been reported, one study finding little change in LCBF but a consistent fall in LCBV following surgery,[28] whereas other studies demonstrated an improvement

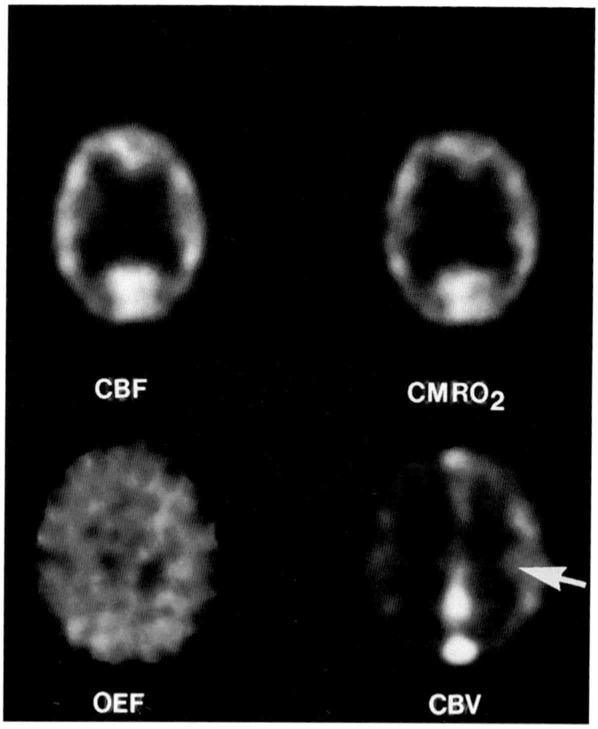

Figure 7–11. PET images of regional cerebral function for a patient with an occluded right internal carotid artery. Cerebral blood flow, arterial oxygen extraction, and oxygen metabolism are all normal. Cerebral blood volume is elevated by 50% in right internal carotid artery territory (*arrow*), the vasodilatation lowering vascular resistance and helping to maintain cerebral blood flow.

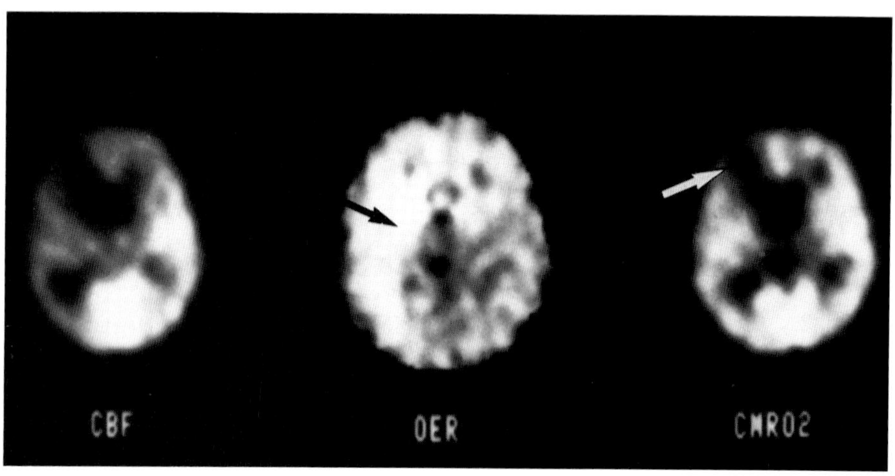

Figure 7–12. PET images of regional cerebral function for a patient with bilaterally occluded carotid arteries and an occluded left vertebral artery. Subject was experiencing transient attacks of right-sided weakness. Cerebral blood flow is reduced in left middle cerebral artery territory, and arterial oxygen extraction has risen to 60% from a normal 40% to maintain the level of cerebral oxygen metabolism. An infarct in the watershed territory between left middle cerebral and anterior cerebral arteries is also present.

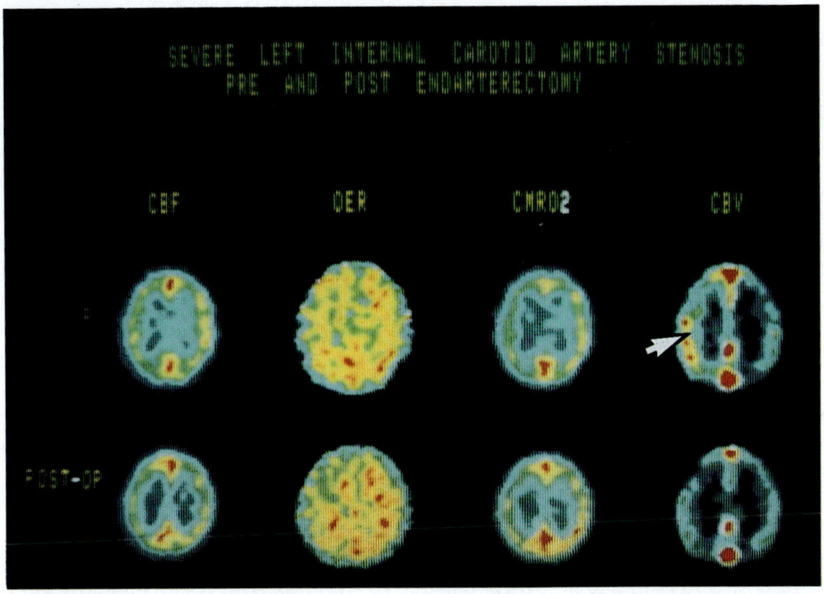

Figure 7 – 13. PET images illustrating the effect of an endarterectomy on the regional cerebral function of a patient experiencing TIAs due to a 95% stenosis of the left internal carotid artery. (*Top row*) Preoperative scans shown reactive vasodilatation in left carotid artery territory, which is helping to maintain cerebral blood flow by reducing vascular resistance. (*Bottom row*) After endarterectomy the reactive vasodilation has resolved as the perfusion pressure has increased.

in LCBF.[27,60,65] Unfortunately, the improvement in LCBF was unsustained on long-term follow-up.[18] Two PET studies demonstrated no significant change in $LCMRO_2$ following EC-IC bypass, although a third study[65] reported a consistent increase in cerebral metabolism following revascularization. Because all the patients studied with PET in this third series had an adequate cerebral arterial oxygen supply prior to their surgery, the mechanism for the observed increase in their cerebral oxygen metabolism following revascularization remains unclear.

In patients with carotid occlusion and an elevated LOEF (that is, with a reduced arterial oxygen reserve), EC-IC bypass generally has led to a satisfactory return of arterial oxygen extraction to normal 40 percent levels.[28,60] Unfortunately, the patients with an elevated LOEF, while having the most to gain from revascularization, were also most at risk of infarction during the bypass procedure. Two such patients in one study developed perioperative infarcts.[28] Although EC-IC bypass may be justified on hemodynamic grounds in patients with a diminished oxygen reserve, it is clearly a high-risk procedure.

The foregoing considerations may in part explain the poor results obtained by the EC-IC bypass cooperative study, which found that revascularization was of no clinical benefit in patients with carotid artery disease.[19] In this study, which examined a heterogeneous patient group, there was a 3% incidence of serious perioperative stroke in the patients who underwent revascularization. The incidence of perioperative stroke in the subgroup of patients with bilateral carotid artery occlusion was not specifically stated.

So far, no results of functional studies on the effect of endarterectomies on cerebral perfusion have been reported. Preliminary results suggest that, like EC-IC bypass, this procedure results in a rise in LCBF; LCBV where vascular reserve is impaired.[27] There is clearly still a need for a controlled trial to examine the effect of revascularization on patients with carotid artery disease who have an impaired vasodilatory and oxygen reserve demonstrated by functional imaging. Initial, uncontrolled, retrospective data suggest that in those patients with carotid stenosis and impaired vascular reserve demonstrated with PET, EC-IC bypass leads to no improvement in the annual incidence of ipsilateral cerebral infarction.[61a]

ASSESSMENT OF THE ISCHEMIC STATE

Ischemia is present when tissue demand for substrates exceeds their supply. At this point the cerebral arterial oxygen extraction reaches 100%; that is, brain oxygen metabolism becomes flow-dependent. The evolution of cerebral infarction has been studied with PET.[35,46,73] A raised LOEF may be present for days or even weeks after the onset of ischemia (Fig. 7–14*A*), but generally the LOEF falls to subnormal levels within 48 hours of the ictus, indicating that tissue infarction has occurred (Fig. 7–14*B*). Following infarction, tissue oxygen utilization ($LCMRO_2$) is low, but blood flow can be either high or low. When LCBF is inappropriately high, the venous blood appears arterialized and a state of "luxury perfusion" is said to be present. Because LCBF is so variable in the subacute phase of infarction, it is an inappropriate parameter to follow when monitoring stroke recovery. It is also inappropriate to treat many infarcts in the first few weeks with regimens designed to increase LCBF, such as hemodilution and vasodilators, because a state of luxury perfusion is frequently present (Fig. 7–15). This is confirmed by a recent study that failed to observe any benefit in patients with acute strokes treated with hemodilution.[66] The only valid parameter to monitor when determining the response of infarction to therapy is regional cerebral metabolism (that is, $LCMRO_2$ or LCMRGlc).

An important clinical application of PET is the study of evolving strokes. When infarction presents as a progressive syndrome, it is possible to determine with PET whether a state of impaired oxygen reserve is present—that is, whether LOEF is focally raised. If this is the case, then a revascularization procedure theoretically would be justifiable on hemodynamic grounds. To date, revascularization procedures and pharmacologic maneuvers to increase the cerebral perfusion of infarcts where a raised LOEF has been demonstrated have failed to raise their cerebral metabolism, although the LCBF has risen and the LOEF has returned to normal levels.[27,38,73] It is likely, therefore, that these regions were already infarcted and not truly ischemic in the sense defined earlier. In spite of their impaired oxygen reserve, patients with these particular infarcts were still able to derive an adequate arterial oxygen supply for the remaining viable tissue by raising the fraction of oxygen extracted from the albeit impaired arterial oxygen supply.

Hydrogen 1-MRS and ^{31}P-MRS have been used to study stroke. Animal models of ischemia have shown that tissue levels of ATP and phosphocreatine become depleted within minutes of infarction.[11] Human infarcts, studied hours to days after the ictus, have had either low or normal ratios of phosphocreatine to ATP, though absolute levels of these high-energy phosphates have not been reported. Unfortunately, to date no studies have been reported of levels of ATP and phosphocreatine in patients with early infarcts, where the LOEF has been shown to be elevated. It is consequently impossible to be sure at present whether the oxygen being extracted from the arterial supply in such early infarcts is being metabolized to produce high-energy phosphates, or is simply uncoupled, serving no useful metabolic purpose. If the latter situation prevails, revascularization procedures would be of little utility.

The metabolic and perfusion thresholds for infarction have been inferred from PET studies.[46,59] When focal levels of $LCMRO_2$ are less than 1.3 mL O_2/100 mL of tissue per minute, infarcted tissue rarely recovers. In a rat model of is-

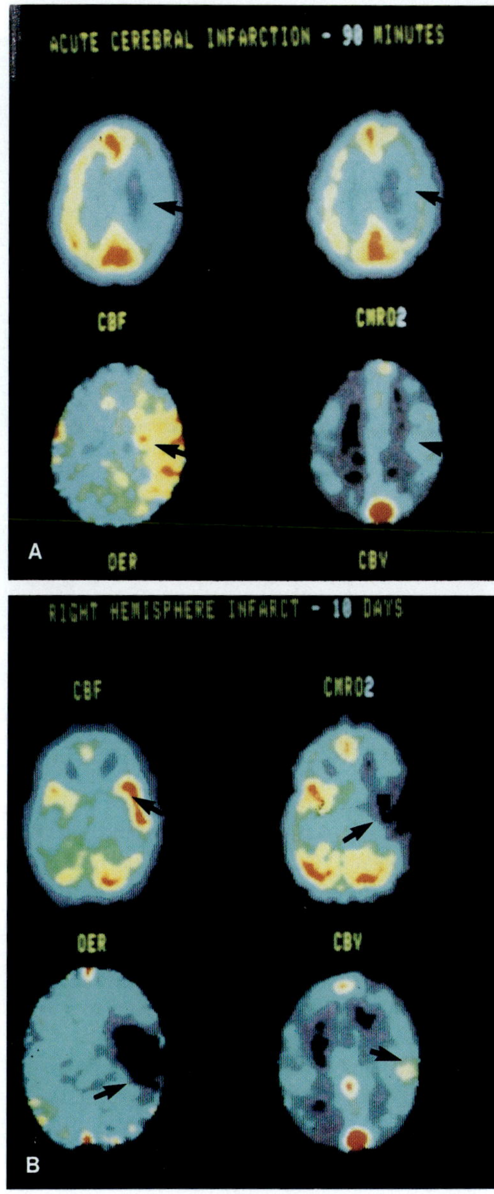

Figure 7–14. (*A*) PET images of regional cerebral function 90 minutes after the sudden onset of a left hemiparesis due to cerebral ischemia. Blood flow has fallen to 25% of that of the contralateral side in the right middle cerebral territory. Arterial oxygen extraction has risen from a normal 40% to 90% in an unsuccessful attempt to maintain cerebral oxygen metabolism. Vasodilatation in right middle cerebral artery territory is also evident. (*B*) Same subject 10 days later. Infarction is now completed and both cerebral oxygen metabolism and arterial oxygen extraction have fallen to near zero in right middle cerebral artery territory. Luxury perfusion is present, cerebral blood flow being inappropriately high in the infarcted territory for the level of cerebral oxygen metabolism present.

chemia, levels of ATP and phosphocreatine are maintained until cerebral blood flow falls below 20 mL/100 mL per minute.[16] At lower CBF values, ATP and phosphocreatine levels fall within minutes, lactate levels rise, and the pH falls.

There are few published data on the effect of transient ischemic attacks on cerebral function. Do patients with TIAs have truly reversible metabolic deficits or does limited neuronal death occur? A PET study of a patient recovering from a migraine attack that resulted in a homonymous hemianopia showed focally raised LOEF in the contralateral occipital lobe. The LOEF had returned to normal when the subject was restudied 2 weeks later.[39] If migraines and TIAs both involve focally decreased cerebral perfusion, it is likely that TIAs also are associated with focally raised

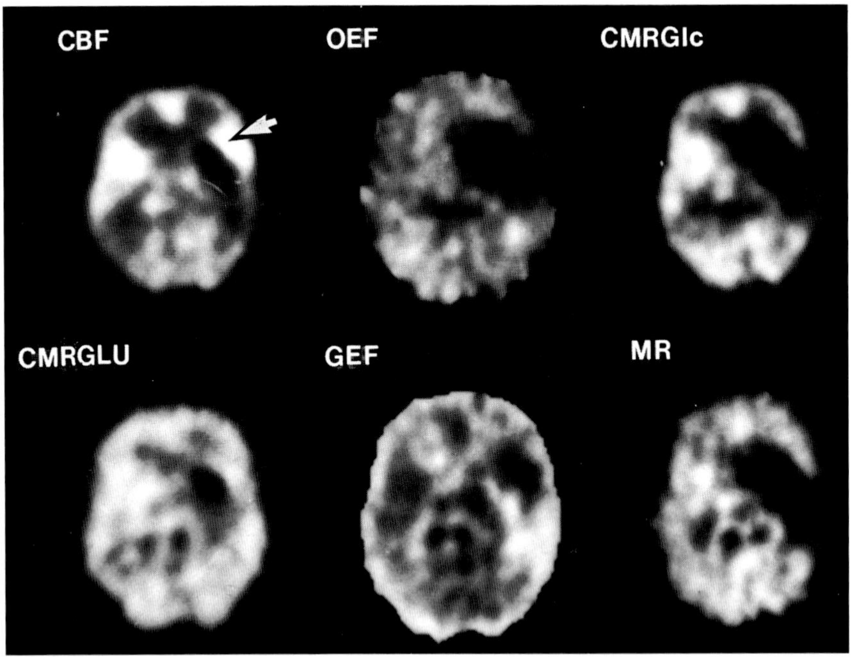

Figure 7–15. PET images of regional cerebral function for a patient with a 2-week-old infarct in right middle cerebral artery territory. Reduced cerebral artery metabolism and arterial oxygen extraction are evident in right middle cerebral artery territory. Luxury perfusion is also seen (*arrow*). Glucose metabolism is preserved and arterial glucose extraction is raised in affected territory as the infarcted tissue preferentially uses aerobic glycolysis. As a consequence, the metabolic molar $CMRO_2$:CMRGlc ratio (MR) has fallen from a normal 5.6 to around 2 in infarcted territory.

LOEF. This postulate, however, still requires demonstration with further PET studies on TIA patients.

A number of studies have examined glucose metabolism in cerebral infarcts, and some have compared oxygen and glucose metabolism.[6,29,35,75] In patients studied within 48 hours of the onset of their symptoms, two patterns of metabolism were found. The majority of subjects had a reduced LCBF, raised LOEF, and a coupled reduction of $LCMRO_2$ and LCMRGlc, suggesting that a state of tissue ischemia was present with generally reduced tissue metabolism.[35] In a minority of subjects, frank infarction had already occurred; normal levels of LCBF, reduced levels of LOEF and $LCMRO_2$, and normal levels of LCMRGlc were present. These findings suggest that in frankly infarcted tissue, preferential glycolysis in the presence of an adequate oxygen supply (that is, aerobic glycolysis) is taking place. Other studies comparing oxygen and glucose metabolism in infarcts older than 48 hours have confirmed the presence of preferential aerobic glycolysis (see Fig. 7–15), the $LCMRO_2$: LCMRGlc ratio being approximately 2 instead of the normal 5.6.[6,29,75] Whether this preferential aerobic glycolysis in established infarcts represents glial and macrophage metabolism or impaired neuronal metabolism remains to be determined. It has been elegantly demonstrated[42] using ^{18}FDG, that PET is a more sensitive method than x-ray CT scanning for detecting infarction. The level of LCMRGlc in infarcts was correlated with the patient's eventual prognosis.[42]

Studies of regional cerebral pH (LpH) during cerebral infarction have used the positron-emitting weak acid tracer ^{11}C-DMO. If patients are studied with PET within 48 hours of onset of ischemia, those who still have a focally low LCBF and raised LOEF (that is, where completed infarction has not yet occurred) have a low LpH in the affected territory.[35] Subjects who show the pattern of metabolism of completed infarction—a low LOEF and $LCMRO_2$ with a variable LCBF—have an LpH that is normal or alkaline. In infarcts that are older than 48 hours, the LpH is invariably normal or alkaline, LpH being inversely correlated with LOEF[69] (Fig. 7–16). These findings suggest that in established infarction, where preferential aerobic glycolysis is occurring, any increased lactate production is adequately buffered or cleared locally, and does not lead to a relative acidosis.

The regional hematocrit in microvasculature reflects the caliber of the vessels, being reduced as vessels become smaller. Regional cerebral hematocrit can be measured quantitatively by both PET and SPECT and is roughly 70% of the hematocrit in large systemic vessels in both gray and white matter.[43] In infarcted brain tissue, regional hematocrit is reduced.[13,47] Although to date no such studies have been published, in theory it should be possible to assess the caliber of the microvasculature of patients at risk from multi-infarct disease, such as hypertensive and diabetic patients, by measurement of their cerebral hematocrit. In this way the effectiveness of their antihypertensive and diabetic treatment could be assessed.

LOCAL AND DISTANT EFFECTS OF CEREBRAL INFARCTION

The volume of regional altered function, as demonstrated by PET and SPECT, consistently has been shown to be far greater than the volume of infarction present on x-ray CT scans in patients with strokes.[1,42] Lacunar infarcts, which may be clinically silent, and microvascular disease associated with hypertension and diabetes, can produce wide-ranging reductions in $LCMRO_2$ and may be associated with dementia.[64,74] It is clear from PET that,

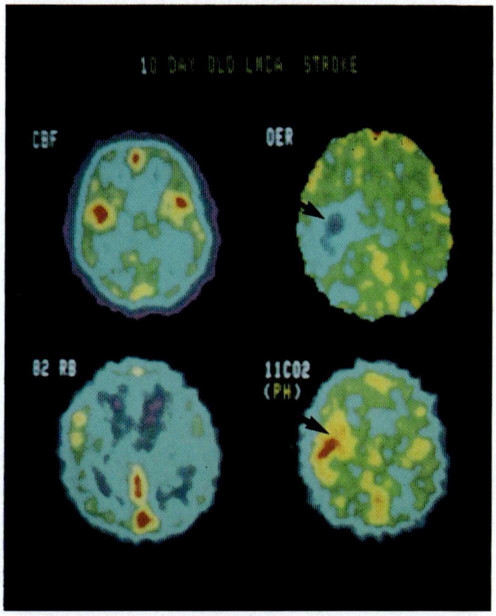

Figure 7–16. Functional images of a 10-day-old left temporal infarct. There is luxury perfusion with a raised CBF and low OEF. The ^{82}Rb scan shows little BBB disruption. The $^{11}CO_2$ pH scan shows that the infarct is alkaline relative to normal brain tissue.

following the onset of ischemia, the deeper cerebral structures infarct first. In eight strokes studied within 36 hours of onset,[73] the highest levels of LOEF were found in the superficial cortex, the basal ganglia generally showing completed infarction. Such findings are probably a consequence of the anatomy of the cerebral microvasculature, the cortex being well supplied by short perforating vessels from anastomoses on the brain surface, whereas the deeper structures are less well supplied by long, penetrating vessels.[58] The same study found no evidence for an "ischemic penumbra" around infarcted tissue; that is, there was no evidence of a rim of brain tissue surrounding the infarct with a maintained $LCMRO_2$ but a high arterial oxygen extraction.

In addition to their local effects, infarcts can produce distant effects on regional cerebral function. Hemispheric infarcts produce a coupled fall in metabolism and blood flow in both cerebellar hemispheres, the function of the contralateral cerebellar hemisphere being most depressed.[4,46,49] This phenomenon has been termed *crossed cerebellar diaschisis* and is likely to result from decreased activity in the corticopontocerebellar efferent tracts (Fig. 7–17). The significance of this phenomenon is unclear, since it does not appear to be associated with clinical signs of cerebellar dysfunction and is frequently reversible. Hemispheric infarcts also have been said to be associated with hypofunction of the contralateral hemisphere, but recently doubt has been cast on this viewpoint.[74] Changes in overlying cortical function are well described in association with thalamic infarcts, again presumably reflecting the reduced activity in thalamocortical efferent fibers.[17] PET provides a potential means of examining the functional connections of the various cerebral structures by illustrating the patterns of altered regional cerebral function following discrete infarcts. It also provides a means of examining the pattern of recovery of the brain when a stroke has occurred, and of determining whether "plasticity" of the brain enables different areas of cortex to take over the functions of the infarcted tissue.

THE ROLE OF NEUROIMAGING IN THE MANAGEMENT OF CEREBROVASCULAR DISEASE

Asymptomatic Carotid Artery Occlusions and Stenoses

Frequently, patients with peripheral vascular disease, or with coronary artery disease requiring bypass grafting, are found on screening to have asymptomatic carotid bruits or significant (>60%) but asymptomatic stenoses of their carotid arteries. Such situations cause the following clinical questions to arise: (1) Are asymptomatic carotid bruits of clinical significance? (2) Should patients with significant carotid artery disease undergo endarterectomies before their coronary or peripheral-artery bypass grafting to lessen the chances of a CVA occurring during bypass surgery?[21]

X-ray CT and MRI brain scanning can help to answer these questions by screening for regions of clinically silent infarction. If infarcts are present within the territory of the stenosed carotid artery, an embolic etiology is more likely, whereas watershed infarctions are more likely to be associated with poor hemodynamic reserve. Frequently, both situations exist concurrently. The finding of clinically silent infarcts would sway one towards performing a prophylactic endarterectomy, although to date no randomized, controlled studies have been published supporting the use of this procedure before bypass surgery.[21] A multicenter trial[19] has failed to demonstrate any benefit from EC-IC bypass in this situation.

The hemodynamic reserve of the microcirculation in the territory of asymptomatic stenosed or occluded ca-

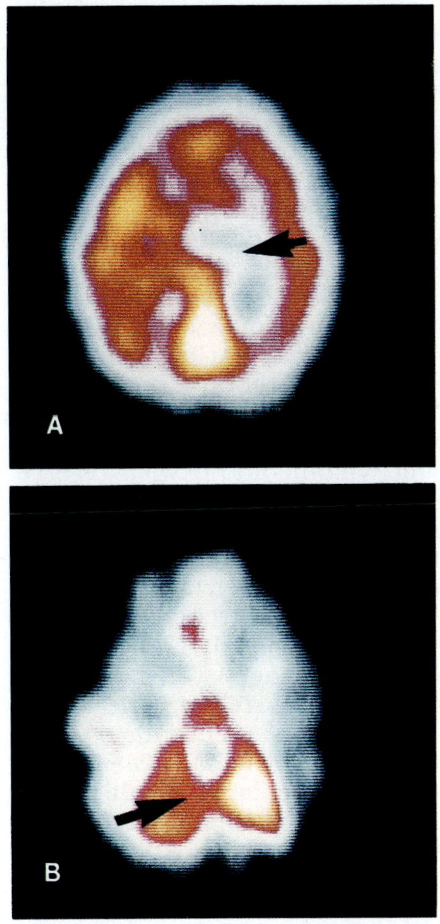

Figure 7–17. (*A*) SPECT images of CBF in a patient with a right thalamic hematoma, using the tracer HIPDM. Reduced blood flow is seen in the thalamus and surrounding structures. (*B*) Reduced CBF in the contralateral cerebellar hemisphere of the same subject, illustrating the phenomenon of crossed cerebellar diaschisis. (Images courtesy of D Perani, Ospedale San Raffaelo, Rome.)

rotid arteries can be assessed with PET or SPECT to measure LCBF:LCBV ratios. Similarly, ^{133}Xe washout, PET, or SPECT can be used to measure the CO_2 or acetazolamide reactivity of LCBF. Measurement of the LOEF with PET also discloses the oxygen reserve. If the hemodynamic or oxygen reserve is compromised, a theoretical rationale for performing a prophylactic endarterectomy on stenosed carotid arteries (or a prophylactic EC-IC bypass on occluded arteries) exists prior to coronary bypass surgery. So far, however, no formal trials of prophylactic revascularization have been carried out on patients with carotid artery disease who have had their functional reserves assessed. Preliminary data suggest that in patients with impaired hemodynamic and oxygen reserve, EC-IC bypass improves cerebral perfusion.[5,28,60,65] Unfortunately, those patients with impaired oxygen reserve—those most at risk from infarction—were also those who were most at risk of having a stroke perioperatively during revascularization.[28]

Symptomatic Carotid Artery Occlusions and Stenoses

Much of the discussion in the previous section also applies to the treatment of diseased carotid arteries associated with TIAs or cerebral infarction. No adequate trials of the effect of endarterectomy on the prognosis of patients with symptomatic carotid artery stenosis have been published.[21] The multicenter EC-IC bypass trial[19] failed to show a benefit from revascularization in patients with carotid artery disease, but unfortunately failed to analyze one particular subgroup of interest, patients with bilateral carotid occlusions and continuing TIAs. A recent report[72] suggested that this subgroup has a 13% per annum chance of developing an infarct. As discussed earlier, a rational approach to the question of revascularization in patients with symptomatic carotid artery disease would be to assess the hemodynamic and oxygen reserve in affected territories in these subjects. If these reserves are compromised, then the patients could be entered into a formal revascularization trial. In patients with symptomatic carotid artery disease but normal hemodynamic reserve on functional imaging, anti-platelet-aggregation agents remain the mainstay of treatment. Current data[3] suggest that 300 mg of aspirin daily is effective in reducing vascular mortality and nonfatal vascular events, and has a low incidence of side effects. Anticoagulation is indicated only if a stroke-in-evolution appears to be occurring, or if a cardiac or intra-arterial source of emboli is present. Repeated phlebotomy or hemodilution to lower hematocrit, and so increase cerebral blood flow, is of unproven value.

Treatment of Acute Cerebral Infarction

MR spectroscopy suggests that within hours of infarction irreversible neuronal damage occurs unless reperfusion can be achieved.[67] After 48 hours the majority of infarcts enter a state of luxury perfusion, with PET studies showing an inappropriately high LCBF for their level of oxygen metabolism.[35,46,73] As such, the treatment of stroke patients in their subacute phase with revascularization procedures or pharmacologic methods designed to increase blood flow would appear to be inappropriate. Even where regional cerebral oxygen extraction has remained persistently elevated after completed infarction, revascularization procedures and pharmacologic intervention, while increasing LCBF, have failed to produce any useful increase in oxygen utilization.[27,38,73]

One situation that awaits clarification is whether revascularization could be beneficial in patients with a stroke-in-evolution and an elevated LOEF. Patients with a stroke-in-evolution should have urgent PET scanning to assess the hemodynamics of the affected territory. If hemodynamic and oxygen reserves are normal, anticoagulation rather than a revascularization procedure is indicated. An impaired oxygen reserve would be an indication to proceed to angiography. If a critical stenosis or occlusion of the extracranial circulation is demonstrated, then it would be reasonable to proceed to endarterectomy or angioplasty in the case of a stenosis, or a bypass procedure where occlusion is present.

The role of structural imaging in acute infarction is primarily diagnostic. X-ray CT scanning is insensitive but nonetheless useful for excluding a hemorrhage, whereas MRI will detect infarcts within hours of their onset.[11] Unfortunately, if edema, BBB breakdown, or both are present, it may be difficult to distinguish acute infarction from inflammatory pathology or cerebral neoplasia on radiologic appearances alone. Usually within a few days, however, the radiologic appearances become distinct as the edema associated with infarction begins to resolve. A major role of structural imaging is in the detection of cerebral hemorrhage. X-ray CT is more sensitive than MRI initially unless special phase-sensitive MRI sequences are used, but MRI is far superior for the detection of hemorrhages that are older than 24–48 hours, and may also detect vascular abnormalities.[54] A frequent dilemma is whether to employ anticoagulation therapy in a patient with a cardiac source of emboli who has recently sustained a cerebral infarct. A recent prospective study[40] showed that secondary hemorrhage occurred in 43% of cerebral infarcts within the first 4 weeks of the event. Hemorrhage was most common in large infarcts with mass effect, and usually occurred within the first 2 weeks. In such patients it may be prudent to withhold anticoagulation initially, and to perform serial x-ray CT brain scans.

REFERENCES

1. Ackerman, RH, Alpert, NM, Correia, JA, Grotta, JC, Fallick, JT, Chang, JY, Brownell, GL, and Taveras, JM: Correlation of positron emission scans with CT scans and clinical course. Acta Neurol Scand (Suppl 72) 60:230–231, 1979.
2. Aisen, AM, Gabrielsen, TO, and McCune, WJ: MR imaging of systemic lupus erythematosus involving the brain. AJNR 6:197–201, 1985.
3. Secondary prevention of vascular disease by prolonged antiplatelet treatment. Antiplatelet trialists' collaboration. Br Med J 296:320–331, 1988.
4. Baron, JC, Bousser, MG, Comar, D, and Castaigne, P: Crossed cerebellar diaschisis in human supratentorial brain infarction. Trans Am Neurol Assoc 105:459–461, 1981.
5. Baron, JC, Bousser, MG, Rey, A, Guillard, A, Comar, D, and Castaigne, P: Reversal of "misery perfusion syndrome" by extra-intracranial arterial bypass in hemodynamic cerebral ischaemia. Stroke 12:454–459, 1981.
6. Baron, JC, Rougemont, D, Soussaline, F, Bustany, P, Crouzel, C, Bousser, MG, and Comar, D: Local interrelationships of cerebral oxygen consumption and glucose utilization in normal subjects and in ischemic stroke patients: A positron tomography study. J Cereb Blood Flow Metabol 4:140–149, 1984.
7. Bell, BA, Symon, L, and Branstom, NM: CBF and time thresholds for the formation of ischemic cerebral edema, and the effect of reperfusion in baboons. J Neurosurg 62:31–41, 1985.
8. Bradley, WG, Waluch, V, Brant-Zawadzki, M, Yadley, RA, and Wycoff, RR: Patchy, periventricular white matter lesions in the elderly: A common observation during NMR imaging. Noninvasive Med Imag 1:35–41, 1984.
9. Brant-Zawadzki, M, Berry, I, Osaki, L, Brasch, R, Murovic, J, and Norman, D: Gd-DTPA in clinical MR of the brain. 1. Intra-axial lesions. AJNR 7:781–788, 1986.
10. Brant-Zawadzki, M, and Kucharczyk, W: Vascular disease: Ischaemia. In Brant-Zawadzki, M, and Norman, D (eds): Magnetic Resonance Imaging of the Central Nervous System. Raven Press, New York, 1987, pp 221–234.
11. Brant-Zawadzki, M, Pereira, B, Weinstein, P, Moore, S, Kucharczyk, W, Berry, I, McNamara, M, and Derugin, N: MRI of acute experimental ischaemia in rats. AJNR 7:7–11, 1986.
12. Brooks, DJ, Lammertsma, AA, Beaney, RP, Leenders, KL, Buckingham, PD, Marshall, J, and Jones, T: Measurement of regional cerebral pH in human subjects using continuous inhalation of $^{11}CO_2$ and positron emission tomography. J Cereb Blood Flow Metabol 4: 458–465, 1984.
13. Brooks, DJ, Lammertsma, AA, Beaney, RP, Turton, DR, Marshall, J, and Jones, T: Measurement of regional cerebral hematocrit in man using ^{11}CO, ^{11}C-methyl-albumin and positron emission tomography. In Lechner, H, Meyer, JS, Reivich, M, and Ott, E (eds): Cerebrovascular Disease 5. World Federation of Neurology. 12th Salzburg Conference. Excerpta Medica, Amsterdam.
14. Brooks, DJ, Leenders, KL, Head, G, Marshall, J, Legg, NJ, Jones, T: Studies on regional cerebral oxygen utilization and cognitive function in multiple sclerosis. J Neurol Neurosurg Psychiatr 47:1182–1191, 1984.
15. Brown, MM, Wade, JPH, Bishop, CCR, and Ross Russell, RW: Reactivity of the cerebral circulation in patients with carotid occlusion. J Neurol Neurosurg Psychiatr 49:800–904, 1986.
16. Crockard, HA, Gadian, DG, Frackowiak, RSJ, Proctor, E, Allen, K, Williams, SR, Ross Russell, RW: Acute cerebral ischaemia: Concurrent changes

in cerebral blood flow, energy metabolites, pH, and lactate, measured with hydrogen clearance and ^{1}H and ^{31}P nuclear magnetic resonance spectroscopy. II. Changes during ischaemia. J Cereb Blood Flow Metabol 7:394–402, 1987.

17. D'Antona, R, Baron, JC, Pantano, P, Serdaru, M, Bousser, MG, and Samson, Y: Effects of thalamic lesions on cerebral cortex metabolism in humans. J Cereb Blood Flow Metabol (Suppl 1) 5:S457–S458, 1985.
18. Di Piero, V, Lenzi, GL, Collice, M, Triulzi, F, Gerundini, P, Perani, D, Savi, AR, Fieschi, C, and Fazio, F: Long-term noninvasive single photon emission computed tomography monitoring of perfusional changes after EC-IC bypass surgery. J Neurol Neurosurg Psychiatr 50:988–996, 1987.
19. EC-IC Bypass Study Group: Failure of extracranial-intracranial bypass to reduce the risk of ischemic stroke: Results of an international randomised trial. N Engl J Med 313:1191–1200, 1985.
20. Edelman, RR, Johnson, K, Buxton, R, Shoukimas, G, Rosen, BR, Davis, KR, and Brady, TJ: MR of haemorrhage: A new approach. AJNR 7:751–756, 1986.
21. Carotid endarterectomy: Three critical evaluations. Stroke 18:987–989, 1987. Editorial.
22. Enzmann, DR, Butt, RH, Lyons, BE, Buxton, JL, and Wilson, DA: Natural history of experimental intracerebral hematoma: Sonograph, computed tomography, and neuropathology. AJNR 2: 517–526, 1981.
23. Fazio, F, Lenzi, GL, Gerundini, P, Collice, M, Gilardi, MC, Colombo, R, Taddei, G, Del Maschio, A, Piacentini, M, Kung, HF, and Blau, M: Tomographic assessment of regional cerebral perfusion using intravenous I-123 HIPDM and a rotating gamma camera. J Comput Assist Tomogr 8:911–921, 1984.
24. Frackowiak, RSJ: The pathophysiology of human cerebral ischaemia: A new perspective obtained with positron emission tomography. Quart J Med 57:713–727, 1985.
25. Frackowiak, RSJ, Lenzi, GL, Jones, T, and Heather, JD: Quantitative measurement of regional cerebral blood flow and oxygen metabolism in man using ^{15}O and positron emission tomography: Theory, procedure and normal values. J Comput Assist Tomogr 4: 727–736, 1980.
26. Gibbs, JM, Wise, RJS, Leenders, KL, and Jones, T: Evaluation of cerebral perfusion reserve in patients with carotid artery occlusion. Lancet I:310–314, 1984.
27. Gibbs, JM, Wise, RJS, Mansfield, AO, Ross Russell, RW, Thomas, DJ, and Jones, T: Cerebral circulatory reserve before and after surgery for occlusive carotid disease. J Cereb Blood Flow Metabol 5:S19–S20, 1985.
28. Gibbs, JM, Wise, RJS, Thomas, DJ, Mansfield, AO, and Ross Russell, RW. Cerebral hemodynamic changes after extracranial-intracranial bypass surgery. J Neurol Neurosurg Psychiatr 50:140–150, 1987.
29. Gjedde, A, Weinhard, K, Heiss, W-D, Kloster, G, Deimer, NH, Herholz, K, and Pawlik, G: Comparative regional analysis of 2-fluorodeoxyglucose and methylglucose uptake in brain of four stroke patients, with special reference to the regional estimation of the lumped constant. J Cereb Blood Flow Metabol 5:163–178, 1985.
30. Gomori, JM, Grossman, RI, Goldberg, HI, Hackney, DB, Zimmerman, RA, and Bilanuik, LT: Occult cerebral vascular malformations: High-field MR imaging. Radiology 158:707–713, 1986.
31. Gomori, JM, Grossman, RI, Hackney, DB, Goldberg, HI, Zimmerman, RA, and Bilanuik, LT: Intracranial hematoma: Imaging by high-field MR. Radiology 157:87–93, 1985.

31a. Gomori, JM, Grossman, RI, Hackney, DB, Goldberg, HI, Zimmerman, RA, and Bilanuik, LT: Variable appearances by subacute intracranial hematomas on high-field spin echo MR. AJR 150:171–178, 1987.

32. Gordon, RE, Hanley, PE, Shaw, D, Gadian, DG, Radda, GK, Styles, P, Bore, PJ, and Chan, L: Localisation of metabolites in animals using ^{31}topical magnetic resonance. Nature 287:736–738: 1980.

33. Gotoh, O, Asano, T, Koide, T, and Takakura, K: Ischemic brain oedema following occlusion of the middle cerebral artery in the rat. 1: The time courses of the brain water, sodium, and potassium contents and blood-brain barrier permeability to I-125 albumin. Stroke 16:101–109, 1985.
34. Grubb, RL, Phelps, ME, and Raichle, ME: The effects of arterial blood pressure on the regional cerebral blood volume by x-ray fluorescence. Stroke 4: 390–399, 1973.
35. Hakim, AM, Pokrupa, RP, Villanueva, J, Diksic, M, Evans, AC, Thompson, CJ, Meyer, E, Yamamoto, YL, and Feindel, WH: The effect of spontaneous reperfusion on metabolic function in early human cerebral infarcts. Ann Neurol 21:279–289, 1987.
36. Harper, AM: Autoregulation of cerebral blood flow: Influence of the arterial blood pressure on the blood flow through the cerebral cortex. J Neurol Neurosurg Psychiatr 29:398–403, 1966.
37. Hellman, RS, Collier, BD, Tikofsky, RS, Kilgore, DP, Daniels, DL, Haughton, VM, Walsh, PR, Cusick, JF, Saxena, VK, Palmer, DW, and Isitman, AT: Comparison of single-photon emission computed tomography with ^{123}I-iodoamphetamine and xenon-enhanced computed tomography for assessing regional cerebral blood flow. J Cereb Blood Flow Metabol 6:747–755, 1986.
38. Herold, S, Frackowiak, RSJ, and Neil-Dwyer, G: Studies on cerebral blood flow and oxygen metabolism in patients with established cerebral infarcts undergoing omental transposition. Stroke 18:46–51, 1987.
39. Herold, S, Gibbs, JM, Jones, AKP, Brooks, DJ, Frackowiak, RSJ, and Legg, NJ. Oxygen metabolism in migraine. J Cereb Blood Flow Metabol 5 (Suppl):S445–S446, 1985.
40. Hornig, CR, Dorndof, W, and Agnoli, AL: Haemorrhagic cerebral infarction: A prospective study. Stroke 17:179–185, 1986.
41. Kistler, JP, Buonanno, FS, De Witt, LD, Davis, KR, Brady, TJ, and Fisher, CM: Vertebral-basilar posterior cerebral territory stroke: Delineation by proton nuclear magnetic resonance imaging. Stroke 15:417–426, 1984.
42. Kushner, M, Reivich, M, Fieschi, C, Silver, F, Chawluk, J, Rosen, M, Greenberg, J, Burke, A, and Alavi, A: Metabolic and clinical correlates of acute ischemic infarction. Neurology 37: 1103–1110, 1987.
43. Lammertsma, AA, Brooks, DJ, Beaney, RP, Turton, DR, Kensett, MJ, Heather, JD, Marshall, J, and Jones, T: In vivo measurement of regional cerebral hematocrit using positron emission tomography. J Cereb Blood Flow Metabol 4:317–322, 1984.
44. Lammertsma, AA, Wise, RJS, Heather, JD, Gibbs, JM, Leenders, KL, Frackowiak, RSJ, Rhodes, CG, and Jones, T. The correction for the presence of intravascular oxygen-15 in the steady state technique for measuring regional oxygen extraction ratio in the brain. 2: Results in normal subjects, brain tumor, and stroke patients. J Cereb Blood Flow Metabol 3:425–431, 1983.
45. Le Bihan, D, Breton, E, Lallemand, D, Grenier, P, Cabanis, E, and Laval-Jeantet, M: MR imaging of intravoxel incoherent motions: Application to diffusion and perfusion in neurologic disorders. Radiology 161:401–407, 1986.
46. Lenzi, GL, Frackowiak, RSJ, and Jones, T: Cerebral oxygen metabolism and blood flow in human cerebral ischemic infarction. J Cereb Blood Flow Metabol 2:321–335, 1982.
47. Loutfi, I, Frackowiak, RSJ, Myers, MJ, and Lavender, JP: Regional brain hematocrit in stroke by single photon emission computed tomography imaging. Am J Physiol Imag 2:10–16, 1987.
48. Marcy, VR, and Walsh, FA: Correlation between cerebral blood flow and ATP content following tourniquet-induced ischaemia in cat brain. J Cereb Blood Flow Metabol 4:362–367, 1984.
49. Martin, WRW, and Raichle, ME: Cerebellar blood flow and metabolism in cerebral hemisphere infarction. Ann Neurol 14:168–176, 1983.
50. McMurdo, SK Jr, Brant-Zawadzki, M,

Bradley, WG Jr, Chang, GY, and Berg, BO: Dural sinus thrombosis study using intermediate field strength MR imaging. Radiology 161:83–86, 1986.

51. McNamara, MT: Paramagnetic contrast media for magnetic resonance imaging of the central nervous system. In Brant-Zawadzki, M, and Norman, D (eds): Magnetic Resonance Imaging of the Central Nervous System. Raven Press, New York, 1987, pp 97–105.

52. Moon, KL Jr, Brant-Zawadski, M, Pitts, LH, and Mills, CM. Nuclear magnetic resonance imaging of CT-isodense subdural hematomas. AJNR 5:319–322, 1984.

53. Nordstrom, DM, West, SG, Andersen, PA: Basal ganglia calcifications in central nervous system lupus erythematosus. Arthritis Rheum 28:1412–1416, 1985.

54. Normand, D: Vascular disease: Haemorrhage. In Brant-Zawadzki, M and Norman, D (eds): Magnetic Resonance Imaging of the Central Nervous System. Raven Press, New York, 1987, pp 209–220.

55. Peress, NS, Kane, WC, and Aronson, SM. Central nervous system findings in a tenth decade autopsy population. In Ford, DE (ed): Neurobiological Aspects of Maturation and Aging. Progress in Brain Research Series 40. Elsevier, New York, 1973, pp 482–483.

56. Phelps, ME, Huang, SC, Hoffman, EJ, Sokoloff, L, and Kuhl, DE. Tomographic measurement of local glucose metabolic rate in humans with (F-18) 2-fluoro-2-deoxy-D-glucose: Validation of method. Ann Neurol 6:371–388, 1979.

57. Phelps, ME, Mazziotta, JC, and Huang, SC: Study of cerebral function with positron computed tomography. J Cereb Blood Flow Metabol 2:113–162, 1982.

58. Plets, C: Macroscopic and microscopic anatomy of cerebral circulation. In Minderkound, JM (ed): Cerebral Blood Flow: Basic Knowledge and Clinical Implications. Excerpta Medica, Amsterdam, 1981, pp 1–19.

59. Powers, WJ, Grubb, RL, Darriet, D, and Raichle, ME: Cerebral blood flow and cerebral metabolic rate of oxygen requirements for cerebral function and viability in humans. J Cereb Blood Flow Metabol 5:600–608, 1985.

60. Powers, WJ, Martin, WRW, Herscovitch, P, Raichle, ME, and Grubb, RL: Extracranial-intracranial bypass surgery: Hemodynamic and metabolic effects. Neurology 34:1168–1174, 1984.

61. Powers, WJ, Press, GA, Grubb, RL, Gado, M, and Raichle, ME: The effect of hemodynamically significant carotid artery disease on the hemodynamic status of the cerebral circulation. Ann Intern Med 106:27–35, 1987.

61a. Powers, WJ, Tempel, LW, and Grubb, RL: Influence of cerebral haemodynamics on stroke risk: One year follow-up of 30 medically treated patients. Ann Neurol 25:325–330, 1989.

62. Pykett, IK, Buonanno, FS, Brady, RJ, and Kistler, JP: True three-dimensional nuclear magnetic resonance neuroimaging in ischemic stroke: Correlation of NMR, x-ray CT and pathology. Stroke 14:173–177, 1983.

63. Raichle, ME, Martin, WRW, Herscovitch, P, Mintun, MA, and Markham, J: Brain blood flow measured with intravenous $H_2{}^{15}O$. II: Implementation and validation. J Nucl Med 24:790–798, 1983.

64. Rougemont, D, Baron, JC, Lebrun-Grandie, P, Bousser, MG, Cabanis, E, and Laplane, D: Debit sanguine cerebral et extraction d'oxygene dans les hemiplegies lacunaire. Rev Neurol 139: 277–282, 1983.

65. Samson, Y, Baron, JC, Bousser, MG, Ray, A, Derlon, JM, David, P, and Comoy, J: Effects of extra-intracranial arterial bypass on cerebral blood flow and oxygen metabolism in humans. Stroke 16:609–616, 1985.

66. Scandinavian Stroke Study Group: Multicenter trial of hemodilution in acute ischemic stroke. I. Results in the total patient population. Stroke 18: 691–699, 1987.

67. Siesjo, BK: Brain Energy Metabolism. John Wiley & Sons, New York.

68. Sipponen, JT: Use of techniques: Visualization of brain infarction with nuclear magnetic resonance imaging. Neuroradiology 26:387–391, 1984.

69. Syrota, A, Castaing, M, Rougemont, D,

Berridge, M, Baron, JC, Bousser, MG, and Pocidalo, JJ: Tissue acid-base balance and oxygen metabolism in human cerebral infarction studied with positron emission tomography. Ann Neurol 14:419–428, 1983.

70. Vermess, M, Bernstein, RM, Bydder, GM, Steiner, RE, Young, IR, and Hughes, GRV: Nuclear magnetic resonance (NMR) imaging of the brain in systemic lupus erythematosus. J Comput Assist Tomogr 7:461–467, 1983.

71. von Schulthess, GK, and Higgins, CB. Blood flow imaging with MR: Spin-phase phenomena. Radiology 157: 687–695, 1985.

72. Wade, JPH, Wong, W, Barnett, HJM, Vandervoort, P. Bilateral occlusions of the internal carotid arteries. Presenting symptoms in 74 patients and a prospective study of 34 medically treated patients. Brain 110:667–682, 1987.

73. Wise, RJS, Bernardi, S, Frackowiak, RSJ, Legg, NJ, and Jones, T: Serial observations on the pathophysiology of acute stroke: The transition from ischaemia to infarction as reflected in regional oxygen extraction. Brain 106: 197–222, 1983.

74. Wise, RJS, Gibbs, JM, Frackowiak, RSJ, Marshall, J, and Jones, T: No evidence for transhemispheric diaschisis after human cerebral infarction. Stroke 17:853–860, 1986.

75. Wise, RJS, Rhodes, CG, Gibbs, JM, Hatazawa, J, Frackowiak, RSJ, Palmer, AJ, and Jones, T. Disturbance of oxidative metabolism of glucose in recent human cerebral infarcts. Ann Neurol 14:627–637, 1983.

76. Yonas, H, Wolfson, SK, Gur, D, Latchaw, RE, Good, WF, Leanza, R, Jackson, DL, Jannetta, PJ, and Reinmuth, OM: Clinical experience with the use of xenon-enhanced CT blood flow mapping in cerebral vasacular disease. Stroke 15:443–450, 1984.

77. Young, IR, and Bydder, GM: Demonstration of perfused flow in the brain using phase mapping. Soc Magn Res Med Book of Abstracts. SMRM, San Francisco, 1987, p 863.

Chapter 8

MOVEMENT DISORDERS

John C. Mazziotta, M.D., Ph.D.

HUNTINGTON'S DISEASE
PARKINSON'S DISEASE
PROGRESSIVE SUPRANUCLEAR PALSY (PSP)
WILSON'S DISEASE
DYSTONIA
TARDIVE DYSKINESIA
MISCELLANEOUS DISORDERS

The movement disorders constitute a widely divergent collection of neurologic afflictions. They have in common the pathophysiologic involvement of motor systems to produce either excessive or deficient motor activity. Many of these disorders have minimal or inconsistent neuropathologic abnormalities, despite obvious and profound clinical signs and symptoms. In spite of ever-increasing knowledge of the anatomy, physiology and biochemistry of both the pyramidal (i.e., corticospinal) and extrapyramidal components of the motor system, an understanding of the fundamental networks that become deranged to produce the various movement disorders has remained elusive. Neuropharmacologic approaches have led to relief or reduction of symptoms for a number of the movement disorders and to some biochemical insights into their possible bases.

Various classification schemes have been proposed for the movement disorders, including genetic, anatomic, pharmacologic, and clinical approaches. The clinical approach is most often used. With this approach, movement disorders can be divided into those with excessive, and those with deficient, motor activity. Those with deficits in motor activity include the hypokinetic and rigid disorders best typified by Parkinson's disease. The hyperkinetic movement disorders, characterized by an excess of movements, include myoclonus, ballismus, chorea, athetosis, and dystonia. Huntington's disease is an example of this group. Even this simple segregation is of limited use, however, since in these prototypical examples themselves, both deficient and excessive motor activity can coexist. That is, rigid Parkinson's patients typically have a hyperkinetic tremor, while end-stage Huntington's disease patients develop rigidity.

Obviously, the optimal categorization scheme would be based on pathophysiology. Although some insights into this approach are currently available, there is too little information to develop such a scheme. Excellent texts and reviews of the clinical, pharmacologic, and theoretical features of the movement disorders are available.[125–128,131,158]

Even a cursory review of the literature indicates that movement disorders have a fundamental biochemical basis. Drugs can both cause symptoms (e.g., neuroleptic-induced Parkinson's disease or tardive dyskinesia), improve symptoms (levodopa correction of parkinsonian bradykinesia), or exaggerate symptoms (levodopa-enhanced chorea in Huntington's disease). Thus, a combined biochemical and anatomic approach to the movement disorders should be the most useful in understanding their fundamental mechanisms and the resultant approaches to their treatment or amelioration.

Whereas a number of the movement disorders are known to be primary inherited degenerative (e.g., Huntington's disease, Wilson's disease) or idiopathic (e.g., Parkinson's) diseases of the nervous system, the effects of drugs or other processes (e.g., metabolic, toxic) may produce symptoms that mimic their appearance (for example, neuroleptic- and tumor-induced Parkinson's symptoms).[39,210,212,217]

Structural neuroimaging techniques (pneumoencephalography, angiography, x-ray computed tomography [CT]) allow visualization of gross pathologic changes of structures during life that parallel postmortem changes. An example would be caudate atrophy seen with pneumoencephalography, or x-ray CT in Huntington's disease. Similarly, these structural imaging techniques can identify structural lesions, such as cerebral infarction or tumors, that produce signs and symptoms that mimic idiopathic degenerative movement disorders. Few new insights into the basic disease mechanisms have come from these structural approaches, however.

Biochemical neuroimaging studies, especially when combined with high-spatial-resolution anatomic studies, provide the best opportunity to identify normal and abnormal neural networks that control motor activity and their failure in disease states. Methodologies that provide such data include positron emission tomography (PET) (see Chapter 3), single photon emission computed tomography (SPECT) (see Chapter 4) and high-field magnetic resonance imaging (MRI) (see Chapter 2). PET and SPECT have been used to trace biochemical pathways in vivo in the human brain. The former can provide information about hemodynamics, metabolism, pH, and both pre- and postsynaptic neurotransmission[29,54,131,138] (see Chapter 3). High-field MRI imaging can be used to examine local magnetic field disturbances caused by ferromagnetic ion deposition (e.g., iron, copper) in the brain, thought to be a factor in certain movement disorders (e.g., Hallervorden-Spatz and Wilson's diseases).

For many of the movement disorders, the basal ganglia have been implicated as a crucial set of structures that either degenerate or participate in the signs and symptoms manifested by patients.[158,159] In classic neuroanatomic terms, the basal ganglia consist of the subcortical nuclei that are embryologically derived from the telencephalon and include the caudate nucleus, putamen, globus pallidus, claustrum, and amygdala. The substantia nigra, subthalamic nucleus and the ventrolateral and ventroanterior nuclei of the thalamus are important connecting structures and components of the extrapyramidal motor system. The amygdala and claustrum are not considered part of this latter system. Collectively, the caudate nucleus and the putamen are known as the striatum, while the putamen and the globus pallidus are known as the lenticular nuclei. In the broadest sense, the basal ganglia constitute a highly complex, integrated, and interconnected system with major inputs from cortical and subcortical areas and outputs to the thalamus and subthalamus.[158] A better understanding of the circuitry, interconnections, and physiology of the basal ganglia undoubtedly will lead to new insights and improved treatments for the movement disorders.

To understand both the clinical features and neuroimaging approaches to diseases of the basal ganglia, it is important to understand the fundamental neurochemistry of the interconnections of these systems. The corticostriatal pathways are excitatory and glutamatergic. The striatonigral and striatopallidal pathways are inhibitory and both GABAergic and peptidergic (e.g., enkephalin, substance P, somatostatin and neuropeptide Y). The nigrostriatal pathway is dopaminergic. Connections between the globus pallidus and the thalamus are inhibitory and GABAergic. Less well documented are the pathways of the subthalamus leading to the globus pallidus. These are presumed to be excitatory and glutamatergic. The neuropharmacology of movement disorders reflects this complex and integrated neurochemical network. Approaches to functional imaging of this neurochemical network (e.g., PET and SPECT) will take advantage of our knowledge of these pathways and their functional effects on target sites in the brain.

Gross structural abnormalities of the basal ganglia can be observed with x-ray CT or MRI. As noted earlier, the deposition of ferromagnetic ions in the basal ganglia can be observed with high-field MRI, while hemodynamic and metabolic properties can be identified with PET and possibly SPECT. PET has been used to look at the effects of therapeutic drugs, neurotransmitters, and ligands at pre- and postsynaptic sites throughout the basal ganglia. Many of these studies, however, are lacking postmortem verification of abnormalities seen in vivo. Of great current interest will be the use of animal models of movement disorders where both structure and function can be manipulated in situations that are either ethically or logistically untenable in human subjects.

HUNTINGTON'S DISEASE

Clinical and Pathologic Features

Huntington's disease is a slowly progressive, hyperkinetic movement disorder characterized by chorea, dementia, and psychiatric symptoms.[85,129] The disease is inherited in an autosomal dominant fashion[35] and the defective gene has been localized to the short arm of chromosome 4 through the use of molecular biological approaches.[71] The age of onset varies widely, but typically occurs during the third and fourth decades of life.

The early clinical symptoms include disorders of ocular motility (altered saccades and pursuits, diminished fixation and impaired optokinetic nystagmus), loss of fine motor control, and diminished rapid alternating movements.[223] This progresses to chorea, which becomes more severe as the disease advances. In the late stages of the disease, typically 10 to 15 years after onset, chorea is gradually replaced by dystonia and hypokinetic rigidity. Dysphagia is typical of the terminal phases of the illness.[190] The average life span after diagnosis is 15 to 20 years.

Dementia, personality disorders, and psychiatric symptoms occur in Huntington's disease and typically are more disabling to the patient than are the motor aspects of the disorder. Frequently, patients and their family members will indicate that psychological, psychiatric, or personality changes preceded the onset of the involuntary movements.[129,130]

A juvenile-onset form of the disease (i.e., onset before age 20) also occurs and is characterized by rigidity and dystonia rather than chorea. Seizures are also more common in the juvenile than in the adult form.

The brunt of the pathologic changes in the brains of patients dying of Huntington's disease is in the striatum. Severe neuronal loss and gliosis typify the changes in this structure.[211] In the terminal phase, neuropathologic changes also occur diffusely throughout the brain but most prominently in the globus pallidus, motor nuclei of the thalamus, and frontal cortex.[1] The striatal cell loss is selective and is most severe for the medium-sized spiny neurons.[130] Spared are the aspiny neurons, which contain somatostatin and neuropeptide Y.[52,130] Abnormalities in dendritic processes have been observed in the striatum in patients with early disease.[68] These changes begin in the dorsal medial caudate nucleus and spread toward the ventral lateral putamen.

The differential diagnosis of patients

presenting with acquired chorea includes, along with Huntington's disease, chorea secondary to and following rheumatic fever (Sydenham's chorea), pregnancy (chorea gravidum), systemic lupus erythematosus, tardive dyskinesia, acanthocytosis, hyperthyroidism, drug effects (phenytoin or birth control pills), and benign hereditary chorea. Huntington's disease can usually be identified clinically by the presence of the triad of chorea, dementia, and autosomal dominant inheritance. Clinical presentations where family history is unobtainable or prior neuroleptic use is an issue can be diagnostically the most difficult.

Pneumoencephalography and X-Ray CT

As early as 1936,[66] pneumoencephalography was used to demonstrate the focal caudate atrophy known to exist pathologically in advanced Huntington's disease patients. The reports demonstrated the loss of the convex shape that the normal caudate nucleus produces in the frontal horn in the lateral ventricle (Fig. 8–1). Atrophy of these nuclei result in a focal enlargement of the anterior horns of the lateral ventricles, with an increased caudate-to-septum distance.[17,62,66] No correlations were identified between these ventricular enlargements and duration of illness, severity of chorea, or degree of cognitive deficits.[17,62]

The advent of x-ray CT provided a noninvasive means of identifying caudate and generalized cerebral atrophy in Huntington's disease patients during life (Fig. 8–2). In the last decade a large number of reports have refined and quantified the focal and generalized atrophic changes associated with Huntington's disease through the use of

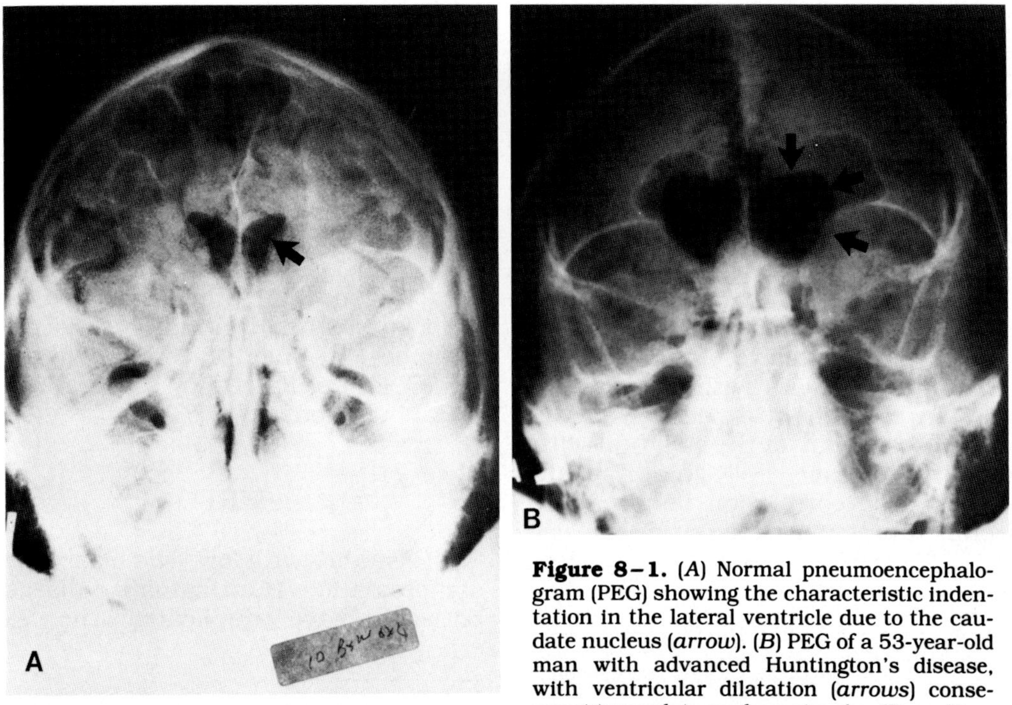

Figure 8–1. (*A*) Normal pneumoencephalogram (PEG) showing the characteristic indentation in the lateral ventricle due to the caudate nucleus (*arrow*). (*B*) PEG of a 53-year-old man with advanced Huntington's disease, with ventricular dilatation (*arrows*) consequent to caudate nucleus atrophy. (From Hayden,[85] with permission.)

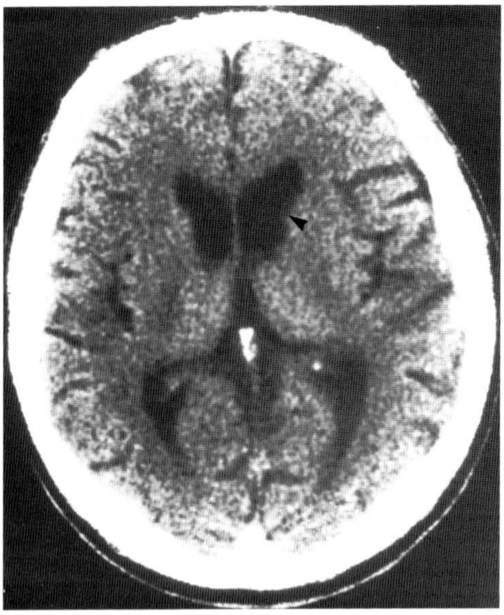

Figure 8–2. CT in Huntington's disease. Note flattening of the ventricular surface of the caudates and their atrophy.

x-ray CT.* Various indices were developed to quantify caudate nucleus changes. In general, these have referenced the separation of the medial surfaces of the two caudate nuclei (bicaudate diameter [CC]) to various other structures identifiable on x-ray CT images. These reference structures have included the width of the frontal horns (FH) or the outer table of the skull (OTcc) at the same angle, level, and position as the bicaudate measurement.† Some investigators have used the maximum internal diameter of the skull as the reference value.[110,153,202] The intercaudate distance (in either absolute terms or referenced to other brain dimensions) increases with disease progression, as might be expected from the relentless atrophy of the striatum with advancing disease.[181,189] There appears to be a good correlation between the overall functional capacity of the patient and the absolute or relative intercaudate distance.[183,189,202] Normal subjects have bicaudate distances in the range of 12.5[8] to 15 mm.[153] Symptomatic Huntington's disease patients have values in excess of 21 mm.[8,110,153,202] FH/CC ratios are typically greater than 2.3[8,151,153] in controls, whereas symptomatic Huntington's disease patients have values ≤ 2.0.‡

Differences in the tomographic angle and level used for patient scanning can affect these measured values and ratios. The characteristic ventricular shape and the large difference in values between normal controls and advanced Huntington's patients, however, usually result in the use of x-ray CT for only confirmatory diagnostic information. Patients with early symptoms[202] and individuals who are offspring of symptomatic patients (at-risk individuals) have normal x-ray CT studies.[151,153,181] Although easily distinguishable clinically, patients with obstructive hydrocephalus can have flattening of the caudate nuclei and absolute or relative bicaudate indices similar to patients with symptomatic Huntington's disease.[110]

X-ray CT also has been useful in defining the generalized cerebral atrophy that occurs in advanced Huntington's disease. In addition, some adult subjects have atrophy of the brainstem and cerebellum, more typical of juvenile cases.[14,81] Finally, x-ray CT studies have been useful in identifying structural lesions that produce chorea not associated with Huntington's disease. Such lesions include cerebral infarction[179] and unilateral or bilateral subdural hematomas.[9,64,100]

MRI

MRI studies with low-field magnets of symptomatic Huntington's disease patients have duplicated the ex-

*References 8,14,81,110,151,153,181,183, 189,202,208,209.

†References 8,14,81,110,151,153,181,202, 209.

‡References 8,140,151,153,181,202,209,221.

perience noted earlier with x-ray CT, demonstrating striatal atrophy.[27,42,101,123,182,191] In a study of 13 choreic and 7 rigid Huntington's patients using spin echo pulse sequences,[180,182] both groups had evidence of caudate atrophy, but the rigid patients selectively had an increase in signal intensity in the putamen.

MRI imaging with high-field magnets (1.5 T) has provided additional information on Huntington's disease. While caudate atrophy is still identifiable, low signal intensity on T_2-weighted images has been seen in the globus pallidus[101] and the striatum.[42] Other studies[42] indicate a decrease in signal intensity in the striatum early in the disease and then an increase in signal intensity in the structure in the late stages of the disorder (Fig. 8–3). Proposed as an explanation for this phenomenon is that iron, early in th disease, causes loss of signal intensity, but late-stage gliosis compensates and overwhelms this earlier effect and results in a relative increase in signal intensity. These authors indicated that signal intensity was also reduced in T_2-weighted images for the substantia nigra, dentate nuclei of the cerebellum, and red nuclei of the midbrain.[42] Initial spectroscopic nuclear magnetic resonance (NMR) information has demonstrated a twofold to threefold increase in phosphoethanolamine from post-mortem tissue obtained from Huntington's disease brains and studied at 4.7 and 14.1 T.[165] Although the significance of this finding is uncertain, it represents an early attempt to use NMR spectroscopic methods to evaluate Huntington's disease brain tissue.

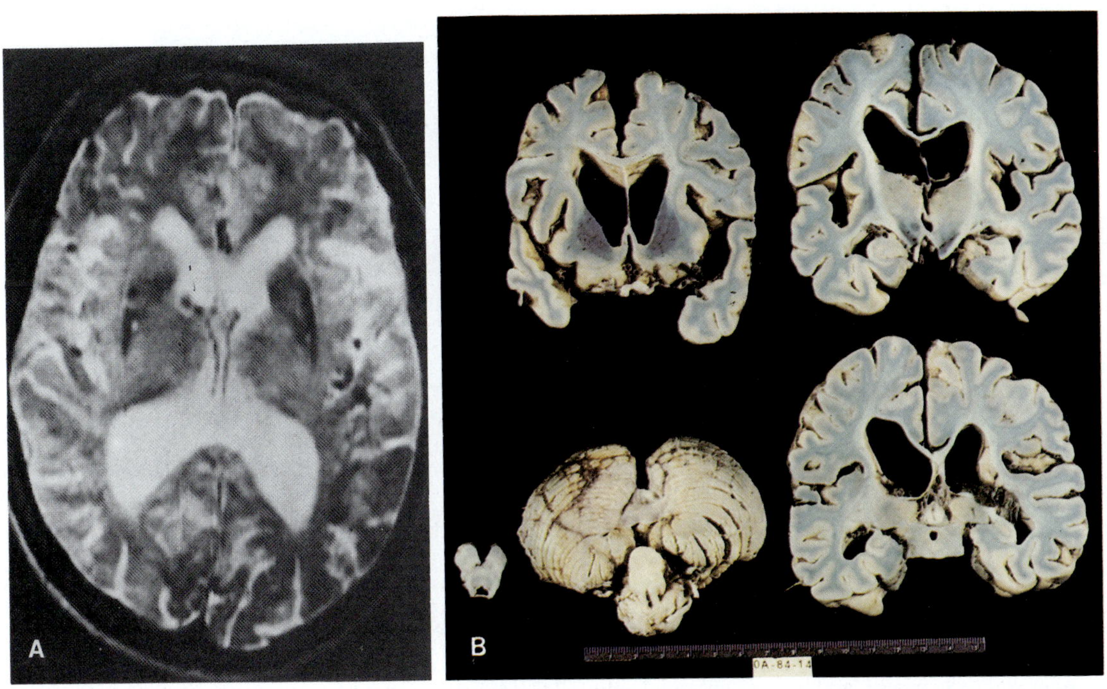

Figure 8–3. (*A*) T_2-weighted (TR 2500, TE 80) MR image. Abnormal enlargement of the lateral ventricles with abnormally prominent hypointensity in the caudate and putamen compared to the globus pallidus suggesting excessive iron accumulation in the striatum in a 42-year-old male with typical, familial Huntington's disease. (*B*) Perls' stain for ferric iron. Prominent ventriculomegaly, caudate atrophy, and striatal iron accumulation consistent with Huntington's disease. (From Drayer,[42] p. 25, with permission.)

PET

METABOLIC AND HEMODYNAMIC IMAGING

At present there are no systematic evaluations of Huntington's disease patients using SPECT. PET, however, has been used to study an increasingly large number of symptomatic Huntington's disease patients since the initial PET study[107] reported in 1982 (Fig. 8–4). The findings in that report have been substantiated and refined by subsequent studies. In general, glucose metabolism is reduced in the striatum of symptomatic Huntington's disease patients irrespective of whether striatal atrophy is grossly detectable by x-ray CT.* Only a few studies of blood flow and oxygen utilization have been performed in Huntington's disease patients, but these also indicate a reduction in these variables comparable to that seen for glucose metabolism.[118,143] SPECT studies of cerebral perfusion also indicate reduced values in the striatum.[111,193] The finding of reduced striatal metabolism seems to occur whether the symptoms are predominantly motoric or psychiatric.[58,84,107,140,222] Because reduced striatal glucose utilization occurs even in subjects with little or no atrophy demonstrated on x-ray CT, it is not a reflection of a reduction in the size of the structure and secondary partial-volume effects.[142]

So far, few correlations have been reported between the reduction in striatal glucose metabolism and clinical signs, symptoms, or their duration.[84,107]

*References 34,83,84,107,140,201,220–222.

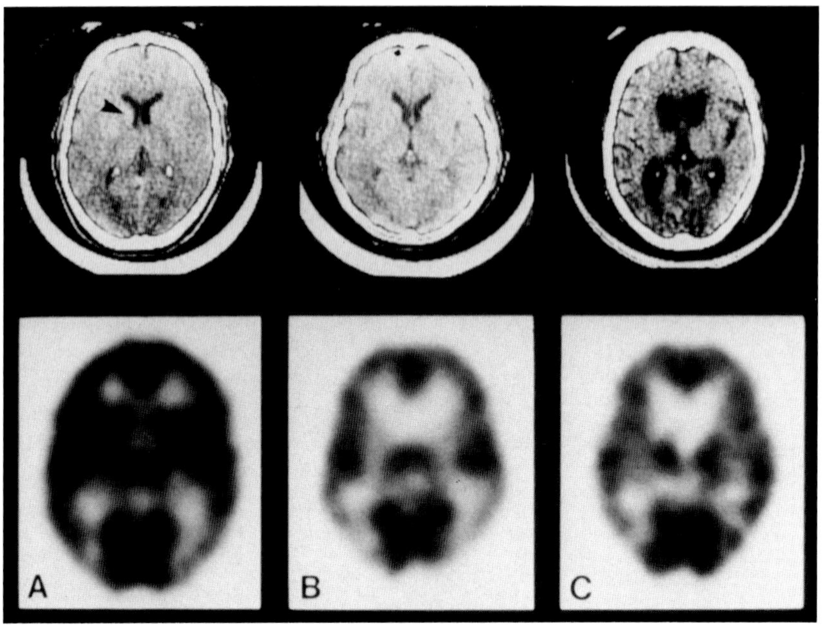

Figure 8–4. Atrophy and glucose metabolism in Huntington's disease demonstrated by X-ray CT (*top row*) and PET images, which were obtained using FDG. (*A*) Normal individual demonstrating the structural and metabolic appearance of the normal caudate nucleus (*arrow*) and putamen. (*B*) Patient with early clinical Huntington's disease, demonstrating the normal structural appearance of the caudate nucleus on X-ray CT, but profound hypometabolism for glucose in the PET study. (*C*) Patient with late Huntington's disease, demonstrating both structural (cortical and subcortical atrophy) and functional abnormalities of the caudate and putamen, bilaterally. Such studies demonstrate that the functional abnormalities of the basal ganglia (as measured by glucose metabolism) in patients with early HD precede structural cell loss sufficient to produce changes in the CT. (From Kuhl, et al,[107] p. 431, with permission.)

Young and co-workers[222] did find a correlation between caudate metabolic rate and patients' total functional capacity, learning and memory abilities, and general motor abnormalities with the exception of dystonia.[222] These investigators indicated that, like the sequence of histopathologic changes in Huntington's disease,[68] changes in putamenal metabolism were not as sensitive or early as changes in caudate metabolism.[222] They did, however, demonstrate that putamenal metabolism was better correlated to motor symptoms than was caudate metabolism.

A number of reports have indicated that there is a trend toward, or in fact a significant increase in, thalamic metabolism in symptomatic Huntington's disease patients. It is postulated that this increase may result from disinhibition of pallidal-thalamic circuits that are under striatal control.[158] Testing of this hypothesis will have to await imaging instruments with higher spatial resolution, which will allow for specific examination of the metabolic activity of the divisions of the globus pallidus and motor nuclei of the thalamus.

Cerebral cortical metabolism in symptomatic Huntington's disease patients is normal,[107,202] but a decrease in frontal cortical glucose or oxygen metabolism has been reported, particularly in patients with disease durations in excess of 8 years.[107,118] It is possible that some of the effect is secondary to frontal cortical atrophy.

Thus, striatal hypometabolism appears to be a sensitive indicator of functional change in symptomatic Huntington's disease patients, regardless of the type of symptoms displayed.* Striatal hypometabolism is not specific for Huntington's disease, however. It is also seen in chorea-acanthocytosis,[166] Wilson's disease,[82] benign hereditary chorea,[134,206] and Lesch-Nyhan syndrome[156] (Table 8–1). Similarly, non-Huntingtonian chorea may occur without reductions in striatal metabolism or perfusion. Examples of the latter situation have been reported with chorea secondary to systemic lupus erythematosus.[72] Finally, choreiform movements are seen in tardive dyskinesia despite the fact that these patients have elevated glucose utilization in the lenticular nuclei.[154,155]

*References 58,84,107,140,201,220,222.

Table 8–1 BASAL GANGLIA GLUCOSE METABOLISM AND INVOLUNTARY MOVEMENTS

Magnitude vs. Normals	***Disorders***
Decreased	Benign hereditary chorea[134,206] Huntington's disease[83,107,134,140,222] Chorea acanthocytosis[166] Lesch-Nyhan syndrome[156] Wilson's disease[82]
No change	Systemic lupus erythematosus[72]
Increased	Tardive dyskinesia[154,155]

IMAGING STUDIES OF PRESYNAPTIC AND POSTSYNAPTIC DOPAMINERGIC NEURONS

Presynaptic dopaminergic function has been evaluated with PET and ^{18}F-labeled levodopa (fluorodopa),[118,205] but because of the limited number of patients studied, these results should be considered preliminary. Striatal fluorodopa uptake and retention were no different from those in controls when evaluated in symptomatic choreic Huntington's disease patients. The single patient reported with rigid juvenile Huntington's disease had a reduction in putamenal fluorodopa uptake, with normal values for the caudate.[205]

Limited data are available from PET studies that evaluate postsynaptic D_2 dopamine receptors with ^{11}C-labeled N-methylspiperone (MSP).[77,118,215] These preliminary studies demonstrate reductions in the apparent numbers of receptors of this class in the striatum of Huntington's disease patients. These in vivo dopamine studies fit well with the known striatal pathology of Huntington's disease. Since nigrostriatal pathways are intact, presynaptic synthesis of dopamine from levodopa and its storage should be unimpaired. This has been substantiated by the finding of normal or even elevated levels of dopamine in the striatum at postmortem examination.[16,85,130] Loss of intrinsic striatal neurons, presumably those with dopaminergic receptors, would result in a decrease in this receptor population following the death of striatal cells. This is also in keeping with postmortem studies.[171] Figure 8–5 demonstrates a PET study of a single patient with symptomatic Huntington's disease who was evaluated for striatal perfusion, metabolism, and both presynaptic and postsynaptic dopaminergic activity.

METABOLIC EVALUATION OF PRESYMPTOMATIC (AT-RISK) SUBJECTS

Because of the consistent finding of striatal hypometabolism in even the earliest symptomatic Huntington's disease patients, similar measurements were explored in asymptomatic offspring of affected parents.* In the original study,[107] just over one third (6/15) of the asymptomatic at-risk individuals had caudate hypometabolism that was more than two standard deviations

*References 34,58,83,118,139,140,219,221.

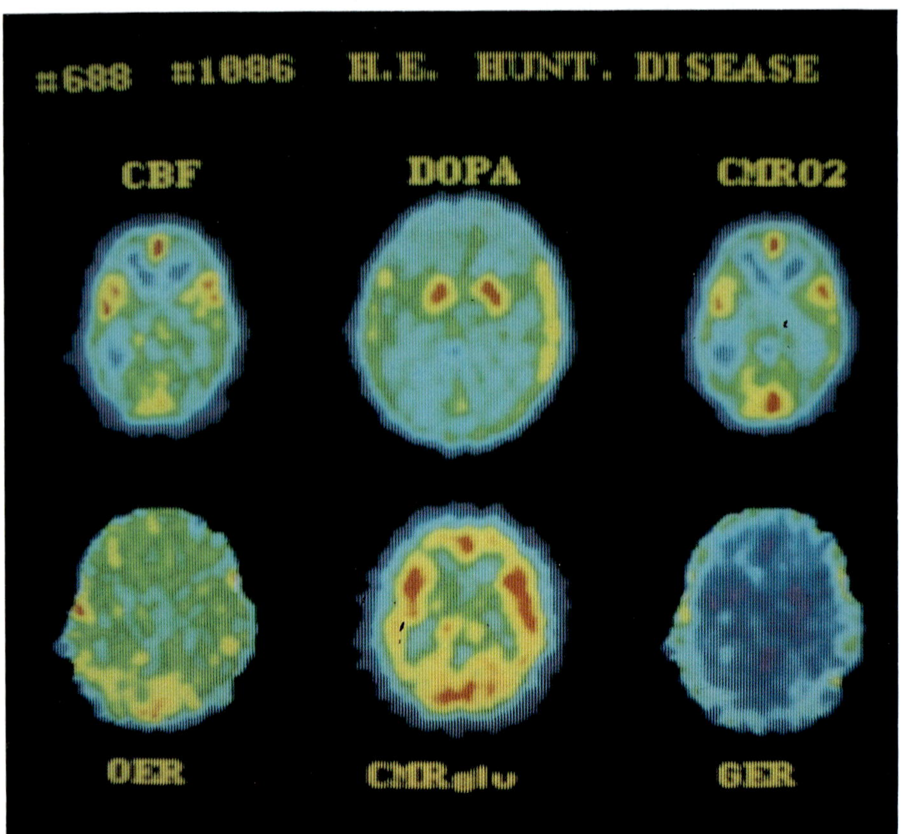

Figure 8–5. Blood flow (CBF), metabolism ($CMRO_2$ = oxygen metabolism, CMRglu = glucose metabolism), and presynaptic dopamine (^{18}F-fluoro-L-DOPA) systems in Huntington's disease. Despite reduced and matched reductions of striatal blood flow and glucose and oxygen metabolism, presynaptic dopamine integrity (i.e., nigrostriatal tract) is intact. (From Leenders, et al.,[118] p. 74, with permission.)

below the level of control subjects. In a subsequent study from the same institution,[140] a similar fraction (18/58) of at-risk subjects was found to have reductions in caudate glucose metabolism that were outside the 95% confidence limits for inclusion in the control group (Fig. 8–6). It is presumed that these individuals, with reductions in caudate glucose metabolism in the absence of clinical symptoms, carry the HD gene and will eventually develop symptomatic Huntington's disease.[140] Four of these 18 individuals have, in fact, developed clinical symptoms at intervals ranging from 1 to 3 years since their last normal PET study. None of the 40 individuals in the presumed normal group have, as yet, gone on to develop clinical Huntington's disease (Fig. 8–7*A*). In a similar and confirmatory report[83] of 13 at-risk individuals picked from 4 large families, about one third (4/13) had caudate hypometabolism[83,84] (Fig. 8–7*B*).

In contrast to these results is a report[221] indicating that caudate glucose metabolism was normal, both qualitatively and quantitatively, in 29 at-risk subjects whose mean age was 28 ± 5 years. The researchers concluded that reduced caudate glucose metabolism observed with PET follows rather than precedes, clinical symptoms.[219,221]

This study, however, employed an at-risk group whose mean age was considerably younger than that of subjects in the other two studies. If glucose metabolism in the caudate declines just before the onset of clinical symptoms, studies of at-risk groups whose mean age is younger will have fewer Huntington's disease gene carriers with caudate hypometabolism. Thus, a biological explanation for the disparate results exists. In addition, the threshold for diagnos-

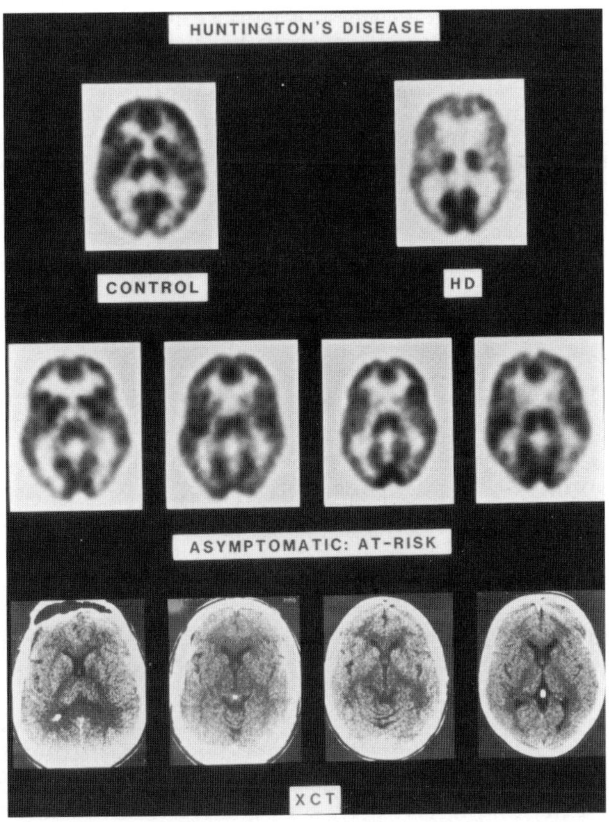

Figure 8–6. PET and x-ray CT in Huntington's disease. Upper left image demonstrates the typical, normal appearance of glucose metabolism at a tomographic level that passes through the heads of the caudate nuclei, the thalamus, and the visual cortex in a control subject. The upper right image is from a symptomatic patient with Huntington's disease. Note the marked reduction in metabolism in the caudate nuclei. The middle and bottom rows of images are from four subjects who were asymptomatic (chorea-free) but at risk for Huntington's disease. X-ray CT studies (*bottom row*) were normal for all four subjects. The metabolic activity of the caudate nuclei, as determined with PET (*middle row*), demonstrates graded changes ranging from a normal appearance (leftmost image) to one closely resembling that seen in symptomatic patients (rightmost image). (Glucose metabolism in the caudate nuclei for these at-risk subjects is indicated by the letters A, B, C, and D [from left to right] in Fig. 8–7*A*.) All PET studies were performed using the NeuroECAT device. (From Mazziotta, et al,[140] p. 359, with permission.)

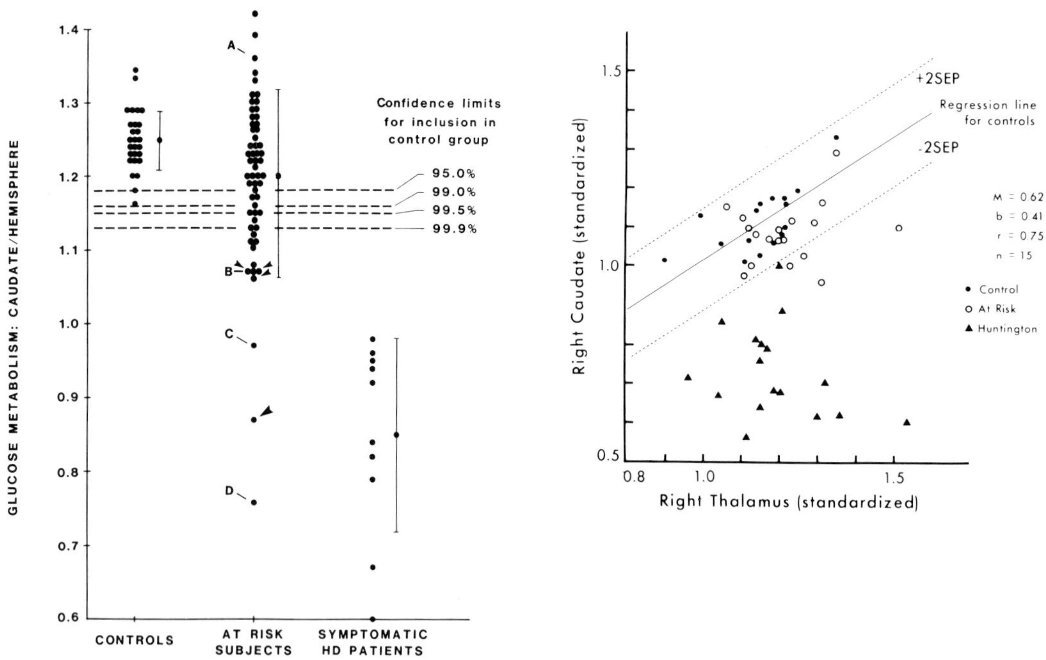

Figure 8–7. (*A*) Caudate glucose metabolism expressed as a ratio of the caudate to the hemispheric metabolic rate (cd/hem) in symptomatic patients with Huntington's disease, persons at risk for the disease, and normal controls. Error bars indicate ± 1 SD. Notice the complete separation of values for the control and symptomatic Huntington's disease groups. Although the mean value for the at-risk group is similar to that for the controls, values for a number of subjects fell well outside the control distribution for this ratio and, in fact, overlapped with values for persons in the symptomatic Huntington's disease group (i.e., the distribution of values for the at-risk group is skewed unidirectionally toward lower values). A threshold for the cd/hem metabolic ratio of 1.15 separates persons at risk into two subgroups so that those above this threshold have a 99.5 percent confidence limit of being included in the control distribution. The labels A,B,C, and D indicate the cd/hem metabolic values for the four at-risk subjects whose PET studies are shown in Figure 8–6. Arrowheads indicate subjects at risk who were studied in an asymptomatic state but in whom clinical symptoms of Huntington's disease developed approximately 2 to 4 years after their PET evaluation. (From Mazziotta, et al.,[140] p. 360, with permission.) (*B*) Standardized right caudate and thalamic glucose metabolic values for control, at-risk, and symptomatic Huntington's disease patients, along with regression line for the normal controls. The graph shows separation of symptomatic patients from controls and also identifies 4 of 14 at-risk subjects whose values are more than 2 SEP below controls. SEP = standard error of prediction; r = correlation between the thalamic and caudate values; M = slope of the regression line; b = y-intercept of the regression line; n = number of subjects. (From Clark, et al.,[34] p. 760, with permission.)

ing patients as clinically symptomatic may have been lower in the study reporting normal caudate metabolism in all at-risk subjects.[83] Also of note is the fact that the variance in the control data of the negative study[221] is substantially larger than that reported in either of the positive studies,[34,83,140] and this would tend to mask positive findings.[141]

PET results of glucose metabolism have been compared to genetic linkage marker studies[71,83,139] as depicted in Figure 8–8. Whereas the majority of outcomes match between the PET and genetic data, the disparate results are of interest. Subjects who have a high probability (> 90%) of having the Huntington's disease gene by linkage marker criteria, but who have normal caudate glucose metabolism, may represent false-positive genetic results due to recombination, false-negative results due to delay in development of caudate hypometabolism, or a combination of the two. Those who have caudate hypometabolism and a low probability for hav-

PET		G8 Marker +	G8 Marker -
PET	+	4	4
PET	-	5	10

PET		D4S43 Marker +	D4S43 Marker -
PET	+	5	2
PET	-	5	9

Figure 8–8. Caudate glucose metabolic versus genetic linkage results in subjects at risk for Huntington's disease. Note that the concordance between genetic and PET results improves when a genetic linkage marker closer to the Huntington's disease gene is used (i.e., D4S43 versus G8).

ing the Huntington's disease gene may represent false-negative genetic results owing to recombination, false-positive PET results owing to the choice of a threshold too low to define caudate hypometabolism, or combinations of the two. Issues relating PET and genetic-linkage results will be elucidated by studying larger numbers of subjects with the two methodologies and by following at-risk individuals to the point of development of clinical symptoms.

The value of PET in Huntington's disease is emphasized by the following facts: symptomatic Huntington's disease patients have caudate hypometabolism; all previously asymptomatic at-risk individuals who have developed clinical symptoms of Huntington's disease have had, in the presymptomatic state, caudate hypometabolism 1 to 4 years before symptom onset; and no at-risk individual with presumed normal caudate metabolism has yet been reported to have developed clinical symptoms.

Thus, glucose metabolism and other physiologic variables may be useful in identifying gene carriers and confirming the diagnosis of Huntington's disease when family history, clinical data, or genetic informativeness is lacking. Lastly, the opportunity to monitor noninvasively and objectively the rate of change of glucose metabolism in symptomatic or presymptomatic Huntington's disease patients provides a unique opportunity to monitor experimental therapies for this disorder. The best candidate for experimental therapy to delay the onset of symptoms in Huntington's disease is a subject with the abnormal gene who is presymptomatic. Identification of such an individual can now occur through the combined use of linkage marker studies and PET. Knowledge about the rate of change of glucose metabolism or other physiologic variables in the striatum could be used as a baseline from which to compare experimental therapies aimed at slowing the rate of degeneration in this structure. Such information could indicate whether a given experimental therapy is beneficial, deleterious, or ineffective in altering the course of the disease.[140]

Future Prospects

The identification of spared striatal neuronal populations[130] and their evaluation in controlled experimental environments (e.g., tissue culture),[99] provides an opportunity to develop selective probes for early pathophysiologic changes in Huntington's disease through PET or SPECT. Markers of the N-methyl-D-aspartate receptors[99,218] are currently in a developmental phase and will provide a valuable link between such basic science research and clinical observations.

Postmortem studies of patients dying from Huntington's disease have demonstrated increased GABA and benzodiazepine receptors in the globus pallidus, with decreased muscarinic receptors in that structure.[160] All these receptor types are reduced in the striatum.[160] Thus, the combined use of probes such as those for the measurement of protein synthesis, acetylcholine (e.g., ^{11}C-scopalamine), benzodiazepine/GABA (e.g., ^{11}C-flumazenil) and NMDA[218] receptor ligands will be important new neuroimaging tools in the study of Huntington's disease. Of equal importance will be the continued comparisons of at-risk individuals whose PET data can be compared to clinical outcome and genetic linkage marker results. The deposition of ferromagnetic ions and the spectroscopic identification of biochemical striatal abnormalities by means of MRI may also prove to be valuable tools in understanding the pathophysiology of Huntington's disease, its genetic expression in the brain, and avenues towards its treatment or prevention.

PARKINSON'S DISEASE

Clinical and Pathologic Features

Parkinson's disease is classically described as a neurodegenerative disorder resulting from the degeneration and death of dopaminergic neurons in the pars compacta of the substantia nigra and locus ceruleus. It is thought that clinical symptoms begin after the majority ($\geq$ 80%) of these cells have died.[97] Parkinsonian symptoms consist of rigidity, bradykinesia, difficulty in initiating and stopping movements, and resting tremor. Typically, patients describe an insidious onset. Clinically, a typical patient will move slowly, walk with a stooped posture without associated arm movements, have an expressionless face, be hypophonic, and have a 7–9-cycle-per-second tremor at rest of the upper extremities, most notable in the fingers. Detailed descriptions of the clinical symptoms and neuropathologic findings have been provided in numerous recent reviews.[47,49,127,128]

The study of Parkinson's disease, its related syndromes, its treatments, and their side effects with neuroimaging techniques has taken a dramatic turn in recent years. The advent of high-field MRI, PET, and SPECT has built upon data from functional studies pioneered through the use of ^{133}Xe cerebral blood flow measurements. These recent studies are in contrast to structural evaluations of the brain in Parkinson's disease patients employing pneumoencephalography and x-ray CT. These earlier studies were of use in identifying the rare and unusual patient presenting acutely or subacutely with parkinsonian features as the result of cerebral infarction,[210] subdural hematomas,[104] intracranial tumors,[39,115,212,217] or globus pallidus damage as a result of carbon monoxide intoxication.[98] Outside of these unusual findings, structural imaging studies in Parkinson's disease are either normal or show some degree of generalized atrophy.

Functional imaging techniques allow for the identification of focal biochemical changes in Parkinson's disease, which may include the deposition of brain iron, altered uptake and retention of precursors to dopamine, and changes in postsynaptic receptor numbers in the basal ganglia. Such techniques also allow for correlating these findings with postmortem human specimens and with animal models (e.g., 6-hydroxydopamine and 1-methyl-4-phenyl-1,2,3,6-tetrahydropyridine [MPTP]) of Parkinson's disease.

With the power of functional imaging come the complexities associated with studying a dynamic, ongoing set of biochemical and pathophysiologic mechanisms. First, Parkinson's disease can be considered as part of a wide spectrum of disorders with parkinsonian features (e.g., unilateral Parkinson's disease, bilateral Parkinson's disease, nigrostriatal degeneration, multisystem atrophy, progressive supranuclear palsy, and toxin exposures). In addition, inconsistencies in patient selection, severity and duration of disease, concurrent medications, and side effects of medications make comparison of results between studies difficult and decrease the likelihood that biologically relevant findings of low magnitude will be identified between laboratories studying the same problem without standardization. Despite these problems, biochemical and functional neuroimaging studies of Parkinson's disease patients provide an exciting and wide range of new information about the pathophysiology of this complex set of disorders.

X-Ray CT

Before the advent of x-ray CT, pneumoencephalography demonstrated that patients with Parkinson's disease either had grossly normal brain anatomy or had mild-to-moderate degrees of generalized cerebral atrophy. Large series of patients[187] were evaluated with pneumoencephalograms as part of the approach to stereotactic thalamotomy used for treatment of the disorder before the advent of levodopa. These studies demonstrated generalized atrophy in the majority of patients evaluated.[187]

X-ray CT has refined this information somewhat. Cerebral atrophy is more obvious in younger (24–49 years) patients with Parkinson's disease[184,200] than in older patients, in whom the disease may be indistinguishable from normal aging.[197,200] Although there is no focal pattern of atrophy that is diagnostic or specific for Parkinson's disease, sites of maximal tissue loss have been reported in the mesial frontal lobe and in the area surrounding the third ventricle.[200]

X-ray CT has been used to determine whether patients with Parkinson's disease who have dementia show more atrophy than those without dementia.[70] Generally, demented patients with Parkinson's disease have a greater degree of cerebral atrophy than do age-matched controls[197] (see Chapter 9). There is no consensus, however, as to whether there is a correlation between the degree or severity of dementia and the amount of atrophy seen on x-ray CT. Some investigators report this correlation[47,49] and others do not.[108] It has been suggested that some aspects of cognitive impairment (e.g., digit span, verbal learning, and visual memory) are correlated with ventricular enlargement but not with cortical atrophy in Parkinson's disease.[170] X-ray CT and, more recently, MRI have been and continue to be used for the preoperative[94] and postoperative[27] evaluation of candidates for stereotactic thalamotomy for parkinsonian tremor.

As noted earlier, rare patients presenting with acute or subacute symptoms of Parkinson's disease who have not been exposed to neuroleptics can benefit from structural imaging studies. Such studies may reveal an underlying cause for a rapidly progressive Parkinsonian syndrome (Fig. 8–9). Such causes include infarction of the basal ganglia;[210] bilateral pallidal lesions following hypotension, hypoxia, or carbon monoxide poisoning;[98] subdural hematoma; and intracranial tumors, which may be either supratentorial[115,212,217] or infratentorial.[39]

MRI

MRI findings in patients with Parkinson's disease can be divided into two groups depending on whether high- or low-field-strength magnets were used for imaging. Results from low-field-strength magnets, in general, parallel the reports from structural imaging with x-ray CT. Typical of these studies is the finding of generalized atrophy[27] and no changes in signal intensity on either spin echo or inversion recovery pulse sequences for cortex or basal ganglia.[123] A single report describes an increase in T_1 duration in patients with Parkinson's disease for the lenticular nuclei irrespective of whether the patients were or were not demented.[13] The same authors did find a correlation between T_1 duration and the severity of dementia in Parkinson's patients for the right frontal, left occipital, and bilateral parietal white matter. The de-

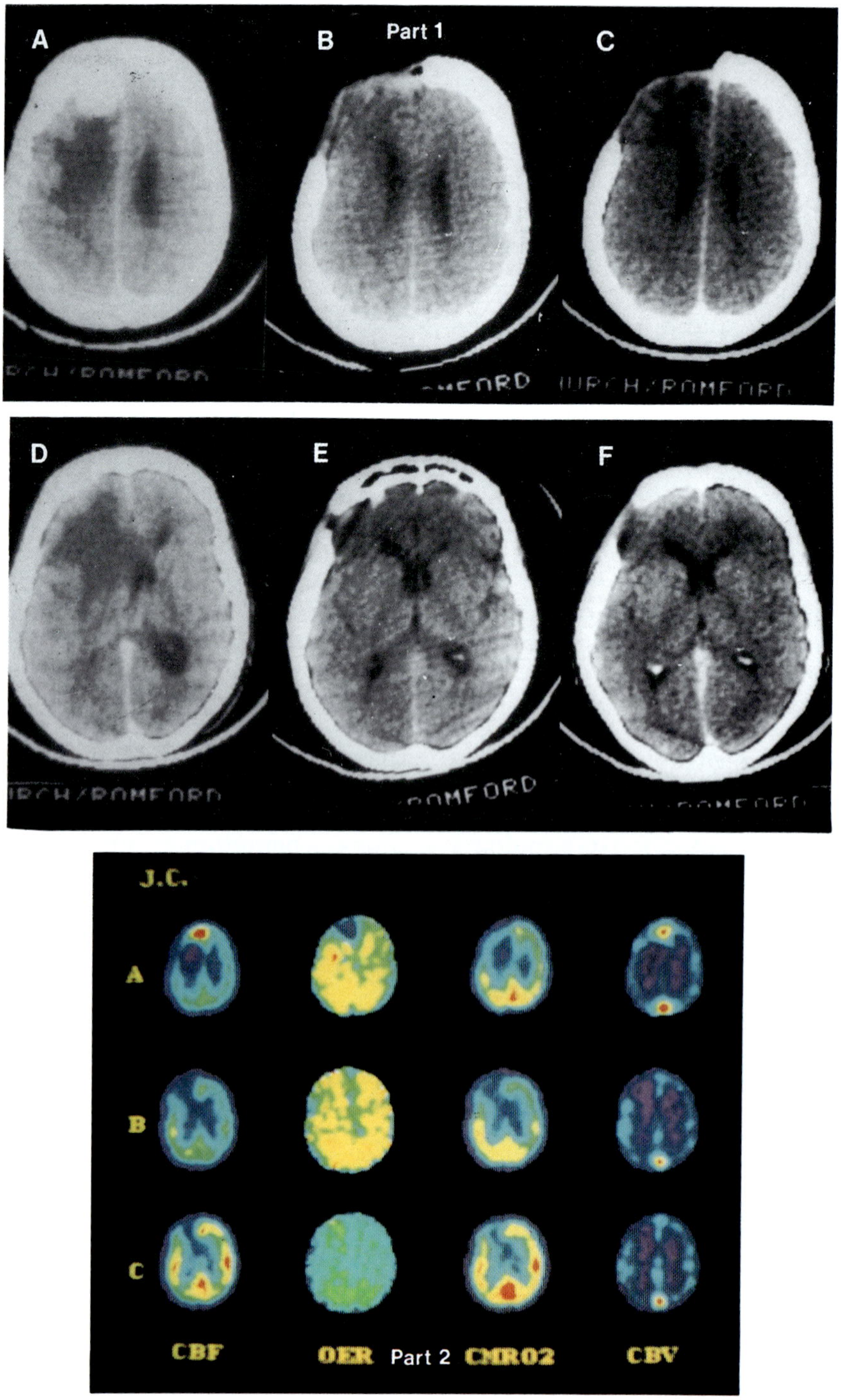

Figure 8–9. Tumor-induced parkinsonism. (*Part 1*) X-ray CT images (after contrast enchancement) through the level of the tumor (*A,B,C*) and through the basal ganglia (*D,E,F*) before surgery (*A,D*), 2 weeks after (*B,E*), and 4 months (*C,F*) after surgery. Before surgery, a left frontal meningioma is seen with edema in the white matter of the left frontal lobe (*A*), extending into the left basal ganglia region (*D*), with considerable midline shift. After surgery, the edema and midline shift have largely disappeared, although some regions with lower attenuation are still present in the anterolateral part of the left frontal lobe. (From Leenders, et al.[115] p. 1075, with permission.) (*Part 2*) PET images at the level of the tumor, (*row A*) before surgery, (*B*) at 2 weeks and (*C*) 4 months after surgery. Each image within a row shows a different function within the same plane: CBF, OER, $CMRO_2$, and CBV, respectively. The absolute value of each function is coded in a linear color scale (code is identical in the three images for each function). The top of each image corresponds to the frontal region of the brain and the left side to the left hemisphere. The left frontal meningioma has a high CBF and CBV, a decreased $CMRO_2$, and an extremely low OER. After surgery, a defect in $CMRO_2$ and CBF is seen at the previous tumor site with a normalized OER. Globally, a marked rise in CBF is demonstrated (*row C*), with a moderate increase in $CMRO_2$. The OER decreases accordingly. (From Leenders, et al., [115] p. 1076, with permission.)

mented patients were matched with nondemented Parkinson's patients for disease duration and severity.[13]

High-field-strength MRI studies have demonstrated focal changes in Parkinson's disease patients. In addition to generalized and frontal atrophy,[42] initial reports[40] with high-field-strength magnets and T_2-weighted images revealed decreased signal intensity in the globus pallidus, red nuclei, substantia nigra, and posterior lateral putamen (Figs. 8–10, 9–5*A*,*B*). It appears, at present, that the most sensitive pulse sequence for demonstrating these changes involves gradient echo images.[42] It is speculated that this decrease in signal intensity is related to iron deposition in these structures, as has been demonstrated in postmortem brain using Perl's stain.[23,42,176] This loss of signal intensity could be due to local disruption of the magnetic environment (i.e., magnetic susceptibility) induced by elevated concentrations of ferromagnetic ions.[42] Ions that have this property include iron, copper, cobalt, manganese, and chromium. Loss of signal intensity in this set of structures in Parkinson's disease could be due to excessive iron accumulation; accumulation of hematin, neuromelanin, and lipofuscin; declining dopamine concentrations; or some combination of these factors.[42]

Drayer and associates[42] (personal communication, 1989) evaluated three groups of patients with parkinsonian features. These groups included patients with: (1) Parkinson's disease with good therapeutic responses to levodopa; (2) progressive supranuclear palsy; and (3) multisystem atrophy. The latter group can be defined as patients with Parkinson's disease plus autonomic failure, ataxia, and pyramidal symptoms.[167,196] They clinically overlap with patients having nigro-striatal degeneration syndrome and olivopontocerebellar atrophy. In this latter group there was a decrease in signal intensity in the putamen (see Fig. 8–10) that was not consistently seen with the other groups.[42] This signal decrease

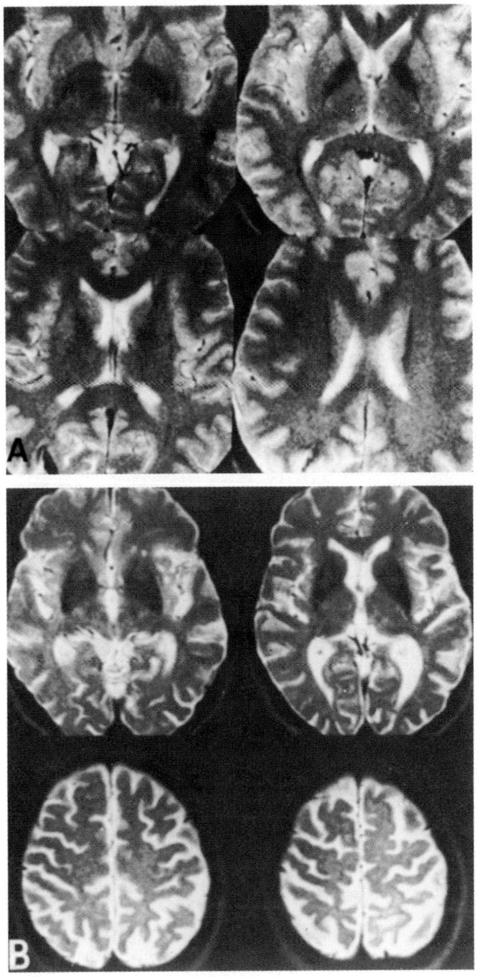

Figure 8–10. Normal adult versus drug-unresponsive Parkinson's patient (T_2-weighted images [TR 2500, TE 80]). (*A*) Normal (age 58). Hypointensity (ferritin, nonheme iron) is maximal in the globus pallidus. Incidental note is made of a small cavernous angioma (hemosiderin) at the right parieto-occipital gray-white junction. (*B*) Drug-unresponsive Parkinson's patient (age 58). The hypointensity in the putamen is abnormally prominent, equivalent to that in the globus pallidus. The cortical sulci are enlarged, and a few hyperintensities are seen in the globus pallidus (état criblé with perivascular atrophic demyelination). (From Drayer, et al.,[42] p. 20, with permission.)

was particularly obvious in the posterior putamen[24,157] and has been related to the severity of rigidity in multisystem atrophy patients. No relationship has been found with overall parkinsonian features, bradykinesia, or tremor. Patients with pure dysautonomia have normal T_1- and T_2-weighted images with high-field MRI.[24]

In patients with Parkinson's disease, the distance between the substantia nigra and the red nuclei is decreased.[42] This change is thought to result from atrophy of the pars compacta of the substantia nigra, deposition of iron in the area, or deposition of other pigments listed above.[42] Similarly, small areas of increased white-matter signal intensity (e.g., internal capsule, cerebral-hemisphere white matter) have been identified in Parkinson's disease patients more often than in controls.[42] These changes are probably vascular in nature, but it is unknown whether they are related to the dementia found in some patients with Parkinson's disease. Studies using NMR spectroscopy in human subjects have been initiated and may result in additional biochemical information helpful in understanding this disorder.[25]

PET and SPECT

CEREBRAL BLOOD FLOW (CBF)

Numerous studies have been made evaluating CBF in patients with Parkinson's disease. Methods used for measuring CBF have included the administration of ^{133}Xe with the detection of radioactivity from individual probes surrounding the head, SPECT and PET. A review of all this information results in a rather inconsistent picture, perhaps due to differences in methods, patient selection, duration of illness, presence or absence of dementia, and the amount and type of medications used by the patients in the studies. Despite this, when CBF measurements obtained with all modalities are evaluated, it is clear that most investigators find a reduction (9.5%–20%) in hemispheric or global cerebral blood flow* in patients with Parkinson's disease versus normal controls. Even this generalization has its exceptions; a few studies have demonstrated no difference in global CBF between age-matched normal subjects and patients with Parkinson's disease.[86,146]

Tomographic techniques have provided more localized information about cerebral blood flow. Reports of CBF measured with SPECT[86] indicate an 18% decrease in flow in the striatum contralateral to the affected limbs in patients with hemi–Parkinson's disease. Similarly, PET studies have demonstrated reduced flow in the basal ganglia contralateral to the affected limbs in a patient with hemi–Parkinson's disease syndrome induced by a meningioma.[115] One group[163] found a reduction in flow in the globus pallidus contralateral to the affected limbs in patients with bradykinesia but no tremor, with the reverse situation—an increase in pallidal blood flow—in hemi–Parkinson's disease patients who had tremor but no bradykinesia.

Normal young subjects studied with methods to measure CBF tend to have higher frontal than parietal-occipital blood flow. CBF has been found to be decreased, however, in mesial frontal cortex contralateral to the affected limbs in hemi–Parkinson's disease.[163] This finding was unchanged by treatment with levodopa. A loss of this "normal CBF hyperfrontality" has been observed in Parkinson's disease patients[11,48] and does not seem to be accounted for by selective frontal cortical atrophy.[48]

In general, correlations between CBF and duration of Parkinson's disease, severity of symptoms, and dementia are lacking.[65,67,112,122,145] An exception is a single SPECT study that reported CBF inversely related to duration of disease.[86]

A number of reports have related tremor to blood flow or metabolism in the globus pallidus in Parkinson's disease patients. In a single case report of a patient with severe unilateral resting tremor,[92] a decrease in CBF (22%) and

*References 19,65,67,93,112,121,145,214.

oxygen metabolism (18%) (relative to the hemisphere ipsilateral to the tremor) was found in the parietal cortex of the hemisphere contralateral to the tremor. This patient then underwent a ventrolateral thalamotomy.[92] Following surgery, CBF in the parietal cortex increased as tremor decreased. In addition, these authors noted that CBF was elevated in the globus pallidus of three out of four unilateral Parkinson's disease patients that they studied with the same techniques.

Pallidal hypermetabolism also has been demonstrated with PET studies of glucose metabolism[45,133,174] as well as in 2-deoxyglucose determinations of glucose metabolism in animal models of Parkinson's disease produced either with 6-hydroxydopamine* or MPTP.[36,148,168,186] Pallidal hypermetabolism appears, however, to be the ramification of many sources of damage to either pyramidal or extrapyramidal systems. It has occurred following the nigral lesions noted earlier, and also with motor cortex ablations.[63] Thus, these changes in pallidal metabolism and blood flow, while interesting, will require further evaluation to determine their specificity to Parkinson's disease and its related syndromes.

Finally, with regard to tremor in Parkinson's disease, no increases in CBF were observed in sensorimotor cortex contralateral to limbs affected by tremor, whereas normal volunteers who mimicked the Parkinsonian tremor did have such increases.[163] Whether the difference between the voluntary and involuntary movement has to do with the level of neuraxis where the movement is generated (i.e., subcortical in the Parkinson's disease patients) remains to be determined.

CEREBRAL METABOLISM

One might hypothesize, from the known nigrostriatal degeneration of Parkinson's disease, that glucose metabolism would be reduced in the striatum of patients with the disorder secondary to dopaminergic deafferentation. It could be further speculated that this hypothetical reduction in striatal metabolism would be corrected by administration of exogenous levodopa. These hypotheses have not been supported. Studies of glucose metabolism and oxygen utilization are, in fact, quite similar to the CBF data reviewed above. That is, global reductions in glucose utilization have been observed[105,161] without either left-right or frontal-posterior cortical asymmetries when compared to age-matched controls.[105] The pattern of metabolism is normal, without a relative reduction in striatal glucose utilization (Fig. 8–11). As noted earlier, a number of studies have demonstrated increased metabolism in the globus pallidus.[45,133,136,174]

Why is it that glucose metabolism is normal in the deafferented striatum of patients with Parkinson's disease? To understand the answer to this question requires some knowledge of how glucose metabolism relates to neuronal function. In simplistic terms, glucose metabolism is most closely linked to synaptic activity in the normal adult brain and is found in its highest levels in synaptic terminals rather than in cell bodies.[137a] Thus, glucose metabolism is largely a reflection of synaptic activity. Although the highest density of dopaminergic synapses is in the striatum, these transmitter-specific synapses represent only a small fraction of the total synapses in that structure. Hence, with a probe that measures all synaptic activity, such as glucose metabolism, this small fractional loss of dopaminergic input cannot be detected selectively. This idea is supported by 2-deoxyglucose studies in animal models of Parkinson's disease where only small (2%–9%) reductions in striatal glucose metabolism have been observed.[102,103,185,216] Measurements specific to the functional integrity of dopaminergic synapses should be and have been (see below) dramatically altered by

---

*References 102,103,178,185,216

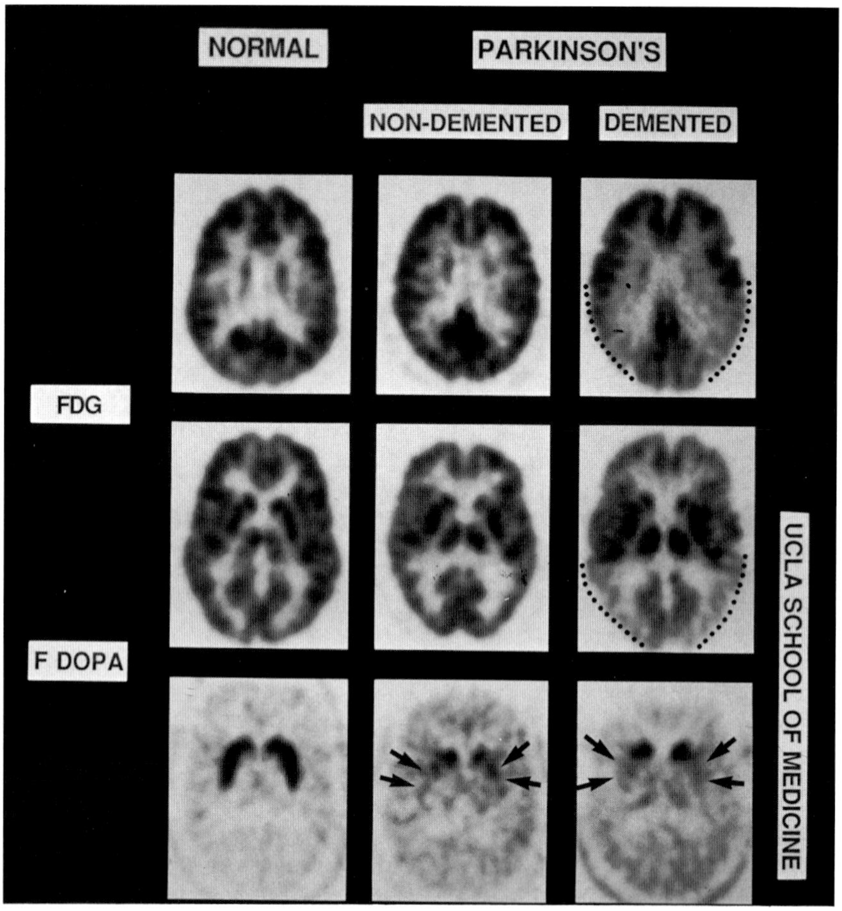

Figure 8–11. PET studies in Parkinson's disease. Top two rows show PET examinations using FDG to measure glucose metabolism, whereas the bottom row has images of ^{18}F-labeled fluorodopa (FD, F-DOPA) to determine presynaptic dopamine integrity. The left column is of a normal elderly volunteer. The center and right columns are Parkinson's patients (*right*) with and (*center*) without dementia. Notice that FD uptake is reduced in the striata of the Parkinson's patients, especially in the putamen. Glucose metabolism is normal in pattern in nondemented Parkinson's patients, but in those with dementia, biparietal-temporal hypometabolism can be seen (see Fig. 9–5*C* and *D*) in a pattern indistinguishable from that seen in Alzheimer's disease (see Fig. 9–4*C*).

the neuropathologic process that produces Parkinson's disease.

The opportunity to evaluate dementia in Parkinson's disease with PET measures of glucose metabolism has been fruitful. A single Parkinsonian patient was studied before and after the development of mild-to-moderate dementia.[105] When studied in the demented state, the patient had a reduction in parietal cortical metabolism (parietal/caudate-thalamus ratio reduced 39%) (see Figs. 8–11, 9–5*C*,*D*). More recent work[106,161] indicates that cortical metabolic changes in Parkinson's disease may be related to the dementing process. Biparietal reductions in glucose metabolism noted in demented patients with Parkinson's disease parallel the distribution of findings seen in demented patients with Alzheimer's disease and are not found in nondemented patients with Parkinson's disease.[106] Further studies will have to be performed to verify this initial and intriguing finding.

The results of the studies described above, however, demonstrate how functional imaging studies identify patterns of altered function that are associated with specific diseases. The concurrence of two diseases in the same patient could be identified in areas of change that are disease-specific. Thus, important insights into any potential overlap between the dementia of Parkinson's and Alzheimer's disease could be investigated with this approach. Confirmatory autopsy studies or more specific probes (such as cholinergic) will be needed to determine the relationship of Parkinson's disease patients with dementia to those with Alzheimer's disease.

EFFECTS OF LEVODOPA

Considerable effort has gone into the evaluation of the functional effects produced by therapeutic doses of levodopa administered either acutely or chronically. However, problems of experimental design and patient selection make comparisons between such studies hazardous. Confounding issues that may cause disparate results include disease severity and duration, differences in levodopa doses between studies, the use of carbidopa, different time intervals between levodopa administration and measurement, delays between plasma peaks in levodopa concentration and clinical responses, and induction of side effects by the medication (e.g., chorea).

In animals, dopamine agonists cause dose-dependent increases (40%–50%) in CBF. Only one study of CBF has been reported in normal humans given levodopa in which stable xenon x-ray CT was used to estimate CBF.[93] The authors found a global 13% reduction in CBF following an acute dose of levodopa. In patients with Parkinson's disease, most reports indicate no change in global CBF[145,146,163] following acute levodopa administration. In patients with unilateral Parkinson's disease studied with PET, no changes in CBF were reported following doses of approximately 200 mg of levodopa plus carbidopa.[163] However, generalized increases in flow (13% in the cortex and 20% in the basal ganglia) were found in patients with bilateral Parkinson's disease following larger (300–1250 mg) doses of levodopa given acutely.[121] Thus, the dose of levodopa and severity of illness may be important variables in the generalized flow response seen with administration of this drug.

SPECT has been used to evaluate the side effects (e.g., chorea) of levodopa administration upon CBF.[19,86] In studies that compared striatal CBF before and after levodopa administration, a difference was found between patients having a therapeutic versus an adverse response to the drug. In the former case, CBF decreased 13%–15% in the striatum, but in the latter case CBF increased 20%.[19,86] Therefore, in addition to dose of the drug and severity of illness, the generation or induction of side effects from the medication also may cause functional changes in basal ganglia and other structures of the brain that serve as confounding issues and avenues for experimental investigation.

In studies in which acute versus chronic levodopa effects have been examined, patients on long-term levodopa therapy (i.e., months) return to baseline flow values even if elevations in flow were seen acutely after administration of the compound.[121]

Thus, it is likely that levodopa and other dopaminergic agonists exert an acute and direct vasodilatory effect with global increases in flow, as has been previously documented in primate studies.[144] This response can be seen acutely in human subjects[121] if the dose is high enough. Local effects (e.g., striatal) may vary in proportion to dose, disease duration, and induction of side effects and have yet to be fully elucidated.

FLUORINE-18–LABELED LEVODOPA (FLUORODOPA) STUDIES

Fluorine-18–labeled levodopa, known as fluorodopa (FD), was first evaluated in primates and humans by Garnett and colleagues.[59,61] This quickly led to its use in patients with Parkinson's disease.* Metabolism of

*References 57,60,74,119,132,136,149.

this compound is described in Figure 8–12. FD is a substrate for dopa-decarboxylase and is thought to be decarboxylated to fluorodopamine within dopaminergic nerve terminals (see Chapter 3). Modeling and interpretation of data from FD studies is complicated by a number of factors.[132] Systemically metabolized FD generates 3-0-methyl-6-FD; this process can be enhanced by the use of carbidopa (see Fig. 8–12). Both this metabolite and the parent FD compound are thought to be transported across the BBB by the neutral amino acid transport system. Transport also can be altered by other neutral amino acids, as has been demonstrated in man with PET.[120] The effect of carbidopa in FD-PET studies is also a factor currently being evaluated.[87,132]

These problems make it difficult to monitor the behavior of FD in the brain, so that precise quantitative information from studies thus far performed is lacking. Nevertheless, the pattern of change in disease syndromes and alterations in the magnitude of FD uptake and retention in the brain have been of interest, if only in the qualitative sense, in patients with Parkinson's disease and related disorders.[132]

FD uptake in the normal brain is maximal in striatum, as would be expected by its high concentration of presynaptic dopaminergic nerve terminals. FD uptake in the striatum is uniform in young subjects and may have a gradient of decreasing retention from anterior to posterior with aging.[57]

In patients with Parkinson's disease, whole-brain FD uptake, its peak activity, and rate of decline are no different from normal age-matched controls.[119] This finding is consistent with the idea that initial levodopa transport and uptake is not altered in this disorder. The distribution and degree of uptake, however, is different in the Parkinson's disease striatum.[57,60,119,132,136,149] Reduction in FD uptake is maximal in the putamen when compared to the caudate. Patients who have signs and symptoms bilaterally have matched reductions in FD uptake and retention in both striata. Patients with hemi-Parkinson's disease have reductions that are maximal in the striatum contralateral to the side of clinical symptoms. In

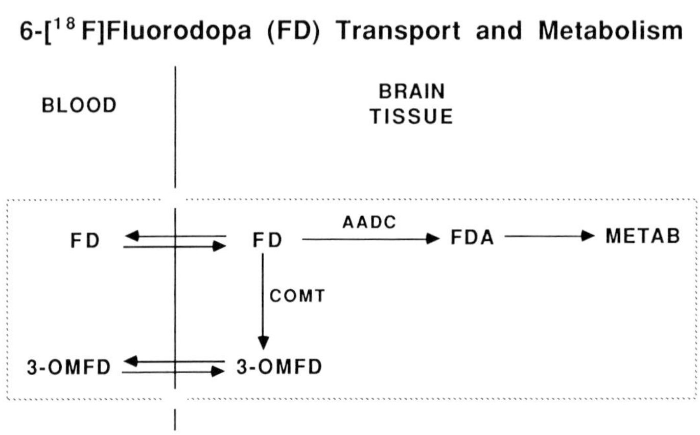

Figure 8–12. Metabolic pathway for the transport and metabolism of ^{18}F-fluorodopa. FD is transported from the blood into brain tissue and can be converted either to fluorodopamine (FDA) by aromatic amino acid decarboxylase (AADC) or to 3-0-methyl fluorodopa (3-OMFD) by catechol-O-methyl transferase (COMT). 3-OMFD is also produced in non–central nervous system tissue and may be transported into brain tissue from the blood, as indicated in the lower line of the diagram. Finally, fluorodopamine is further metabolized in tissue or is stored (not shown) in presynaptic terminals of dopaminergic cells. Tracer kinetic models (see Chap. 3) that describe the neurochemistry of dopamine transport, storage, and metabolism must take into account these various, and at times competing, pathways in order to describe rigorously the behavior of labeled fluorodopa introduced into both healthy subjects and patients.

patients with normal striatal glucose metabolism, FD uptake and retention has been found to be reduced in the patterns noted above when both studies have been performed in the same patients[136] (see Fig. 8–11).

Attempts to correlate FD uptake and retention with signs and symptoms are underway. An initial report[74] indicates that the severity of tremor is correlated with the reduction in FD activity in the putamen, while tremor, rigidity, and bradykinesia are correlated with reductions in caudate FD activity.

Reductions in striatal FD activity have been found in subjects exposed to MPTP who had minimal clinical signs and symptoms of Parkinsonism and normal x-ray CT and MRI studies.[28,137] The magnitude of these reductions was intermediate between findings in patients with idiopathic Parkinson's signs and symptoms and those of age-matched normal controls (Fig. 8–13). Similarly, ipsilateral and unilateral reductions in FD activity have been reported in primates receiving unilateral carotid MPTP administrations.[75]

The lowest levels of FD activity have been observed in patients with advanced disease and "on/off" symptoms.[119,152] These fluorodopa studies probably measured the capacity of the striatum to convert fluorodopa to fluorodopamine and that the final images probably measured stored fluorodopamine. Advanced patients with the "on/off" phenomenon had the most severe restriction to striatal dopaminergic storage and thus the lowest FD activity. If one were to rank, in decreasing order, clinical disease severity and decreasing FD uptake, the following list would result: normal control subjects, subjects exposed to but not symptomatic from MPTP, idiopathic Parkinson's disease patients with a good therapeutic response to levodopa, and advanced Parkinson's disease patients with "on/off" phenomenon.

Thus, reduced FD activity may be a very specific if not pathognomonic marker of Parkinson's disease, in both symptomatic and perhaps "presymptomatic" subjects. The methodological issues about its use and its evaluation in large series of carefully selected patient groups make it an interesting and active area of current PET research. Other agents taken up by dopaminergic terminals will be developed in the future and may provide quantitative data.

Perhaps the most exciting area in Parkinson's research has been in the transplantation of fetal substantia nigra cells into the affected striata of patients. PET with FD has been a key measurement variable demonstrating the functional dopaminergic activity of these grafts.[53a,122a,122b]

NEURORECEPTORS

Three specific dopaminergic systems have been studied with PET in the human and nonhuman primate striatum, both in patients with Parkinson's disease and in MPTP-exposed subjects. The three receptor classes include postsynaptic dopamine D_2 receptors, postsynaptic D_1 receptors, and presynaptic reuptake receptors. Early reports of PET investigations of these systems in patients with Parkinson's disease[56,76,77] and following MPTP exposure[164] are still preliminary and inconsistent in their results, but nonetheless interesting. An increase in postsynaptic dopaminergic receptors has been reported in a single human case of MPTP exposure studied with PET and ^{18}F-spiperone,[164] and in the MPTP primate model studied with PET and ^{11}C-labeled raclopride.[114] Both these compounds are postsynaptic D_2 dopamine receptor ligands. In contrast to these results is a study using ^{76}Br-spiperone in a primate given multiple doses of MPTP and serially studied with PET.[79] In this situation, receptor density estimated with PET was reduced. This reduction was confirmed at postmortem, in addition to evidence that 80 percent of the pars compacta cells had been destroyed. It appears that these early results will help lead the way to determining what role postsynaptic receptors play in parkinsonian symptoms and side effects of treatment. At present, however, too few

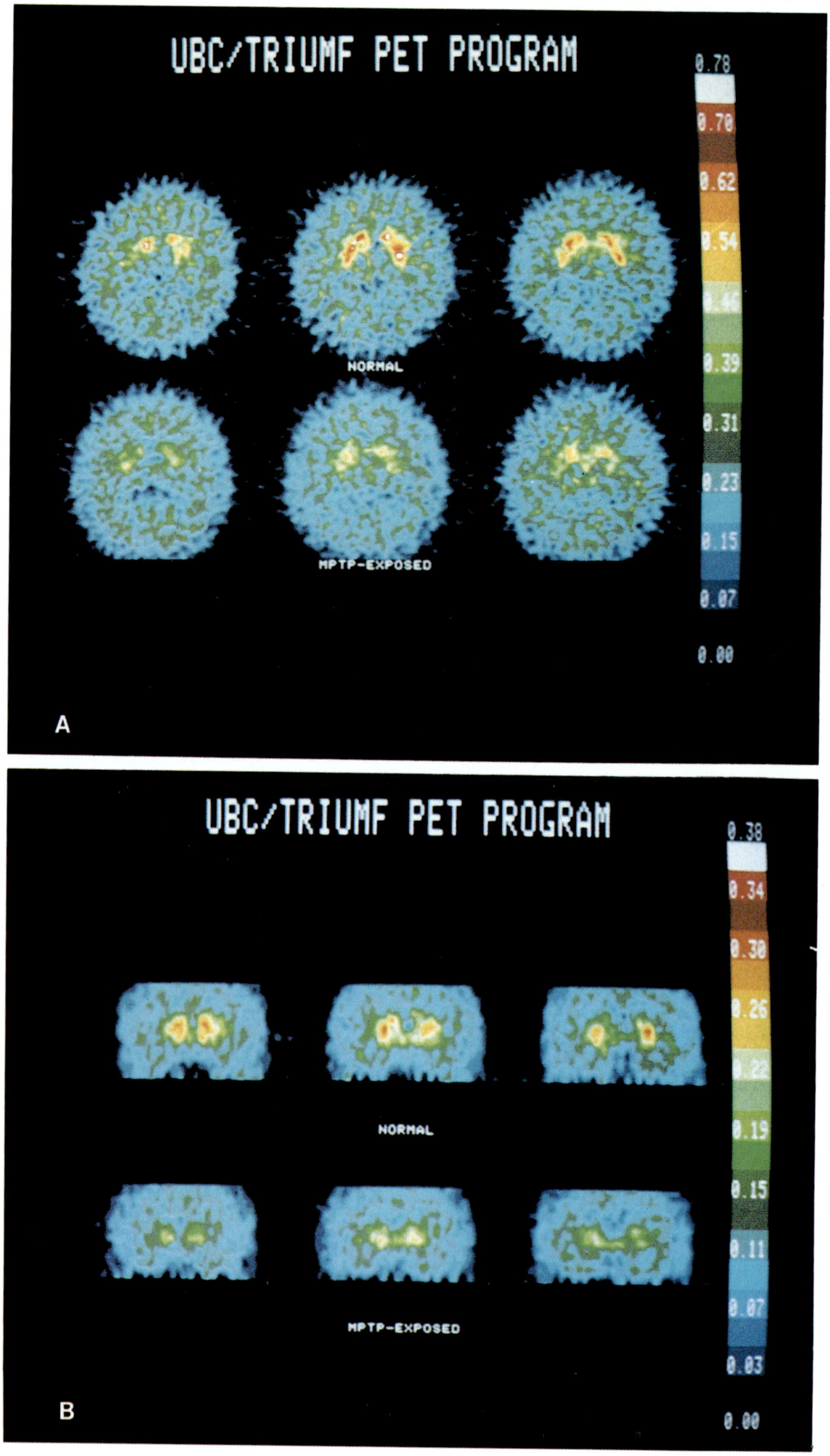

Figure 8–13. Fluorine 18-labeled fluorodopa in human MPTP exposure and normal controls. (*A*) Axial sections from three contiguous levels of a normal subject and an MPTP-exposed subject. (*B*) Coronal sections from the same normal and exposed subject.

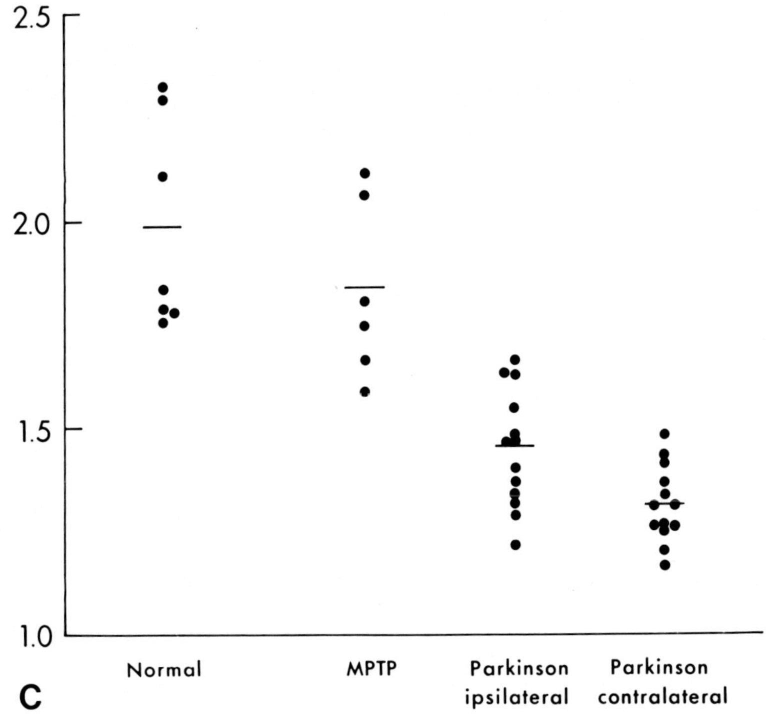

Figure 8–13. *Continued.* (*C*) Putamen/cerebellum activity ratios from normal subjects, MPTP-exposed subjects, and patients with asymmetric PD. Values ipsilateral and contralateral to the most severely affected limbs are indicated for the PD patients. The mean for each group is indicated. (From Martin, et al.,[136] p. 320,322, with permission.)

data are available for conclusions to be drawn.

Equally preliminary but exciting are results of studies that examine presynaptic dopaminergic reuptake receptors with either ^{11}C-labeled nomifensine[114] or postsynaptic D_2 receptors with ^{11}C-labeled SCH-23390 for the assessment of these systems in primates receiving unilateral carotid MPTP. These results parallel those noted above with FD; that is, unilateral reductions in presynaptic receptor site binding were observed ipsilateral to the side of MPTP administration and contralateral to the side of the parkinsonian symptoms in primates[73] (Fig. 8–14).

Future Prospects

Thus, many avenues of investigation are now open in Parkinson's disease and its related syndromes. These include the use of high-field MRI to evaluate selective atrophy and ferromagnetic ion deposition. Similarly, functional studies with PET and SPECT of flow, metabolism and both presynaptic and postsynaptic dopaminergic function are bearing fruit. It is likely that a better understanding of the pathophysiology of Parkinson's disease will emerge from these studies, as well as an understanding of the mechanism of action and side effects induced by treatment with either levodopa or other dopamine agonists.

PROGRESSIVE SUPRANUCLEAR PALSY

Clinical and Pathologic Features

Progressive supranuclear palsy (PSP) was originally described by Steele,

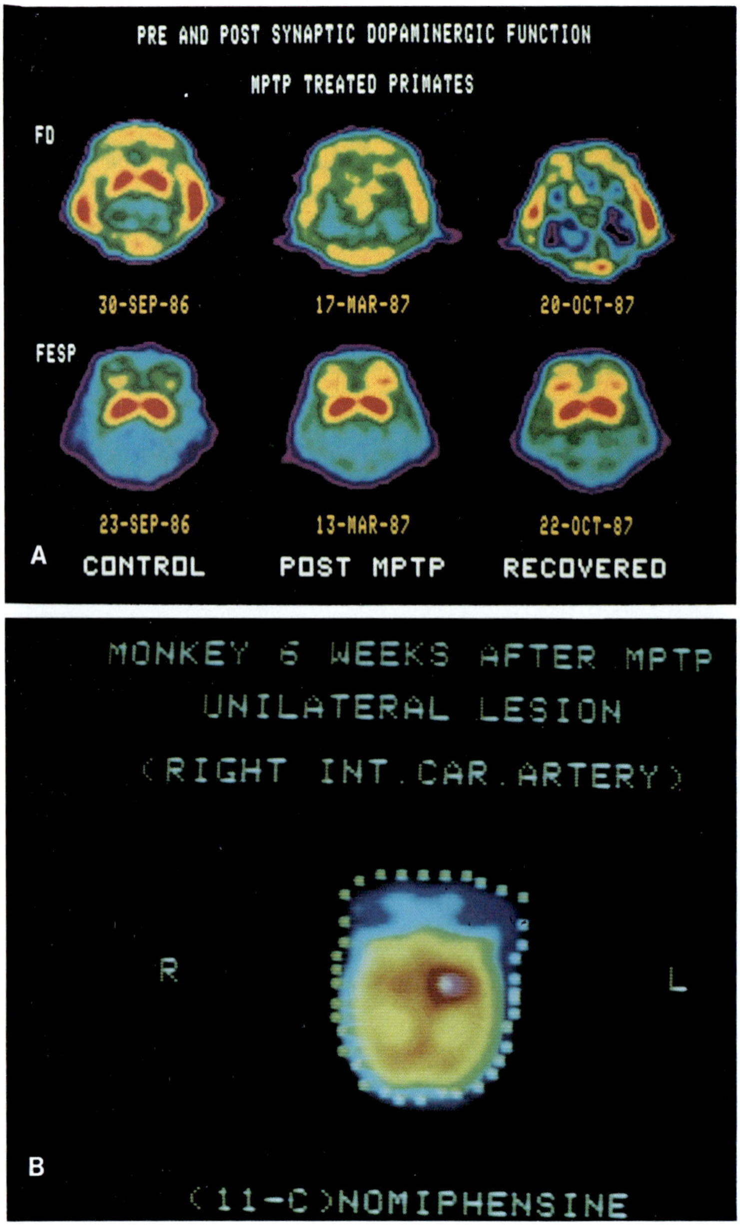

Figure 8–14. Pre- and postsynaptic dopamine function after MPTP exposure in the monkey, as measured with PET and (*A, top row*) ^{18}F-fluoro-L-DOPA (FD), (*A, bottom row*) ^{18}F-fluoroethylspiperone (FESP), and (*B*) ^{11}C-nomifensine. (*A*) Intravenous MPTP. Identical animal studied a total of six times (three times each with FD and FESP). Left column is prior to MPTP, center column is post-MPTP with acute Parkinsonian signs, and right column is after clinical recovery. FD activity in striatum is absent after MPTP and does not appear to return despite clinical recovery. Postsynaptic D_2 receptor binding with FESP appears unaltered by both MPTP exposure and clinical state. (*B*) ^{11}C-nomifensine binds to presynaptic dopamine reuptake receptors and declines in the right striatum of this monkey after ipsilateral carotid MPTP. This finding parallels the decrease in presynaptic FD uptake (*A, top row, center and right images*) after MPTP and supports the fact that MPTP destroys presynaptic nigrostriatal inputs to the caudate and putamen. Such studies demonstrate the ability of PET to examine the in vivo neuropharmacology of a select neurotransmitter system in an animal model of a movement disorder. (Courtesy of Leenders, et al.[114])

Richardson, and Olszewski in 1964.[199] The disorder typically begins in the sixth or seventh decade of life and the duration of illness ranges from 2 to 12 years. Clinical signs include rigidity, which is more prominent axially than in the extremities, bradykinesia, supranuclear gaze palsies, pseudobulbar palsy, and dementia (see also Chapter 9). Some patients manifest cerebellar and corticospinal tract signs as well as personality change. A clinical hallmark of PSP is paralysis of vertical gaze, particularly in the downward direction.

The neuropathologic features of PSP include mild-to-moderate atrophy of the brainstem and, at times, of the cerebellum on gross inspection. Histopathology demonstrates neuronal cell loss, gliosis, granulovascular degeneration and neurofibrillary tangles. These histologic changes are most prominent in the tectum and tegmentum of the midbrain and upper pons. Structures with lesions in this distribution also include the red nuclei, substantia nigra, reticular formation, locus ceruleus, colliculi, and the periaqueductal gray matter. Other structures with histologic changes include the globus pallidus, subthalamic nuclei, vestibular nuclei and the dentate nuclei of the cerebellum.[3,88,89,127]

Gross structural changes of PSP were first demonstrated in living subjects with pneumoencephalography[10] (Fig. 8–15). These findings, obtained with midsagittal optical tomography from pneumoencephalograms, demonstrated severe atrophy of the midbrain

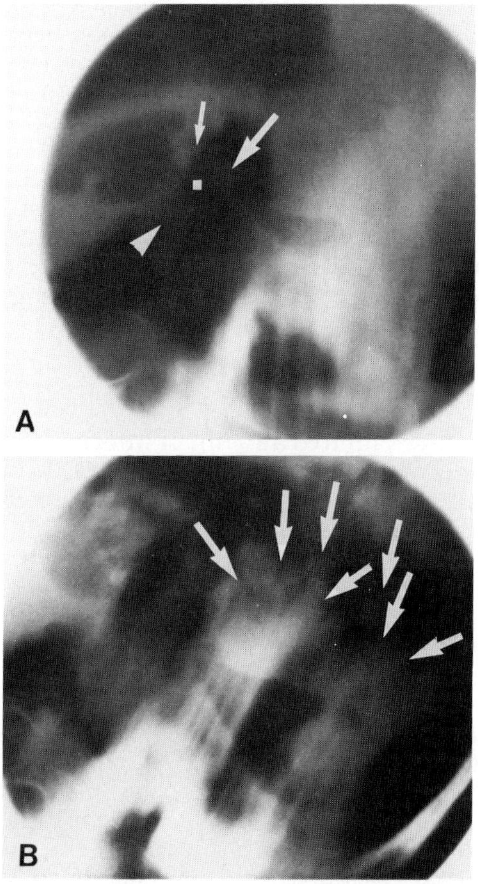

Figure 8–15. Pneumoencephalography (midsagittal tomogram) in progressive supranuclear palsy, demonstrating atrophy of the midbrain and cerebellum. (*A*) Midbrain atrophy. Distance between interpeduncular cistern (*arrowhead*) and aqueduct (*dot*) is reduced secondary to midbrain tegmental atrophy. Superior tectum (*thin arrow*) is more atrophic than the inferior tectum (*thick arrow*). (*B*) Cerebellar atrophy noted as an increase in the size of the cerebellar sulci and reduced folia (*arrowheads*). (Courtesy of J Bentson, UCLA).

tegmentum as well as atrophy of the superior colliculi that was distinct from and in excess of atrophic changes of this brain region in normal subjects, Parkinson's disease patients, or patients with other posterior fossa degenerative diseases.[10]

X-Ray CT

X-ray CT findings in PSP parallel the gross neuropathologic findings seen at postmortem.[5,44,78] These findings consist of atrophy of the midbrain, pons, dentate nuclei of the cerebellum and, to some degree, the cerebellar hemispheres.[5,78] Specifically noted is an increase in aqueductal size, as well as the size of the quadrigeminal, ambient, and crural cisterns.[5] A mild increase in the supratentorial ventricular system is also typically seen.[5,78] Specifically, an increase in the width of the posterior portion of the third ventricle has been reported and is thought to be secondary to posterior thalamic atrophy.[5] Notable on x-ray CT and MRI is thinning of the quadrigeminal plate.[5,96]

The x-ray CT findings in PSP appear to be specific enough that, when combined with the typical clinical picture, they provide reasonable and valuable confirmatory evidence for the diagnosis.

MRI

Only a limited amount of information is presently available about MRI in PSP[44,96] (see Fig. 9–7*A,B*). In studies with low-field-strength magnets, findings parallel those noted above with x-ray CT.[96] This is true with both inversion recovery and spin echo techniques. Of note is a report[44] in which 58 patients with PSP were evaluated with either x-ray CT or low-field-strength MRI. Nineteen (33%) of the patients had either clinical or radiologic evidence consistent with cerebrovascular disease. These patients typically had multiple infarcts identified in the brainstem, internal capsule, basal ganglia, or centrum semiovale. This is in contrast to a smaller fraction (13%) of patients having cerebrovascular findings and pure Parkinson's disease. The authors concluded that some of the cardinal features of PSP may also be caused by cerebral infarction. They felt that multi-infarct patients who mimic the PSP syndrome could be differentiated by the clinical history of prior strokes, the presence of focal dystonia, hemiparesis, and intention tremor. Autopsy verification of such results has yet to be reported.

There are no current reports of MRI studies in PSP patients using high-field-strength magnets. Such studies should prove interesting, since changes in signal intensity between patients with pure Parkinson's disease and multisystem atrophy (described in the section on Parkinson's disease) have been reported.[42]

PET

No studies have been reported to date using SPECT to study PSP; PET, however, has been used in a number of investigations for the determination of cerebral blood flow, glucose and oxygen metabolism, and neurotransmitter/receptor integrity for the dopaminergic system.[6,7,37,53,116,117]

These studies have demonstrated global reductions in cerebral oxygen[116,117] and glucose[53] metabolism that are maximal in the superior frontal cortex[37,53,116,117] (Figs. 8–16*A*, 9–7*C,D*). Cerebral blood flow reductions have also been found in a similar distribution, though of lesser magnitude, in one study.[116] Temporal cortical hypometabolism has also been reported.[116] Patients evaluated with PET typically did not have cerebral cortical atrophy on x-ray CT. While one study demonstrated a correlation between the severity of the metabolic changes and the duration of illness,[116,117] another study reported no correlation between metabolic changes and the severity of signs or symptoms.[37] It is uncertain whether the metabolic changes are a result of

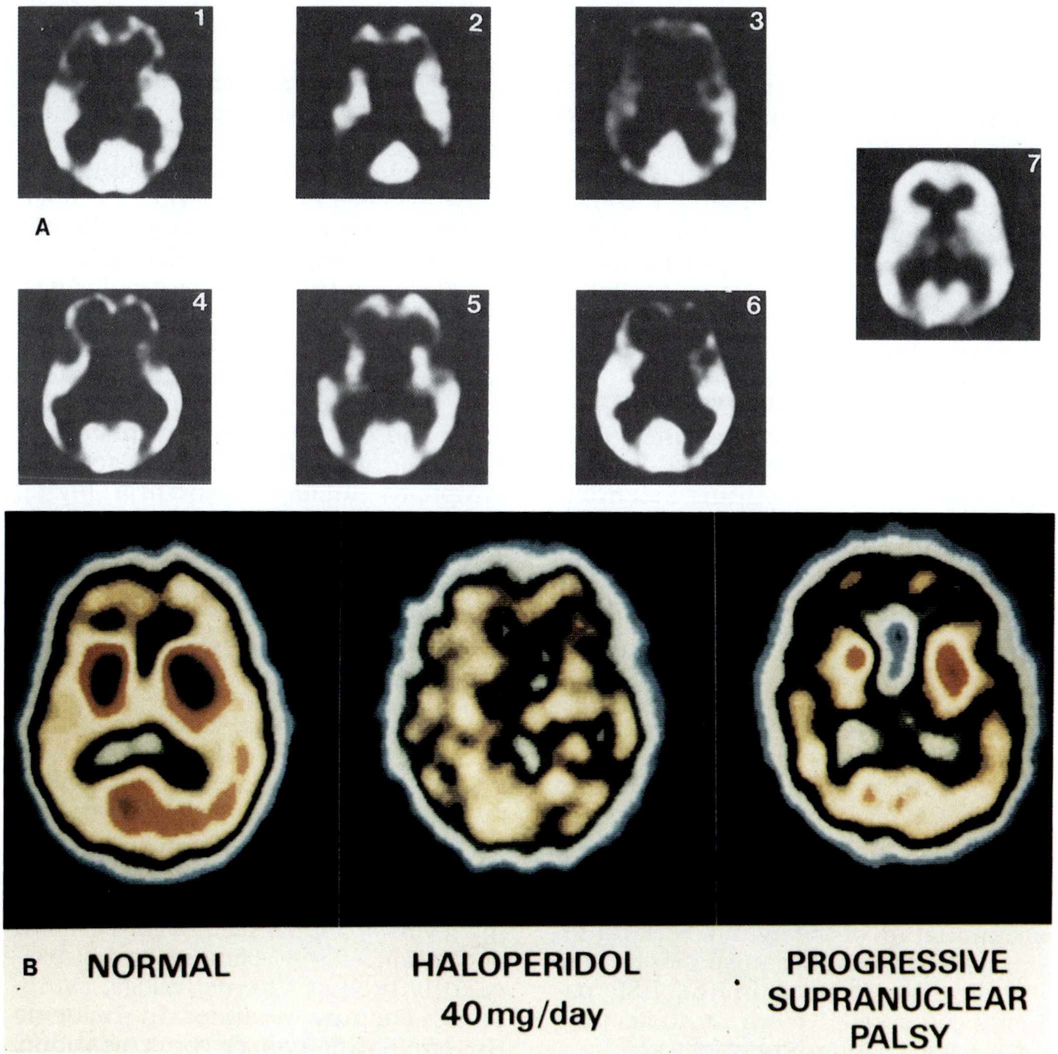

Figure 8–16. PET studies in progressive supranuclear palsy. (*A*) PET images of glucose metabolism at an upper thalamic level in six patients with PSP (*images 1–6*) and one control subject (*image 7*). In these images, anterior is up and left is to the left of the reader; lighter shades of gray indicate higher metabolism. These images are not cross-scaled, so differences in mean metabolic rate among patients are not apparent; this mode of display, however, allows visual assessment of the regional metabolic pattern. Compared with image 7, which is normal, every patient with PSP has an altered metabolic pattern, with marked bifrontal hypometabolism; posterior (occipital) regions appear relatively hypermetabolic. (From D'Antona, et al,[37] p. 789, with permission.) (*B*) Illustrative PET images at the level of the basal ganglia showing the distribution of ^{76}Br-bromospiperone 4.5 hours after intravenous injection in (*left*) a normal control, (*center*) a schizophrenic patient treated with large oral doses of neuroleptics (haloperidol 40 mg/day, and (*right*) a patient with progressive supranuclear palsy. The images are normalized to the mean radioactivity concentration present in the cerebellum in each case. Increasing radioactive concentrations relative to cerebellum range from blue (low levels) to brown (high levels) across a blue-green-yellow-red-brown color scale. High radioactive concentration can be seen in the striatum of the control subject, as a result of specific binding of ^{76}Br-bromospiperone to dopamine (D_2) receptors. In the patient (*center*) loaded with therapeutic amounts of unlabeled neuroleptics, the featureless image indicates the striatal D_2 receptors were occupied and, hence, no specific binding of ^{76}Br-bromospiperone could be obtained. In the patient (*right*) with progressive supranuclear palsy, decreased accumulation of ^{76}Br-bromospiperone in striatum is readily apparent, indicating partial loss of dopamine receptors (X-ray CT of this patient did not show significant ventricular enlargement). (From Baron, et al.,[6] p. 134, with permission.)

primary neuronal loss in these cortical zones or a product of disconnection from subcortical regions.[37] Changes in the nucleus basalis have been reported in PSP, whereas nucleus basalis lesions are not a component of Parkinson's or Huntington's disease, in which frontal cortical metabolism is either minimally changed or not affected in mildly to moderately symptomatic patients. Thus, the nucleus basalis lesions of PSP may be an important part of the cortical abnormalities in this disorder.

The integrity of dopaminergic systems in PSP has been examined with PET. In a single study using ^{18}F-labeled levodopa, accumulation and retention of the compound in the striatum (referenced to the cortex) was found to be significantly reduced.[116,117] This is in keeping with the concept that nigrostriatal projection pathways are damaged in this syndrome. In a different set of studies,[6,7] ^{76}Br-labeled bromospiperone was used as an index of striatal postsynaptic D_2 receptor integrity (see Fig. 8–16*B*). In seven PSP patients who were relatively unresponsive to levodopa or other dopamine agonists, this compound was used to determine striatal-to-cerebellar ratios of uptake and accumulation of the ligand. Striatal retention of labeled bromospiperone was significantly reduced in the PSP patients compared to controls, in keeping with prior postmortem studies.[175]

This preliminary evidence would support a presynaptic dopaminergic lesion as well as a postsynaptic dopaminergic D_2-receptor abnormality in the striatum. Such evidence is in keeping with current theories that attempt to explain the lack of responsiveness of PSP patients to dopamine agonist compounds. The binding of spiperone and its analogs in the striatum may be dopamine agonist–dependent in vivo.[33] Thus, presynaptic pathway lesions may have effects previously not considered or observed on the functional postsynaptic D_2 receptors in the striatum, measured in either animal models of nigrostriatal pathology or in postmortem examinations of patients with naturally occurring lesions.

WILSON'S DISEASE

Clinical and Pathologic Features

Hepatolenticular degeneration (Wilson's disease) is an inherited, autosomal recessive, degenerative disorder involving abnormal copper deposition in the liver and the brain, particularly in the lenticular nuclei. On initial presentation, one third of patients have hepatic-related symptoms. Many of those who initially present with neurologic signs and symptoms have a history of earlier attacks of jaundice. Signs and symptoms include dysarthria (97%), dystonia (65%), difficulties with rapid alternating movements (58%), rigidity (52%), gait disturbance (42%), and flapping tremor of the extremities (arms greater than legs, 32%).[198] Patients also have typical Kayser-Fleischer corneal rings.

While the principal biochemical abnormality in Wilson's disease has yet to be determined, low serum ceruloplasmin, high serum copper levels, and increased urinary amino-acid and copper excretion are typical of untreated patients. It is presumed that high circulating levels of copper lead to the cerebral deposition of this element and subsequently produce the neurologic symptoms. Therapy is aimed at reducing the circulating copper concentrations, leading to a negative copper balance.[198] Such treatment may prevent symptoms in individuals at risk, and may reverse symptoms in patients with established clinical neurologic dysfunction.

Neuropathologically, the lenticular nuclei bear the brunt of changes associated with Wilson's disease. In addition to this site, damage occurs in the red nuclei, dentate nuclei, brainstem, frontal cortex, and caudate nuclei. The pathologic changes range from gross cavitary lesions to microscopic focal degeneration most typically found in the middle one third of the putamen, frequently spreading anteriorly and, at times, including the caudate. Cerebral cortical changes are frequently seen in the frontal lobe.[198] Thus, Wilson's disease is a neurodegenerative disorder with progressive symptoms. The primary site of abnormality is the lenticular nuclei.

Most studies using neuroimaging methods to evaluate patients with Wilson's disease have been conducted with the patients on medical therapy. The clinical differential diagnosis of Wilson's disease includes many of the entities described in the section for Huntington's disease; the most common psychiatric misdiagnoses are depression, personality disorder, schizophrenia, and panic attacks.[198] The disorder may be mistaken for other neurologic diseases, particularly other movement disorders involving the basal ganglia, or multiple sclerosis. The hepatic symptoms of Wilson's disease may be misidentified as cirrhosis or hepatitis.[198]

X-Ray CT

Atrophic changes in the lenticular nuclei and striata were reported in the 1930s[66] from pneumoencephalography studies. These studies demonstrated an increased size of the anterior horns of the lateral ventricles in a bilaterally symmetric fashion.[66] X-ray CT gave a much more complete picture of the distributed sites of lesions found in Wilson's disease, and these results correlated more closely with the neurologic findings.*

In patients with symptomatic Wilson's disease, x-ray CT findings parallel neuropathologic abnormalities. Most patients with central nervous system disease have abnormal x-ray CT studies,[80] with normal studies reported only rarely ($\leq 5\%$).[213] Areas of low attenuation occur in regions of brain degeneration. These can take the form of diffuse attenuation reductions involving basal ganglia, thalamus, or dentate nuclei,[95,172,188,213] or bilateral slit-like low densities typically found in the putamen.[172,173] Most authors report generalized atrophy of the brain involving the lenticular nuclei, caudate nuclei, cerebral cortex, brainstem, and cerebellum.[80,95,109,150,172,213] Focal changes occur not only in the basal ganglia, but also in the thalamus and internal capsule.[172,188] Enhancement is not seen following the administration of iodinated contrast material.

Increases in ventricular size as well as subcortical white matter lesions[172,188,213] are typically reported in Wilson's disease.[95,213] The subcortical white matter lesions most typically are seen in the frontal lobe.[213]

The x-ray CT finding of bilateral focal lenticular lesions can be seen with both degenerative and toxic states. As well as in Wilson's disease,[127,198] focal low-attenuation lesions of the putamen can be seen in association with dystonia in Leigh's disease, stroke, and tumor. They also may follow exposure to carbon monoxide or methanol,[31a] cerebral hypoxia (secondary to narcotic overdoses or birth injury), or cerebral infarction in sickle cell disease.[95,213]

Attempts have been made to correlate the clinical signs and symptoms of Wilson's disease with the site and magnitude of x-ray CT lesions. The results are inconsistent; some authors find no correlations,[80] while others find a high correlation.[95] Similarly, some authors find no relationship between the findings with imaging and the medical treatment of Wilson's disease with copper chelating agents,[80] while others find dramatic improvements with resolution of focal changes and atrophy.[213] These latter authors[213] indicate that this increase in neuronal tissue volume is unlikely to be secondary to neuronal regeneration but probably reflects either gliosis or regrowth of the neuropil.[213] One case report demonstrates substantial improvement in the x-ray CT appearance of a patient's brain following liver transplantation.[173] Most authors agree that x-ray CT imaging in Wilson's disease does not provide a direct prognostic index predicting response to medical therapy.[213] All patients should have the opportunity to be treated medically, irrespective of the severity of the lesions seen by x-ray CT.

*References 2,80,95,109,150,172,173,188, 213.

Finally, patients with purely hepatic symptoms of Wilson's disease have been studied with cranial x-ray CT. Again, inconsistencies exist. Some investigators report that all such patients have normal cerebral anatomy,[95,150] while others report one or more lesions despite the absence of clinical signs and symptoms of neurologic disease.[213]

MRI

Because focal and distributed lesions are known from neuropathologic studies to occur in Wilson's disease, MR scanning was applied to this disorder soon after it became available.* Evidence that ferromagnetic element deposition in the brain would result in magnetic susceptibility changes and a loss of signal intensity on T_2-weighted images with high-strength magnetic fields was another motivation to evaluate copper deposition in brains of patients with Wilson's disease.[176] In general, abnormalities seen with high-field-strength magnets consist of signal loss on T_2-weighted images, seen most prominently in the putamen[38] but also in the caudate nucleus and globus pallidus.[38,198] Decreases in signal intensity can be seen in the lenticular, dentate, and red nuclei.

Studies with low-field-strength magnets demonstrate decreases in signal intensity on T_1-weighted images in the lenticular nuclei[38,42] as well as in the caudate nucleus and thalamus. These images also demonstrate cerebral atrophy in advanced cases. Low-field-strength T_2 images are notable for increased signal intensity in the lenticular nuclei,[2,27,42,113,124,198] caudate nucleus,[2,27,124,198] thalamus, brainstem and dentate nuclei.[2,113,198] White matter lesions of the centrum semiovale have been reported.[2,38]

The great majority of patients with neurologic signs and symptoms of Wilson's disease who have been studied with MRI have had abnormalities on their examinations.[198] Patients with the purely hepatic form of this disorder and no neurologic signs and symptoms may also have MRI abnormalities.[113,198] As with other imaging techniques, attempts have been made to correlate neurologic signs and symptoms with lesions seen with MRI.[2,198] These investigations have demonstrated a reasonable but imperfect correlation. In one such study,[198] dystonia was correlated with lesions in the putamen, while dysarthria was related to lesions in both the putamen and caudate nuclei. In addition, these authors reported a single patient with severe tremor and dysmetria who had cerebellar dentate nuclei lesions on MRI.[198] In patients with no evidence of neurologic, hepatic, or ocular signs of Wilson's disease,[198] MRI has been normal.

Finally, the relationship of therapy with clinical outcome has been studied with MRI in a single report.[22] These authors indicated that there was transient worsening of neurologic signs and symptoms following the initiation of D-penicillamine treatment, possibly due to the mobilization of large hepatic copper stores. During this period, new cerebral lesions were detected by MRI.[22] To date, no systematic study of correlations between MRI findings and either prognosis or response to clinical or surgical (liver transplantation) therapies has been conducted.

PET and SPECT

To date there are no SPECT studies in patients with Wilson's disease. Only one PET study has been performed, in which FDG was used to determine glucose metabolism[82] (Fig. 8–17). In this single report of four patients,[82] of whom three were on medical therapy and one had only minimal (unilateral upper extremity intention tremor) signs, diffuse reductions in glucose metabolism were noted. These changes were seen in the cerebral hemispheres, particularly frontal and parietal cortex, caudate and lenticular nuclei, and frontal and parietal white matter. In the entire group, the

*References 2,22,27,38,42,113,123,124,176, 198.

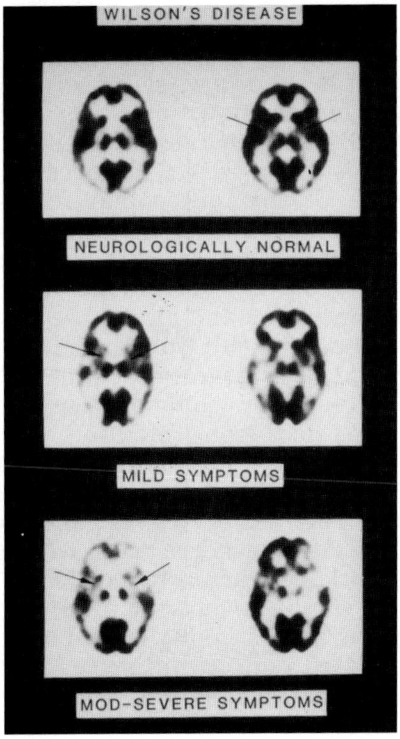

Figure 8–17. PET-FDG studies in Wilson's disease. All these patients have diagnosed Wilson's disease. The top-image pair (images on left are 8 mm above those on right) shows mild reductions in glucose metabolism of the lenticular nuclei (*arrows*), even though the individual was neurologically asymptomatic. The center and bottom image sets are from neurologically affected patients. The degree of lenticular hypometabolism appears to parallel the severity of symptoms. In all subjects, caudate metabolism is better preserved than in patients with Huntington's disease (see Figs. 8–4 to 8–6). The patient at the bottom also has hypometabolic areas involving the right thalamus, temporal, and frontal cortices. (From Hawkins, et al.,[82] p. 1708, with permission.)

thalamus appeared to be metabolically spared and no structural abnormality of that region was seen by x-ray CT.[82] The metabolic abnormalities were consistently symmetric. The zone of maximal hypometabolism occurred in the lenticular nuclei. This is in contrast to patients with Huntington's disease, in whom the initial and maximal changes are seen in the caudate nuclei.[107,140] The one patient with minimal neurologic symptoms who was studied had higher metabolic values than the three more symptomatic patients.[82] It remains to be determined to what degree clinical symptoms, prognosis, detection of at-risk individuals, and monitoring of therapy can be evaluated with PET or SPECT. As noted in other neurologic diseases, however, the PET findings demonstrated abnormalities in a wider range and greater number of structures than did structural imaging studies, either as performed in individual patients[82] or as reported in the literature.

DYSTONIA

Clinical and Pathologic Features

The dystonias represent a heterogeneous collection of neurologic movement disorders. Dystonia itself is actually a sign that can be a component of an evolving disease process and of a variety of specific neurologic disorders (e.g., Parkinson's disease, Huntington's disease, and Hallervorden-Spatz disease). In the temporal sense, dystonia is the slowest (i.e., longest duration) of the involuntary movements and is often manifested by static fixed postures. Typically, the patient experiences awkward postures of a given part of the body. These may be focal, involving the upper extremity (e.g., writer's cramp), neck (torticollis), larynx (spastic dysphonia), or face (Meige's syndrome). The distribution of dystonia may be more extensive, including half the body (hemidystonia), or it may be generalized.

Dystonia may be inherited (e.g., dystonia musculorum deformans) or occur sporadically. Similarly, dystonic symptoms may occur on an idiopathic basis or may be secondary to specific lesions of the nervous system such as trauma[21,147] or infarction.[55] When dystonias are secondary to structural lesions, the sites of these lesions are typically in the lenticular nuclei. Hornykiewicz and colleagues have demonstrated postmortem abnormalities of adrenergic activity in the basal ganglia.[87a] This report represents one of the few examples of a neuropathologic localization, neurotransmitter deficiency, or other biochemical abnormality for any of the dystonias despite the obvious and often incapacitating symptoms and signs demonstrated by these patients.

X-Ray CT

Although x-ray CT is normal in idiopathic dystonic syndromes, dystonia caused by stroke[55,69] or trauma[21,147] can be seen in association with either low attenuation[55,69] or calcification[21,147] of the putamen[55,69] or caudate nuclei.[21,147] In addition, thalamic atrophy has been reported.[69] In patients with unilateral secondary dystonias, structural lesions are located in the striatum contralateral to the affected limbs.[21,26,55,69,147] If the dystonic symptoms are bilateral, then the structural lesions are bilateral as well,[55] such as in conditions that reduce substrate availability to the brain in general (e.g., hypoxia, hypoperfusion, or carbon monoxide intoxication), resulting in bilateral lenticular nucleus low-attenuation regions. In patients with dystonia secondary to Wilson's disease or Leigh's disease (subacute necrotizing encephalomyelopathy), x-ray CT usually demonstrates lesions of the putamen.[127]

It should be emphasized, however, that the identification of a structural lesion on x-ray CT is the exception rather than the rule in dystonia. Patients with idiopathic generalized or focal dystonia typically have no abnormalities on x-ray CT studies.

MRI

In the dystonias caused by gross structural brain lesions, MRI findings parallel those described above for x-ray CT.[26,55] Typical findings include decreased signal intensity for lenticular structures on T_1-weighted images and increased signal intensity on T_2-weighted images, typified by that seen in the lenticular nuclei following hypoxia.[42] In the primary and idiopathic dystonias (e.g., spastic dysphonia, Meige's syndrome, torticollis, and writer's cramp) no MRI abnormalities have yet been defined.[42]

The inherited, predominantly childhood disorder known as Hallervorden-Spatz disease includes dystonic postures among its typical features. Other features of this autosomal recessive disorder include rigidity, spasticity and expressionless facies. Iron-containing pigments have been found in and around neurons and glia of the medial globus pallidus.[41,42] Studies of iron uptake and disappearance using a narrow-field-of-view collimator and ^{59}Fe demonstrated iron retention in the basal ganglia.[207] With high-field MRI and T_2-weighted images, decreased signal intensity has been found bilaterally in the globus pallidus, red nuclei, and substantia nigra[42] (Fig. 8–18). This loss of signal is thought to be due to magnetic susceptibility effects induced by elevated concentrations of iron in these structures.

As noted earlier, dystonia is a typical sign in Wilson's disease. MRI abnormalities include cavitation of the striatum with increased signal intensity on T_2-weighted images and decreased signal intensity on T_1-weighted images.[42] Severity of dystonia has been correlated with the presence of lesions detected by MRI in the putamen of patients with Wilson's disease.[198]

PET

Since no SPECT studies of dystonia have been reported, this discussion will be limited to results obtained with PET. Studies of cerebral metabolism in patients with primary or secondary hemidystonias have demonstrated decreased metabolic rates, although the sites and magnitudes of these changes have been variable.* When found, these changes have been either in sensorimotor cortex[91] or in the striatum† contralateral to the symptomatic side of the

*References 91,162,204; personal and unpublished observations.

†References 162,204; personal and unpublished observations.

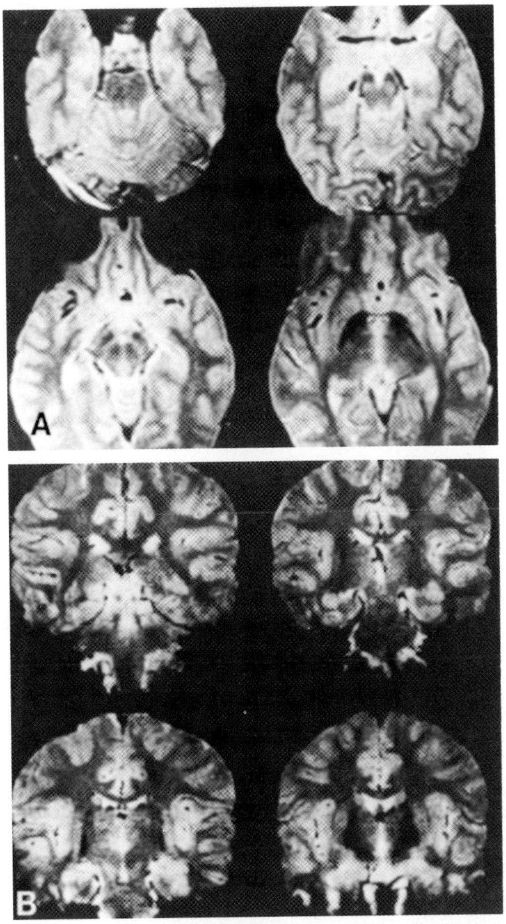

Figure 8–18. Hallervorden-Spatz disease. A 10-year-old female with typical clinical presentation and deteriorating neurologic status. (*A*) T_2-weighted spin echo (TR 2500, TE 80) axial MR images. Markedly prominent hypointensity in the globus pallidus, with less prominence in the red nucleus and pars reticulata of the substantia nigra. Although these are sites of normal iron localization in adults, the degree of hypointensity is severely abnormal for a 10-year-old and is consistent with the distinctive iron pigmentation seen pathologically in this disorder. (*B*) T_2-weighted gradient echo (TR 610, TE 40, flip angle 20°) coronal MR images. Excellent visualization of the abnormal hypointensity in the globus pallidus and medial putamen due to iron pigmentation. This abnormality in iron concentration is better seen on the gradient echo images due to their superb sensitivity to ferritin (i.e., magnetic susceptibility effects). (From Drayer, et al.,[42] p. 26, with permission.)

body. These patients typically have had normal gross anatomic brain structure as determined by x-ray CT or angiography.

A single patient with hand and foot dystonia secondary to cerebral infarction of the contralateral putamen that was visible on x-ray CT and MRI was evaluated with PET using FD.[55] Decreased retention of FD in the putamen contralateral to the affected limbs was observed. The authors felt that these findings demonstrated an alteration in putamenal function with loss of normal control between the striatum and the globus pallidus. They felt that the latter structure was activated by the subthalamus in situations where putamenal input was disrupted.[55]

The idiopathic focal dystonia of head and neck musculature known as torticollis has been studied with PET to measure local glucose metabolism.[203,204] In 16 such patients, metabolic rates were normal. Compared with normal control subjects who voluntarily assumed the dystonic neck posture, however, alterations in glucose metabolic correlations between the basal ganglia and thalamus were found (i.e., lack of significant correlations between the lenticular nuclei or caudate and the thalamus).[203,204]

To date, neuroimaging studies of patients with dystonic symptoms have produced limited insights into the pathophysiology of these disorders. The most consistent finding across both functional and structural imaging techniques is the observation that abnormalities in lenticular nuclear structures are associated with dystonic postures of the contralateral body. Neurotransmitter-specific agents (e.g., cholinergic and adrenergic) may prove more fruitful in elucidating the functional alterations of these heterogeneous disorders.

TARDIVE DYSKINESIA

Tardive dyskinesia is a syndrome typified by, but not limited to, oro-buccal-lingual dyskinesa, dystonia, and facial grimacing. It typically occurs in patients who have been exposed to neuroleptic medication, but can occur in the absence of previous use of these classes of drugs. Most patients have the underlying diagnosis of schizophrenia, which confounds the ability to separate findings related specifically to the movement disorder. Various theories have been proposed to explain these abnormal movements but none have been proved.

There is reasonable consensus that in such patients the brain is devoid of gross structural abnormalities when examined after death.[32] This finding has been substantiated by x-ray CT studies, which show no focal abnormalities.[4,18,20,90] Increased ventricular size occasionally has been noted,[4] but this may be a confounding finding, since a fraction of schizophrenic patients without tardive dyskinesia also have increased ventricular size. Thus, this finding may not be specifically related to tardive dyskinesia.

Only a single MRI study[12] has thus far been reported in medicated schizophrenic patients with and without tardive dyskinesia. This evaluation utilized a low-field-strength magnet and T_1-weighted images. No difference was found between patients and controls, but a difference was found between schizophrenics with and without tardive dyskinesia. The latter group had an increased T_1 duration in the basal ganglia.[12] The significance of this finding awaits confirmation and elaboration.

No SPECT studies have been performed in patients with tardive dyskinesia. PET has been used to examine this syndrome with measures of both glucose metabolism[154,155] and postsynaptic D_2 dopamine receptor binding.[30] In a study of medicated schizophrenic male patients with tardive dyskinesia, glucose metabolic rate was increased in the globus pallidus, precentral motor cortex, thalamus, and cerebellar cortex bilaterally[154,155] (Fig. 8–19). Striatal metabolic rates were normal. There was no correlation between the in-

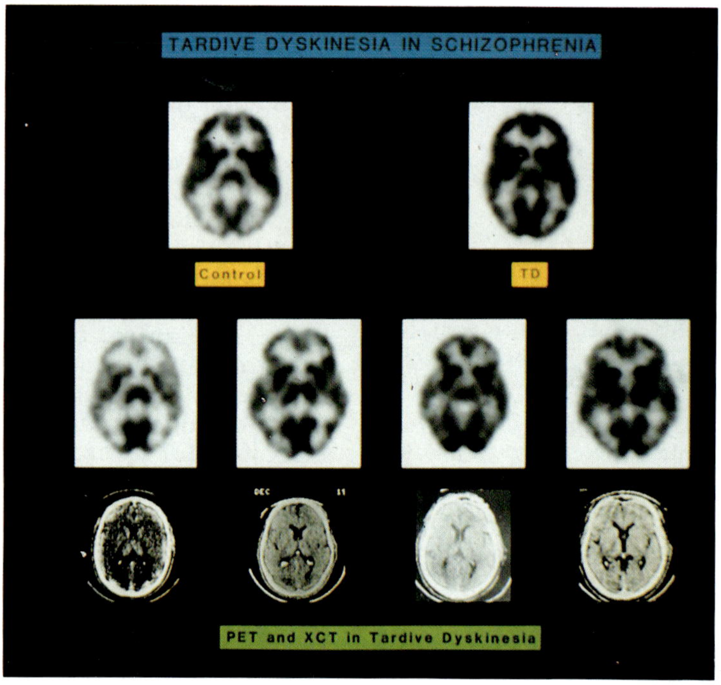

Figure 8–19. Glucose metabolism determined with PET in schizophrenic patients with tardive dyskinesia (TD) compared to control subjects and to schizophrenic patients without tardive dyskinesia. Those with TD have relative increases in glucose metabolism of the lenticular nuclei. Images in the top row are of a (*left*) normal control and a (*right*) TD patient. The center row shows the range of lenticular hypermetabolism seen in TD; the bottom row shows the normal x-ray CT studies of the subjects whose PET scans are shown in the middle row. (Courtesy of JJ Pahl, UCLA School of Medicine.)

creased metabolic rate in the structures noted above and the duration or severity of the symptoms of tardive dyskinesia.[154,155] This finding demonstrates that choreiform movements can occur with metabolic rates that are elevated in the lenticular nuclei (as in tardive dyskinesia[154,155]), decreased in the striatum (as has been seen in Huntington's disease,[84,107,140,222] Lesch-Nyhan syndrome,[156] chorea-acanthyocytosis,[166] or benign hereditary chorea,[134]) or normal in basal ganglia structures (e.g., chorea in systemic lupus erythematosus,[72] Parkinson's disease patients with chorea from excess therapeutic levodopa) (see Table 8–1).

A single study[30] has been published showing changes in striatal D_2 dopamine receptor binding examined with PET and ^{76}Br-labeled spiperone. Seven patients with tardive dyskinesia and either behavioral disorder (n = 1) or atypical depressions (n = 6) were evaluated. Patients who were studied at least 9 days after neuroleptics were discontinued were compared with age-matched controls. Both groups were evaluated for the ratio of concentrations of the tracer in the striatum to that in the cerebellum at $4\frac{1}{2}$ hours after administration of the compound.[30] The results were identical for controls and the tardive dyskinesia patients. These results do not support the hypothesis that tardive dyskinesia is caused by an excess number of postsynaptic D_2 receptor sites. The confounding effects of the associated psychiatric syndromes and the brief medication withdrawal, however, raise questions that await further study.

It seems likely that the availability of compounds to evaluate both presynaptic dopamine neurotransmission (e.g., fluorodopa[59,61] or ^{11}C-labeled SCH-23390 for presynaptic dopamine D_1 receptors[50]) and postsynaptic D_2 receptors[50,51] will allow a more thorough evaluation of the presynaptic and postsynaptic balance in the dopaminergic system in patients with tardive dyskinesia.

MISCELLANEOUS DISORDERS

The preceding discussion of movement disorders has focused on those with the most significant human data available from both structural and functional imaging techniques. Isolated reports of patients having even more limited neuroimaging evaluations do not provide enough information for discussion at this time. These other movement disorders include palatal myoclonus,[195] hemiballismus,[15,46,177] essential tremor,[43] and Gilles de la Tourette's syndrome.[192]

CONCLUSION

Future studies of movement disorders with neuroimaging techniques will have great advantages over those performed to date. A comprehensive evaluation of specific diseases or movement disorder syndromes in clinically homogeneous patients can now be performed using a battery of structural and functional neuroimaging approaches. The exquisite anatomic spatial resolution of MRI can be combined with the neuropharmacologic and physiologic measurements available through PET and, perhaps, SPECT. Such studies may identify not only the site of abnormalities but also their biochemical defects. High-field-strength MRI can be used to localize abnormally high concentrations of ferromagnetic ions in brain structures that may be part of the pathophysiologic process in a number of disorders (e.g., Wilson's disease, Parkinson's disease, Hallervorden-Spatz disease) (Table 8–2). PET has been and will continue to be used to look at presynaptic and postsynaptic dopaminergic function in a variety of movement disorders that have had this neurotransmitter system implicated in their pathophysiology.

Modern neuroimaging techniques provide the first opportunity to evaluate with high spatial resolution both the structure and function of the central

Table 8–2 HIGH-FIELD-STRENGTH MRI OF BRAIN IRON IN PATIENTS WITH MOVEMENT DISORDERS

		Thalamus	*Striatum*	*Substantia Nigra, Pars Compacta*	*Globus Pallidus*	*Substantia Nigra Reticulata*	*Dentate*	*Red N.*
Normal	<10 yr	1	1	1	1–2	1	1	1
	15–65 yr	1	2	1	3	3	3	3
	>70 yr	1	3	1	3	3	3	3
Huntington's disease		1	1–4	1	3	3	3	3
Parkinson's disease	Drug-responsive	1	2–3	1–3	3	3	3	3
	Drug-unresponsive	1	4	3	3–4	3–4	3	3
	PD+, Nigro Str degen, OPCA, Shy-Drager	1	5	3	3–4	3–4	3	3
Dystonias	Torticollis, inherited	1	2	1	3	3	3	3
	Anoxia, Kerns Sayre, Wilson's	1	1	1	1–3	3	1–3	3
Hallervorden-Spatz		1	3	?1	5	4	3	4

T_2-weighted imaging of movement disorders with high-magnetic-field (1.5 T) MRI (TR 2500, TE 80). Values given in range of 1 (increased signal) to 5 (decreased signal). A value of 3 is considered normal. Increasing concentrations of ferromagnetic material decreases signal because of magnetic susceptibility effects. Brain iron is low in children. (Adapted from Drayer, et al[40–42] with permission.)

nervous system in patients with movement disorders. This can lead to a structurally and pathophysiologically based differential diagnosis of a given sign across movement disorders. An example of this would be chorea (see Table 8–1). Similarly, this approach can be applied to dystonia and bradykinesia. In addition, since all current neuroimaging approaches can be used both in the human condition and in animal models of these disorders, they provide the best opportunity to identify and validate animal models of these syndromes.

Neuroimaging techniques have been and will be used not only to categorize patients but also to follow the effects of therapy, whether routine therapy such as the use of levodopa in patients with Parkinson's disease (as evaluated with fluorodopa and PET), or experimental therapies such as might be applied in Huntington's disease.

Structural and functional neuroimaging techniques will be used to confirm diagnoses. For example, in patients with adult-onset chorea who have unknown family histories and possible past exposure to neuroleptics, PET could be used to differentiate Huntington's disease from tardive dyskinesia, the former having striatal hypometabolism and the latter having lenticular hypermetabolism. In a similar fashion, Parkinson's disease may be separated from its more complex and associated syndromes through the use of high-field MRI imaging or PET studies with levodopa and postsynaptic dopamine-binding compounds.

Measurements of metabolism and other physiologic processes can be used to monitor pathophysiologic processes as they unfold in movement disorders, particularly in the inherited ones that have an insidious course and complex symptomatology (e.g., Huntington's disease). When performed on presymptomatic individuals, such information, in and of itself or in combination with genetic data available from molecular biological approaches, can be used to predict which individuals carry the defective gene.

An overwhelming amount of information has been reported about movement disorders in the last decade, in contrast to the paucity of information that structural imaging techniques provided about these complex syndromes in the previous seven decades. It is anticipated that the hitherto unavailable structural and functional neuroimaging approaches to the movement disorders will increase this rapid rise in information about abnormal sites and pathophysiology. In the future, these approaches will be used to categorize patients into subgroups that are not identifiable on clinical grounds, and to expand the fund of information available to select both and monitor the medical and surgical therapy of the movement disorders.

ACKNOWLEDGMENTS

The author wishes to acknowledge the generous participation of all investigators who shared their results and illustrations. In addition, special thanks to Maureen Chang and Maggie Marquez in the preparation of the manuscript and to Lee Griswold for the preparation of illustrative materials. This work was supported in part by DOE cooperative agreement #DE-FC03-87ER60615, NIMH grant R01-MH-37916, NIH grants R01-6M-248388 and P01-NS-15654, and a grant from the Hereditary Disease Foundation.

REFERENCES

1. Adams, JH, Corsellis, JAN, and Duchen, LW (eds): Neuropathology. John Wiley & Sons, New York, 1984.
2. Aisen, AM, Martel, W, Gabrielsen, TO, Glazer, GM, Brewer, G, Young, AB, and Hill, G: Wilson disease of the brain: MR imaging. Radiology 157:137–141, 1985.
3. Albert, ML, Feldman, RG, and Willis, AL: The "subcortical dementia" of progressive supranuclear palsy. J Neurol Neurosurg Psychiatr 37:121–130, 1974.

4. Albus, M, Naber, D, Muller-Spahn, F, Douillet, P, Reinertshofer, T, and Ackenheil, M: Tardive dyskinesia: Relation to computer-tomographic, endocrine, and psychological variables. Biol Psych 20:1082–1089, 1985.
5. Ambrosetto, P, Michelucci, R, Forti, A, and Tassinari, CA: CT findings in progressive supranuclear palsy. J Comput Assist Tomogr 8 (3):406–409, 1984.
6. Baron, JC, Maziere, B, Loc'h, C, Cambon, H, Sgouropoulos, P, Bonnet, AM, and Agid Y: Loss of striatal [^{76}Br]bromospiperone binding sites demonstrated by positron tomography in progressive supranuclear palsy. J Cereb Blood Flow Metabol 6:131–136, 1986.
7. Baron, JC, Maziere, B, Loc'h, C, Sgouropoulos, P, Bonnet, AM, and Agid, Y: Progressive supranuclear palsy: Loss of striatal dopamine receptors demonstrated in vivo by positron tomography. Letter to the Editor. Lancet 2:1163–1164, 1985.
8. Barr, AN, Heinze, WJ, Dobben, GD, Valvassori, GE, and Sugar, O: Bicaudate index in computerized tomography of Huntington's disease and cerebral atrophy. Neurology 28:1196–1200, 1978.
9. Bean, SC and Ladisch, S: Chorea associated with a subdural hematoma in a child with leukemia. J Pediatr 90:255–256, 1977.
10. Bentson, JR and Keesey, JC: Pneumoencephalography of progressive supranuclear palsy. Radiology 113:89–94, 1974.
11. Bes, A, Guell, A, Fabre, N, Arne-Bes, MC, and Geraud, G: Effects of dopaminergic agonists (piribediland bromocriptine) on cerebral blood flow in parkinsonism (abstr). J Cereb Blood Flow Metabol (Suppl 1) 3:S490, 1983.
12. Besson, JAO, Corrigan, FM, Cherryman, GR, and Smith, FW: Nuclear magnetic resonance brain imaging in chronic schizophrenia. Br J Psychiatry 150:161–163, 1987.
13. Besson, JAO, Mutch, WJ, Smith, FW, and Corrigan, FM: The relationship between Parkinson's disease and dementia. Br J Psychiatry 147:380–382, 1985.
14. Bianco, F, Bozzao, L, Rizzo, PA, and Morocutti, C: Cerebellar atrophy in Huntington's disease. Acta Neurol (Napoli) 36:425–428, 1981.
15. Biller, J, Graff-Radford, NR, Smoker, WRK, Adams, HP, and Johnston, P: MR imaging in "lacunar" hemiballismus. J Comput Assist Tomogr 10:793–797, 1986.
16. Bird, ED: Chemical pathology of Huntington's disease. Annu Rev Pharmacol Toxicol 20:533–551, 1980.
17. Blinderman, EE, Weidner, W, and Markham, CH: The pneumoencephalogram in Huntington's chorea. Neurology 11:601–607, 1964.
18. Bogerts, B, Meertz, E, and Schonfeldt-Bausch, R: Basal ganglia and limbic system pathology in schizophrenia. Arch Gen Psychiatry 42:784–791, 1985.
19. Bottcher, J and Henriksen, L: Regional cerebral blood flow in parkinsonism measured by 133-xenon inhalation and emission computerized tomography. Effects on regional cerebral blood flow after levodopa. Acta Neurol Scand (Suppl 90) 65:284–285, 1982.
20. Brainin, M, Reisner, Th, and Zeitlhofer, J: Tardive dyskinesia: Clinical correlation with computed tomography in patients aged less than 60 years. J Neurol Neurosurg Psychiatr 46:1037–1040, 1983.
21. Brett, EM, Sheehy, MP, and Marsden, CD: Letter to the Editor. J Neuro Neurosurg Psychiatr 44:460, 1981.
22. Brewer, GJ, Terry, CA, Aisen, AM, and Hill, GM: Worsening of neurologic syndrome in patients with Wilson's disease with initial penicillamine therapy. Arch Neurol 44:490–493, 1987.
23. Brittenham, GM, Farrel, DE, Harris, JW, Feldman, ES, Danish, EH, Muri, WA, Tripp, JH, and Bellon, EM: Magnetic-susceptibility measurement of human iron stores. N Engl J Med 307:1671–1675, 1982.
24. Brown, RT, Polinsky, R, Di Chiro, G, Pastakia, B, Wener, L, and Simmons, JT: MRI in autonomic failure. J Neurol Neurosurg Psychiatr 50:913–914, 1987.
25. Bueri, JA, Levine, SR, Welch, KMA, Smith, MB, Ewing, JR, Helpern, JA, Bruce, RC, and Kensora, TG: Cerebral

phosphate metabolism in Alzheimer and Parkinson dementia measured by ^{31}P-NMR spectroscopy. Neurology (Suppl 1) 37:160, 1987.

26. Burton, K, Farrell, K, Li, D, and Calne, DB: Lesions of the putamen and dystonia: CT and magnetic resonance imaging. Neurology 34:962–965, 1984.

27. Bydder, GM, Steiner, RE, Young, IR, Hall, AS, Thomas, DJ, Marshall, J, Pallis, CA, and Legg, NJ: Clinical NMR imaging of the brain: 140 cases. AJNR 139:215–236, 1982.

28. Calne, DB, Langston, JW, Martin, WRW, Stoessl, AJ, Ruth, TJ, Adam, MJ, Pate, BD, and Schulzer, M: Letter to the Editor. Nature 317:246, 1985.

29. Cambon, H, Baron, JC, Boulenger, JP, Loc'h, C, Zarifian, E, and Maziere, B: In vivo assay for neuroleptic receptor binding in the striatum. Positron tomography in humans. Br J Psychiatry 151: 824–830, 1987.

30. Cambon, H, Bonnet, AM, Dubois, B, Loc'h, C, Duquesnoy, Y, Maziere, B, and Baron, JC: A ^{76}Br-bromospiperone PET study of tardive dyskinesia (abstr). J Cereb Blood Flow Metabol (Suppl 1) 7:S365, 1987.

31. Chawluk, J, Mesulam, MM, Hurtig, H, Kushner, M, Weintrub, S, Saykin, A, Rubin, N, Alavi A, and Reivich, M: Positron emission tomographic studies in slowly progressive aphasia without generalized dementia (abstr). Ann Neurol 16 (1):136, 1984.

31a. Chen, J, Schneiderman, J, Wortzman, G: Methanol poisoning: Bilateral putamenal and cerebellar cortical lesions. J Comput Assist Tomogr 15 (3):522–524, 1991.

32. Christensen, E, Moller, JE, and Faurbye, A: Neuropathological investigation of 28 brains from patients with dyskinesia. Acta Psychiatr Scan 46:14–23, 1970.

33. Chugani, DC, Ackermann, RF, and Phelps, ME: In vivo [3-H]spiperone binding: Evidence for accumulation in corpus striatum by agonist-mediated receptor internalization. J Cereb Blood Flow Metabol 8:291–303, 1988.

34. Clark, CM, Hayden, MR, Stoessl, AJ, and Martin WRW: Regression model for predicting dissociations of regional cerebral glucose metabolism in individuals at risk for Huntington's disease. J Cereb Blood Flow Metabol 6:756–762, 1986.

35. Conneally, PM: Huntington's disease: Genetics and epidemiology. Am J Hum Genet 36:506–526, 1984.

36. Crossman, AR, Mitchell, IJ, and Sambrook MA: Regional brain uptake of 2-deoxyglucose in N-methyl-4-phenyl-1,2,3,6-tetrahydropyridine (MPTP)-induced parkinsonism in the Macaque monkey. Neuropharmacol 24(6):587–591, 1985.

37. D'Antona, R, Baron, JC, Samson, Y, Serdaru, M, Viader, F, Agid, Y, and Cambier, J: Subcortical dementia: Frontal cortex hypometabolism detected by positron tomography in patients with progressive supranuclear palsy. Brain 108:785–799, 1985.

38. De Haan, J, Grossman, RI, Civitello, L, Hackney, DB, Goldberg, HI, Bilaniuk, LT, and Zimmerman, RA: High-field magnetic resonance imaging of Wilson's disease. J Comput Tomogr 11:132–135, 1987.

39. DeVera Reyes, JA: Parkinsonian-like syndrome caused by posterior fossa tumor. J Neurosurg 33:599–601, 1970.

40. Drayer, BP, Olanow, CW, and Burger, P: High field strength magnetic resonance imaging in patients with Parkinson's disease. Neurology (Suppl 1) 36:309, 1986.

41. Drayer, BP: Brain iron permits MRI of movement disorders. Diag Imag Nov: 308–314, 1987.

42. Drayer, BP: Magnetic resonance imaging and brain iron: Implications in the diagnosis and pathochemistry of movement disorders and dementia. Barrow Neurologic Institute Quarterly 3(4):15–30, 1987.

43. Dubinsky, R and Hallett, M: Glucose hypermetabolism of the inferior olive in patients with essential tremor (abstr). Ann Neurol 22(1):118, 1987.

44. Dubinsky, RM and Jankovic, J: Progressive supranuclear palsy and a multi-infarct state. Neurology 37:570–576, 1987.

45. Dubinsky, RM, Brown, RT, Polinsky, RJ, and DiChiro, G: Regional brain glucose hypometabolism in multiple sys-

tem atrophy (abstr). Neurology 38:330, 1988.

46. Dubinsky, RM, Greenberg, M, Hallet, M, DiChiro, G, and Baker, M: Metabolism of the basal ganglia in hemiballismus. Ann Neurol 22:145, 1987.

47. Duvoisin, RC: Diseases of the extrapyramidal system. In Rosenberg, RN (ed): The Clinical Neurosciences. Churchill Livingstone, New York, 1983, p 441.

48. Fabre, N, Adam, P, Geraud, G, Guell, A, Roulleau, J, and Bes, A: Correlations between CBF and CT scan in parkinsonism, J Cereb Blood Flow Metabol (Suppl 1) 3:S516, 1983.

49. Fahn, S: Management of Parkinson's disease at different stages of illness. Clin Neuropharmacol 5(1):S1–S43, 1982.

50. Farde, L, Halldin, C, Stone-Elander, S, and Sedvall, G: PET analysis of human dopamine receptor subtypes using ^{11}C-SCH 23390 and ^{11}C-raclopride. Psychopharmacol 92:278–284, 1987.

51. Farde, L, Wiesel, FA, Halldin, C, and Sedvall, G: Central D_2-dopamine receptor occupancy in schizophrenia patients treated with antipsychotic drugs. Arch Gen Psychiatry 45:71–76, 1988.

52. Ferrante, RJ, Kowall, NW, Beal, MF, Richardson, EP, Bird, ED, and Martin, JB: Selective sparing of a class of striatal neurons in Huntington's disease. Science 230:561–563, 1985.

53. Foster, NL, Gilman, S, Berent, S, Morin, EM, Brown, MB, and Koeppe, RA: Cerebral hypometabolism in progressive supranuclear palsy studied with positron emission tomography. Ann Neurol 24:399–406, 1988.

53a. Freed, C, Breeze, R, Rosenberg, N, Scheck, S, et al: Transplantation of human fetal dopamine cells for Parkinson's disease. Arch Neurol 47:505–512, 1990.

54. Frey, KA: Cerebral positron emission tomography: Pre and postsynaptic neurotransmitter studies. In Am Acad Neurol Course on PET and SPECT 218:39–51, 1988.

55. Fross, RD, Martin, WRW, Li, D, Stoessl, AJ, Adam, MJ, Ruth, TJ, Pate, BD, Burton, K, and Calne, DB: Lesions of the putamen: Their relevance to dystonia. Neurology 37:1125–1129, 1987.

56. Frost, JJ, Uhl, GE, Wong, DF, Preziosi, TJ, Dannals, RF, Ravert, HT, and Wagner, HN: Dopamine receptor alteration in asymmetrical and symmetical parkinsonism measured by positron emission tomography. Ann Neurol 16(1):128–129, 1984.

57. Garnett, ES, Firnau, G. Lang, AE, and Nahmias, C: Temporal changes in striatal dopamine distribution in control subjects and patients with Parkinson's disease (abstr). J Cereb Blood Flow Metabol (Suppl 1) 7:S367, 1987.

58. Garnett, ES, Firnau, G, Nahmias, C, Carbotte, R, and Bartolucci, G: Reduced striatal glucose consumption and prolonged reaction time are early features in HD. J Neurol Sci 65:231–237, 1984.

59. Garnett, ES, Firnau, G, and Nahmias, C: Dopamine visualized in the basal ganglia of living man. Nature 305:137–138, 1983.

60. Garnett, ES, Nahmias, C, and Firnau, G: Central dopaminergic pathways in hemi-parkinsonism examined by positron emission tomography. Can J Neurol Sci 11:174–179, 1984.

61. Garnett, S, Firnau, G, Nahmias, C, and Chirakal, R: Striatal dopamine metabolism in living monkeys examined by positron emission tomography. Br Res J 280:169–171, 1983.

62. Gath, I and Vinja, B: Pneumoencephalographic findings in Huntington's chorea. Neurology 18:991–996, 1968.

63. Gilman, S, Dauth, GW, Frey, KA, and Penney, JB: Experimental hemiplegia in the monkey: Basal ganglia glucose activity during recovery. Ann Neurol 22:370–376, 1987.

64. Gilmore, PC and Brenner, RP: Chorea: A late complication of subdural hematoma. Neurology 29:1044–1045, 1979.

65. Globus, M, Mildorf, B, and Melamed, E: rCBF changes in Parkinson's disease: Correlation with dementia. J Cereb Blood Flow Metabol (Suppl 1) 3:S508, 1983.

66. Goodhart, SP, Balser, BH, and Bieber, I: Encephalographic studies in cases of

extrapyramidal disease. Arch Neurol Psychiatry 35:240–252, 1936.
67. Granerus, AK, Nilsson, NJ, Suurkula, M, and Svanborg, A: Cerebral blood flow in Parkinson's syndrome. Adv Neurol 40:403–405, 1984.
68. Graveland, GA, Williams, RS, and DiFiglia, M: Evidence for degenerative and regenerative changes in neostriatal spiny neurons in Huntington's disease. Science 227:770–773, 1985.
69. Grimes, JD, Hassan, MN, Quarrington, AM, and D'Alton, J: Delayed-onset posthemiplegic dystonia: CT demonstration of basal ganglia pathology. Neurology 32:1033–1035, 1982.
70. Growdon, JH and Corkin, S: Cognitive impairments in Parkinson's disease. Adv Neurol 45:383–392, 1986.
71. Gusella, JF, Wexler, NS, Conneally, PM, Naylor, SL, Anderson, MA, Tanzi, RE, Watkins, PC, Ottina, K, Wallace, MR, Sakaguchi, AY, Young, AB, Shoulson, I, Bonilla, E, and Martin, JB: A polymorphic DNA marker genetically linked to Huntington's disease. Nature 306:234–238, 1983.
72. Guttman, M, Lang, AE, Garnett, ES, Nahmias, C, Firnau, G, Tyndel, FJ, and Gordon, AS: Regional cerebral glucose metabolism in SLE chorea: Further evidence that striatal hypometabolism is not a correlate of chorea. Movement Disorders 2(3):201–210, 1987.
73. Guttman, M, Ruth, T, and Calne, DB: SCH-23390 PET scans show reduced D-1 dopamine receptor binding in unilaterally MPTP lesioned monkeys (abstr). Neurology 38:259, 1988.
74. Guttman, M, Stoessl, J, Peppard, Martin, WRW, Ruth, T, Adam, MJ, Pate, BD, Tsui, JK, and Mak, E: Correlation between clinical findings and 6-(18F) fluorodopa PETs in Parkinson's disease (abstr). Neurology (Suppl 1) 37:329, 1987.
75. Guttman, M, Yong, VW, Kim, SU, Calne, DB, Martin, WRW, Barwick, S, Walsh, E, Adam, MJ, Ruth, TJ, and Pate, BD: Asymptomatic unilateral MPTP lesions visualized in vivo by fluorodopa positron emission tomographic scans in cynomolgus monkeys (abstr). Ann Neurol 22(1):172, 1987.
76. Hagglund, J, Aquilonius, SM, Bergstrom, K, Eckernas, SA, Hartvig, P, Lundqvist, H, Langstrom, B, Malmborg, P, and Nagren, K: Regional kinetics of [C-11]methylspiperone in the brain studied by positron emission tomography in patients with Parkinson's disease. Adv Neurol 45:99–101, 1986.
77. Hagglund, J, Aquilonius, SM, Eckernas, SA, Hartvig, P, Lundqvist, H, Gullberg, P, and Langstrom, B: Dopamine receptor properties in Parkinson's disease and Huntington's chorea evaluated by positron emission tomography using C-11 N-methylspiperone. Acta Neurol Scand 75:87–94, 1987.
78. Haldeman, S, Goldman, JW, Hyde, J, Pribram, HFW: Progressive supranuclear palsy, computed tomography, and response to antiparkinsonian drugs. Neurology 31:442–445, 1981.
79. Hantraye, P, Loc'h, C, Tacke, U, Riche, D, Stulzaft, O, Doudet, D, Guibert, B, Naquet, R, Maziere, B, and Maziere, M: "In vivo" visualization by positron emission tomography of the progressive striatal dopamine receptor damage occurring in MPTP-intoxicated non-human primates. Life Sci 39: 1375–1382, 1986.
80. Harik, SI and Post, MJD: Computed tomography in Wilson's disease. Neurology 31:107–110, 1981.
81. Hattori, H, Takao, T, Ito, M, Nakano, S, Okuno, T, and Mikawa, H: Cerebellum and brain stem atrophy in a child with Huntington's disease. Comp Radiol 8(1):53–56, 1984.
82. Hawkins, RA, Mazziotta, JC, and Phelps, ME: Wilson's disease studied with FDG and positron emission tomography. Neurology 37:1707–1711, 1987.
83. Hayden, MR, Hewitt, BS, Stoessl, AJ, Clark, C, Ammann, W, and Martin, WRW: The combined use of positron emission tomography and DNA polymorphisms for preclinical detection of Huntington's disease. Neurology 37: 1441–1447, 1987.
84. Hayden, MR, Martin, WRW, Stoessl, AJ, Clark, C, Hollenberg, S, Adam, MJ, Ammann, W, Harrop, R, Rogers, J, Ruth, T, Sayre, C, and Pate, BD: Posi-

tron emission tomography in the early diagnosis of Huntington's disease. Neurology 36:888–894, 1986.

85. Hayden, MR: Huntington's chorea. Springer-Verlag, New York, 1981.

86. Henriksen, L, and Boas, J: Regional cerebral blood flow in hemi-Parkinsonian patients. Emission computerized tomography of inhaled 133-xenon before and after levodopa. Acta Neurol Scand 71:257–266, 1985.

87. Hoffman, JM, Luxen, A, Bahn, MM, Barrio, JR, Huang, SC, Mazziotta, JC, and Phelps, ME: Carbidopa pretreatment in 6-[F-18]L-Dopa PET studies: Is it useful? J Cereb Blood Flow Metab (Suppl 1) 7:S363, 1987.

87a. Hornykiewicz, O, Kish, S, Becker, L, Farley, I, Shannak, K: Brain neurotransmitters in dystonia musculorum deformans. N Engl J Med 315(6):347–353, 1986.

88. Ishino, H and Otsuki, S: Frequency of Alzheimer's neurofibrillary tangles in the cerebral cortex in progressive supranuclear palsy (subcortical argyrophilic dystrophy). J Neurol Sci 28:309–316, 1976.

89. Ishino, H, Ikeda, H, and Otsuki, S: Contribution to clinical pathology of progressive supranuclear palsy (subcortical argyrophilic dystrophy). On the distribution of neurofibrillary tangles in the basal ganglia and brain-stem and its clinical significance. J Neuro Sci 24:471–481, 1975.

90. Jeste, DV, Wagner, RL, Weinberger, DR, Rieth, KG, and Wyatt, RJ: Evaluation of CT scans in tardive dyskinesia. Am J Psychiatry 137 (2):247–248, 1980.

91. Junck, L, Gilman, S, Hichwa, RD, Young, AB, Markel, DS, and Ehrenkaufer, LE: PET study of local cerebral glucose metabolism in idiopathic torsion dystonia (abstr). Neurology (Suppl 1) 36:182–183, 1986.

92. Katayama, Y, Tsubokawa, T, Tsukiyama, T, and Hirayama, T: Changes in regional cerebral blood flow and oxygen metabolism following ventrolateral thalamotomy in Parkinson syndromes as revealed by positron emission tomography. Appl Neurophysiol 49:76–85, 1986.

93. Kawamura, J, Gotoh, F, Ebihara, S, Hata, T, Takashima, S, and Terayama, Y: Local cerebrovascular reactivities in Parkinson's disease (abstr). J Cereb Blood Flow Metabol (Suppl 1) 7:S372, 1987.

94. Kelly, PJ, Aslskog, JE, Goerss, SJ, Daube, JR, Duffy, JR, and Kall, BA: Computer-assisted stereotactic ventralis lateralis thalamotomy with microelectrode recording control in patients with Pakinson's disease. Mayo Clin Proc 62:655–664, 1987.

95. Kendall, BE, Pollock, SS, Bass, NM, and Valentine, AR: Wilson's disease clinical correlation with cranial computed tomography. Neuroradiol 22:1–5, 1981.

96. Kinkel, WR, Kinkel, PR, Jacobs, L, Hopkins, LN, and Bates, V: Serial magnetic resonance imaging of the evolution of cerebral ischemia and infarction (abstr). Neurology (Suppl 1) 35:136, 1985.

97. Kish, SJ, Shannak, K, and Hornykiewicz, O: Uneven pattern of dopamine loss in the striatum of patients with idiopathic Parkinson's disease. New Engl J Med 318:876–880, 1988.

98. Klawans, HL, Stein, RW, Tanner, CM, and Goetz, CG: A pure Parkinsonian syndrome following acute carbon monoxide intoxication. Arch Neurol 39: 302–304, 1982.

99. Koh, JY, Peters, S, and Choi, DW: Neurons containing NADPH-deaphorase are selectively resistant to quinolinate toxicity. Science 234:73–76, 1986.

100. Kotagal, S, Shuter, E, and Horenstein, S: Chorea as a manifestation of bilateral subdural hematoma in an elderly man. Arch Neurol 38:195, 1981.

101. Kozachuk, W, Salanga, V. Conomy, J, and Smith, A: MRI (magnetic resonance imaging) in Huntington's disease. Neurology (Suppl 1) 36:310, 1986.

102. Kozlowski, MR and Marshall, JF: Plasticity of ^{14}C-2-deoxy D-glucose incorporation into neostriatum and related structures in response to dopamine neuron damage and apomorphine

replacement. Brain Res 197:167–183, 1980.

103. Kozlowski, MR and Marshall, JF: Recovery of function and basal ganglia ^{14}C-2-deoxyglucose uptake after nigrostriatal injury. Brain Res 259:237–248, 1983.

104. Krul, JMJ and Wokke, JHJ: Bilateral subdural hematoma presenting as subacute Parkinsonism. Clin Neurol Neurosurg 89(2):107–109, 1987.

105. Kuhl, DE, Metter, JE, and Riege, WH: Patterns of local cerebral glucose utilization determined in Parkinson's disease by the [F-18]fluoro-deoxyglucose method. Ann Neurol 15:419–424, 1984.

106. Kuhl, DE, Metter, JM, Benson, FD, Ashford, JW, Riege, WH, Fujikawa, DG, Markham, CH, Mazziotta, JC, Maltese, A, and Dorsey, DA. Similarities of cerebral glucose metabolism in Alzheimer's and parkinsonian dementia. J Cereb Blood Flow Metabol 5(1):S169–S170, 1985.

107. Kuhl, DE, Phelps, ME, Markham, CH, Metter, EJ, Riege, WH, and Winter, J: Cerebral metabolism and atrophy in Huntington's disease determined by 18-FDG and computed tomographic scan. Ann Neurol 12:425–434, 1982.

108. Kuhl, DE, Small, GW, Riege, WH, Fujikawa, DG, Metter, EJ, Benson, DF, Ashford, JW, Mazziotta, JC, Maltese, A, and Dorsey, DA: Cerebral metabolic patterns before the diagnosis of probable Alzheimer's disease (abstr). J Cereb Blood Flow Metabol (Suppl 1) 7:S406, 1987.

109. Kvicala, V, Vymazal, J, and Nevsimalovas, S: Computed tomography of Wilson's disease. AJNR 4:429–430, 1983.

110. Lang, C: Is direct CT caudatometry superior to indirect parameters in confirming Huntington's disease? Neuroradiol 27:161–163, 1985.

111. Lassen, NA: Single photon emission computed tomography. In Mazziotta, JC, Gilman, S, (eds): Clinical Brain Imaging. FA Davis, Philadelphia, 1989, 1992.

112. Lavy, S, Melamed, E, Cooper, G, Bentin, S, and Rinot, Y: Regional cerebral blood flow in patients with Parkinson's disease. Arch Neurol 36:344–348, 1979.

113. Lawler, GA, Pennock, JM, Steiner, RE, Jenkins, WJ, Sherlock, S, and Young, IR: Nuclear magnetic resonance (NMR) imaging in Wilson disease. J Comput Assist Tomogr 7(1):1–8, 1983.

114. Leenders, KL, Aquilonius, SM, Bergstrom, K, Hartvig, P, Lundqvist, H, Tedroff, J, Bjurling, P, Gee A, Nagren, K, and Langstrom, B: Unilaterally MPTP-lesioned Rhesus monkey studied with PET using dopaminergic tracers (abstr). Neurology (Suppl 1) 37:338, 1987.

115. Leenders, KL, Findley, LJ, and Cleeves, L: PET before and after surgery for tumor-induced parkinsonism. Neurology 36:1074–1078, 1986.

116. Leenders, KL, Frackowiak, RSJ, and Lees, AJ: Progressive supranuclear palsy (PSP) studied with positron emission tomography (PET) (abstr). Neurology (Suppl 1) 37:113, 1987.

117. Leenders, KL, Frackowiak, RSJ, and Lees, AJ: Steele-Richardson-Olzewski (SRO) syndrome (supranuclear palsy) studied with positron emission tomography (PET) (abstr). J Cereb Blood Flow Metabol (Suppl 1) 7:S397, 1987.

118. Leenders, KL, Frackowiak, RSJ, Quinn, N, and Marsden, CD: Brain energy metabolism and dopaminergic function in Huntington's disease measured in vivo using positron emission tomography. Movement Disorders 1 (1):69–77, 1986.

119. Leenders, KL, Palmer, AJ, Quinn, N, Clark, JC, Firnau, G, Garnett, ES, Nahmias, C, Jones, T, and Marsden, CD: Brain dopamine metabolism in patients with Parkinson's disease measured with positron emission tomography. J Neurol Neurosurg Psychiatr 49:853–860, 1986.

120. Leenders, KL, Poewe, WH, Palmer, AJ, Brenton, DP, and Frackowiak, RSJ: Inhibition of [F-18] fluorodopa uptake into human brain by amino acids demonstrated by positron emission tomography. Ann Neurol 20:258–262, 1986.

121. Leenders, KL, Wolfson, L, Gibbs, JM,

Wise, RJS, Causon, R, Jones, T, and Legg, NJ: The effects of L-dopa on regional cerebral blood flow and oxygen metabolism in patients with Parkinson's disease. Brain 108:171–191, 1985.

122. Lenzi, GI, Jones, T, Reid, JL, and Moss, S: Regional impairment of cerebral oxidative metabolism in Parkinson's disease. J Neurol Neurosurg Psychiatr 42:59–62, 1979.

122a. Lindvall, O, Rehnerona, S, Brundin, P, Gustavii, B, et al: Human fetal dopamine neurons grafted into the striatum in two patients with severe Parkinson's disease. Arch Neurol 46:615–631, 1989.

122b. Lindvall, O, Brundin, P, Widner, H, et al: Grafts of fetal dopamine neurons survive and improve motor function in Parkinson's disease. Science 247:574–577, 1990.

123. Lukes, SA, Aminoff, MJ, Crooks, L, Kaufman, L, Mills, C, and Newton, TH: Nuclear magnetic resonance imaging in movement disorders. Ann Neurol 13(6):690–691, 1983.

124. Luxenberg, MN: Magnetic resonance imaging diagnosis of hepatolenticular degeneration. Arch Ophthalmol 105: 277, 1987.

125. Marsden, CD and Fahn, S (eds): Movement Disorders. Butterworth Scientific, London, 1981.

126. Marsden, CD: Neurotransmitters and CNS disease. Lancet 1141–1146, 1982.

127. Marsden, CD: The mysterious motor function of the basal ganglia. Neurology 32(5):514–539, 1982.

128. Marsden, CD: The pathophysiology of movement disorders. Neurol Clin North Am 2:435–459, 1984.

129. Martin, J: Huntington's disease: New approaches to an old problem. Neurology 34:1059–1072, 1984.

130. Martin, JB and Gusella, JF: Huntington's disease: Pathogenesis and management. N Engl J Med 315(20):1267–1276, 1986.

131. Martin, WR: Positron emission tomography in movement disorders. Can J Neurol Sci 12:6–10, 1985.

132. Martin, WRW, Adam, MJ, Ruth, TJ, Stoessl, RJ, Ammann, W, Bergstrom M, Harrop, R, Laihinen, A, Rogers, JG, Sayre, CI, Pate, BD, and Calne, DB: The study of dopa metabolism in man with positron emission tomography (abstr). Neurology (Suppl 1) 35:115, 1985.

133. Martin, WRW, Beckman, JH, Calne, DB, Adam, MJ, Harrop, R, Rogers, JG, Ruth, TJ, Sayre, CI, and Pate, BD: Cerebral glucose metabolism in Parkinson's disease. Can J Neurol Sci 11:169–173, 1984.

134. Martin, WRW, Hayden, MR, Suchowersky, O, Beckman, J, Adam, M, Ammann, W, Bergstrom, M, Harrop, R, Rogers, J, Ruth, T, Sayre, C, and Pate, BD: Striatal metabolism in Huntington's disease and in benign hereditary chorea. Ann Neurol 16(1):126, 1984.

135. Martin, WRW, Stoessl, AJ, Adam, MJ, Ammann, W, Bergstrom, M, Harrop, R, Laihinen, A, Rogers, JG, Ruth, TJ, Sayre, CI, Pate, BD, and Calne, DB: Positron emission tomography in Parkinson's disease: Glucose and DOPA metabolism. Adv Neurol 45:95–98, 1986.

136. Martin, WRW, Stoessl, AJ, Adam, MJ, Grierson, JR, Ruth, TJ, Pate BD, and Calne, DB: Imaging of dopamine systems in human subjects exposed to MPTP. In MPTP: A Neurotoxin Producing a Parkinsonian Syndrome. Academic Press, San Diego, Calif, 1986, pp 315–325.

137. Martin, WRW: PET: Applications in patients with movement disorders. Am Acad Neurol Course on PET and SPECT 218:93–104, 1988.

137a. Mata, M, Fink, D, Gainer, H, et al: Activity-dependent energy metabolism in rat posterior pituitary primary reflects sodium pump activity. J Neurochem 34:213–215, 1980.

138. Mazziotta, JC and Phelps, ME: Positron emission tomography studies of the brain. In Phelps, ME, Mazziotta, JC, and Schelbert, HR (eds): Positron Emission Tomography and Autoradiography: Principles and Applications for the Brain and Heart. Raven Press, New York, 1986, pp 493–579.

139. Mazziotta, JC, Pahl, JJ, Phelps, ME, Baxter, LR, Riege, WH, Hoffman, JM, Huang, SC, Gusella, J, Hyslop, P,

Schwab, R, Selin, C, Sumida, R, Kuhl, DE, Wapenski, J, Conneally, M, and Markham, CH: Presymptomatic evaluation of subjects at risk for Huntington's disease (HD): PET and DNA polymorphism studies (abstr). J Cereb Blood Flow Metabol (Suppl 1) 7:S366, 1987.

140. Mazziotta, JC, Phelps, ME, Pahl, JJ, Huang, SC, Baxter LR, Riege, WH, Hoffman, JM, Kuhl, DE, Lanto, AB, Wapenski, JA and Markham, CH: Reduced cerebral glucose metabolism in asymptomatic subjects at risk for Huntington's disease. N Engl J Med 316:357–362, 1987.

141. Mazziotta, JC, Phelps, ME, Pahl, JJ, Huang, SC, Baxter, LR, Hoffman, JM, Markham, CH, Riege, WH, and Lanto, AB: Studies of persons at risk for Huntington's disease. N Engl J Med 317:382–384, 1987.

142. Mazziotta, JC, Phelps, ME, Plummer, D, and Kuhl, DE: Quantitation in positron emission computed tomography: 5. Physical–anatomical effects. J Comput Assist Tomogr 5(5):734–743, 1981.

143. Mazziotta, JC, Wapenski, J, Phelps, ME, Riege, WH, Baxter, LR, Fullerton, A, Kuhl, DE, Selin, C, and Sumida, R: Cerebral glucose utilization and blood flow in Huntington's disease: Symptomatic and at-risk subjects. J Cereb Blood Flow Metabol (Suppl 1) 5:S25–S26, 1985.

144. McCulloch, J and Edvinsson, L: Cerebral circulatory and metabolic effects of Piribedil. Eur J Pharmacol 66:327–337, 1980.

145. Melamed, E, Mordechai, G, and Mildworf, B: Regional cerebral blood flow in patients with Parkinson's disease under chronic levodopa therapy: Measurements during "on" and "off" response fluctuations. J Neurol Neurosurg Psychiatr 49:1301–1304, 1986.

146. Melamed, E, Lavy, S, Cooper, G, and Bentin, S: Regional cerebral blood flow in parkinsonism. J Neurol Sci 38:391–397, 1978.

147. Messimy, R, Diebler, C, and Metzger, J: Dystonie de torsion du membre superieurgauche probablement consecutive a un traumatisme cranien. Rev Neurol 133(3):199–206, 1977.

148. Mitchell, IJ, Cross, AJ, Sambrook, MA, and Crossman, AR: Neural mechanism mediating 1-methyl-4-phenyl-1,2,3,6-tetrahydropyridine-induced parkinsonism in the monkey: Relative contributions of the striatopallidal and striatonigral pathways as suggested by 2-deoxyglucose uptake. Neurosci Letters 63:61–65, 1986.

149. Nahmias, C, Garnett, ES, Firnau, G, and Lang, A: Striatal dopamine distribution in Parkinsonian patients during life. J Neurol Sci 69:223–230, 1985.

150. Nelson, RF, Guzman, DA, Grahovac, Z, and Howse, DCN: Computerized cranial tomography in Wilson's disease. Neurology 29:866–868, 1979.

151. Neophytides, AN, DiChiro, G, Barron, SA, and Chase, TN: Computed axial tomography in Huntington's disease and persons at risk for Huntington's disease. Adv Neurol 23:185–191, 1979.

152. Nutt, JG, Woodward, WR, Hammerstad, JP, Carter, JH, and Anderson, JL. The "on/off" phenomenon in Parkinson's disease. Relationship to levodopa absorption and transport. N Engl J Med 310:483–488, 1984.

153. Oepen, G and Osterlag, Ch: Diagnostic value of CT in patients with Huntington's chorea and their offspring. J Neuroradiol 225:189–196, 1981.

154. Pahl, JJ, Mazziotta, JC, Cummings, J, Bartzokis, G, Marder, S, Schwab, R, Sumida, R, Kuhl, DE, Baxter, LR, and Phelps, ME: Positron emission tomography in tardive dyskinesia and Huntington's disease: LCMRGlc in two patient populations with chorea (abstr). J Cereb Blood Flow Metabol (Suppl 1) 7:S373, 1987.

155. Pahl, JJ, Mazziotta, JC, Bartzokis, G, Cummings, J, Altschuler, L, Mintz, J, Marder, SM, and Phelps, ME: Personal communication, 1989.

156. Palella, TD, Hichwa, RD, Ehrenkaufer, RL, Rothley, JM, McQuillan, MA, Young, AB, and Kelley, WN: 18-F Fluoro-deoxyglucose PET scanning in HPRT deficiency. Am J Hum Genet 37:A70, 1985.

157. Pastakia, B, Polinsky, R, DiChiro, G, Simmons, JT, Brown, R, and Wener, L: Multiple system atrophy (Shy-Drager

syndrome): MR imaging. Radiology 159:499–502, 1986.

158. Penney, JB and Young, AB: Speculations on the functional anatomy of basal ganglia disorders. Annu Rev Neurosci 6:73–94, 1983.
159. Penney, JB and Young, AB: Striatal inhomogeneities and basal ganglia function. Movement Disorders 1:3–15, 1986.
160. Penney, JB and Young, AB: Quantitative autoradiography of neurotransmitter receptors in Huntington's disease. Neurology 32:1391–1395, 1982.
161. Peppard, RF, Martin, WRW, Guttman, M, Walsh, EM, Carr, GD, Phillips, AG, Grochowski, E, Okada, J, Tsui, JKC, Mak, E, Ruth, T, Adam, MJ, and Calne, DB: The relationship of cerebral glucose metabolism to cognitive deficits in Parkinson's disease (abstr). Neurology 38:364, 1988.
162. Perlmutter, JS and Raichle, ME: Pure hemidystonia with basal ganglion abnormalities on positron emission tomography. Ann Neurol 15:228–233, 1984.
163. Perlmutter, JS and Raichle, ME: Regional blood flow in hemiparkinsonism. Neurology 35:1127–1134, 1985.
164. Perlmutter, JS, Kilbourn, MR, Raichle, ME, and Elsch, MJ: Positron emission tomographic demonstration of upregulation of radioligand receptor binding in human MPTP-induced parkinsonism (abstr). J Cereb Blood Flow Metabol (Suppl 1) 7:S371, 1987.
165. Pettegrew, JW, Kopp, SJ, Dadok, J, Minshew, NJ, Feliksik JM, and Glonek, T: Chemical characterization of a prominent phosphorylmonoester resonance in animal, Huntington, and Alzheimer brain: Phorphorus-31 and hydrogen-1 nuclear magnetic resonance analysis at 4.7 and 14.1 tesla. Ann Neurol 16 (1):136–137, 1984.
166. Phillips, PC, Brin, MF, Fahn, S, Greene, PE, Sidtis, JJ, Ragassa, J, Krol, G, Moeller, JR, Sergi, ML, and Rottenberg, DA: Abnormal regional cerebral glucose metabolism in choreo-acanthocytosis: An F-18-fluoro-deoxyglucose positron emission tomographic study. Neurology (Suppl 1) 37:211, 1987.
167. Polinsky, RJ, Kopin, IJ, Ebert, MH, and Weise, V: Pharmacologic distinction of different orthostatic hypotension syndromes. Neurology 31:1–7, 1981.
168. Porrino, LJ, Burns, RS, Crane, AM, Kopin, IJ, and Sokoloff, L: Measurement of local cerebral glucose metabolism in a primate model of Parkinson's disease (abstr). J Cereb Blood Flow Metabol (Suppl 1) 5:S167, 1985.
169. Porrino, LJ, Palombo, E, Crane, AM, Jehle, JW, Ho, VW, Bankiewicz, KS, Kopin, IJ, and Sokoloff, L: Metabolic mapping of a primate model of hemiparkinsonism (abstr). J Cereb Blood Flow Metabol (Suppl 1) 7:S375, 1987.
170. Portin, R, Raininko, R, and Rinne, UK: Neuropsychological disturbances and cerebral atrophy determined by computerized tomography in parkinsonian patients with long-term levodopa treatment. Adv Neurol 40:219–227, 1984.
171. Reisine, TD, Fields, JZ, Bird, ED, Spokes, E, and Yamamura, HI: Characterization of brain dopaminergic receptors in Huntington's disease. Commun Psychopharmacol 2:79–94, 1978.
172. Ropper, AH, Hatten, HP, and Davis, KR: Computed tomography in Wilson's disease: Report of 2 cases. Ann Neurol 5:102–103, 1979.
173. Rothfus, WE, Hirsch, WL, Malatack, J, and Bergman, I: Improvement of cerebral CT abnormalities following liver transplantation in a patient with Wilson's disease. J Comput Assist Tomogr 12(1):138–140, 1988.
174. Rougemont, D, Baron, JC, Collard, P, Bustany, P, Comar, D, and Agid, Y: Local cerebral glucose utilization in treated and untreated patients with Parkinson's disease. J Neurol Neurosurg Psychiatr 47:824–830, 1984.
175. Ruberg, M, Javoy-Agid, F, Hirsch, E, Scatton, B, Hauw, JJ, Duyckaerts, J, Serdaru, M, Morel-Maroger, A, and Agid, Y: Aminergic, cholinergic, and gabaergic systems in the brain of patients with progressive supranuclear palsy. Ann Neurol 18:523–529, 1985.
176. Runge, VM, Clanton, JA, Smith, FW, Hutchison, J, Mallard, J, Partain, CL, and James, AE: Nuclear magnetic reso-

nance of iron and copper disease states. AJR 141:943–948, 1983.

177. Rutledge, JN, Hilal, SK, Silver, AJ, Defendini, R, and Fahn, S: Study of movement disorders and brain iron by MR. AJNR 8:397–411, 1987.

178. Sagar, JM and Snodgrass, SR: Effects of substantia nigra lesions of forebrain 2-deoxyglucose retention in the rat. Brain Res 185:335–348, 1980.

179. Saris, S: Chorea caused by caudate infarction. Arch Neurol 40:590, 1983.

180. Sax, DS and Buonanno, S: Putaminal changes in spin-echo magnetic resonance imaging signal in bradykinetic/rigid forms of Huntington's disease. Neurology (Suppl 1) 36:311, 1986.

181. Sax, DS and Menzer, L: Computerized tomography in Huntington's disease (abstr). Neurology 27:388, 1977.

182. Sax, DS, Buonanno, FS, Kramer, C, Miatto, O, Kistler, JP, Martin, JB, and Brady, TJ: Proton nuclear magnetic resonance imaging in Huntington's disease. Ann Neurol 18(1):142, 1985.

183. Sax, DS, O'Connell, B, Butters, N, Menzer, L, Montgomery, K, and Kayne, HL: Computed tomographic, neurologic, and neuropsychological correlates of Huntington's disease. Int J Neurosci 18:21–36, 1983.

184. Schneider, E, Becker, H, Fischer, PA, Grau, H, Jacobi, P, and Brinkman, R: The course of brain atrophy in Parkinson's disease. Arch Psychiatry 227:89–95, 1979.

185. Schwartz, WJ: A role for the dopaminergic nigrostriatal bundle in the pathogenesis of altered brain glucose consumption after lateral hypothalamic lesion. Evidence using the ^{14}C-labeled deoxyglucose technique. Brain Res 158:129–147,

186. Schwartzman, RJ and Alexander, GM: Changes in the local metabolic rate for glucose in the 1-methyl-4-phenyl-1,2,3,6-tetrahydropyridine (MPTP) primate model of Parkinson's disease. Brain Res 358:137–143, 1985.

187. Selby, G: Cerebral atrophy in Parkinsonism. J Neurol Sci 6:517–559, 1968.

188. Selekler, K, Kansu, T, and Zileli, T: Computed tomography in Wilson's disease. Arch Neurol 38:727–728, 1981.

189. Shoulson, I: Huntington's disease: Functional capacity in patients treated with neuroleptic and antidepressant drugs. Neurology 31:1333–1335, 1981.

190. Shoulson, I: Huntington's disease. In Asbury, AK, McKhann, GM, and McDonald, WI (eds): Diseases of the Nervous System. WB Saunders, Philadelphia, 1986, pp 1258–1267.

191. Simmons, JT, Pastakia, B, Chase, TN, and Schults, CW: Magnetic resonance imaging in Huntington's disease. AJNR 7:25–28, 1986.

192. Singer, HS, Wong, DF, Tiemeyer, M, Whitehouse, P, and Wagner, HN: Pathophysiology of Tourette syndrome: A positron emission tomographic and postmortem analysis (abstr). Ann Neurol 18)3:416, 1985.

193. Smith, FW, Besson, JAO, Gemmell, HG, and Sharp, PF: The use of technetium-99m-HMPAO in the assessment of patients with dementia and other neuropsychiatric conditions. J Cereb Blood Flow Metabol 8:S116–S122, 1988.

194. Sokoloff, L: Metabolic Probes of Central Nervous System Activity in Animals and Man. Magnes Lecture Series, Vol 1. Sinaur, Sunderland, Mass, 1984.

195. Sperling, MR and Hermann, C: Syndrome of palatal myoclonus and progressive ataxia: Two cases with magnetic resonance imaging. Neurology 35:1212–1214, 1985.

196. Spokes, EGS, Bannister, R, and Oppenheimer, DR: Multiple system atrophy with autonomic failure. J Neurol Sci 43:59–82, 1979.

197. Sroka, N, Elizan, TS, Elizan, S, Yahr, MD, Burger, A, and Mendoza, MR: Organic mental syndrome and confusional states in Parkinson's disease. Arch Neurol 38:339–342, 1981.

198. Starosta-Rubenstein, S, Young, AB, Kluin, K, Hill, G, Aisen, AM, Gabrielsen, T, and Brewer, GJ: Clinical assessment of 31 patients with Wilson's disease. Arch Neurol 44:365–370, 1987.

199. Steele, J, Richardson, J, Olszewski, J: Progressive supranuclear palsy. Arch Neurology 10:333–359, 1964.

200. Steiner, I, Gomori, JM, and Melamed, E: Features of brain atrophy in Parkin-

son's disease. Neuroradiol 27:158–160, 1985.
201. Stober, T, Beil, C, Thielen, T, Emser, W, Pawlik, G, and Heiss, WD: Isoniazid therapy in Huntington's disease: Clinico-electrophysiologic-metabolic correlation. Neurology (Suppl 1) 36:311, 1986.
202. Stober, T, Wussow, W, and Schimrigk, K: Bicaudate diameter: The most specific and simple CT parameter in the diagnosis of Huntington's disease. Neuroradiol 26:25–28, 1984.
203. Stoessl, AJ, Martin, WRW, Clark, C, Adam MJ, Ammann, W, Beckman, JH, Bergstrom, M, Harrop, R, Rogers, JG, Ruth, TJ, Sayre, CI, Pate, BD, and Calne, DB: PET studies of cerebral glucose metabolism in idiopathic torticollis. Neurology 36:653–657, 1986.
204. Stoessl, AJ, Martin, WRW, Clark, CM, Pate, BD, and Calne, DB: Glucose metabolic relations in torticollis and voluntary head rotation (abstr). Neurology (Suppl 1) 37:123, 1987.
205. Stoessl, AJ, Martin, WRW, Hayden, MR, Adam MJ, and Ruth, TJ: Dopamine in Huntington's disease: Studies using positron emission tomography (abstr). Neurology (Suppl 1) 36:310, 1986.
206. Suchowersky, O, Hayden, MR, Martin, WRW, Stoessl, AJ, Hildebrand AM, and Pate, BD: Cerebral metabolism of glucose in benign hereditary chorea. Movement Disorders 1(1):33–44, 1986.
207. Swaiman, KF, Smith, SA, Trock, GL, and Siddiqui, AR: Sea-blue histiocytes, lymphocytic cytosomes, movement disorder and ^{59}Fe-uptake in basal ganglia: Hallervorden-Spatz disease or ceroid storage disease with abnormal isotope scan? Neurology 33:301–305, 1983.
208. Terrance, CF and Rao, G: Neuropathologic correlation of computerized tomography in Huntington's disease. South Med J 73:817–819, 1980.
209. Terrence, CF, Delaney, JF, and Alberts, MC: Computed tomography for Huntington's disease. Neuroradiol 13: 173–175, 1977.
210. Tolosa, ES and Santamaria, J: Parkinsonism and basal ganglia infarcts. Neurology 34:1616–1618, 1984.
211. Vonsattel, JP, Myers, RH, Stevens, TJ, Ferrante, RJ, Bird, ED, and Richardson, EP: Neuropathological classification of Huntington's disease. J Neuropathol Exp Neurol 44(6):559–577, 1985.
212. Wakai, S, Nakamura, K, Niizaki, K, Masakatsu, N, Nishizawa, T, Yokoyama, S, and Katayama, S: Meningioma of the anterior third ventricle presenting with Parkinsonism. Surg Neurol 21:88–92, 1984.
213. Williams, FJ and Walshe, JM: Wilson's disease: An analysis of the cranial computerized tomographic appearances found in 60 patients and the changes in response to treatment with chelating agents. Brain 104:735–752, 1981.
214. Wolfson, LI, Leenders, KL, Brown, LL, and Jones, T: Alterations of regional cerebral blood flow and oxygen metabolism in Parkinson's disease. Neurology 35:1399–1405, 1985.
215. Wong, DF, Links, JM, Wagner, HN, Folstein, SE, Suneja, S, Dannals, RF, Ravert, HT, Wilson, AA, Tune, LE, Pearlson, G, Folstein, MF, Bice, A, and Kuhar, MJ: Dopamine and serotonin receptors measured in vivo in Huntington's disease with C-11 N-methylspiperone PET imaging. J Nucl Med 26(5):107, 1985.
216. Wooten, GF and Collins, RC: Metabolic effects of unilateral lesion of the substantia nigra. J Neurosci 1(3):285–291, 1981.
217. Yebenes, JG, Gervas, JJ, Iglesias, J, Mena, MA, Martin del Rio, R, and Somoza, E: Biochemical findings in a case of parkinsonism secondary to brain tumor. Ann Neurol 11:313–316, 1982.
218. Young AD, Greenamyer, JT, Hollingsworth, Z, Albin, R, D'Amato, C, Shoulson, I, and Penney, JB: NMDA Receptor losses in putamen from patients with Huntington's disease. Science 241:981–983, 1988.
219. Young, AB, Penney, JB, Markel, DS, Hollingsworth, Z, Teener, J, and Stern, J: Genetic linkage analysis, glucose metabolism and neurological examination: Comparison in persons at risk for Huntington's disease (abstr). Neurology 38:359, 1988.

220. Young, AB, Penney, JB, Markel, DS, Starosta-Rubenstein, S, Rothley, J, and Betley, A: Glucose metabolism in juvenile Huntington's disease: Comparison with adult onset cases (abstr). Neurology 38:360, 1988.
221. Young, AB, Penney, JB, Starosta-Rubenstein, S, Markel, D, Berent, S, Rothley, J, Betley, A, and Hichwa, R: Normal caudate glucose metabolism in persons at risk for Huntington's disease. Arch Neurol 44:254–257, 1987.
222. Young, AB, Penney, JB, Starosta-Rubenstein, S, Markel, DS, Berent, S, Giordani, B, Ehrenkaufer, R, Jewett, D, and Hichwa, R: PET scan investigations of Huntington's disease: Cerebral metabolic correlates of neurologic features and functional decline. Ann Neurol 20:296–303, 1986.
223. Young, AB, Shoulson, I, Penney, JB, Starosta-Rubenstein, S, Gomez, F, Travers, H, Ramos-Arroyo, MA, Snodgrass, R, Bonilla, E, Moreno, H, and Wexler, NS: Huntington's disease in Venezuela. Neurology 36:244–249, 1986.

Chapter 9

DEMENTIA

Ranjan Duara, M.D.

CHARACTERISTICS OF DEMENTIA
DEGENERATIVE DISORDERS AND NORMAL AGING
VASCULAR DISORDERS
NORMAL PRESSURE HYDROCEPHALUS
THE USE OF NEUROIMAGING IN THE DIFFERENTIAL DIAGNOSIS OF DEMENTING CONDITIONS

CHARACTERISTICS OF DEMENTIA

Dementia is a term that implies loss of mental faculties sufficient to interfere with social and occupational functioning. The criteria for determining the presence of dementia have recently been the subject of intense scrutiny. In DSM-III-R[48] the American Psychiatric Association defines the features of dementia as some combination of personality changes and alteration in overall intellectual ability, abstraction, judgment, memory, and language, and the presence of agnosias and apraxias.

Clinical Symptoms and Signs

Memory impairment is generally the most easily quantifiable deficit in patients with mild dementia. Characteristically, a deficit of recent (short-term) memory is most prominent, although remote (long-term) memory deficits occur as well and are almost invariable as the dementia worsens. Language disorders, especially naming deficits,[6] occur frequently in dementia, and can be assessed by a variety of neuropsychologic tests, in addition to the clinical examination. Visuospatial disorientation and visuoconstructive deficits are common and may be the initial cause of such symptoms as getting lost in familiar surroundings. Simple tests of graphomotor praxis such as writing a sentence, or drawing a clock-face or a flower are often sufficient to demonstrate deficits in these areas of functioning. Psychiatric symptoms are not uncommon in the demented patient,[165] with depression, anxiety and paranoia more likely to occur in the earlier stages of the disorder, and agitation and hallucinations in the intermediate and late stages.

Dementia has been subdivided by some clinicians into cortical and subcortical types. This cortical-subcortical dichotomy has been somewhat controversial[197] but it does have experimental support.[21,29,145] Cortical dementia includes abnormalities of neocortical function such as aphasia, apraxia, and agnosia, in addition to a prominent memory deficit. In subcortical dementia the memory impairment is typically mild and neocortical functions are intact; inattention and slowing of cognition are prominent features. Pseudodementia refers to a condition where the symptoms associated with dementia are prominent, the signs are relatively mild, and the disorder is entirely ascribable to a psychiatric condition, usually depression.

The course of dementing disorders may vary. An acute onset of dementia is usually associated with delirium, which implies an alteration in the state of consciousness as well as impairment of mental faculties. Depending on the underlying disease process, dementia can be either insidious and slowly progressive (the most common presentation), or a rapidly evolving condition. A stepwise deterioration and fluctuating course are suggestive of a vascular etiology (multiple cerebral infarcts). Dementia can be reversible if the underlying disease is responsive to treatment (as in chronic subdural hematoma, normal pressure hydrocephalus, or benign tumor), and if significant permanent brain damage has not taken place.

Pathophysiology

The brain is remarkably heterogeneous, both morphologically and functionally. A discrete disorder involving only a small part of the structure of the brain may produce substantial functional disturbances, as, for example, occur with substantia nigra lesions (motor dysfunction) or destruction of the medial dorsal nucleus of the thalamus (short-term memory dysfunction). On the other hand, a relatively large volume of the brain may be lost with minimal functional consequences, as occurs with normal aging.[45] Structure-function relationships in the brain, therefore, are very complex. A strategy for gaining an understanding of these relationships may be to examine, as far as is possible, the consequences of disease on subdivisions of structure (e.g., cortical gray matter versus subcortical white matter; left hemisphere versus right hemisphere; frontal versus parietal or temporal regions) and subdivisions of function (e.g., neocortical-type functions such as language, praxis, or gnosis versus nonneocortical functions such as short-term memory). Just as neuropsychologic, neurologic or psychiatric methods can be used to identify subtypes of a dementing disease, so, too, can neuroimaging techniques. Subtyping dementias with neuroimaging techniques may be useful in identifying correlations with specific clinical or behavioral subtypes. Such an approach may thereby elucidate aspects of the pathophysiology of dementia.

Etiology

The etiology of dementia can be broadly classified into causes primarily *within* or *outside* the nervous system. Table 9–1 lists some important causes of dementia and gives the relative incidence of each type. Disease within the nervous system, as implied by the classification of cortical and subcortical dementia, can involve primarily the cortex or subcortical gray and/or white matter. Examples of predominantly cortical dementias include Alzheimer's and Pick's diseases and some forms of multi-infarct dementia. Progressive supranuclear palsy was the original disorder described as a subcortical dementia, but it has been suggested that certain forms of multi-infarct dementia (lacunar state and Binswanger's disease); Parkinson's, Huntington's, or Wilson's disease; normal pressure hydrocephalus; and multiple sclerosis may also fall into this category. This classification is likely to pertain only to the early stages of each of these diseases, as widespread involvement of the brain is likely to occur in the later stages of both types of dementia.

Causes of dementia primarily outside of the nervous system include excessive use of drugs and alcohol; hypothyroidism; Vitamin B_{12} deficiency; chronic infections such as syphilis, cryptococcosis, and tuberculosis; anoxic-ischemic encephalopathy, such as after cardiac arrests or anesthetic accidents; and the remote effects of carcinoma, particularly small-cell carcinoma of the lung.

Table 9–1 ETIOLOGIES OF DEMENTIA

Primary Cerebral Disorders (Presenting with Dementia Syndrome)				**Systemic Disorders Affecting the Brain (Presenting with Dementia Syndrome)**	
Cortical Dementia (80%)		***Subcortical Dementia (10%–15%)***			
Alzheimer's disease	(50%–60%)*	Progressive supranuclear palsy	(1%)	Drugs and alcohol	(5%–10%)
Pick's disease	(1%)	Parkinson's disease	(15)	Endocrine disorders,	(<1%)
Creutzfeldt-Jakob disease	(<1%)	Huntington's disease	(<1%)	particularly hypothyroidism	(<1%)
Multi-infarct dementia (cortical infarcts	(5%)	Wilson's disease	(<1%)	Vitamin B_{12} deficiency	(<1%)
		Multiple sclerosis	(<1%)	Remote effects of cancer	(<1%)
		Multi-infarct dementia	(10%)	Chronic infections (syphilis,	(<1%)
		(Binswanger's disease; lacunar state)	(1%)	cryptococcosis, tuberculosis, AIDS)	(<1%)
		Normal-pressure hydrocephalus		Collagen vescular disease	
				Anoxic-ischemic encephalopathy	

Percentages within parentheses are the estimates of the relative incidence of each condition obtained from published clinical and pathologic surveys.[20,119,151,152,176,182,190]

*An additional 15%–20% of cases have mixed (Alzheimer's and multi-infarct) forms of dementia.

DEGENERATIVE DISORDERS AND NORMAL AGING

Normal Aging

X-RAY CT STUDIES

X-ray CT studies conducted on large numbers of normal individuals from young adulthood to late senescence consistently note alterations in ventricular size and subarachnoid space with the aging process, although to varying degrees.[121] For example, one study of 130 subjects[103] demonstrated that CSF volume increased progressively from 40 years of age. Other researchers[205] found intracranial CSF volume to increase consistently only after the age of 60 years. In both these studies, compartments representing CSF in the ventricular and subarachnoid space were quantified by counting the number of pixels in each space. These volumes were accompanied by a reduction in gray matter volume for cortical and subcortical structures. White matter volume, however, remained unchanged through the age range.

Reports[206] of alterations in the attenuation value (CT number or Hounsfield unit) in the white matter of the centrum semiovale were not confirmed by other studies.[30,177] The x-ray CT scan may show patchy areas of reduced attenuation in the white matter of "normal" elderly individuals.[83,187] The incidence of these lesions in normals increases with age;[83] although not demented, subjects with such lesions are cognitively and neurologically inferior to those without them.[187]

MRI STUDIES

Figures 9–1 (*A*, *B*) and 9–2 (*A*,*B*) demonstrate the changes that occur with normal aging as shown by MRI. Although a method of measuring intracranial fluid volume has been described,[38] no reported MRI studies have yet demonstrated changes with age. Because the CSF-brain boundary is seen well in both x-ray CT and MRI, however, there is no reason for the results to be different. Measurement of white matter volume is relatively easy in MR images, and one preliminary report suggests no change in volume of white matter with age.[51]

In normal individuals, MRI often reveals focal crescentic or semicircular areas of increased intensity on T_2-weighted scans, capping of the frontal and occipital horns of the lateral ventricles, or pencil-thin bands of hyperintensity along the borders of the body of the lateral ventricles.[189] With age, these changes increase slightly in width; between the third and ninth decade they are found in almost 90% of individuals.[207] The histologic correlate of these changes is astrocytic gliosis, perhaps resulting from seepage of CSF into the parenchyma.

Some normal individuals above age 55 show other areas of increased signal intensity on T_2-weighted scans. These white matter lesions clearly increase in incidence with age and with the presence of cerebrovascular disease, particularly hypertension,[8,84] but their functional significance is unclear. The lesions are patchy, sometimes punctate, nodular or confluent areas in the centrum semiovale and the subcortical white matter of the frontal, parietal, temporal, and occipital lobes. The pathologic bases for these findings are arteriosclerosis, dilated perivascular spaces, vascular ectasia, and gliosis.[7] Preliminary studies[54] examining the metabolic consequences of MRI-defined subcortical white matter signal changes have not found corresponding deficits on fluorodeoxyglucose (FDG) PET scans.

Normal aging is also associated with the progressive accumulation of iron in the brain, especially in the globus pallidus, red nucleus, zona reticulata of the substantia nigra, the subthalamic nucleus of Luys, and the dentate nucleus of the cerebellum. This distribution of iron content is seen in normal elderly individuals as dark areas on T_2-weighted MRI scans using high mag-

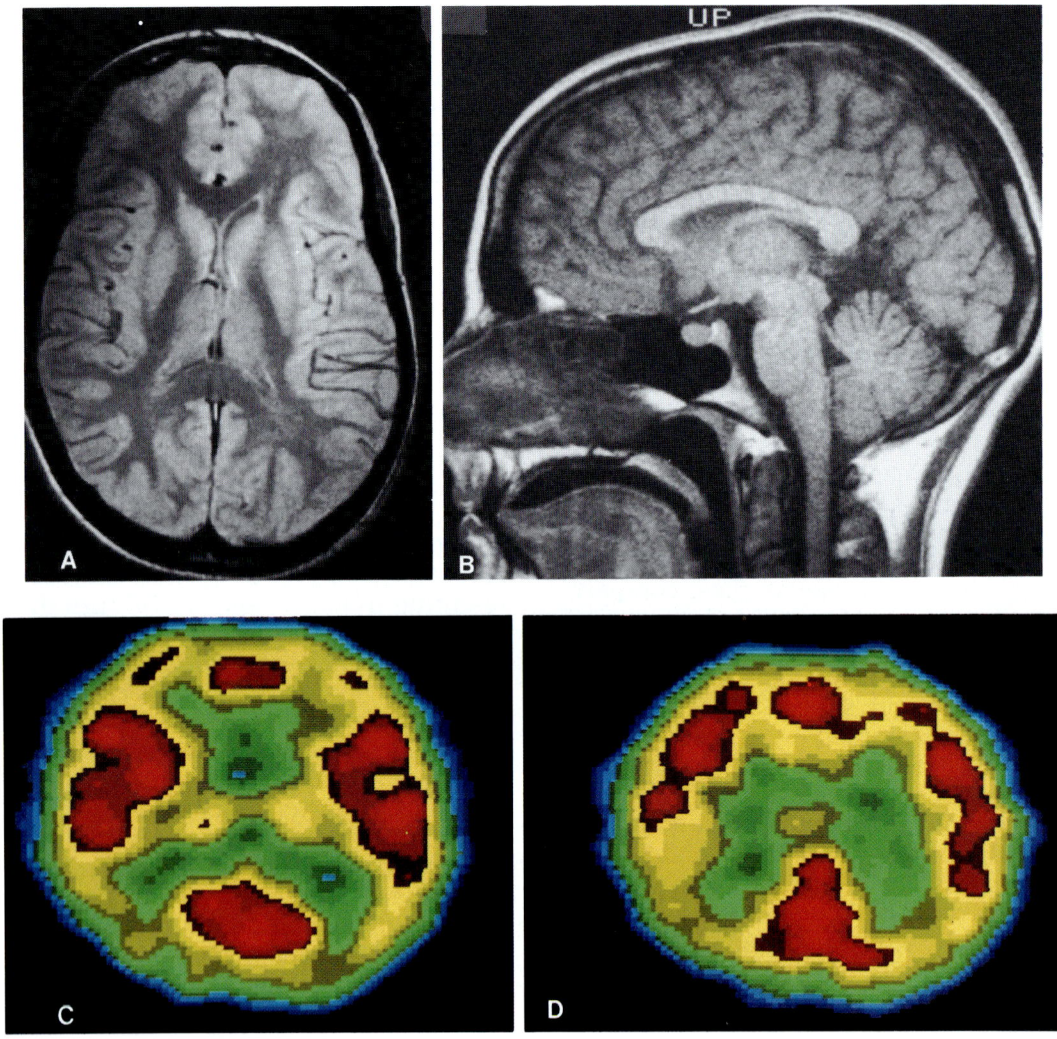

Figure 9–1. Normal young subject. (*A*) MRI horizontal section at the level of the basal ganglia (TR 2500, TE 25, 1.5 T). Note small ventricular size and lack of increased periventricular signal around frontal horns. (*B*) MRI midsagittal section (TR 3000, TE 17, 1.5 T). Note small ventricular and cortical sulcal size. (*C*) PET at basal ganglia level. (All PET studies were performed on a PETT V scanner with 15-mm resolution, using ^{18}F-fluorodeoxyglucose as the tracer.) (*D*) PET at the superior parietal and frontal levels.

netic fields, because the paramagnetic properties of iron accelerate T_2 relaxation time (see chapters 2 and 10).

PET AND SPECT STUDIES

PET and SPECT scan studies of cerebral blood flow (CBF) in normal human aging show a significant reduction with increasing age.* Cerebral glucose metabolism did not appear age-related in the majority of studies using ^{18}FDG or ^{11}C-deoxyglucose and PET,[45,56,58,94,174,204] although one study[116] reported a significant reduc-

*References 28,47,73,120,140,141,149.

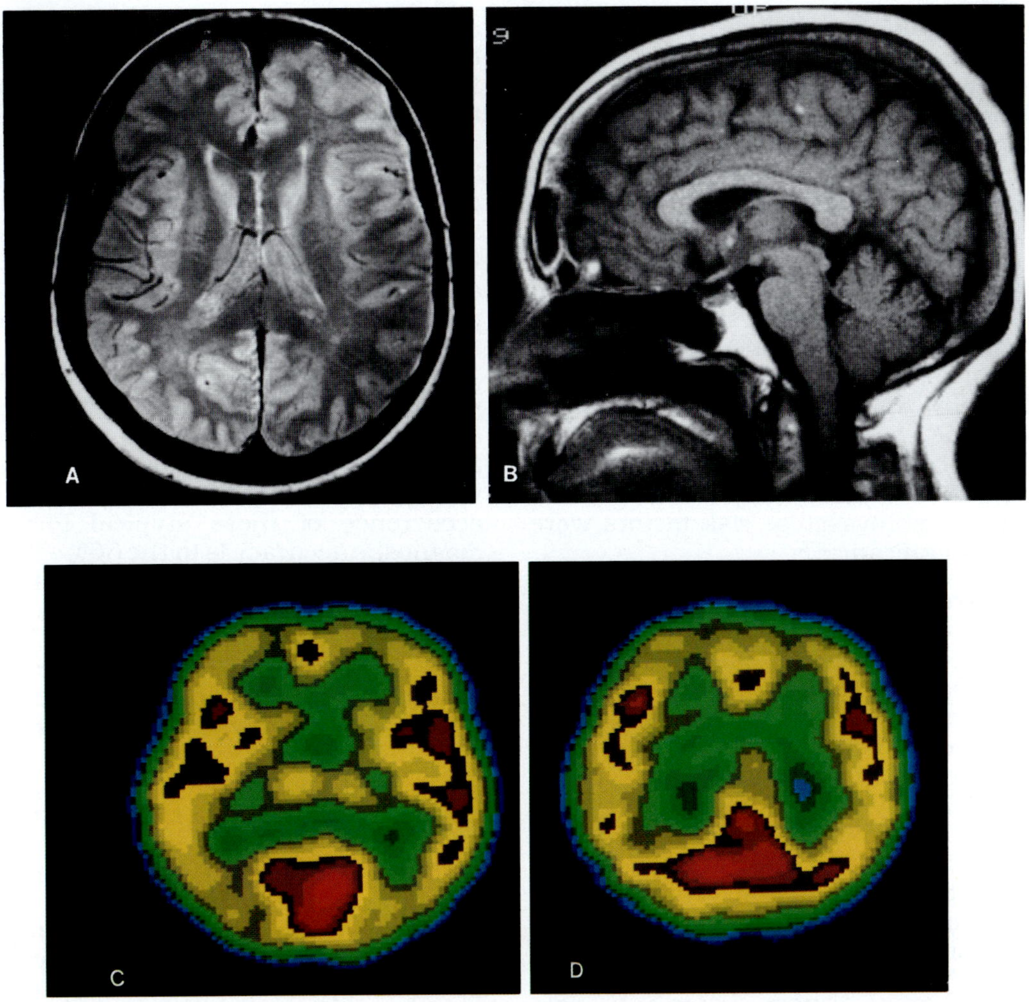

Figure 9–2. Normal elderly subject. (*A*) MRI horizontal section at the level of the basal ganglia (TR 2500, TE 25, 1.5 T). Note slightly increased ventricular size, presence of increased periventricular signal-capping frontal horns. (*B*) MRI midsaggital section (TR 300, TE 17, 1.5 T). Note increased ventricular size, prominence of cortical sulci. (*C*) PET at basal ganglia level. (*D*) PET at superior parietal and frontal level. Note relative frontal hypometabolism compared to young normal.

tion in cerebral metabolic rate for glucose (CMRGlc). Studies with oxygen metabolism ($CMRO_2$) are also inconsistent, with some showing a reduction,[73,124,153] and one showing no reduction with age.[120] Two studies[174,204] showed that when the effects of brain atrophy are accounted for, the age-related decrement in CMRGlc is eliminated.

The ratio of frontal to occipital metabolism tends to decrease with age[3,116,204] (compare parts *C* and *D* of Figs. 9–1 and 9–2). In the "resting" state, most studies demonstrate the highest metabolic rates to be in the calcarine cortex,[3,47,56,116,204] and the right hemisphere tends to have slightly higher metabolic rates or blood flow values than the left hemisphere.[3,47,120,128,155,159] This pattern tends not to change through the age range.[56]

The variability of absolute values of

CBF, $CMRO_2$, and particularly CMRGlc in normal subjects has been a source of concern (see Chapter 3). The variability of CMRGlc increases with advancing age.[56] Different techniques used in many different centers have yielded coefficients of variation of up to 30% in normal subjects. Variability may decrease if individuals are studied when behaviorally activated rather than in the ill-defined resting state,[53] but activation failed to reduce variability of local cerebral blood flow (LCBF) in one study.[10] Among normal subjects, brain volume and extent of cerebral atrophy were found to contribute significantly to the total variance in CMRGlc; age, sex, and cerebrovascular risk factors were not significant.[204]

Atrophy Correction. Because the spatial resolution of current PET and SPECT scanners does not allow definition of the sulci of the cortex, nor delineation of the ventricular margins, metabolically inactive CSF is averaged with metabolically active brain tissue. Global values of CBF, $CMRO_2$, and CMRGlc may be corrected for atrophy by dividing the uncorrected global values by the fraction of intracranial volume occupied by the parenchyma of the brain (as measured by x-ray CT or MRI).[34,98] Such correction increases global values of CBF or $CMRO_2$ by 13% in normal, aged subjects and by 24% in demented subjects;[98] and of CMRGlc by 9% in normal elderly controls and 17% in Alzheimer's patients.[34]

Correction of regional PET measures for the effects of atrophy will be very difficult without computer programs that superimpose corresponding structural images on PET images, to allow automatic atrophy correction for any region of interest.

Alzheimer's Disease

Alzheimer's disease (AD) is a degenerative disorder and the most common neurologic cause of dementia. It presents insidiously with progressive alterations of memory, higher intellectual functions, language, ability to perform skilled movements (praxis), orientation in the environment, and ability to recognize objects, faces, and places (gnosis). It is the classic example of a cortical dementia, although in the later stages of the disease subcortical features (apathy and slowness of response) also become evident, along with extrapyramidal signs (e.g., rigidity), incontinence, and gait apraxia.

Atypical forms of AD are not uncommon and include subtypes with predominant aphasia, visual agnosia, apraxia, right parietal syndromes, or with pure memory loss. In spite of the occurrence of these atypical forms, diagnostic accuracy is in the 66%–90% range,[109] using clinical methods that entail the exclusion of all other known causes of dementia. The NINCDS-ADRDA Workgroup[139] has suggested criteria for the diagnosis of dementia which are currently used widely for research studies.

Neuropathologically, there is no abnormality in AD that is qualitatively different than that seen in some normal aged subjects.[160] Quantitatively, however, there are usually prominent differences. There is marked neuronal loss in the cortex, but especially so in the hippocampus. Senile plaques and neurofibrillary tangles, the most characteristic pathological features of AD, generally occur diffusely in the neocortex, but are most prominent in the hippocampus and amygdala. Other features are granulovacuolar degeneration and Hirano bodies. Neuronal loss and neurofibrillary tangles occur in many subcortical sites as well.

X-RAY CT STUDIES

At least 10 well-controlled x-ray CT studies have been done to evaluate morphologic alterations affecting the ventricles and the sulci in Alzheimer's disease (Table 9–2). These studies are consistent in demonstrating significant alterations, beyond those expected for age, in patients with even the early

Table 9–2 X-RAY CT STUDIES OF ALZHEIMER'S DISEASE AND OTHER DEMENTIAS

		Control		Patients				
Author/Year	***Method of Measurement***	***N***	***$\bar{x}$ Age (yr)***	***N***	***$\bar{x}$ Age (yr)***	***Comments on Subjects***	***Results***	***Comments on Results***
Roberts and Caird,[168] 1976	Maximum ventricular area and sulcal width measurement	17	73 ±7	49	77 ±7	All patients considered to have degenerative dementia. Three grades of dementia.	Ventricular area enlarged in the demented but sulcal area not different.	Correlation of $r = 0.49$ between maximum ventricular area and memory-information test score.
Earnest et al.,[61] 1979	Width of sulci, linear ratios and area of ventricles	30	70 ±5	29	86 ±5	Not a true patient group, some were normals. Not a true control group; some were impaired.	Sulci and ventricles larger in the older and more impaired group.	Correlation up to $r = 0.52$ between psychologic measures and ventricular measures.
deLeon et al.,[44] 1980	Subjective ratings. Linear sulcal and ventricular measurements.	—	—	43	70 ±6	Detailed neurologic and psychiatric evaluation. All considered to have degenerative dementia.	65% of correlations between ventricular rankings and psychiatric test scores were significant. Third ventricle width showed best correlations.	Subjective ranking or rating was superior to linear measurements.
Jacoby and Levy,[106] 1980	Area of ventricle, Evan's ratio and subjective rating of sulci.	50	73 ±6	40	79 ±7	All considered degenerative dementia (but 10 had cerebral infarcts seen on x-ray CT).	All measures showed highly significant differences between subject groups.	Highest correlation between ventricular area and memory. CT indices predicted group membership in 83% of cases.

(Continued)

Table 9–2—*Continued*

Author/Year	Method of Measurement	Control		Patients		Comments on Subjects	Results	Comments on Results
		N	$\bar{x}$ Age (yr)	N	$\bar{x}$ Age (yr)			
Brinkman et al.,[23] 1981	Bifrontal and bicaudate ratios. Area of ventricles, distance from third ventricle to Sylvian fissure (3V-SF), sulcal width measurement.	30	80 ±7	28	60 ±9	All considered degenerative dementia (mild dementia: mean WAIS Verbal IQ = 88.8). Patients significantly younger than controls.	No differences in bicaudate, bifrontal ratios. Age-corrected ventricular area larger in the demented group; 3V-SF significantly less in demented group; sulcal width larger in controls.	Correlations between Verbal and Performance IQ and ventricular area/brain area ratio was $r = 0.53$, and −0.65 respectively. 96% of demented patients and 41% of controls had abnormal findings for at least one measure.
Ito et al.,[103] 1981	Pixel counts of cranial volume, CSF volume, and brain volume	130	20–79			Although all subjects were described as normal, some demented patients clearly were included. Patients were not separated from controls.	Significant increase in CSF volume and decrease in brain volume with age	Brain volume was correlated with a mental status score ($r = -0.43$)
Wu et al.,[201] 1981	Linear measurements and subjective rating of ventricular and sulcal size	31	50–77	24	50–77	Controls had neurologic symptoms, were not demented, and had no focal lesions on x-ray CT. Patients were not separated out in any of the analyses.	Highest correlation between x-ray CT and behavioral measures was that of orientation and bicaudate index ($r = -0.52$).	With the exception of the sulcal measures, all other x-ray CT measures correlated significantly with at least one behavioral measure.

Gado et al.,[80] 1982	Pixel counts for ventricles, subarachnoid space, and cranial cavity. Linear indices and subjective ratings also obtained.	27	65–83	20	65–81	Controls described as healthy. Patients clinically diagnosed to have mild AD.	Volumetric measures were clearly better than linear measures in separating demented patients from controls, although both gave significant results for ventricular and subarachnoid space.	An unspecified degree of overlap was found between controls and patients using any of the x-ray CT measures.
Wilson et al.,[198] 1982	Linear and subjective ratings of ventricular and sulcal size. X-ray CT density measures in 14 brain regions.	38	69	42	69	Controls were healthy. All patients were clinically diagnosed to have AD.	On a composite score patients had more atrophy than did controls. High degree of overlap was noted between groups (not quantified). None of the x-ray CT density measures was different between groups.	Wechsler Memory Scale scores were correlated with atrophy ($r = -0.39$) only for the combined patient and control group.
Soininen et al.,[183] 1982	Linear measures of ventricular and sulcal size	85	75 ±7	76	77 ±6	Controls healthy and neurologically normal. Using Hachinski scores, 57 patients had AD and 19 had multi-infarct dementia (MID).	Demented patients showed significant increases over controls in all measures. Overlap was noted particularly between mildly demented and control groups. AD patients had larger ventricles than MID patients.	Psychological test scores correlated with ventricular but not sulcal measures of atrophy. Highest correlation ($r = -0.49$) was between the frontal horn index and activities-of-daily-living score.

(*Continued*)

Table 9–2—*Continued*

Author/Year	Method of Measurement	Control		Patients		Comments on Subjects	Results	Comments on Results
		N	$\bar{x}$ Age (yr)	N	$\bar{x}$ Age (yr)			
Eslinger et al.,[65] 1984	Area measurement of frontal horns, third ventricles, and bodies of lateral ventricles and interhemispheric fissure.	26	75 ±6	26	75 ±6	Controls described as unequivocally normal on clinical, x-ray CT and neuropsychologic criteria. Patients clinically diagnosed as degenerative (46%), vascular (15%), and miscellaneous (39%) dementias.	Demented patients differed from controls in third and lateral ventricle and frontal horn measurements. Highest behavioral correlations were with x-ray CT measures of bodies of lateral ventricles ($r = 0.63$).	Correct classification into normal or dementia groups was 73%, 83% and 92% using x-ray CT only, neuro-psychologic only, and combined CT and neuro-psychologic criteria, respectively.
Albert et al.,[4] 1984	Area measurements of CSF space and linear measures of ventricular size. Tissue density (CT number) measures also done.	10	57 (53–64)	8	58 (53–64)	Controls were described as free of systemic disease. Patients were clinically diagnosed as having presenile dementia of the Alzheimer's type. All	Fluid volume in the bodies of the lateral ventricles was significantly greater in demented patients than in controls	Highest correlation between behavioral measures and area of bodies of lateral ventricles was $r = -0.68$.

						patients were considered to have mild dementia.	and correctly predicted group membership in 89% of subjects. No tissue density differences were noted.	
Yerby et al.,[203] 1985	Area measurement of CSF (subarachnoid and ventricular) space and ratio of brain to intracranial space (CT ratio).	—	—	117	75 (54–94)	Patients were clinically diagnosed as AD alone (60%), AD with depression (14%), depression alone (13%), and other diagnoses (13%).	Age accounted for 11% and diagnostic category accounted for only 4% of the total variance in CT ratios.	CT ratio could not separate those with and without dementia. Correlations of CT and neuropsychologic measures was poor, particularly in demented subjects.
LeMay et al.,[123] 1986	Perceptual ratings (0–4 scale) for atrophy in 13 regions by 3 neuroradiologists; and linear measurements.	22	65	24	67	Healthy controls. Patients were all diagnosed to have AD, but degree of dementia was not stated.	Perceptual rating, which was superior to linear measures, correctly classified over 80% of subjects. Specific temporal lobe atrophic changes discriminated up to 90% of subjects correctly.	The size of the suprasellar cistern, and the width of the interhemispheric fissure and Sylvan fissures were the best discriminators.

stages of AD. There is general agreement that for the purposes of quantitation, linear measures are inferior to area or volumetric measures of ventricular enlargement. In assessing morphologic changes of ventricle size and cortical atrophy, perceptual ratings by experienced observers have been shown to be quite sensitive and reliable.[123] This last point is important from a clinical standpoint, in that most neurologists or radiologists do not make detailed measurements routinely from x-ray CT scans. There is general agreement that x-ray CT scan measures of cortical atrophy, as assessed by an increase in the subarachnoid space, are unreliable and insensitive to the changes in AD.[44,65,201] Loss of gray-white matter discriminability in AD has been reported[82] but has not yet been confirmed. CT measures of attenuation in Hounsfield or other units have not shown any consistent differences between AD and control subjects, although one study[4] initially reported lower CT numbers in patients with senile dementia.

In spite of statistically significant greater ventricular and sulcal size in AD patients compared with age-matched controls, the discrimination between these two subject groups cannot be made with a high degree of certainty. Particularly in the earlier stages of AD, a great deal of overlap exists between normal and AD patients in the degree of brain atrophy. Many cognitively normal elderly subjects have enlargement of ventricles or relatively prominent cortical atrophy, and many patients with mild AD have unimpressive atrophic features. Therefore, an x-ray CT scan demonstrating cerebral atrophy in any one patient does not assist in the clinical evaluation of possible dementia. The history, examination, and assessment of the behavior of the patient remain the most important evidence in determining the presence of dementia. In spite of the poor separation of the findings in normal aging and AD, the x-ray CT scan is of great utility in excluding certain causes of dementia other than AD (e.g., multi-infarct dementia, cerebral tumor, subdural hematoma, and normal pressure hydrocephalus).

X-ray CT scan studies, summarized in Table 9–2, have demonstrated a gross overall relationship between quantitative measures of loss of brain tissue and behavioral deterioration. Brain atrophy does not explain more than 40% to 45% of the variance in behavioral measures, however. For example, studies of demented patients, or combined normal and demented patients, have shown correlation coefficients of 0.29–0.65 between x-ray CT measures of brain atrophy and psychologic function.[44,61,65,103,106,201] Methodologic factors, such as the validity of linear measurements in the brain as indices of volumetric change, and the reliability and validity of psychologic measures as indices of brain function, may have contributed to a weakening of morphology-behavior correlations in the brain.

Because dementia is a heterogenous syndrome, patients with AD and with multi-infarct dementia ideally have not been lumped together in an analysis of structure-function relationships.[65] AD itself may be heterogenous, however, and there may be specific subtypes distinguishable clinically and with neuroimaging approaches, with corresponding distinct cognitive subtypes. Behavioral heterogeneity in AD is well known.[18,135] Associations of behavioral subtypes of AD with the rate of progression of the disease or genetic forms of the disease have been described.[22,35] The relationship of any of these behavioral subtypes to specific neuroimaging-neuroanatomic features would be of great interest, but this remains to be defined. For example, asymmetry of ventricles and of cortical atrophy in AD has not been alluded to in any of the quantitative studies described in Table 9–2. In a review of x-ray CT changes in dementing disease, LeMay[121] singles out only Pick's disease as showing asymmetrical atrophy. In clinical practice, however, obvious asymmetry of ventricles and of cortical atrophy is observed frequently in patients with probable AD.

In recent x-ray CT and MRI studies, it has been emphasized that changes in periventricular white matter in cases clinically diagnosed as having AD occur frequently.[64,66,169,187] These periventricular white matter lucencies are more common in demented subjects than in age-matched controls.[64,83] When patients with AD are classified on the basis of the occurrence of periventricular white matter lucencies on x-ray CT scans, those with such lucencies perform worse on cognitive tests than those without,[187] and the severity of the dementia is correlated with the extent of the white matter lucencies. Many patients with clinical features of AD and with lucencies on x-ray CT have been found at autopsy to have AD.[63,83,129,194] Corresponding to the white matter lucencies demonstrated on x-ray CT, pathologic abnormalities that have been described in these brain regions include demyelination, axonal loss, hyalinization and fibrous thickening of medullary arterioles, and cystic degeneration.[83,129]

MRI STUDIES

MRI is more sensitive than x-ray CT to the changes that occur in the brains of patients with dementia.[64,83,110] The abnormalities that are especially amenable to definition by MRI are periventricular and subcortical white matter lesions, atrophy of gray matter structures such as the hippocampus and amygdala, and enlargement of basal cisterns and the Sylvian fissure[110] (Fig. 9–3*A*,*B*). In T_2-weighted images, areas of high signal intensity affecting hippocampal and Sylvian cortex have also been described in AD patients.[66]

A comprehensive study of neuropathologic alterations and postmortem MR relaxation times of white matter in patients with AD[24,63] demonstrated that incomplete white matter infarction was encountered in 60% of patients. This infarction was characterized by loss of myelin, axons, and oligodendrogial cells, mild reactive astrocytic gliosis, and hyaline fibrosis of arterioles in the deep white matter. These pathologic changes gradually decreased in severity as the cortex was approached. In parallel to these pathologic changes, prolongation of T_1 and T_2 relaxation times occurred. The MR imaging characteristics that would correspond to these T_1 and T_2 changes would be decreased signal intensity in T_1-weighted and increased intensity in T_2-weighted images in a predominantly periventricular distribution. One group of researchers[64] noted that the MRI showed periventricular "white matter changes" in about one third of their cases with AD. They did not study normal controls, however, so it is not known whether these periventricular changes were in excess of that expected for age.

The high sensitivity of MRI for detecting changes in the brain has been both an asset and a source of confusion. The profusion of abnormalities seen on MRI often leaves the clinician unable to categorize a patient because of the present lack of adequate data regarding the normal accompaniments of aging and the specific MRI features of multi-infarct dementia. The additional information contributed by MRI studies in AD patients has not yet resulted in an increase in the specificity of diagnosis. Thus, at the present time, both x-ray CT and MRI are used primarily for excluding other causes of dementia in the diagnosis of Alzheimer's disease.

Nevertheless, a recent study has shed some light on this problem. Fazekas and colleagues[66] described the MRI findings in patients with clinically diagnosed probable and possible Alzheimer's disease and compared them with patients diagnosed to have multi-infarct dementia. A "halo" of periventricular hyperintensity frequently was found in AD patients (Fig. 9–4). This halo is characterized by a smooth margin and is significantly more extensive than the hyperintensity found in controls. Hence the increase in high-sig-

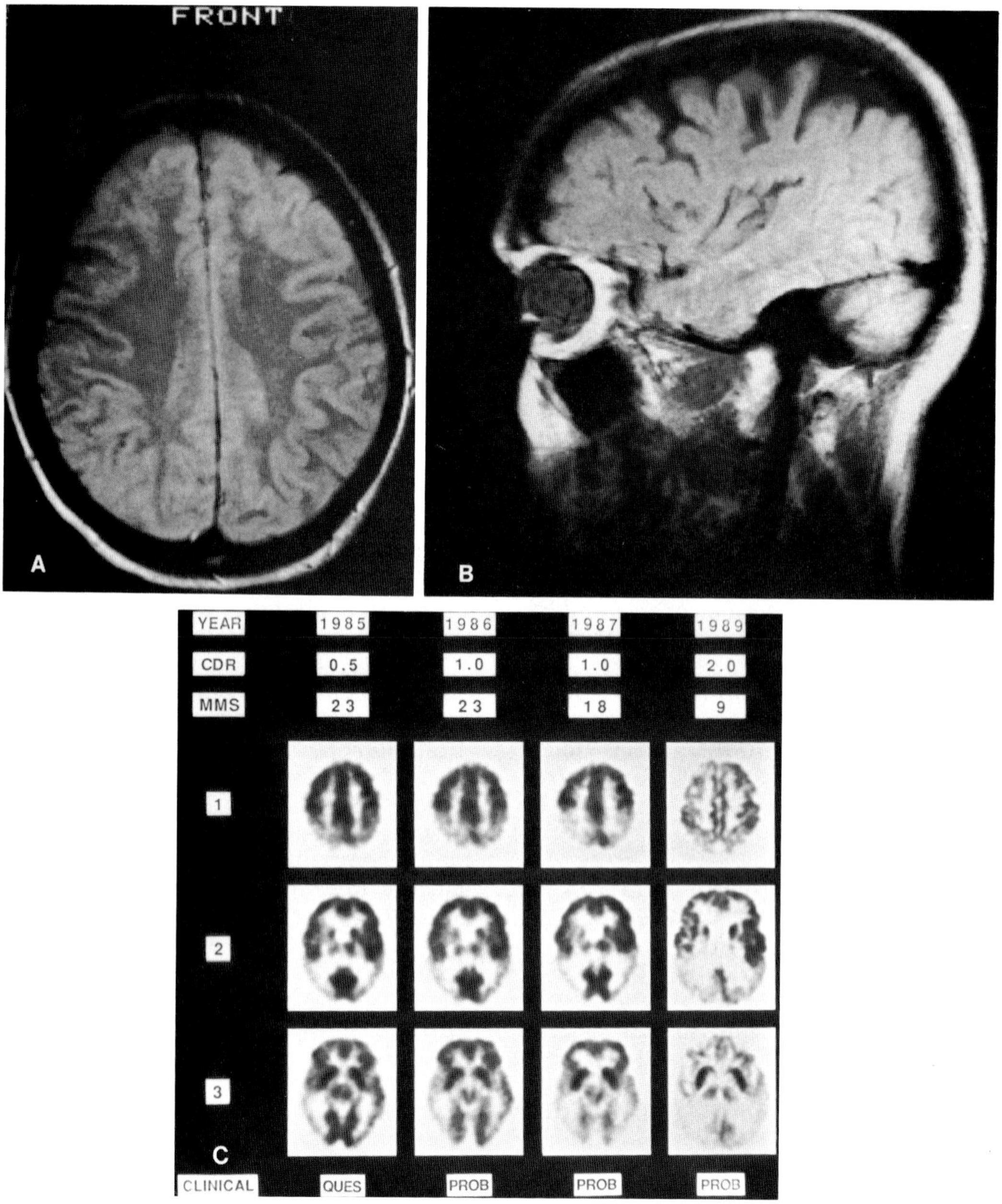

Figure 9–3. Alzheimer's disease. (*A*) MRI horizontal section (TR 2500, TE 25, 1.5 T). Note increase in sulcal size. (*B*) MRI midsagittal section (TR 300, TE 17, 1.5 T). Note prominence of cortical sulci with evident gyral atrophy at the vertex and superior parietal region. (*C*) PET at basal ganglia level. Note decrease in metabolism in association cortices of parietotemporal and frontal regions, relative sparing of occipital, basal ganglia regions. (*D*) PET superior parietal and frontal region level. Note predominant parietal metabolic deficits.

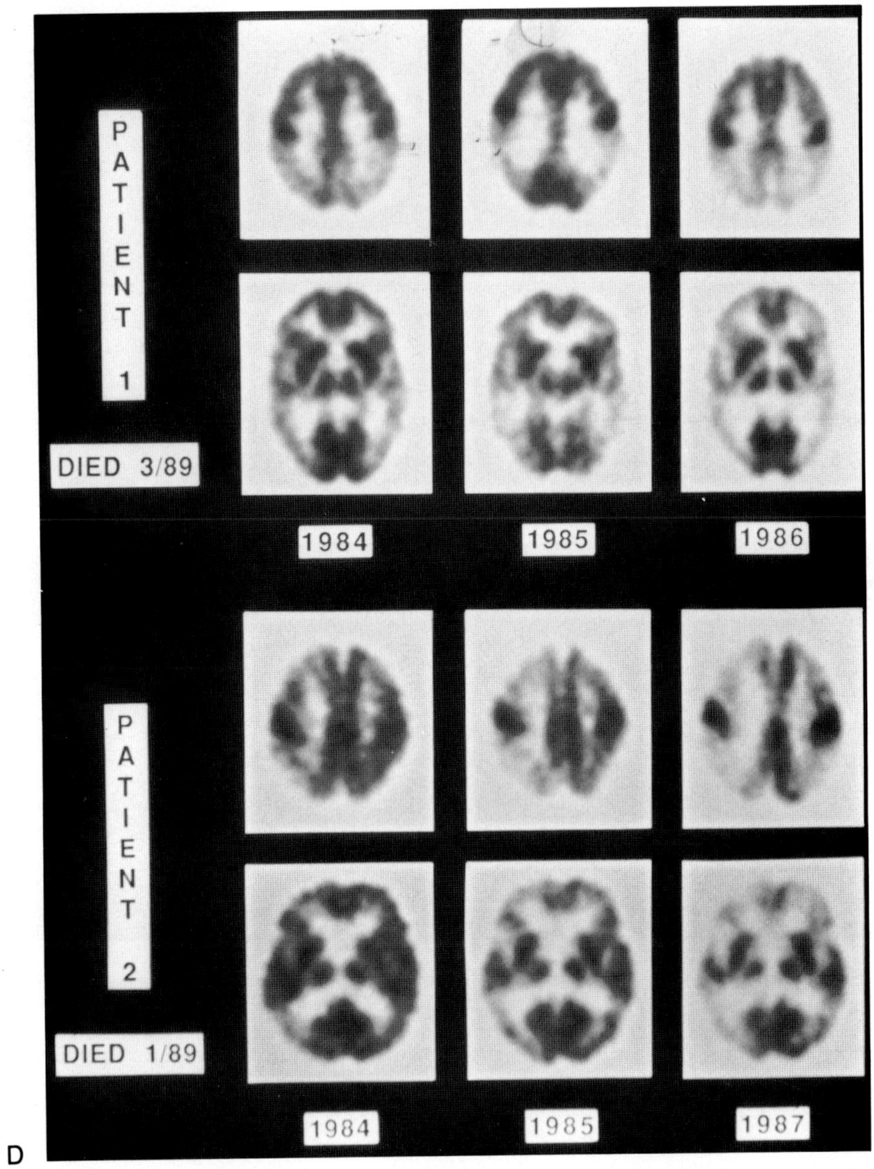

Figure 9-3. *Continued.* (*C*) PET images demonstrate the serial progression of changes in glucose metabolism in a single patient with clinically probable Alzheimer's disease, studied four times between 1985 and 1989. The patient's Clinical Dementia Rating scale (CDR) and Mini-Mental State score (MMS) demonstrate increasing dementia. In these and other images, the left hemisphere is on the reader's left, and black represents the highest metabolic rate. In 1985, decrements in glucose metabolism are seen bilaterally in the superior parietal cortex. These spread to involve superior temporal cortical zones and the entire parietal neocortex by 1987. In 1989, all neocortical areas, including prefrontal cortex, are hypometabolic relative to the less affected sensory-motor cortices, striata, and thalamus. Note also that between 1987 and 1989 the patient experienced a small cerebral infarction affecting the optic radiations leading to the left occipital lobe, which resulted in markedly lower metabolism in the left occipital lobe compared to the right (rows 2 and 3). (*D*) Serial PET studies of glucose metabolism in two patients with autopsy confirmation of Alzheimer's disease. The spatial extent of glucose hypometabolism increases sequentially, beginning in the superior portions of the parietal lobe and extending to the superior temporal and frontal cortices. The thalami, striata, and the auditory, visual, sensorimotor, and cingulate cortices are relatively spared. Hypometabolic zones affect both hemispheres, but the degree of reduction is symmetric in patient 1 and asymmetric (left < right) in patient 2.

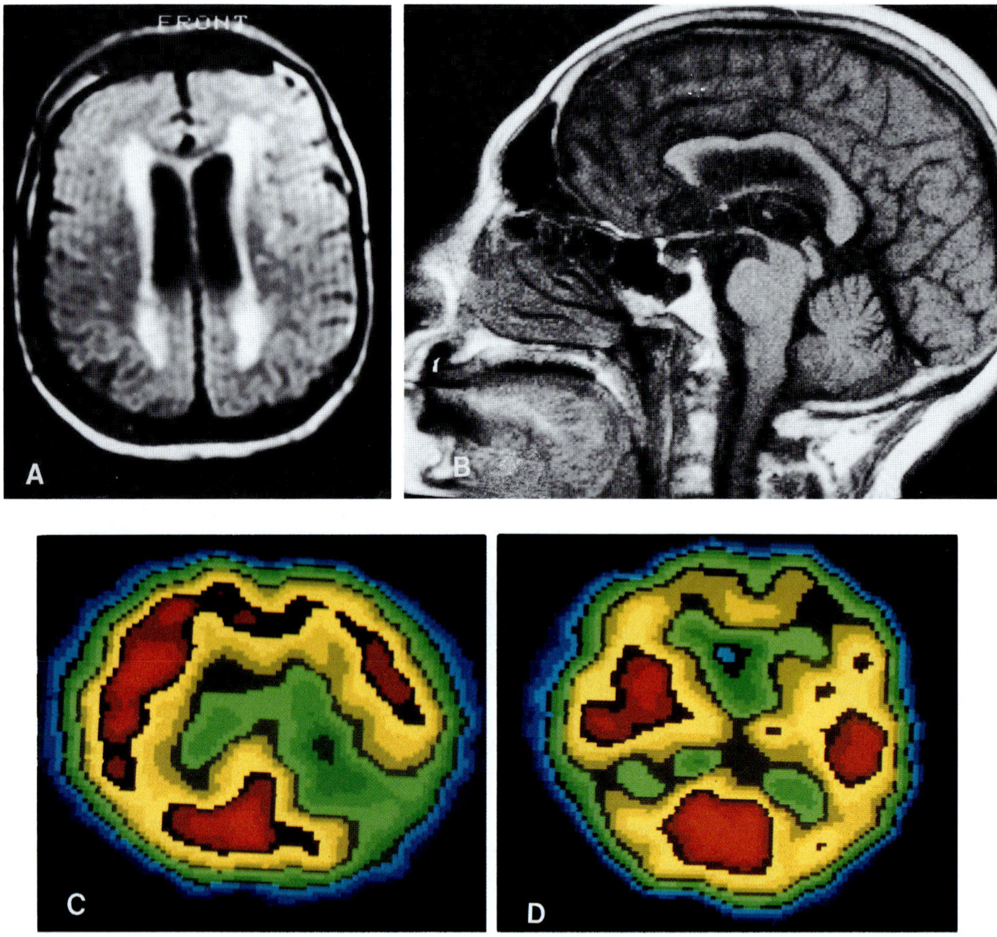

Figure 9–4. Alzheimer's disease. (*A*) MRI horizontal section (midventricular level) (TR 2500, TE 25, 1.5 T). Prominent periventricular white-matter changes (increased signal) extending into the white matter of the frontal and parieto-occipital lobes. (*B*) MRI midsagittal section (TR 300, TE 17, 1.5 T). Note relative thinning of corpus callosum, but normal brainstem (pontine tegmentum, aqueduct of Sylvius, and fourth ventricle size). (*C*) PET at high ventricular level. Note marked asymmetry in parietal metabolism. (*D*) PET at midventricular level. Note greater frontal than parietal metabolic deficits.

nal-intensity area in the immediate vicinity of the ventricles can be associated with AD alone, without any component of vascular dementia. Another type of lesion outside of the immediate periventricular area comprises punctate or partially confluent deep-white-matter foci of hyperintensity, which are fairly frequently found in controls as well as in AD and MID patients. The existence of these foci does not imply vascular dementia. On the other hand, extensive, irregular periventricular hyperintensity and widespread confluent areas of deep-white-matter hyperintensity were found only in cases of multi-infarct or mixed dementia.

PET STUDIES

Although the gross morphologic changes in the brain in the early stages of Alzheimer's disease are subtle and variable as judged by x-ray CT and MRI scanning, alterations in function are more evident. Because a variety of functional parameters in the brain can be examined using PET and SPECT (see Chapters 3 and 4), these methods should be ideal in depicting abnormalities very early in the course of Alzheimer's disease. Moreover, function in the brain can be evaluated under a variety of behavioral and pharmacologic conditions. The optimal condition for functional abnormalities in AD may be different in different subtypes or stages of the disease. Very little work has been done thus far in exploiting such functional states to study AD, so as to enhance metabolic or blood flow deficits. Manipulating the functional conditions of a PET study also may be useful in clarifying some aspect of the pathophysiology of AD.

Table 9–3 lists studies done in the "resting state" to study Alzheimer's disease by PET. With the exception of a study by Frackowiak and coworkers,[74] who used ^{15}O-labeled molecular oxygen and carbon dioxide to study cerebral blood flow, oxygen extraction ratio, and oxygen consumption, all the other studies have been done using ^{18}F-labeled fluorodeoxyglucose (FDG). The earlier studies[13,46,67,74] focused on alterations in absolute metabolic rate in AD patients, whereas later studies examined the regional pattern of change in metabolism.

In general, an inverse correlation has been found between absolute metabolic rates and the severity of dementia; that is, the more severe the dementia, the lower were the global glucose and oxygen metabolic rates and the cerebral blood flow. The extent of reduction in metabolic rate in severe dementia has been reported to be from 31%[74] to 49%.[13] In the mild and moderate stages of AD, however, often no significant reduction in absolute metabolic rate has been found.[40,57,95] Many studies have addressed the regional alterations in metabolic rate and the right-left asymmetries in metabolic rate that have been observed in patients with AD (see Figs. 9–3, 9–4*C,D*). The pattern that has consistently been reported in AD is one of regional deficits in the association neocortices (e.g., parietotemporal, prefrontal) and relative sparing of primary sensory and motor cortices, such as peri-Rolandic and medial occipital, as well as the basal ganglia, thalamus, and cerebellar hemispheres (Fig. 9–4 *C, D*) (see Fig. 9–3). Association cortex hypometabolism in AD has usually been reported to affect the parietotemporal regions to a greater extent and earlier in the course of the disease than frontal regions. In Down's syndrome patients, who are known invariably to have the neuropathology of AD by the age of 40 years, metabolic deficits similar to those described in AD have been found to occur when progressive dementia occurs.[178]

The finding of asymmetric metabolic deficits in AD was somewhat surprising when initially reported because the degenerative changes were understood to be relatively diffuse. In fact, it was expected that asymmetric metabolic deficits would be a differentiating feature of multi-infarct dementia.[13] It has been reported that in AD, asymmetric metabolic deficits appear early in the disease course and the side of predominant involvement correlates with the dominant neuropsychologic deficit that is found. Patients with predominant language deficits manifest predominant left-sided metabolic deficits and those with dominant visuoconstructive deficits manifest predominant right-sided metabolic deficits.[71,95] Moreover, it appears that metabolic asymmetries may occur before, and predict the pattern of, "neocortically mediated" neuropsychologic deficits.[96]

The pathophysiology of the metabolic deficits in AD has been the source of some speculation. Two major possibilities exist. First, that pathology in the neocortical association areas in parietal, temporal, and frontal regions gives rise to the metabolic deficits in these same regions. Second, that pathology in other brain regions is manifested primarily as deficits in association neocortical regions, because of transneuronal functional disconnection (diaschisis) effects. Evidence in support of the first hypothesis is that the distribution of neuronal loss in the neocortex of AD patients is similar to the distribution of metabolic deficits, particularly in the early stages of the disease.[25,75] The lack of prominent metabolic deficits in me-

Table 9–3 POSITRON EMISSION TOMOGRAPHY IN DEMENTIA

		Control		Patients				
Author/Year	***Type of Study***	***N***	***$\bar{x}$ Age (yr)***	***N***	***$\bar{x}$ Age (yr)***	***Comments on Subjects***	***Results***	***Comments on Results***
Ferris et al.,[67] 1980	^{18}F-FDG (glucose metabolism)	3	63 ±7	7	73 ±5	Healthy controls. Patients were diagnosed as having mild (2), moderate (3) and moderate-severe (2) Alzheimer's disease.	Metabolic rate in frontal, temporal cortices and caudate, thalamus in patients was 33–37% below control values.	Control group was too small for adequate comparison. Analysis was preliminary. Correlation between behavioral decline and metabolic decline was found.
Frackowiak et al.,[74] 1981	Blood flow, oxygen metabolism, and oxygen extraction ratio	14	61 ±8	22	66 ±9	Healthy controls. Patients were diagnosed as degenerative (13) or vascular (9) dementia; severity was moderate (11) and severe (11).	Degenerative and vascular patients had a parallel reduction of LCBF and $LCMRO_2$, with the parietal region being most affected (−33%). Occipital regions were least affected (−19%).	Asymmetries were not studied; however, those with severe aphasia had greater left temporal $LCMRO_2$ reduction. Correlation found between dementia severity and flow/metabolism reduction.
deLeon et al.,[46] 1983	Glucose metabolism	22	66 ±7	24	73 ±7	Healthy controls. Patients were diagnosed as having AD.	Reductions of 17% (caudate) to 24% (parietal) found in AD patients. Membership in AD or control groups could be predicted in 80% of subjects, by regional metabolic rates.	Correlations of up to 0.73 found between memory tests and regional metabolism. Asymmetries were not specifically examined.

Friedland et al.,[78] 1983	Glucose metabolism	6	64 ±8	10	65 ±7	Healthy controls. Patients diagnosed as having AD.	Prominent asymmetries in some, but anterior-posterior differences were consistent in AD. Frontal/temporoparietal ratio was 1.00–1.04 in controls and 1.34–1.54 in AD patients.	This study highlighted the regional temporoparietal metabolic deficits in AD and emphasized asymmetries as well. Relative sparing of occipital metabolism also noted.
Foster et al.,[71] 1983	Glucose metabolism			13	59	Clinically diagnosed to have AD. Three had prominent language deficit and four had predominant visuoconstructive apraxia.	Metabolic deficits of 19% (left temporo-parietal) in the aphasic patients and 31% (right parietal) in apraxic patients.	Correlation between language performance and left temporal metabolism (r = 0.71) and between visuoconstructive tests and right parietal metabolism was as high as $r = 0.81$.
Benson et al.,[13] 1983	Glucose metabolism	16		11		Controls were not described. Eight patients had AD (Hachinski scores less than 4). Three had MID ("high" Hachinski scores), but with normal x-ray CT scans.	AD patients had 49% and MID patients had 35% reduction in metabolic rate. In AD and MID, parietotemporal association cortex was most affected and primary visual cortex was least affected.	Authors state that in contrast to the frontoparietal association cortex deficits in AD, there is a variable pattern in MID. (Subject number is small and reliability of diagnosis in MID group is unclear).

(Continued)

Table 9–3—*Continued*

Author/Year	Type of Study	Control N	Control $\bar{x}$ Age (yr)	Patients N	Patients $\bar{x}$ Age (yr)	Comments on Subjects	Results	Comments on Results
Chase et al.,[33] 1984	Glucose metabolism	5	57 ±2	17	61 ±2	Patients diagnosed to have AD ("minimal" to severe dementia). All subjects received WAIS IQ subtests. Correlations done on the control and patient groups together.	WAIS IQ scores correlated with overall metabolism ($r = 0.68$). Verbal IQ correlated best with left temporal ($r = 0.76$) and performance IQ with right parietal metabolism ($r = 0.70$).	WAIS Arithmetic subtests correlated best with left inferior parietal–superior temporal metabolism, whereas digit span correlated best with anterior and superior frontal metabolism bilaterally.
Friedland et al.,[76] 1984	Glucose metabolism	7	63 ±3	2	63& 64	Mild and moderate AD. Patients also had x-ray CT and MRI evaluation.	MRI and x-ray CT showed only symmetrical ventricular enlargement in one patient, and symmetrical ventricular enlargement and cortical atrophy in the other. Both patients had predominant right sided temporo-parietal metabolic deficits.	Author concludes that PET is superior to MRI and x-ray CT in diagnosis of AD.
Haxby et al.,[95] 1985	Glucose metabolism	26	63 (45–83)	10	64 ±9	Healthy controls. Patients had mild-to-moderate dementia. Ten patients and 10	Temporal, parietal and frontal association cortices showed metabolic deficits and	No difference between patients and controls in absolute metabolic rates. Sensorimotor and

						controls were tested with a syntax comprehension test, a drawing test, and memory tests.	asymmetries in AD patients relative to controls. The direction of these asymmetries was related to asymmetries of language and visuospatial function.	visual cortices showed no deficits, and asymmetry was not greater in these structures than in controls.
Kuhl et al.,[117] 1985	Glucose metabolism	14	—	14	—	Controls not described. Patients consisted of AD (n = 28), Parkinson's dementia (PD) (n = 14) and MID (n = 6). Degree of dementia described as questionable, mild, moderate, and severe.	Parietal/cerebellar metabolic ratio was 0.84 in AD, 0.94 in PD, 1.28 in controls, and 1.29 in MID.	Parietal/cerebellar ratio correlated with severity ($r = 0.69$) and duration ($r = 0.46$) of dementia.
Cutler et al.,[40] 1985	Glucose metabolism	12	58 ±4	1	57	Patient had familial AD (father and paternal great aunt had autopsy-proven AD and two other paternal relatives had dementia). PET scan and psychological testing was repeated twice at 8-mo intervals.	Mild memory loss and normal WAIS IQ subtests were present initially and were not measurably worse subsequently. Metabolic pattern initially normal. Parietal deficits present in second and third scans.	Author shows that very early in the disease metabolic deficits may not be present. Without objective behavioral deterioration, metabolic deficits appeared in subsequent scans.
Alavi et al.,[3] 1986	Glucose metabolism	11	—	17	—	Patients had probable AD.	A tendency to left parietal and left temporal metabolic deficits in mild and moderate patients became significant in severe cases.	Reduction was 17% in the left temporal and 42% in the left inferior parietal regions, in severe AD.

(Continued)

Table 9–3—*Continued*

Author/Year	Type of Study	Control N	Control $\bar{x}$ Age (yr)	Patients N	Patients $\bar{x}$ Age (yr)	Comments on Subjects	Results	Comments on Results
Duara et al.,[57] 1986	Glucose metabolism	29	63 ±10	21	64 ±9	Controls were healthy. Patients had probable AD (10 mild, 7 moderate, and 4 severe cases).	Global metabolism was reduced in severe cases only. In mild AD, deficits occurred in the parietal lobe only, but in moderate and severe cases temporal and frontal lobes were also affected.	Asymmetries occurred in parietal regions only in mild AD and in frontal and parietal regions, in moderate AD. Predominant left temporal deficits were found in severe AD. Five moderate AD patients showed reduction in WAIS IQ without change in metabolism, on follow-up scans.
McGeer et al.,[138] 1986	Glucose metabolism	11	66	14	69	Controls were neurologically normal. Patients had mild (n = 4), moderate (n = 5), and severe dementia (n = 5). MRI or x-ray CT scans were also obtained.	Metabolic rates reduced by 32%, 24%, 20%, and 18% in temporal, frontal, parietal, and occipital cortices, respectively.	Asymmetries occurred in all cortical regions in AD patients, greatest in the temporal. Authors conclude that atrophy could not account for the regional hypometabolism seen.

Haxby et al.,[96] 1986	Glucose metabolism	29	64 ±11	22	65 ±9	Healthy controls. Patients had probable AD (10 mild and 12 moderate cases). Memory, language and visuospatial function were also assessed.	Mild cases had memory deficits and metabolic asymmetries but without any language or visuospatial deficits. Moderate cases showed metabolic asymmetries with appropriate asymmetries of language vs. visuospatial function.	The authors conclude that cortical metabolic dysfunction is evident in early AD, often preceding the appearance of neocortically mediated neuropsychologic dysfunction. In moderate AD, metabolic and neuropsychologic asymmetries are correlated.
Loewenstein et al.,[128] 1987	Glucose metabolism	45	68 ±9	42	73 ±10	Healthy controls. Patients were divided into those with AD (n = 31) and MID (n = 11). MRI-detected lesions were quantified in MID patients.	71% of AD patients had abnormal scans (outside 95% confidence limits for regional asymmetry or hypometabolism). 48% had predominant left and 13% predominant right-sided hypometabolism. 64% of MID patients had abnormal scans; 46% had predominant left and 9% predominant right-sided hypometabolism.	This study quantified the number of patients with abnormal scans for each diagnostic group (AD and MID). In both groups significantly more had left- than right-sided hypometabolism. MRI lesions were not asymmetrical in MID patients.

dial temporal cortex,[69] where the pathology is known to be most severe in early AD, however, goes against this theory. Degeneration in basal forebrain nuclei or in amygdala-hippocampal regions, both of which regions are known to project heavily to association neocortex, could result in disconnection of and hypometabolism in these neocortical regions.

In a single case of AD in whom antemortem PET scan findings of glucose metabolism were correlated with postmortem neuropathologic findings,[137] the left hemisphere, especially in the parietal regions, showed far greater atrophic changes than the right on gross pathology. Metabolism also was reduced asymmetrically, with predominant left-hemisphere hypometabolism. Reduced metabolism correlated best with severity of gliosis and least with the number of plaques in a brain area.

PET has been used to study the blood-brain barrier in AD,[77,173] but no disruption of the barrier has been detected by the methods used. Behavioral activation studies in AD patients[15,53,142] have not as yet yielded any results that have improved diagnostic ability or clarified the pathophysiology of AD.

SPECT STUDIES

Several SPECT imaging studies have been reported in Alzheimer's patients, with either ^{123}I-labeled iodoamphetamine or ^{99m}Tc-labeled HMPAO used to obtain measures of cerebral blood flow (see Chapter 4). These studies have demonstrated the same distribution of deficits as are evident on PET studies of blood flow or glucose metabolism.* The greater availability of SPECT cameras and the lack of the necessity for a local cyclotron to produce the isotopes needed for SPECT studies makes SPECT an attractive alternative to PET for assessment of the functional disturbances in dementia, although the poorer spatial resolution and lack of true quantitation of data remain disadvantages.

*References 17, 32, 37, 97, 108, 110, 150, 156, 179.

Parkinson's Disease

Parkinson's disease is a degenerative disorder and is a major neurologic cause of morbidity in the middle-aged and elderly patient (see Chapter 8). The clinical features are those of resting tremor, rigidity, bradykinesia, and postural changes. Most studies of the behavior of Parkinson's patients demonstrate a certain degree of alteration in performance measures of the IQ, along with slowing of responses (bradyphrenia) and the frequent co-occurrence of depression. These are all elements of a subcortical dementia or cognitive disorder, albeit with the prominent omission of a memory disorder. It is, therefore, difficult to detect the appearance of a mild dementia in the Parkinson's patient. Although frank dementia may ultimately occur in at least 30% of Parkinson's patients,[134] it is unknown whether or not this represents the coincidental development of AD in most of these cases, or a separate and distinct form of dementia.

The typical pathologic findings in Parkinson's disease patients are a reduction in brain weight, cortical cell loss, Lewy bodies in the substantia nigra and locus coeruleus, and substantial loss of cells in the nucleus of Meynert. In a high proportion of cases there are senile plaques, neurofibrillary tangles, and granulovacuolar changes in the hippocampus.

X-RAY CT STUDIES

Although dementia is a relatively common finding in Parkinson's disease patients, only one study has been reported comparing x-ray CT scans of demented to those of nondemented Parkinson's patients.[184] It was found that there was indeed an increase in ventricular size in demented Parkinson's patients compared to the nondemented, who in turn did not have larger ventricles than age-matched normal subjects.

Indices of cortical atrophy and ventricular enlargement on CT scans showed a greater degree of atrophy in Parkinson's patients compared with controls, although severity of atrophy and extrapyramidal symptoms were not correlated.[175] A study[1] of patients with Parkinson's disease with onset before and after age 65 years showed that only the later-onset patients demonstrated cortical atrophy, which was found to affect the frontal regions most prominently. Another study,[186] however, showed that earlier-onset patients (before 50 years) demonstrated the greatest degree of both central atrophy (lateral and third ventricular enlargement) and cortical atrophy. Patients in the 60–79-year age range differed from controls to a lesser extent and only with regards to cortical atrophy. These differing results may reflect the varying proportions of demented patients included in each study. Thus x-ray CT scans are not very revealing in nondemented Parkinson's patients, but should be considered in evaluating the demented patient.

MRI STUDIES

Drayer[49] summarized his experience with high-field MRI studies in patients with Parkinson's disease. He described mild ventricular but prominent sulcal enlargement, and signal hypointensity (on T_2-weighted scans), outside the average range, in the globus pallidus, red nucleus, substantia nigra, dentate nucleus, and putamen (Fig. 9–5*A*,*B*; see also Fig. 8–10). Patients with Parkinson-plus syndromes (multisystem atrophy), including some with dementia, have been described to have particularly prominent signal hypointensity specifically in the putamen,[50,154] whereas in normal, aged individuals and those with idiopathic Parkinson's disease, the hypointensity in the globus pallidus is more prominent than in the putamen. These signal alterations have been found to correspond to the concentration of iron deposited in these structures.[50] Drayer[49] also described above-average subcortical white matter signal hyperintensity on T_2-weighted images in Parkinson's patients. In a preliminary report, Huber and associates[101] used MRI scans to compare age-matched Parkinson's disease patients with and without dementia to normal controls and were unable to show any differences between the controls and the demented and nondemented groups in the extent of generalized atrophy, atrophy of the corpus callosum, thickness of the substantia nigra, or areas of high signal intensity.

PET STUDIES

Parkinson's patients without dementia have been reported to have an 18% reduction in global cerebral glucose metabolism[115] and a 20% reduction in global cerebral blood flow,[199] compared with controls. No consistent focal pattern of deficit has been reported in Parkinson's disease patients,[157] except in those who have concomitant dementia, where parietal lobe reductions in glucose metabolism have been found[115,118] (see Fig. 9–5*C*,*D*; see also Fig. 8–11). These deficits in demented Parkinson's disease patients resemble those seen in Alzheimer's disease. Pathologic studies suggest that the majority of patients with Parkinson's disease and dementia have some concomitant neuropathologic changes of AD.[163]

SPECT STUDIES

A single report of SPECT studies in seven patients with Parkinson's disease revealed diffusely decreased cortical tracer uptake; demented Parkinson's patients, however, were not studied.[162]

Pick's Disease

The clinical presentation of Pick's disease has been considered to have certain typical features by some investigators[39] but not by others.[89] Changes in personality and behavior (such as disordered social conduct, loss of initiative, and disinhibition) generally occur early in the disease course, whereas significant memory and visuospatial dys-

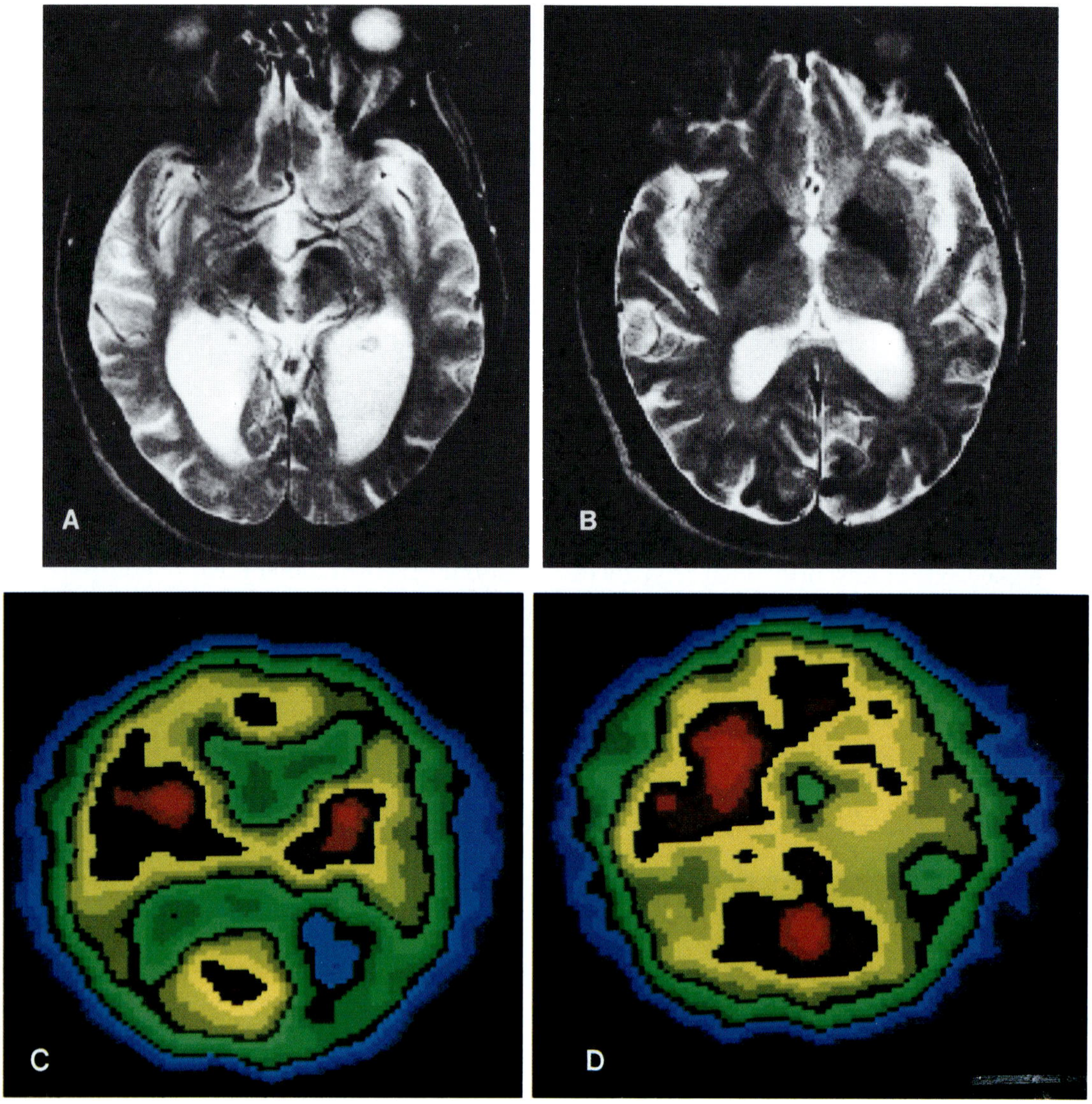

Figure 9–5. Parkinson's dementia. (*A*) MRI (horizontal section, low ventricular level). Note marked increase in the size of the temporal horns. There is reduced signal in the red nucleus and substantia nigra regions from iron deposition. Low signal in substantia nigra merges with the low signal of the cerebral peduncles. (T_2-weighted image using TR 2500, TE 80) (*B*) MRI (horizontal section, basal ganglia level). Note low signal of globus pallidus from iron deposition merging with low signal of the anterior commissure, which can be seen (faintly) crossing the midline. (T_2-weighted image using TR 2500, TE 80 msec.) (*C*) PET (basal ganglia level). Note reduced metabolism in association cortices, especially in one temporal region. (*D*) PET (low ventricular level). Note reduced metabolism in midtemporal regions, more prominent on one side.

function occur relatively late. Aphasic features at the onset are common, and some patients develop components of the Kluver-Bucy syndrome, such as oral exploratory tendencies, sensory agnosia, and hypersexuality. Nevertheless, many patients with Pick's disease are diagnosed as having AD antemortem, and it is likely that a proportion have the typical presentation of AD.[100]

Grossly, the brain typically shows lobar atrophy with primarily frontal and temporal involvement. This pattern of atrophy has been reported occasionally among patients with AD.[181] Histologically, there is marked neuronal loss, marked astrocytic gliosis, inflated neurons, and Pick bodies. The amygdala, in addition to the cortex and basal ganglia, is severely involved.

X-RAY CT STUDIES

Several clinicopathologic studies of Pick's disease have been reported since the introduction of the x-ray CT scanner.* The x-ray CT findings in Pick's disease typically have been those of frontal and temporal atrophy, evidenced by increased width of the frontal interhemispheric space, the Sylvian fissures, and the frontal horns of the lateral ventricles. Groen and Hekster[87] studied 14 adults from 3 generations of a family with autosomal dominant Pick's disease. In 3 clinically affected members, the x-ray CT findings were generalized atrophy, generalized atrophy with frontal predominance, and frontotemporal atrophy, respectively. Of 11 clinically unaffected members at risk, 3 showed frontotemporal atrophy in the fifth decade of life. Age of onset was typically in the sixth and seventh decades of life, in this family.

When typical findings are obtained, x-ray CT appears to be a useful procedure to assist in making the antemortem diagnosis of Pick's disease. A note of caution must be included, however. Two cases[172] were initially and erroneously diagnosed as Pick's disease on x-ray CT because of ventricular and Sylvian fissure enlargement, although both had gait apraxia and incontinence in addition to progressive intellectual impairment, and were otherwise clinically typical cases of normal-pressure hydrocephalus. They both responded well to shunting, with reduction in size of the ventricles and the Sylvian fissures. These cases must be regarded as NPH cases with the x-ray CT appearance of Pick's disease.

MRI STUDIES

Thus far, MRI has not revealed any findings additional to those obtained with x-ray CT in Pick's disease (Fig. 9–6*A*,*B*). It should be possible by MRI to demonstrate the extensive subcortical gliosis that is part of the pathology of Pick's disease. Future studies with T_2-weighted sequences may demonstrate this hypothesized finding.

PET STUDIES

Studies of cerebral blood flow with scalp detectors and ^{133}Xe inhalation predicted the findings that were obtained with PET and SPECT in Pick's disease.[167] A single clinico-pathologic study in a patient with Pick's disease confirmed marked (greater than 50%) reduction of cerebral glucose metabolism in the frontal lobes bilaterally.[111] The frontoparietal ratio was about 26% lower in the Pick's disease case than the control value, more than 30% lower than in 12 patients with AD, and more than four standard deviations from the mean of the AD value. Of particular interest in this study was the finding that reductions in regional cerebral glucose metabolic rate correlated best with degree of gliosis ($r = 0.78$) and correlated least with the number of Pick bodies or inflated neurons ($r = 0.17$)

PET scans on patients with clinically diagnosed Pick's disease also have revealed bilateral or unilateral frontal and anterior temporal metabolic deficits[55] (Fig. 9–6*C*,*D*).

SPECT STUDIES

Neary and colleagues[150] studied nine patients with mental changes suggestive of Pick's disease by SPECT scanning, using the agent ^{99m}Tc-HMPAO. Seven of the nine (78%) showed only frontal-lobe perfusion defects, one showed a parietofrontal abnormality, and one patient showed only posterior defects. These results were very different from those obtained in patients diagnosed as having AD, in whom 14 of 21 patients (67%) had parietal or parie-

*References 39,87,111,113,136,144,146,180, 195.

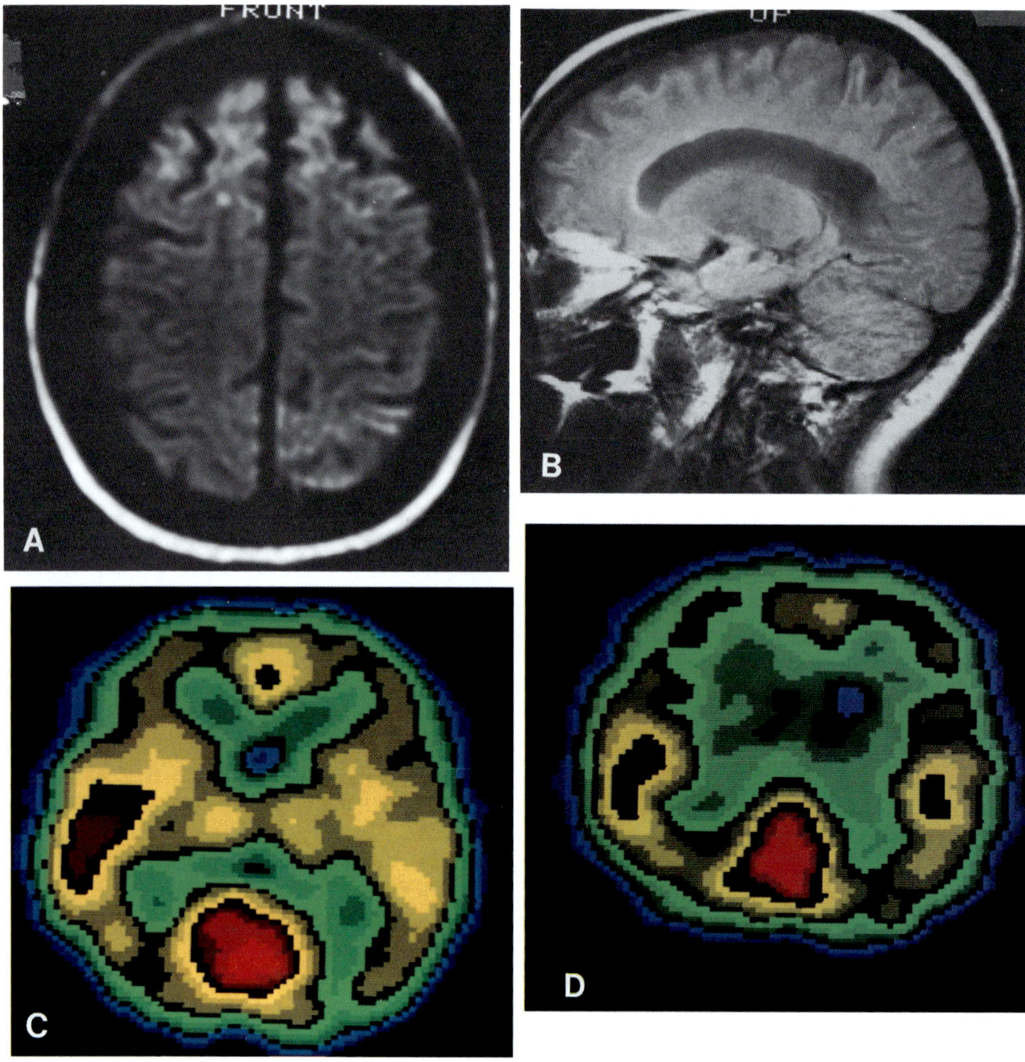

Figure 9–6. Pick's disease. (*A*) MRI horizontal section (TR 2500, TE 25, 1.5 T). Note severe atrophy of anterior frontal region. (*B*) MRI sagittal section (TR 300, TE 17, 1.5 T). Note sulcal prominence predominantly in frontal and temporal regions. (*C*) PET (basal ganglia level). Note that metabolism is reduced primarily in frontal and anterior temporal regions. (*D*) PET (superior frontal/superior parietal level). Note that frontal cortex metabolism is reduced.

tofrontal defects and 3 (14%) had only frontal defects in perfusion.

Hence, SPECT studies of cerebral perfusion generally confirm the impression on x-ray CT, MRI, and PET that primarily anterior cerebral abnormalities in the frontal and temporal lobes are characteristic of Pick's disease.

Progressive Supranuclear Palsy (PSP)

This degenerative disease is diagnosed on clinical grounds on the basis of vertical supranuclear gaze paresis (downward gaze), axial rigidity, gait instability, and slowing of mentation or frank dementia. Neuroimaging methods generally do not contribute towards making the diagnosis, but may be helpful in evaluating the presence of concomitant disease and evaluating the pathophysiology of some features of the disease, especially the dementia. A detailed discussion on the relation of imaging changes to motor symptoms and signs is provided in Chapter 8.

X-RAY CT STUDIES

The most complete description of the x-ray CT changes in PSP have been made by Ambrosetto and coworkers.[5] The findings include brainstem and quadrigeminal plate atrophy, manifested by enlargement of the quadrigeminal cistern, the ambient cisterns, and the interpeduncular fossa, and dilatation of the aqueduct and the fourth ventricle. Because of degeneration of the midline thalamic nuclei, the posterior part of the third ventricle is also dilated, producing a characteristic "skittle" shape to this structure, in horizontal sections. Some investigators[93,105,130] have emphasized the dilatation of the lateral ventricles that also occurs in this disease, while still others[59] have emphasized the frequency with which multiple infarctions on x-ray CT or MRI are evident in patients with PSP (33%), compared with patients with Parkinson's disease (12%). This significantly higher incidence of cerebral infarcts was presumably related to a higher frequency of hypertension, older age at onset of disease, and other stroke risk factors. Nevertheless, extrapolating from these x-ray CT findings, it is possible that a proportion of patients with the clinical syndrome of PSP have this disorder not on the basis of degenerative changes, but because of a multi-infarct state.

MRI STUDIES

Abnormalities of signal intensity are frequently found in PSP patients (Fig. 9–7*A*,*B*). A preliminary report[131] using high-field MRI showed decreased signal intensity on T_2-weighted scans in the pallidum, putamen, thalamus, pars compacta of the substantia nigra, and the superior colliculi. These changes presumably represented increased iron accumulation in these structures and are findings not obtained in patients with idiopathic Parkinson's disease, but are ones seen in patients with multisystem atrophy.

PET STUDIES

Decreased frontal lobe glucose metabolism (see Fig. 9–7) has been reported in PSP.[14,42] Investigators also have shown a loss of striatal dopamine receptors in PSP using PET with radiolabeled ligands[12] (see Fig. 8–16).

In comparing metabolic deficits, Foster and associates[70] showed that in AD the cerebral cortex was most abnormal, followed by thalamic and basal ganglia structures; in PSP, however, there was relatively equivalent hypometabolism of basal ganglia, thalamic and cortical structures. These researchers[72] also have shown that whereas metabolism in the entire cerebral cortex is reduced compared to normals, it is the frontal cortex that is most reduced in PSP (Fig. 9–7*C*,*D*). This pattern is quite different from that seen in AD.

A disorder that can be difficult to distinguish clinically from PSP in its early stage is olivopontocerebellar atrophy (OPCA) (see Chapter 11). In OPCA, metabolism is reduced in the cerebellar hemispheres, the vermis, and the brainstem, regions that are spared in PSP, but normal values are obtained in the thalamus and cortex.[85]

The pathophysiology of frontal cortical hypometabolism in PSP is not well understood. One study[125] showed that patients with bilateral pallidal lesions and behavioral changes have metabolic deficits predominantly in the frontal cortex. Hence, dysfunction in the pallidum may be relevant to the frontal hypometabolism in PSP, perhaps with pallidothalamic and thalamocortical connections mediating the effects.

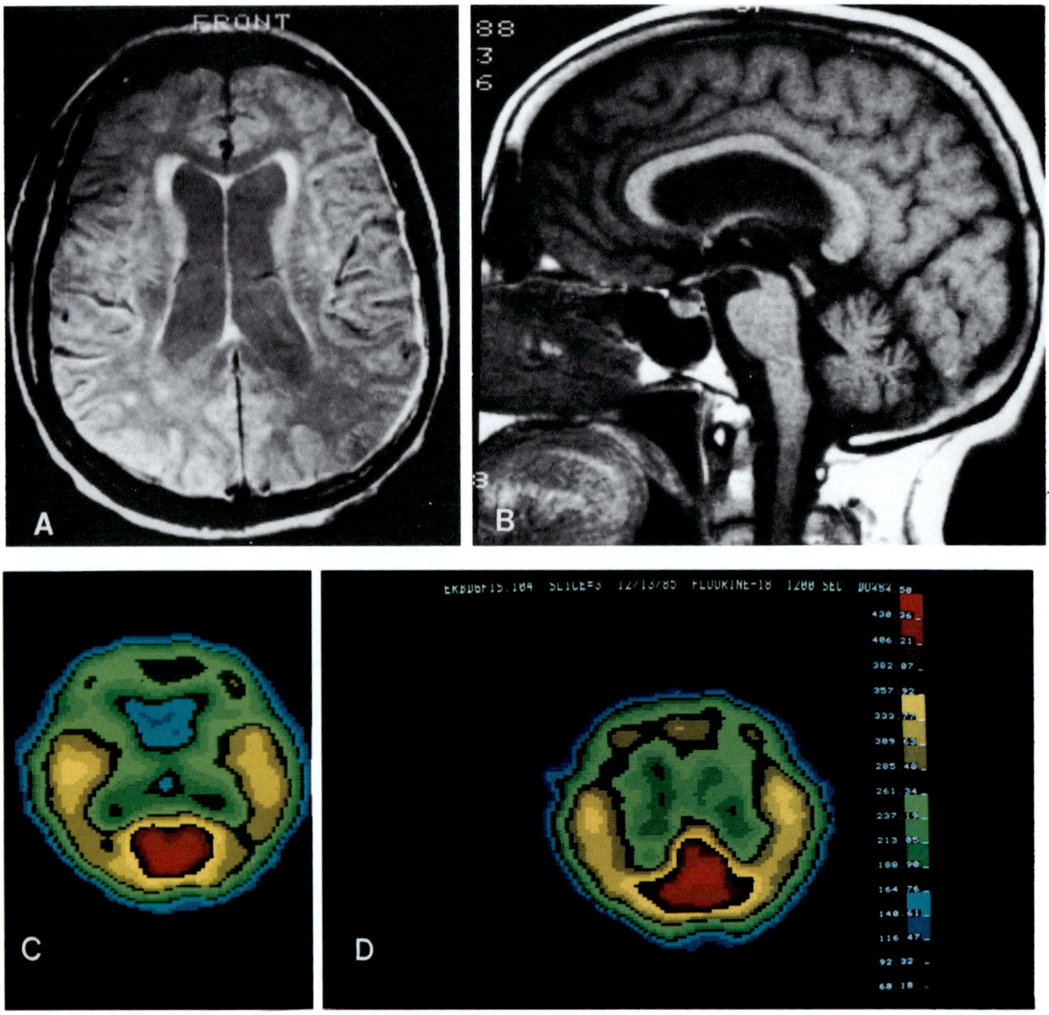

Figure 9–7. Progressive supranuclear palsy. (*A*) MRI (horizontal section at midventricular level) (TR 2500, TE 25, 1.5 T). Note increase in ventricular size, increase in periventricular signal around frontal horns, and a few subcortical signal abnormalities in the right parietal and left frontal regions. (*B*) MRI (midsagittal section) (TR 300, TE 17, 1.5 T). Note increased ventricular size, atrophy of the brainstem, especially pontine tegmentum, midbrain, and medulla. There is increased size of the aqueduct of Sylvius and fourth ventricle. Cerebellar atrophy is also evident. (*C*) PET (basal ganglia level). Note marked reduction of frontal metabolism bilaterally. Basal ganglia metabolism also appears reduced. (*D*) PET at superior frontal–superior parietal level showing frontal hypometabolism.

SPECT STUDIES

Neary's group[150] studied eight patients with PSP and demonstrated that seven (88%) had frontal perfusion deficits, whereas one (12%) had a normal pattern. This result is in keeping with the PET findings.

Neurotransmitter and Neuroreceptor Studies in Degenerative Dementia

A high level of interest exists in using PET and SPECT to study presynaptic and postsynaptic receptor function in dementing disease, because most degenerative dementias have been associated with dysfunction in one or more neuroreceptor systems. These studies are still in their infancy, since quantitative techniques for measuring synthesis of ligands or receptor number, affinity, and occupancy have not yet been perfected. Nevertheless, some interesting studies have been done and are listed below according to the areas to which they pertain.

NORMAL AGING

Presynaptic dopaminergic function has been studied using [^{18}F]6-fluoro-L-dopa (fluorodopa) and PET in normal subjects 22 to 80 years of age.[133] The fluorodopa uptake rate constant was found to be negatively correlated with age.

The binding of D_2 dopamine and S_2 serotonin receptors by [^{11}C]3-N-methylspiperone in the caudate nucleus and frontal cortex, respectively, in man is reduced as a function of age.[200] A study of 22 men and 22 women demonstrated that D_2 dopamine receptor binding, but not S_2 serotonin receptor binding, declined more steeply in men (46%) than in women (25%) over a five-decade age range.

ALZHEIMER'S DISEASE (AD)

Although no consistent alteration in muscarinic receptors has been found in AD in postmortem tissue, a recent report suggests a decrease in muscarinic receptors in six AD patients in parietal cortex, as estimated by binding of ^{123}I-IodoQNB, studied by SPECT.[196] Another SPECT study using ^{123}I-labeled RO16-0154 to study benzodiazepine receptor binding in the brain also showed reduced binding in AD patients. These results may have been obtained, however, because of tissue or synaptic loss in the cortex and will require confirmation with appropriate correction techniques.

PARKINSON'S DISEASE

Presynaptic uptake of dopamine in the striatum has been studied using fluorodopa as a tracer[80,133] (see Chapters 3 and 8). In hemi-Parkinsonism the striatal accumulation of dopamine is reduced in the striatum (especially putamen) on the side opposite the major motor symptoms.[145] One study[62] reported a correlation between fluorodopa uptake rate constants and clinical scores for dementia, as well as scores for bradykinesia, rigidity, tremor, gait disturbance, and left-right motor symmetry.

Postsynaptic receptor changes can be studied using a variety of agents that have been used to quantify D_2 and D_1 receptor density in the striatum. Preliminary reports in Parkinson's patients suggest D_2 receptor supersensitivity, but demented patients were not included in these studies.[158,166]

PROGRESSIVE SUPRANUCLEAR PALSY (PSP)

Postsynaptic dopaminergic D_2 receptor density studied by the agent [^{76}Br] bromospiperone showed a loss of striatal D_2 receptors in PSP.[166] This finding was in contrast to the supersensitivity of D_2 receptors reported above in Parkinson's disease patients.

VASCULAR DISORDERS

The term *multi-infarct dementia* appears self-explanatory: a dementia caused by multiple cerebral infarctions. Since the term was coined in 1974 by Hachinski, Lassen, and Marshall,[90] however, the criteria for the diagnosis of this entity, its incidence in the demented population, and its clinical features have been the subject of increasing debate. The application of various types of imaging devices to define this entity more precisely has provided a wealth of information. The data seem to point to a variety of entities under the umbrella of multi-infarct dementia. Because many patients who have this syndrome do not have sufficient cognitive deficits to warrant the term dementia, *multi-infarct cognitive disorder* rather than multi-infarct dementia may be a more appropriate term.

The existence of the entity of multi-infarct dementia is based upon the studies of Blessed,[16] and of Tomlinson[191] and associates, who showed that in demented old people without the neuropathologic features of AD, a strong correlation existed between the volume of brain "softening" (infarction) and the degree of dementia ($r = 0.68$). Moreover, an aggregate volume of at least 50 ml of softening was required to produce the clinical syndrome of dementia. This vascular dementia was diagnosed on pathologic grounds in 9 out of 50 demented subjects (18%). Unfortunately, this classic study has not yet been replicated.

When this issue is viewed from another perspective, namely, selection of patients because of the presence of infarcts rather than dementia, the results are quite different. In a detailed study of 1042 consecutive adults who came to autopsy,[68] 114 individuals (10.9%) had one or more lacunes in the brain (average: 3.3 lacunes). Contrary to expectation, only 23% had any neurologic symptoms or signs before death. An analysis of those with more than 10 lacunes showed that even in them, "dementia, if present at all, was mild," and there was no clinical evidence of pseudobulbar palsy in these patients. The patients who were most disabled mentally showed cortical infarcts or multiple hemorrhages in addition to the lacunes. Subcortical infarcts are, nevertheless, well known to be capable of producing cognitive disorders, as has been clearly documented.[36,41,79,147] Thus, it seems that in autopsy studies, when patients are selected for antemortem evidence of dementia, about one fifth may be found to have MID, but when patients are selected because of the presence of multiple infarcts, a much smaller fraction will be found to have dementia. Perhaps factoring in the location of these infarcts may account for some of the discrepancy.

Another team of researchers[102] studied the brains of 370 patients who had died with dementia, of whom 91 (25%) were classified as multi-infarct dementia. They were able to classify these cases of multi-infarct dementia into three categories on the basis of the location of the lesions. Twenty-eight cases had large cortical infarcts as the basis for dementia. Another 30 cases had more than 6 lacunes each, with diffuse softening of the white matter, predominantly in the frontal lobes, and with clinical features of subcortical dementia and pseudobulbar palsy. The remainder of the 91 cases had findings that were a mixture of the first two categories.

Binswanger's disease, which coincides pathologically with the subcortical white matter disease cases in this study,[102] is an entity that was rarely diagnosed antemortem until the last decade. A review of the clinical and pathologic features of this disease[9] revealed that it is a very common radiologic entity, even in normal individuals. The disease itself cannot be diagnosed, however, without the occurrence of a dementia or other cognitive and neurologic abnormalities. Pathologically, microscopic vascular changes are invariably present and are most prominent in the arterioles in the white matter, which is diffusely softened except for the subcortical U-fibers.

The existence of the entity of multi-infarct dementia is not in doubt, but it is said to be both underdiagnosed[151] and overdiagnosed.[27] One critical and extensive review of the literature[126] concluded that "assuming that strokes have certain reliable neurological manifestations and that strokes are able to cause dementia, then, when demented patients are noted to have a history consistent with one or more strokes, it may be erroneously reasoned that the one led to the other." From a neuroimaging point of view, it is important to realize that although it is valuable to identify cerebral infarcts in a demented patient, the existence of these infarcts does not mean that they necessarily caused or contributed to the dementia.[26]

On neuroimaging studies, the pattern of regional ischemic involvement allows a classification of MID patients into those with predominantly multiple cortical infarcts (MCI), those with multiple discrete subcortical infarcts, and those with diffuse white matter pathology or Binswanger's disease. In the first group (MCI), frank dementia with a cortical dementia syndrome is likely. In the other two groups, frank dementia is much less likely, but some elements of a subcortical dementia syndrome may be present.

X-ray CT Studies of Multi-infarct Dementia

Because most reports of multi-infarct dementia refer to the entity described above as MCI, the term MID will be used below interchangeably with MCI. The clinical diagnosis of MID is usually dependent on structural (x-ray CT, MRI) evidence of infarcts in the brain. Typical CT criteria for MID include focal low attenuation areas, focal and asymmetric ventricular enlargement, and asymmetric Sylvian fissures. Historically, however, Hachinski and coworkers[91] developed criteria for the diagnosis of MID using an ischemic score (IS) (without including neuroimaging findings). The IS consists of 13 items on a checklist, including abrupt onset, stepwise deterioration, history of hypertension, focal neurologic symptoms, focal neurologic signs, associated atherosclerosis, and so on. In a demented patient, a high score suggested a diagnosis of multi-infarct dementia, whereas a low score suggested AD. On the basis of a small series of patients (n = 14) on whom clinicopathologic correlation was obtained,[170] it has been suggested that the IS could separate, without overlap, AD patients from those with MID or mixed dementia (that is, both AD and MID). Patients with AD had an IS of 5 or less, whereas MID and mixed dementia cases had scores of 7 or greater.

In one study of 58 demented patients,[143] 45 had been classified as AD (n = 28), MID (n = 11) or mixed dementia (n = 6), using the same IS criteria and without including x-ray CT scan findings. The accuracy of clinical diagnosis, on the basis of neuropathologic examination, was 71% for AD, 42% for MID, and 20% for mixed dementia.

Subsequently, a more elaborate study including the use of x-ray CT scans was reported[194] on 65 patients with dementia. An IS of 4 or less, a suggestive history, and an x-ray CT scan that was clear of infarcts were used to diagnose AD. Patients were diagnosed as having MID if they had an IS greater than 4, a history suggestive of cerebrovascular events, and an x-ray CT scan that showed infarcts. Patients with mixed features were labeled as having a mixed dementia. A miscellaneous group, with diagnoses such as PSP or Creutzfeldt-Jakob disease, was also identified. Pathologic verification was most accurate for 39 patients diagnosed as having AD (85% accuracy), and for the six patients diagnosed with miscellaneous conditions (83% accuracy). Of four patients diagnosed to have MID, one did have MID (25% accuracy) and three had mixed dementia (a combination of AD and MID). Of 16 patients diagnosed to have mixed dementia, five (31%) did have this pathologically, while five had AD and four had MID. Thus, it appears that the x-ray CT scan is most useful for improving the accuracy of the diagnosis of AD by separating AD from MID and mixed dementia. Predictably, the x-ray CT scan does not seem to help in distinguishing between MID and mixed dementia.

Other studies have compared the x-ray CT diagnosis to the Hachinski Ischemic Score classification of multi-infarct dementia versus AD. One[164] found that only 38% of patients classified as MID according to the IS (≥6) had x-ray

CT scan criteria for MID. However, if they did have the x-ray CT criteria, there was a 90% chance of also having IS criteria for MID. Another study[127] classified 94 patients with dementia according to the IS. Of 28 patients with IS ≥7 (classified as MID), 17 (61%) had x-ray CT criteria for MID (multiple areas of reduced density attributable to ischemic lesions), whereas 95% of those with x-ray CT criteria also had IS criteria for MID. Hence, the IS is not a very good predictor of the x-ray CT findings, whereas the x-ray CT scan is a much better predictor of the IS.

One group[64] classified patients as having AD (n = 22) and MID (n = 29) on the basis of clinical criteria alone (i.e., without using the x-ray CT scan). They distinguished between cortical and white matter infarcts on x-ray CT scans and found that 18 (62%) of the MID cases had infarcts outside the white matter, whereas none of the AD cases had such infarcts. Cystic infarcts and areas of low attenuation in the white matter were present in 26 (90%) of MID cases, and 1 (5%) of the AD cases. With findings that included a combination of white matter lesions and cortical infarcts, 97% of MID and 95% of AD could be correctly classified according to their clinical criteria. Thus, the correspondence of clinical and x-ray CT criteria for MID may be reasonably good when stringent clinical criteria are used. A recent report[2] suggests, however, that white matter changes in demented patients are not very specific. White matter changes in the cerebral hemispheres on x-ray CT scans were described in 56% of clinically diagnosed AD and 97% of MID patients. Ventricular dilatation (perhaps an index of severity of white matter disease) was correlated with cognitive status in MID but not in AD cases. From the aforementioned studies it may be surmised that clinical criteria, including x-ray CT findings, will not distinguish effectively between pathologically determined MID and mixed dementia[194] but will be more effective in separating AD from MID or mixed dementia.

X-ray CT Studies of Binswanger's Disease

Binswanger's disease was considered rare and was diagnosed only on autopsy before the advent of the x-ray CT scan. Subsequently, it has become a relatively common diagnosis. To quote Kinkel and associates,[112] "There remains a large group of patients, usually in the seventh through ninth decades, who develop an identifiable CT pattern of white matter disease of unknown origin. By CT scans, their lesions appear as bilateral, usually symmetric, areas of decreased density of the periventricular white matter and centra semiovale." Of 23 patients diagnosed on CT scans by these researchers to have Binswanger's disease,[112] 8 had nonspecific complaints such as blurred vision and dizziness and no clinical neurologic deficits. Seven cases presented with motor strokes; most of these were demented as well. Eight patients who presented with dementia also had gait disturbance and motor deficits, including hemiparesis and paraparesis. One of the severely demented patients came to autopsy and was found to have numerous cystic infarcts (1 – 6 mm in diameter) in the centra semiovale, basal ganglia and thalamus; there were early and evolving infarcts in subcortical white matter and gray matter structures. The white matter demonstrated irregular zones of demyelination. Even though the circle of Willis showed minimal atherosclerosis, subcortical arterioles were moderately to severely sclerosed, thus earning the label "subcortical arteriosclerotic encephalopathy (SAE)" (see Chapter 10).

The same investigators[112] distinguished the white matter hypodensities seen in Binswanger's disease from those seen in normal-pressure hydrocephalus (NPH). Although the ventricles are frequently enlarged in Binswanger's disease, the periventricular hypodensities on x-ray CT scans extend further dorsally into the centra semiovale and have a more heterogeneous appearance than in NPH. In some cases, however, the appearances are difficult to tell apart, and in fact the two conditions possibly coexist occasionally.

Other studies on Binswanger's disease[31,171] have reported essentially the same experience. Although many patients with typical x-ray CT findings of Binswanger's disease are not demented or have mild cognitive disturbance, a positive relationship of severity of dementia to extent of x-ray CT changes has been described.[86,192] One interesting CT-pathologic study[129] included 82 patients selected only because they had antemortem x-ray CT examination and subsequently postmortem examination of the brain. Twenty of these patients had the x-ray CT appearance of Binswanger's disease, of whom 18 had histologic evidence of demyelination, axonal loss, and fibrous thickening of the arterial walls in the affected white matter. One patient had metastatic carcinoma, and another, an aqueductal tumor that had produced hydrocephalus; in both these cases the x-ray CT lucency was presumably caused by edema. In 10 patients with normal white matter by x-ray CT, however, there was minimal or no pathologic evidence of Binswanger's disease. Thus, it appears that the diagnosis of Binswanger's disease on x-ray CT scan alone is usually verified on pathologic examination. From a clinician's standpoint, a patient presenting with nonspecific or focal neurologic symptoms, with or without positive neurologic findings, who has the x-ray CT appearance of Binswanger's disease, is likely to be proven to have Binswanger's disease on postmortem examination.

MRI Studies

A profusion of MRI periventricular lesions in patients at risk for stroke, and therefore theoretically at risk for multi-infarct dementia, has been reported consistently. It is unclear, however, whether a critical extent and anatomic distribution of these lesions is associated with the development of dementia. (Fig. 9–8*A*,*B*) Because neuropathologic studies on MID patients with antemortem MR scans have not yet been reported, the ability of these MRI lesions to predict the likelihood of dementia is unknown.

Gerard and Weisberg[84] noted that of patients aged 60 years and above, 10% with no risk factors for stroke, 40% with such risk factors, and 69% with definite evidence of cerebrovascular disease had MRI periventricular high-signal-intensity patterns. Marshall and associates[132] studied postmortem brains by MRI and then by detailed pathologic examination. In 3 of 21 brains there were multiple foci of periventricular hyperintensity on the MR image; these were confirmed histologically to be deep white matter infarcts, but of smaller size than the MR abnormality. The gliosis surrounding these infarcts made them appear larger than their true size on the T_2-weighted MR images. These studies attest to the fact that MRI is highly sensitive to some of the common neuropathologic effects of aging, including white matter infarcts and subsequent gliosis.

In another study[8] of 270 consecutive patients who had MR scans, incidental subcortical MRI lesions were not more frequent or severe in those with an overt diagnosis of dementia than in age-matched, nondemented controls. These researchers, however, did not distinguish between the different types of dementia and did not subtype the white matter lesions. On the other hand, another study[66] classified 16 patients with dementia into those with probable AD (n = 7), possible AD (n = 5), and MID (n = 4). The MRI findings in the MID patients differed from those in the AD group. Patients with MID had two distinguishing features: irregular periventricular hyperintensities extending into the deep white matter, and large confluent areas of deep white matter hyperintensity (DWMH). In AD patients, DWMHs were either punctate or showed only slight evidence of confluence, and periventricular hyperintensities were smooth and halolike in appearance.

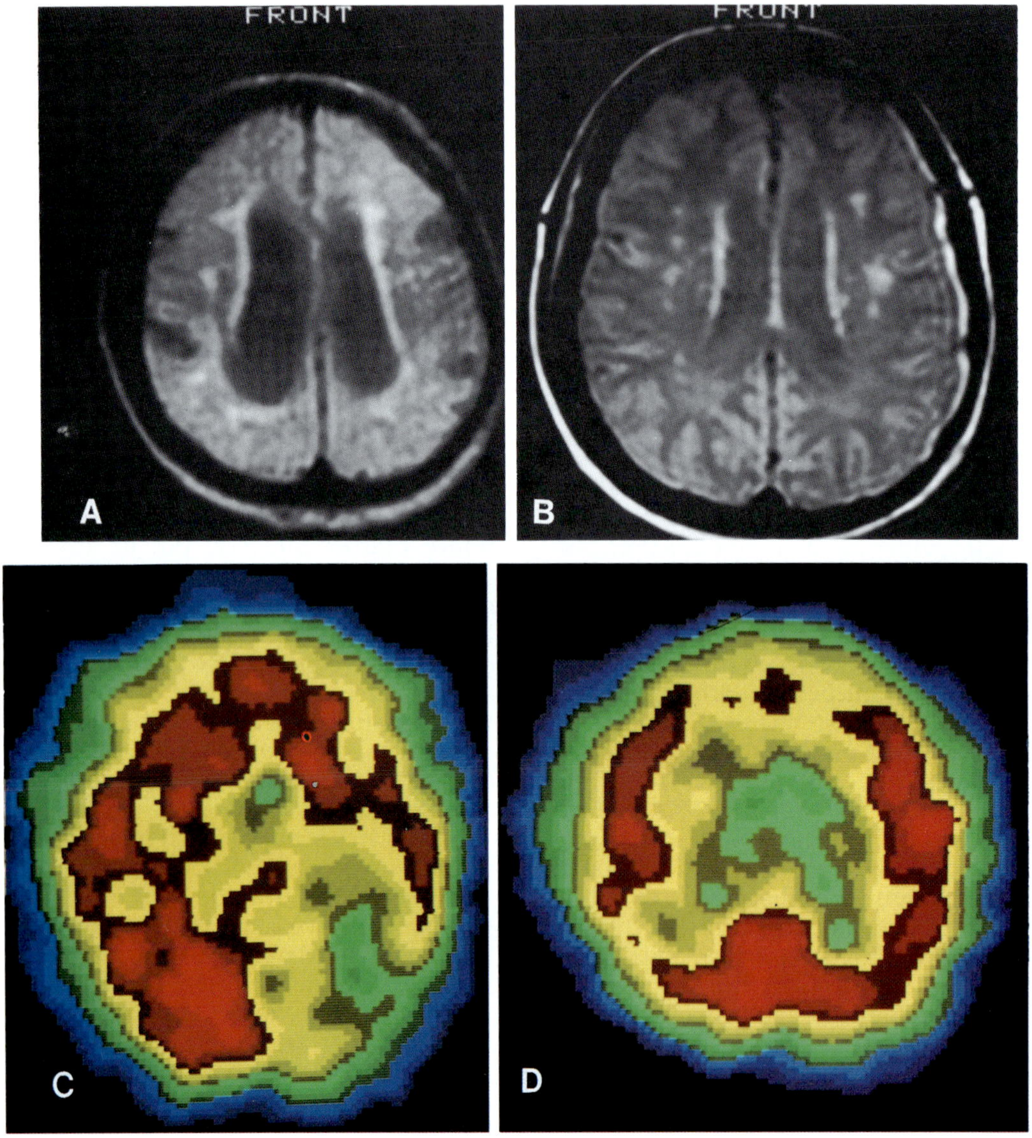

Figure 9–8. Multi-infarct dementia. (*A*) MRI horizontal section at midventricular level (TR 2500, TE 25, 1.5 T). Note multiple old cortical infarcts (low-density areas) and several nodular areas of increased signal in the white matter, representing infarcts. Moderately increased periventricular signal also is seen. (*B*) MRI horizontal section at high ventricular level. Note numerous subcortical white-matter areas with increased signal. (*C*) PET at low ventricular level. Note large area of reduced metabolism in one temporal lobe. (*D*) PET at supraventricular level. Note demarcated regions of bilateral frontal hypometabolism and unilateral parietal hypometabolism.

Other investigators,[64] who did not subdivide white matter changes in MRI into periventricular and deep white matter lesions, concluded that all 29 patients with vascular dementia and only 8 of 22 patients with AD had white matter changes. Another group[99] studied this problem by focusing on patients with known cerebral vascular disease and classifying them into those with and those without dementia. Twenty-four percent of their sample had dementia. The only significant difference on MRI between the demented and nondemented groups was the greater size of the ventricles in demented patients.

The frequency of abnormalities seen in MR scans of demented and nondemented patients has resulted in a blurring of the distinction between MID and AD, a distinction that seems more readily apparent on x-ray CT scans. Opinions currently vary widely with regard to the significance of MRI abnormalities in dementia. With more specific descriptions of the white matter changes in dementing diseases and in normal aging, as well as with future pathologic correlations, the place of MRI in studying dementia is likely to be better understood. The high sensitivity of MRI for cerebral ischemic lesions may also be accompanied by higher specificity for the diagnosis of multi-infarct dementia.

The studies on dementia using MRI have seemingly neglected mention of cortical lesions (MCI cases) in spite of the known sensitivity of MRI in detecting such lesions. This may reflect the relatively low prevalence of MCI cases. Binswanger's disease, on the other hand, is probably overdiagnosed by MRI in demented patients. It is clear that patients with AD have prominent periventricular hyperintense areas on relatively T_2-weighted images, more so than age-matched controls. There is a tendency, then, to classify these patients with AD within the category of Binswanger's disease. In fact, Roman[169] has suggested the label "senile dementia of the Binswanger type." Adopting such a label will most likely only confuse the categorization of dementia. White matter lesions on MRI should be classified into those that are strictly periventricular and smooth (as in normal aging and particularly in AD), those that are irregular and spread diffusely out of the periventricular area towards the cortex (as in Binswanger's disease) (Fig. 9–9*A*,*B*) and those that are multiple, discrete, subcortical white and gray–matter lesions (as in a lacunar state). In the latter two situations, the additional presence of ventricular dilatation may be the marker of a progressive dementing disorder.

PET Studies

In Table 9–3, three studies are listed that have addressed the differences in the PET scan appearances of MID and AD.[13,74,117] Unfortunately, a definitive statement has not been possible regarding reliable differentiating factors in these two conditions. Benson and colleagues[13] state that in MID the pattern of deficits is asymmetric and variable, compared to the symmetric and diffuse deficits in AD cases (see Fig. 9–8*C*,*D*). Frackowiak and coworkers[74] were unable to discover any differentiating factors on PET between patients diagnosed to have vascular or degenerative dementia. Of interest from a pathophysiologic point of view is that the occipital cortex was relatively spared in MID cases as well as AD cases (Fig. 9–9*C*,*D*).

The border zone between the middle and anterior cerebral arteries is a frequent site of cerebral infarction[102] and there is a strong predisposition for hypertension-associated lacunar infarcts to affect the basal ganglia and thalami. Therefore, metabolic deficits that affect frontal and subcortical gray matter structures predominantly may be expected to be the hallmark of MID. Also, the well-known phenomenon of crossed cerebellar hypometabolism (that is, reduced cerebellar metabolism on the side opposite predominant cortical hypometabolism), commonly reported in stroke cases, may be expected to be a common phenomenon in MID cases. One preliminary report[117] indicated that the parietocerebellar ratio was significantly lower in AD than in MID cases, suggesting that parietal metabolism was relatively spared in MID. Duara and coworkers,[52] however, were unable to confirm this finding when they classified PET scan patterns in demented patients into those with frontal and deep gray matter deficits versus those with parietotemporal deficits. They compared these patterns of metabolic deficits to the clinical diagnosis of dementia and were unable to find a statistically significant difference in fre-

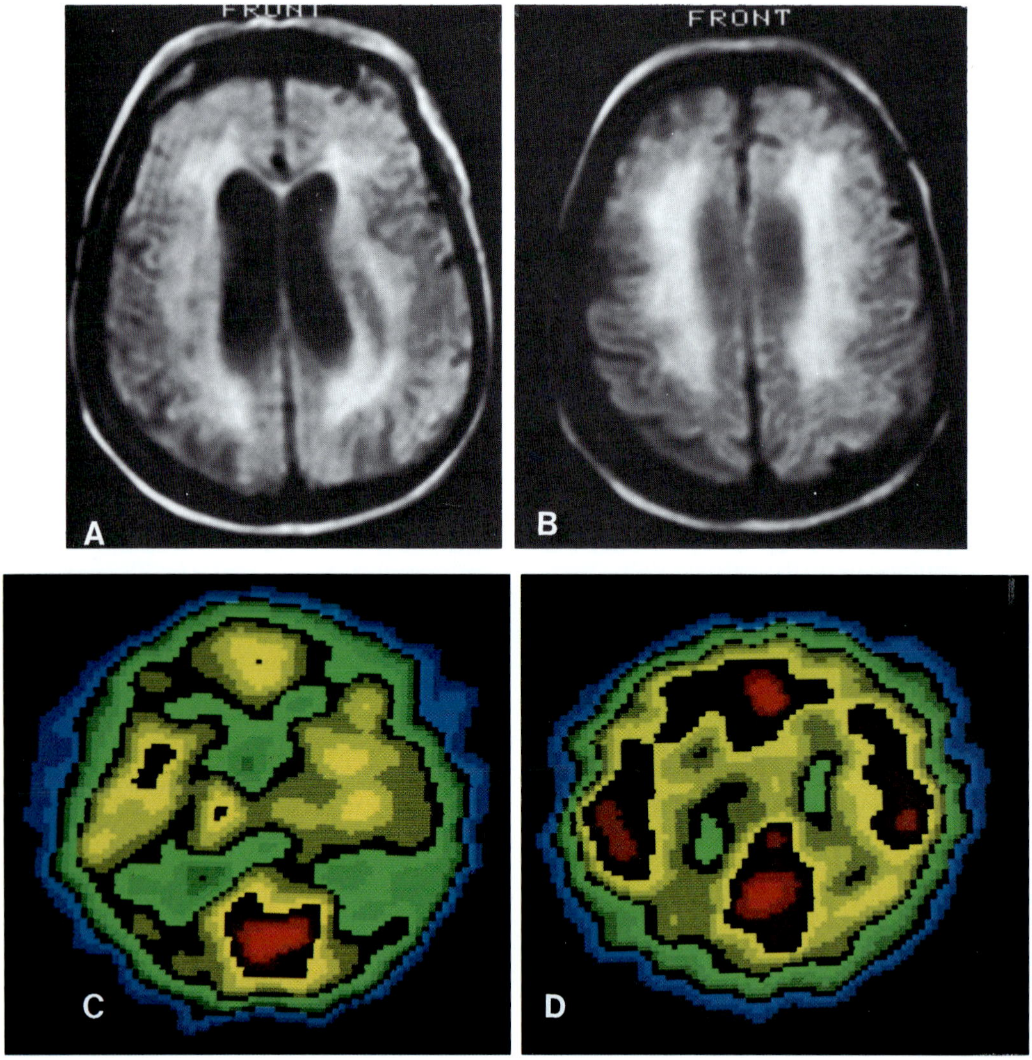

Figure 9–9. Binswanger's disease. (*A*) MRI at midventricular level (TR 2500, TE 25, 1.5 T). Note increase in periventricular signal spreading into the corona radiata and centrum semiovale and extending up to the cortical ribbon in many locations. (*B*) MRI at high ventricular level (TR 2500, TE 25, 1.5 T). Note diffuse increase in signal of the entire white-matter regions of this slice. (*C*) PET (basal ganglia level). Note reduced bilateral frontal and parietal metabolism. Left thalamus also shows reduced metabolism. (*D*) PET (high ventricular level). Note predominantly parietal hypometabolism.

quency of any particular pattern in AD and MID cases. Crossed cerebellar hypometabolism in demented patients,[11] however, was found to be significantly more frequent in MID cases.

SPECT Studies

A group led by Sharp[179] described ^{123}I-isopropyl-amphetamine (IMP) SPECT studies in 13 patients diagnosed as MID on the basis of a Hachinski score greater than eight. No typical pattern of IMP distribution was found and the appearances varied from a near-normal pattern to one with marked focal defects. The majority of the deficits were in posterior parietotemporal and posterior frontal regions, which is similar to what was found in AD cases. Another group [37] correctly identified three patients with MID in their sample on the basis of SPECT findings of asymmetric defects involving the gray matter or both gray and white matter. It seems unlikely, however, that they truly could distinguish defects in the white matter using a SPECT scanner because of the poor spatial resolution of these devices and because regional cerebral flow is relatively low in normal white matter, rendering it anatomically indistinguishable from the lateral ventricles. No other SPECT studies in MID patients have been reported to date.

Regardless of the etiology of dementia, when the pathology is widespread in the brain, the metabolism or perfusion deficits are likely to be diffuse. In several PET studies of stroke patients, the metabolism or blood flow deficits have been found to be much more widespread than the apparent structural deficits on x-ray CT (see Chapter 7). Thus, multiple focal lesions on x-ray CT or MR scans in MID cases are likely to be represented by large confluent cortical deficits on PET or SPECT scans. This may then account for the lack of clear distinguishing factors in the PET or SPECT scan appearances of AD and MID cases.

NORMAL-PRESSURE HYDROCEPHALUS

Normal-pressure hydrocephalus (NPH), described initially by Hakim and Adams,[92] consists of the clinical triad of dementia, gait disorder, and urinary incontinence. Dilatation of the ventricular system with normal CSF pressure on lumbar puncture (i.e., less than 180 mm H_2O) is a feature of the disorder. An entirely satisfactory name for this entity has not yet been found because it has been determined that intermittently CSF pressure may be raised.[188] NPH is an infrequent cause of dementia, with several studies reporting incidence rates of less than 1% of all dementing diseases.[119,190]

Pathologic studies examining patients diagnosed antemortem to have NPH are few and the findings have not been uniform. The common theory of pathogenesis is that bulk CSF flow from the subarachnoid space into the superior sagittal sinus by way of the arachnoid granulations is obstructed, eventually leading to ventricular dilatation. Studies[114,193] have confirmed that on autopsy, meningeal fibrosis with or without changes in the arachnoid granulations occur in most NPH patients. These changes have been associated with prior subarachnoid hemorrhage, central nervous system infections, head trauma, and intracranial surgery. In many instances, however, these pathologic findings had no known cause. Several patients with antemortem diagnoses of NPH have not shown postmortem evidence of meningeal fibrosis and instead have had pathologic evidence of hypertensive cerebrovascular disease with lacunar infarcts, amyloid angiopathy, and even typical AD. The frequent co-occurrence of significant cerebrovascular changes in those cases that also showed meningeal fibrosis has aroused speculation that multiple cerebral lacunar infarcts may predispose to the development of NPH because of reduced tensile strength of the ventricular walls.[60]

The clinical diagnosis of NPH has been based upon the presence of the triad of signs and symptoms, evidence of ventricular dilatation and, usually, evidence from a "confirmatory" procedure such as isotope cisternography, which characteristically shows prolonged ventricular reflux in NPH. Some clinicians use a more elaborate procedure such as long-term epidural pressure recordings or a CSF infusion test for confirmation of diagnosis. The reason for doing these confirmatory tests has been to identify the patients who are most likely to respond to a shunting procedure. It is still unclear, however, that any of these additional tests enhances the ability to predict shunt responsiveness. Although some patients have demonstrated dramatic and rapid improvement of all or most of their symptoms, the overall success rate of a shunting procedure has been reported to be 24% to 75%,[161,185] with a postoperative complication rate of up to 38%.

X-ray CT Studies

Dilatation of the ventricular system is an absolute requirement for the diagnosis of NPH. The extent of dilatation is variable, although it has been suggested that at least a "moderate" degree of ventricular enlargement along with "rounding" of the frontal horns of the lateral ventricles must be present to support the diagnosis.[193] More specifically, LeMay and Hochberg[122] report a frontal horn ratio (ratio of the maximum width of the frontal horns to the external skull diameter at the corresponding level) of 50% as being a feature indicative of NPH. In addition, they emphasize enlargement of the temporal horn tips to 2 mm or more in width. Nevertheless, others[161] could not establish any relationship of ventricular size to response to a shunting procedure, nor could they relate the degree of reduction of ventricular size after shunting to clinical response to the procedure.

Many investigators have required obliteration of the cerebral sulci for the diagnosis of NPH. LeMay and Hochberg[122] state that "the Sylvan fissures and superficial sulci could be seen, although not very wide, in 14 of the 100 patients" with NPH. Vassilouthis[193] observed that obliteration of the sulci at higher levels was sometimes observed in association with dilatation of the subarachnoid spaces, such as Sylvan fissures, at lower levels, perhaps indicating obstruction of the subarachnoid space of the convexity. This author also documented reappearance of cerebral sulci postoperatively. Parenthetically, it should be noted that obliteration of the subarachnoid space unilaterally in experimental animals leads to ipsilateral ventricular dilatation.[88] As was the case for ventricular size, no relationship could be documented between the extent of sulcal enlargement (from none to moderate) and response to a shunting procedure.[161]

The presence of periventricular low-density areas has been regarded to be a feature of NPH. This finding has been considered to be a reflection of transependymal resorption of CSF, a phenomenon known to occur experimentally. This phenomenon may, in fact, account for the reduction of ventricular pressure to normal levels in NPH. Yamada and coworkers[202] have identified a specific low-density pattern that appears in NPH following subarachnoid hemorrhage, consisting of a fan-shaped irregular area of lucency extending from the anterior horns to the frontal pole, which disappears following a shunting procedure. These authors considered the possibility that the seepage of the CSF into frontal white matter may have an independent effect on mentation and also on continence and gait. However, once again other research[161] was unable to document a relationship between either the presence of periventricular lucency or its disappearance after shunting and the response to the shunting procedure.

In summary, x-ray CT studies in NPH are important for documenting the presence of ventricular dilatation. The findings of moderate-to-severe enlargement of frontal horns, obliteration of sulci over the convexity, and presence of periventricular hypodensity are common in NPH cases but do not necessarily predict, by their presence, a good response to a shunting procedure. On the other hand, coexistence of the clinical triad of symptoms and a relatively short duration of symptoms (less than 2 years) generally helps to predict good shunt responses. In general, symptoms of gait disorder and incontinence respond better to a shunt procedure than do the intellectual deficits.

MRI Studies

MRI has certain potential advantages over x-ray CT in the evaluation of NPH (Fig. 9–10 *A,B*). First, because of the freedom from beam hardening artifacts (see Fig. 1–8*A*), assessment of the sub-

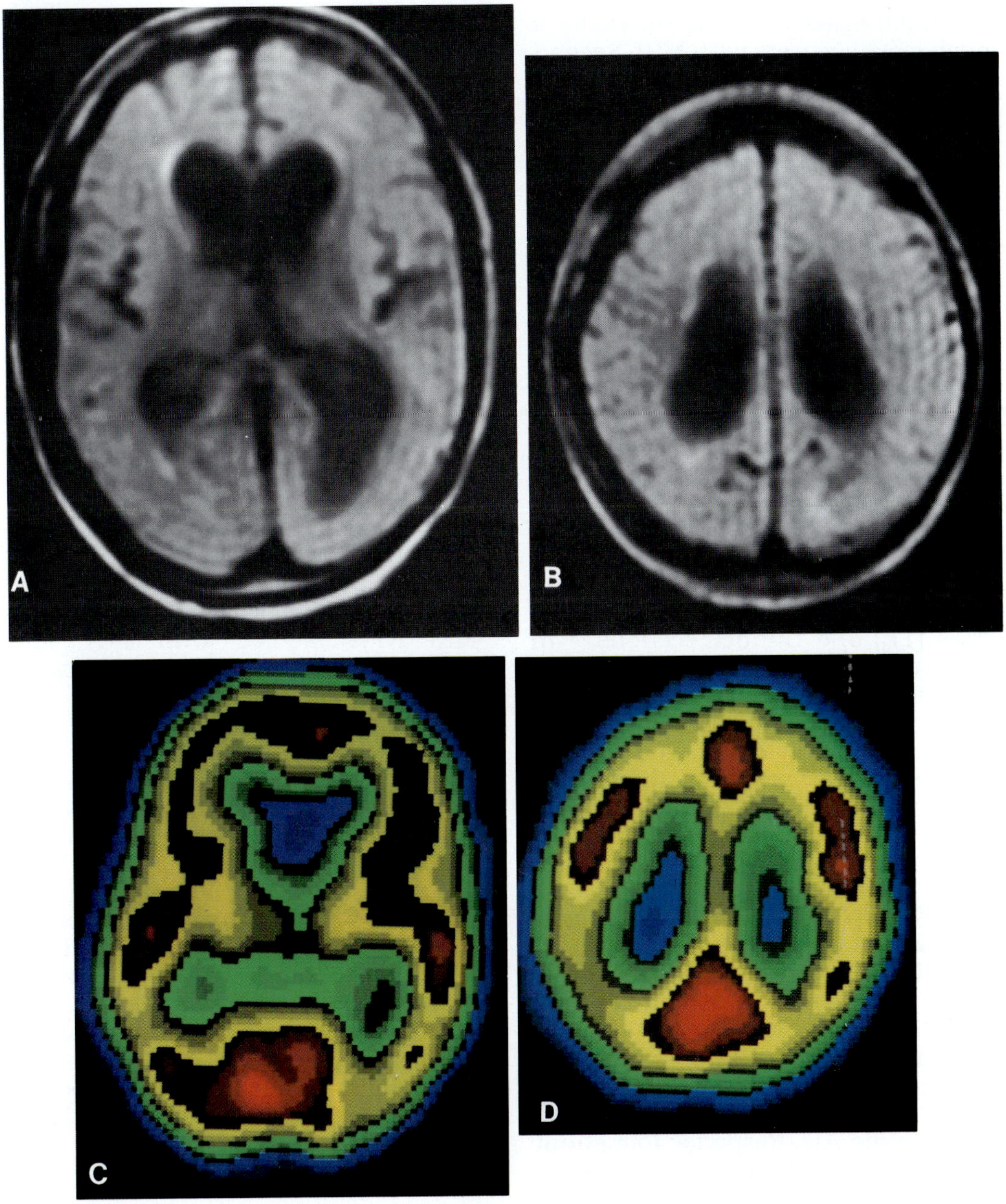

Figure 9–10. Normal pressure hydrocephalus. (*A*) MRI at basal ganglia level (Tr 2500, TE 25, 1.5 T). Note prominent ventricular enlargement. Rounding of frontal horns is evident with surrounding cap of periventricular signal increase. (*B*) MRI at high ventricular level (TR 2500, TE 25, 1.5 T). Note prominence of ventricles with rounding of contours. (*C*) PET (basal ganglia level). Note preserved metabolism in the cortex. Impression of enlarged ventricles is evident in the hypometabolic central regions. (*D*) PET (high ventricular level). Note preserved cortical metabolism with ventricular impression in central regions.

arachnoid space over the convexity is much more accurate with MRI. Second, the periventricular lucencies seen with x-ray CT, presumed to be indicative of transependymal seepage of fluid, can be assessed with much greater sensitivity with MRI. Distinctions may be possible between lesions that result from deep white matter infarctions and those that are contiguous with the ependymal surface and represent fluid. Finally, the flow of CSF in the aqueduct of Sylvius would be expected to be abnormally slow in NPH and can be assessed by the CSF flow void sign. Normally, on T_2-weighted spin echo scans, the signal from CSF in the aqueduct is reduced compared to the signal from the CSF in lateral ventricles because of the increased velocity and turbulence of CSF in the aqueduct. This CSF flow void sign can best be assessed with longer echo times (TE) and thinner sections.[19] In NPH, because of the decrease in compliance of the ventricular walls, pulsatile CSF flow through the aqueduct is more turbulent and accelerated than in nonhydrocephalic cases, even though the bulk flow of CSF through the aqueduct may be reduced. Hence, CSF flow void sign is likely to be more prominent in NPH.

One group[104] performed a comprehensive evaluation of the utility of MRI in NPH and comparison to the use of MRI in other forms of dementia. They found that periventricular signal intensity was greater in NPH than in non-Alzheimer dementia (presumably MID), which in turn had greater signal intensity than did AD. Response to a shunt procedure was "slightly" better in those with a greater degree of periventricular signal intensity. The presence of deep white matter lesions was most strongly related to age. These lesions were more frequently found in demented than in nondemented patients. Although NPH patients had a higher incidence of deep white matter lesions than any other diagnostic group, the response to a shunt procedure was best in those NPH cases without these lesions. This would be the expected finding, given that these deep white matter lesions probably represent a multi-infarct state of the brain. The CSF flow void sign was more prominent in patients with NPH than in any other dementing disorder. These authors did not comment on obliteration of the subarachnoid space of the convexity.

In summary, at this point MRI is more likely than x-ray CT to contribute to the accuracy of the diagnosis of NPH and the prediction of shunt responsiveness in patients with this diagnosis.

PET and SPECT Studies

Perhaps because of the relatively small number of patients who have this disorder, very few studies have been performed on NPH patients with PET or SPECT. In a report on three patients with NPH studied with PET and ^{18}FDG,[107] glucose metabolic rates were reduced significantly compared to controls, but no regional deficit was seen (Fig. 9–10 *C,D*). Although no SPECT studies on NPH cases have been reported to date, the absence of regional deficits may be expected to be found in SPECT scans as well.

PET and SPECT studies may be useful for predicting shunt responsiveness in patients diagnosed to have NPH on the basis of clinical and x-ray CT or MRI findings. The presence of regional metabolic or blood flow deficits may indicate a concurrent disease such as MID or AD, and therefore a low likelihood of a clinically sustained response to a shunt procedure.

THE USE OF NEUROIMAGING IN THE DIFFERENTIAL DIAGNOSIS OF DEMENTING CONDITIONS

Morphologic abnormalities that can cause or contribute to a dementing disorder are most amenable to definition and quantitation by x-ray CT or MRI. For example, after a subarachnoid hemorrhage, hydrocephalus may develop and the size of the lateral ventricle on the x-ray CT scan may suggest why a persistent disorder of mentation is present. In this specific situation, reduction in size of the ventricle after a shunting procedure often coincides with rapid clearing of the cognitive deficit. The same phenomenon is often observed with a subdural hematoma before and after it is evacuated, and x-ray CT or MR scanning can demonstrate the resolution of the morphologic abnormality. Unfortunately, these morphologic abnormalities that are best visualized by x-ray CT or MRI are relatively uncommon causes of dementia. On the other hand, a disease such as Alzheimer's may or may not be associated with morphologic abnormalities such as cortical atrophy and ventricular enlargement, yet the functional deficits can be detected very early in the course of the disease by PET or SPECT scans.

It can be seen that for the most common cause of dementia, AD, functional imaging is far more informative than morphologic imaging. Nevertheless, in all the previously mentioned disorders, a combination of morphologic and functional definition of the brain is useful for establishing the diagnosis and understanding the pathophysiology. An example of a situation where this combined information is very useful is multi-infarct dementia. This condition cannot be effectively diagnosed without x-ray CT or MRI evidence of multiple infarcts. Multiple cerebral ischemic lesions, however, may be found in nondemented elderly individuals, who may sometimes be asymptomatic. A PET or SPECT scan could then be used to determine whether physiologic deficits are also present, thereby suggesting that the morphologic lesions are having a major functional impact in that patient.

The pathophysiology of dementia in any given patient may be complex. Certain disorders such as a frontal meningioma may produce dementia by direct mechanical effects. These effects can be visualized easily by x-ray CT or MR scanning, but secondary vascular effects also may play a part and only be detectable by functional imaging. Ambiguity often exists as to what factors have contributed to the dementia. Morphologic and functional imaging of the brain play very important roles in defining these contributions and thereby may help guide the management of these patients.

Figure 9–11 describes the use of neuroimaging techniques to assist in the diagnosis of some major causes of dementia. Clinical evaluation is the crucial first step—and not infrequently, the only step—required to make the diagnosis (e.g., for medication effects, depression, endocrine disorders). Because of the frequency with which more than one cause for a dementing syndrome may be present, however, the clinician often has to evaluate the patient further. Neuroimaging methods are invariably the next step in the diagnostic process.

Progressive dementing disorders can be classified according to clinical features in many different ways (e.g., subcortical versus cortical dementias, rapidly progressive versus gradually progressive dementias). In Fig. 9–11, the scheme of dividing causes of dementia into those with and those without major motor disorders is used because this method results in about half of all dementias being placed in each subdivision. Therefore, this is a clinically relevant approach to classifying dementias. The term "motor disorder" implies pyramidal, extrapyramidal and cerebellar dysfunction, all of which are very uncommon in AD and Pick's disease, in the mild and even moderate stages. In many of the other causes of dementia listed in Fig. 9–11, motor disorders are the most characteristic features of the disease. In multi-infarct dementia, Creutzfeldt-Jakob disease, and the space-occupying lesions, however, motor dysfunction is frequently present but not necessarily characteristic of the early stages of the disease.

Once a preliminary evaluation has

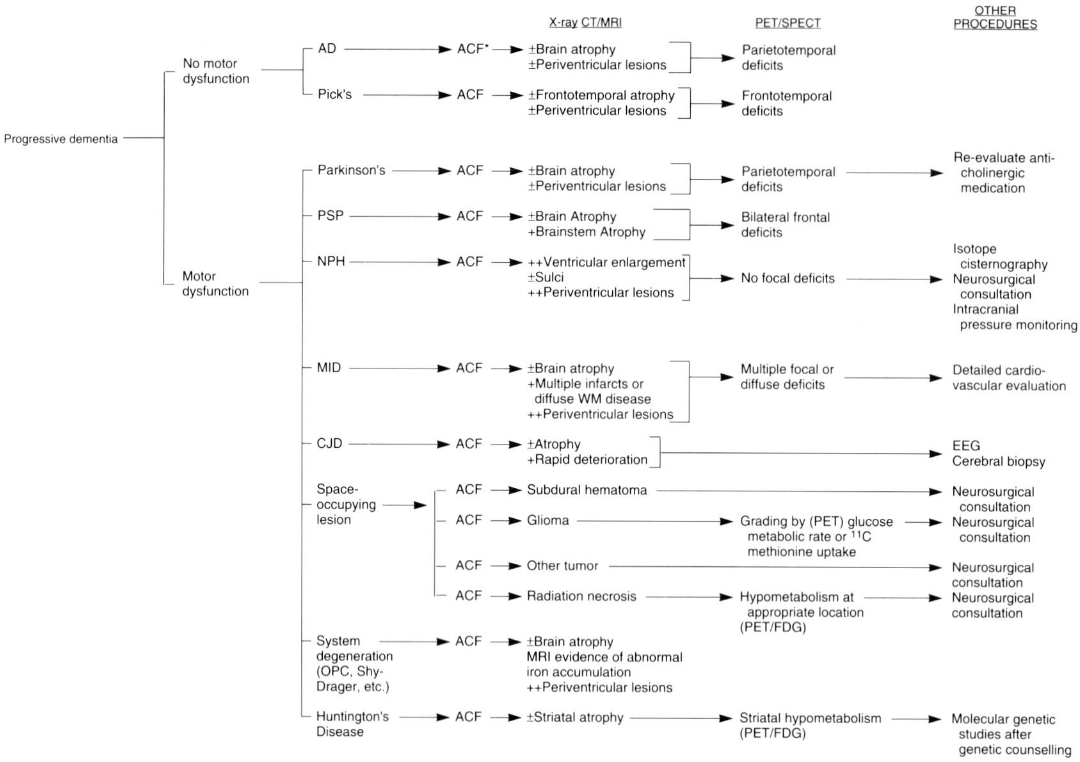

Figure 9–11. Neuroimaging methods in the differential diagnosis of dementia. Prior to the use of neuroimaging methods, clinical evaluation and laboratory tests are used to rule out medication effects, primary depression, endocrine disorders, syphilis, vitamin B_{12} deficiency, remote effects of cancer, Korsakoff's psychosis, post-traumatic state, collagen vascular disease, and, when appropriate, chronic meningoencephalitis (cryptococcosis, tuberculosis, and AIDS). ACF = appropriate clinical findings; AD = Alzheimer's disease; CJD = Creutzfeld-Jakob disease; FDG = fluorodeoxyglucose; MID = multi-infarct dementia; NPH = normal pressure hydrocephalus; OPC = olivoponto cerebellar degeneration; PSP = progressive supranuclear palsy; WM = white matter.

ruled out common and easily diagnosed conditions such as overmedication, hypothyroidism, and primary depression, appropriate clinical findings are the starting point in the evaluation of each diagnostic entity, followed by x-ray CT or MR scans. In some instances the MR scan provides a clear advantage over x-ray CT, as in assessing brainstem atrophy in PSP, or the extent of periventricular lesions and subarachnoid space in NPH; and in obtaining evidence of iron accumulation in systems degenerations. In the case of multi-infarct dementia, MRI may be able to detect many more ischemic lesions than x-ray CT, but the quantitative differences in these lesions in nondemented and demented subjects (if such a difference exists) is presently unclear.

PET and SPECT are particularly useful where the clinical and the x-ray CT/MRI findings are not clearly diagnostic, as is commonly the case. Alzheimer's disease, Pick's disease, and early cases of Huntington's disease are such disorders where CT/MRI studies are often unrevealing. In patients with MID and with NPH, PET and SPECT studies provide very useful additional information which may have therapeutic implications in NPH or provide evidence of the functional significance of CT/MRI lesions in MID.

REFERENCES

1. Adam, P, Fabre, N, Guell, A, Bessoles, G, Roulieau, J, and Bes, A: Cortical atrophy in Parkinson's disease: Correlation between clinical and CT finding with special emphasis on pre-frontal atrophy. AJNR 4:442–445, 1983.
2. Aharon-Peretz, L, Cummings, JL, and Hill, MA: Vascular dementia and dementia of the Alzheimer type: Cognition, ventricular size, and leuko-araiosis. Arch Neurol 45:719–721, 1988.
3. Alavi, A, Dann, R, Chawluk, J, Alavi, J, Kushner, M, and Reivich, M: Positron emission tomography imaging of regional cerebral glucose metabolism. Semin Nucl Med XVI(1):2–34, 1986.
4. Albert, M, Naeser, MA, Levine, HL, and Garvey, AJ: Ventricular size in patients with presenile dementia of the Alzheimer's type. Arch Neurol 41: 1258–1263, 1984.
5. Ambrosetto, P, Michelucci, R, Forti, A, and Tassinari, CA: CT findings in progressive supranuclear palsy. J Comput Assist Tomogr 8(3):406–409, 1984.
6. Appell, J, Kertesz, A, and Fisman, M: A study of language functioning in Alzheimer's patients. Brain Lang 17:73–91, 1982.
7. Awad, I, Johnson, P, Spetzler, R, and Hodak, J: Incidental subcortical lesions identified on magnetic resonance imaging in the elderly. II. Postmortem pathological correlations. Stroke 17:1090–1097, 1986.
8. Awad, I, Spetzler, R. Hodak, J, Awad, C, and Carey, R: Incidental subcortical lesions identified on magnetic resonance imaging in the elderly. I. Correlation with age and cerebrovascular risk factors. Stroke 17:1084–1089, 1986.
9. Babikian, V and Ropper, AH: Binswanger's disease: A review. Stroke 18(1):2–12, 1987.
10. Ball, S, Fox, P, Pardo, J, and Raichle, M: Control state stability for PET brain imaging: Rest versus task (abstr). Neurology (Suppl 1)38:362, 1988.
11. Barker, WW, Loewenstein, DA, Chang, JY, Pascal, S, Smith, D, Boothe, TE, Apicella, A, and Duara, R: FDG/PET studies of crossed cerebellar hypometabolism in dementia (abstr). Neurology (Suppl 1)38:364, 1988.
12. Baron, JC, Comar, D, Zarifian, E, Agid, Y, Crouzel, C, Loo, H, Deniker, P, and Kellershohn, C: Dopaminergic receptor sites in human brain: Positron emission tomography. Neurology 35:16–24, 1985.
13. Benson, DF, Kuhl, DE, Hawkins, RA, Phelps, ME, Cummings, JL, and Tsai, SY: The fluorodeoxyglucose ^{18}F scan in Alzheimer's disease and multi-infarct dementia. Arch Neurol 40:711–714, 1983.
14. Berent, S, Foster, NL, Gilman, S, Hichwa, R, and Lehitnen, S: Patterns of cortical ^{18}F-FDG metabolism in Alzheimer's and progressive supranuclear palsy patients are related to the types of cognitive impairment (abstr). Neurology (Suppl)37:172, 1987.
15. Berman, KF, and Weinberger, DR: Cortical physiological activation in Alzheimer's disease: rCBF studies during resting and cognitive states (abstr). Soc Neurosci Abstr 12:1160, 1986.
16. Blessed G, Tomlinson BE, and Roth, M: The association between quantitative measures of dementia and of senile change in the cerebral grey matter of elderly subjects. Br J Psychiatry 114:797–811, 1968.
17. Bonte, FJ, Ross, ED, Chehabi, HH, and Devous, MD Sr: SPECT study of regional cerebral blood flow in Alzheimer's disease. J Comput Assist Tomogr 10 (4):579–583, 1986.
18. Botwinick, J, Storandt, M, and Berg, L: A longitudinal, behavioral study of senile dementia of the Alzheimer's type. Arch Neurol 43:1124–1127, 1986.
19. Bradley, WG, Jr, Kortman, KE, and Burgoyne, B: Flowing cerebrospinal fluid in normal and hydrocephalic states: Appearance on MR images. Radiology 159:611–616, 1986.
20. Bradshaw, JR, Thompson, JLG, and Campbell, MJ: Computed tomography in the investigation of dementia. Br Med J 286:277–280, 1983.
21. Brandt, J, Folstein, SE, and Folstein, MF: Differential cognitive impairment

in Alzheimer's disease and Huntington's disease. Ann Neurol 23:555–561, 1988.
22. Breitner, JCS and Folstein, MF: Familial Alzheimer's dementia: A prevalent disorder with specific clinical features. Psychol Med 14:63–80, 1984.
23. Brinkman, SD, Sarwar, M, Levin, HS, and Morris, HH III: Quantitative indexes of computed tomography in dementia and normal aging. Radiology 138:89–92, 1981.
24. Brun, A and Englund, E: A white matter disorder in dementia of the Alzheimer type: A pathoanatomical study. Ann Neurol 19:253–262, 1986.
25. Brun, A and Englund, E: The pattern of degeneration in Alzheimer's disease: Neuronal loss and histopathological grading. Histopathology 5:549–564, 1981.
26. Brust, JCM: Dementia and cerebrovascular disease. In Mayeaux, R, and Rosen, WG (eds): The Dementias. Raven Press, New York, 1983, p 131.
27. Brust, JCM: Vascular dementia is overdiagnosed. Arch Neurol 45:799–801, 1988.
28. Butler, RW, Dickinson, WA, Katholi, C, and Halsey, H Jr: The comparative effects of organic brain disease on cerebral blood flow and measured intelligence. Ann Neurol 13:155–159, 1983.
29. Butters, N, Albert, MS, Sax, DS, Miliotis, P, Nagode, J, and Sterste, A: The effect of verbal mediators on the pictorial memory of brain-damaged patients. Neuropsychologia 21:307–323, 1983.
30. Cala, LA, Burns, P, Davis, R, and Jones, R: Alcohol-related brain damage: Serial studies after abstinence and recommencement of drinking. Australian Alcohol/Drug Rev 3:127–140, 1984.
31. Caplan, LR and Schoene, WC: Clinical features of subcortical arteriosclerotic encephalopathy (Binswanger disease). Neurology 28:1206–1215, 1978.
32. Celsis, P, Agriel, A, Puel, M, Rascol, A, and Marc-Vergnes, J-P: Focal cerebral hypoperfusion and selective cognitive deficit in dementia of the Alzheimer types. J Neurol Neurosurg Psychiatr 50:1602–1612, 1987.
33. Chase, TN, Fedio, P, Foster, NL, Brooks, R, Di Chiro, G, and Mansi, L: Wechsler adult intelligence scale performance. Cortical localization by fluorodeoxyglucose F18-positron emission tomography. Arch Neurol 41:1244–1247, 1984.
34. Chawluk, JB, Alavi, A, Dann, R, Hurtig, HI, Bais, S, Kushner, MJ, Zimmerman, RA, and Reivich, M: Positron emission tomography in aging and dementia: Effect of cerebral atrophy. J Nucl Med 28:431–437, 1987.
35. Chiu, HC, Teng, EL, Henderson, VW, and Moy, AC: Clinical subtypes of dementia of the Alzheimer's type. Neurology 35(11):1544–1550, 1985.
36. Ciemens, VA: Localized thalamic hemorrhage: A cause of aphasia. Neurology 20:776–782, 1970.
37. Cohen, MB, Graham, LS, Lake, R, Metter, EJ, Fitten, J, Kulkarni, MK, Sevrin, R, Yamada, L, Chang, CC, Woodruff, N, and Kling, AS: Diagnosis of Alzheimer's disease and multiple infarct dementia by tomographic imaging of Iodine-123 IMP. J Nucl Med 27:769–774, 1986.
38. Condon, BR, Patterson, J. Wyper, D, Hadley, M, Teasdale, G, Grant, R, Jenkins, A, Macpherson, P, and Rowan, J: A quantitative index of ventricular and extraventricular intracranial CSF volumes using MR imaging. Radiology 10(5):784–792, 1986.
39. Cummings, JL and Duchen, LW: Kluver-Bucy syndrome in Pick disease: Clinical and pathologic correlations. Neurology 31:1415–1422, 1981.
40. Cutler, NR, Haxby, JV, Duara, R, Grady, CL, Moore, AM, Parisi, JE, White, J, Heston, L, Margolin, RM, and Rapoport, SI: Brain metabolism as measured with positron emission tomography: Serial assessment in a patient with familial Alzheimer's disease. Neurology 35:1556–1561, 1985.
41. Damasio, AR, Damasio, H, Risso, M, Varney, N, and Gersh, F: Aphasia with nonhemorrhagic lesions in the basal ganglia and internal capsule. Arch Neurol 39:15–20, 1982.
42. D'Antona, R, Baron, JC, Samson, Y, Seraru, M, Viader, F, Agid, Y, and Cam-

bier, J: Subcortical dementia. Frontal cortex hypometabolism detected by positron emission tomography in patients with progressive supranuclear palsy. Brain 108:785–799, 1985.

43. Dastur, DK, Lane, ML, Hansen, DB, Kety, SS, Butler, RN, Perlin, S, and Sokoloff, L: Effects of aging on cerebral circulation and metabolism in man. In Human Aging: A Biological and Behavioral Study, P.H.S. Publication No. 986, US Govt Printing Office, Washington DC, 1963, pp 59–76.
44. DeLeon, MJ, Ferris, SH, George, AE, Reisberg, B, Kricheff, II, and Gershon, S: Computed tomography evaluations of brain-behavior relationships in senile dementia of the Alzheimer's type. Neurobiol Aging 1:69–79, 1980.
45. DeLeon, MJ, George, AE, Ferris, SH, Christman, DR, Fowler, JS, Gentes, C, Brodie, J, Reisberg, B, and Wolf, AP: Positron emission tomography and computerized tomography of the aging brain. J Comput Tomogr 8:88–94, 1984.
46. DeLeon, MJ, Ferris, SH, George, AE, Christman, DR, Fowler, JS, Gentes, CI, Reisberg B, Gee, B, Kricheff, II, Emmerich, M, Yonekura, Y, Brodie, J, Kricheff, II, and Wolf, AP: Positron emission tomography studies of aging and Alzheimer disease. AJNR 4:568–571, 1983.
47. Devous, MD Sr, Stokely, EM, Chehabi, HH, and Bonte FJ: Normal distribution of regional cerebral blood flow measured by dynamic single-photon emission tomography. J Cereb Blood Flow Metabol 6:95–104, 1986.
48. Diagnostic and Statistical Manual of Mental Disorders (DSM-IIIR). American Psychiatric Association, Washington, DC, 1987.
49. Drayer, BP: Imaging of the aging brain: Part I. Normal findings. Radiology 166:785–796, 1988.
50. Drayer, BP, Olanow, W, Burger, P, Johnson, GA, Herfkens, R, and Reiderer, A: Parkinson plus syndrome: Diagnosis using high field MR imaging of brain iron. Radiology 159:493–498, 1986.
51. Duara, R, Yoshii, F, Barker, WW, Apicella, A, Chang, JY, and Sheldon, J: White matter (WM) and gray matter (GM) alterations in aging and dementia by magnetic resonance scanning (abstr). Neurology (Suppl)36:103, 1986.
52. Duara, R, Yoshii, F, Chang, JY, Barker, WW, Apicella, A, and Sheldon, J: PET in the differential diagnosis of dementia (abstr). Neurology (Suppl 1)37:158, 1987.
53. Duara, R, Gross-Glenn, K, Barker, WW, Chang, JY, Apicella, A, Loewenstein, DA, and Boothe, T: Behavioral activation and the variability of cerebral glucose metabolic measurements. J Cereb Blood Flow Metabol 7:266–271, 1987.
54. Duara, R, Barker, WW, Chang, JY, Loewenstein, DA, Apicella, A, Yoshii, F, and Kothari, P: Relationship of cortical and isolated white matter MRI lesions to local cortical metabolism on FDG/PET scans (abstr). Neurology (Suppl 1) 38:399, 1988.
55. Duara, R, Gutterman, A, Loewenstein, D, Eisdorfer, C, Chang, JY, Barker, WW, and Apicella, A: The clinical and PET scan pattern of probable Pick's disease (abstr). Neurology (Suppl 1)38:415, 1988.
56. Duara, R, Grady, C, Haxby, JV, Ingvar, D, Sokoloff, L, Margolin, RA, Manning, RG, Cutler, R, and Rapoport, SI: Human brain glucose utilization and cognitive function in relation to age. Ann Neurol 16:702–713, 1984.
57. Duara, R, Grady, C, Haxby, J, Sundaram, M, Cutler, NR, Heston, L, Moore, A, Schlageter, N, Larson, S, and Rapoport, SI: Positron emission tomography in Alzheimer's disease. Neurology 36:879–887, 1986.
58. Duara, R. Margolin, RA, Robertson-Tchabo, EA, London, ED, Schwartz, M, Renfrew, JW, Koziarz, BJ, Sundaram, M, Grady, C, Moore, AM, Ingvar, DH, Sokoloff, L, Weingartner, H, Kessler, RM, Manning, RG, Channing, MA, Cutler, NR, and Rapoport, SI: Cerebral glucose utilization, as measured with positron emission tomography in 21 resting healthy men between the ages of 21 and 83 years. Brain 106:761–775, 1983.

59. Dubinsky, RM and Jankovic, J: Progressive supranuclear palsy and a multi-infarct state. Neurology 37:570–576, 1987.
60. Earnest, MP, Fahn, S, Karp, JH, and Rowland, LP: Normal pressure hydrocephalus and hypertensive cerebrovascular disease. Arch Neurol 31:262–266, 1974.
61. Earnest, MP, Heaton, RK, Wilkinson, WE, and Manke, WF: Cortical atrophy, ventricular enlargement and intellectual impairment in the aged. Neurology 29:1138–1143, 1979.
62. Eidelberg, D, Moeller, JR, Sidtis, JJ, Dhawan, V, Strother, DC, Ginos, JZ, Cedarbaum, J, Greene, P, Fahn, S, and Rottenberg, DA: The metabolic pathology of Parkinson's disease: Complementary ^{18}F-fluorodopa and ^{18}F-fluorodeoxyglucose PET studies (abstr). Neurology (Suppl 1)39:273, 1989.
63. Englund, E, Brun, A, and Persson, B: Correlations between histopathologic white matter changes and proton MR relaxation times in dementia. Alzheimer Disease and Associated Disorders 1(3):156–170, 1987.
64. Erkinjuntti, T, Ketonen, L, Sulkava, R, Sipponen, N, Vuorialho, M, and Iivanainen, M: Do white matter changes on MRI and CT differentiate vascular dementia from Alzheimer's disease? J Neurol Neurosurg Psychiatr 50:37–42, 1987.
65. Eslinger, PJ, Damasio, H, Braff-Radford, N, and Damasio, AR: Examining the relationship between computed tomography and neuropsychological measures in normal and demented elderly. J Neurol Neurosurg Psychiatr 47:1319–1325, 1984.
66. Fazekas, F, Chawluk, JB, Alavi, A, Hurtig, HI, and Zimmerman, RA: MR signal abnormalities at 1.5 T in Alzheimer's dementia and normal aging. AJNR 8:421–426, 1987
67. Ferris, SH, deLeon, MJ, Wolf, AP, Farkas, T, Christman, DR, Reisberg, B, Fowler, JR, MacGregor, R, Goldman, A, George, AE, and Rampal, S: Positron emission tomography in the study of aging and senile dementia. Neurobiol Aging 1(2):127–131, 1980.
68. Fisher, CM: Lacunes: Small, deep cerebral infarcts. Neurology 15:774–784, 1965.
69. Foster, NL, Hansen, MS, Siegel, GJ, and Kuhl, DE: Medial and lateral temporal glucose metabolism in aging and Alzheimer's disease studied by PET (abstr). Neurology (Suppl 1)38:133, 1988.
70. Foster, NL, Morin, EM, Kuhl, DE, and Gilman, S: Glucose metabolic activity in the basal ganglia and thalamus differs in progressive supranuclear palsy and Alzheimer's disease (abstr). Neurology (Suppl 1)38:369, 1988.
71. Foster, NL, Chase, TN, Fedio, P, Paronas, NJ, Brooks, RA, and Di Chiro, G: Alzheimer's disease: focal cortical changes shown by positron emission tomography. Neurology 33:961–965, 1983.
72. Foster, NL, Gilman, S, Berent, S, Morin, EM, Brown, MB, and Koeppe, RA: Cerebral hypometabolism in progressive supranuclear palsy studied with positron emission tomography. Ann Neurol 24:399–406, 1988.
73. Frackowiack, RSJ, Lenzi, GL, Jones T, and Heather, JD: Quantitative measurement of regional cerebral blood flow and oxygen metabolism in man using ^{15}O and positron emission tomography: theory, procedure, and normal values. J Comput Assist Tomogr 4(6):727–736, 1980.
74. Frackowiack, RSJ, Pozzilli, C, Legg, NJ, Du Boulay, GH, Marshall, J, Lenzi, GL, and Jones, T: Regional cerebral oxygen supply and utilization in dementia: A clinical and physiological study with oxygen-15 and positron tomography. Brain 104:753–778, 1981.
75. Friedland, RP, Brun, A, and Budinger, TF: Pathologic and positron emission tomographic correlations in Alzheimer's disease. Lancet 1:228, 1985.
76. Friedland, RP, Budinger, TF, Brant-Zawadzki, M, and Jagust, WJ: The diagnosis of Alzheimer-type dementia. JAMA 252:2750–2752, 1984.
77. Friedland, RP, Yano, Y, Budinger, TF, Ganz, E, Huesman, RH, Derenzo, SE, and Knittel, B: Quantitative evaluation of blood brain barrier integrity in Alz-

heimer-type dementia: Positron emission tomographic studies with Rubidium-82. Eur Neurol 22(S2):19–20, 1983.

78. Friedland, RP, Budiner, TF, Ganz, E, Yano, Y, Mathid, CA, Koss, B, Ober, BA, Huesman, RH, and Derenzo, SE: Regional cerebral metabolic alterations in dementia of the Alzheimer type: Positron emission tomography with [^{18}F] fluorodeoxy-glucose. J Comput Assist Tomogr 7(4):590–598, 1983.
79. Fromm, D, Holland, AL, Swindell, CS, and Reinmuth, OM: Various consequences of subcortical stroke. Arch Neurol 42:943–950, 1985.
80. Gado, M, Hughes, CP, Danziger, W, Chi, D, Jost, G, and Berg, L: Volumetric measures of the cerebrospinal fluid spaces in demented subjects and controls. Radiology 144:535–538, 1982.
81. Garnett, ES, Nahmias, C, and Firnau, G: Central dopaminergic pathways in hemiparkinsonism examined by positron emission tomography. Can J Neurol Sci 11:174–179, 1984.
82. George, AE, deLeon, MJ, and Ferris, SH: Parenchymal CT correlates of senile dementia: Loss of gray-white discriminability. AJNR, 2:205–213, 1981.
83. George, AE, deLeon, MJ, Gentes, CI, Miller, J, London, E, Budzilovich, GN, Ferris, S, and Chase, N: Leukoencephalopathy in normal and pathologic aging: 1. CT of brain lucencies. AJNR 7:561–566, 1986.
84. Gerard, G and Weisberg, LA: MRI periventricular lesions in adults. Neurology 36:998–1001, 1986.
85. Gilman, S, Markel, DS, Koeppe, RA, Junck, L, Kluin, KJ, Gebarski, SS, and Hichwa, RD: Cerebellar and brainstem hypometabolism in olivopontocerebellar atrophy detected with positron emission tomography. Ann Neurol 23:223–230, 1988.
86. Goto, K, Ishii, N, and Fukasawa, H: Diffuse white-matter disease in the geriatric population. Radiology 141:687–695, 1981.
87. Groen, JJ and Hekster, REM: Computed tomography in Pick's disease: Findings in a family affected in three consecutive generations. J Comput Assist Tomogr 6(5):907–911, 1982.
88. Guinane JE: Why does hydrocephalus progress? J Neurol Sci 32:1–8, 1977.
89. Haase, G: Diseases presenting as dementia. In Wells, C (ed): Dementia. FA Davis, Philadelphia, 1977, pp 27–67.
90. Hachinski, VC, Lassen, NA, and Marshall, J: Multi-infarct dementia: A cause of mental deterioration in the elderly. Lancet July:207–210, 1974.
91. Hachinski, VC, Hiff, LD, Zalkha, E, Du Boulay, GH, McAllister, VL, Marshall, J, Russell, RWR, and Symon, L: Cerebral blood flow in dementia. Arch Neurol 32:632–637, 1975.
92. Hakim, S and Adams, RD: The special clinical problem of symptomatic hydrocephalus with normal cerebrospinal fluid pressure. Observations on cerebrospinal fluid hydrodynamics. J Neurol Sci 2:307–327, 1965.
93. Haldeman, S, Goldman, JW, Hyde, J, and Pribram, HFW: Progressive supranuclear palsy, computed tomography and response to antiparkinsonian drugs. Neurology 31:442–445, 1981.
94. Hawkins, RA, Mazziotta, JC, Phelps, ME, Huang, SC, Kuhl, DE, Carson, RE, Metter, RJ, and Reige, WH: Cerebral glucose metabolism as a function of age in man: Influence of the rate constants in the fluorodeoxyglucose method. J Cereb Blood Flow Metabol 3:250–253, 1983.
95. Haxby, JV, Duara, R, Grady, CL, Cutler, NR, and Rapoport, SI: Relations between neuropsychological and cerebral metabolic asymmetries in early Alzheimer's disease. J Cereb Blood Flow Metabol 5:193–200, 1985.
96. Haxby, JV, Grady, CL, Duara, R, Schlageter, N, Berg, G, and Rapoport, SI: Neocortical metabolic abnormalities precede nonmemory cognitive defects in early Alzheimer's-type dementia. Arch Neurol 43:882–885, 1986.
97. Hellman, RS and Collier, BD: Single photon emission computed tomography: A clinical experience. In Freeman LM, and Weissmann, HS (eds): Nuclear Medicine Annual 1987. Raven Press, New York, 1987, pp 51–101.

98. Herscovitch, P, Auchua, A, Gado, M, Chi, D, and Raichle, M: Correction of positron emission tomography data for cerebral atrophy. J Cereb Blood Flow Metabol 6:120–124, 1986.
99. Hershey, LA, Modic, MT, Greenough, G, and Jaffee, DF: Magnetic resonance imaging in vascular dementia. Neurology 37:29–36, 1987.
100. Heston, LH and Mastri, AR: Age at onset of Pick's and Alzheimer's dementia: Implications for diagnosis and research. J Gerontol 37:422–424, 1982.
101. Huber, SJ, Paulson, GW, Shuttleworth, EC, and Chakeres, D: Magnetic resonance imaging is nonspecific to dementia in Parkinson's disease (abstr). Neurology (Suppl 1)38:329, 1988.
102. Ishii, N, Nishihara, Y, and Imamura, T: Why do frontal lobe symptoms predominate in vascular dementia with lacunes? Neurology 36:340–345, 1986.
103. Ito, B, Hatazawa, J, Yamaura, H, and Matsuzawa, T: Age-related brain atrophy and mental deterioration: A study with computed tomography. Br J Radiol 54:384–390, 1981.
104. Jack, CR Jr, Mokri, B, Laws, ER, Houser, OW, Baker, HL Jr, and Petersen, D: MR findings in normal-pressure hydrocephalus: Significance and comparison with other forms of dementia. J Comput Assist Tomogr 11(6):923–931, 1987.
105. Jackson, JA, Jankovic, J, and Ford, J: Progressive supranuclear palsy: Clinical features and response to treatment in 16 patients. Ann Neurol 13:273–278, 1983.
106. Jacoby, RJ and Levy, R: Computed Tomography in the Elderly. 2. Senile dementia: Diagnosis and functional impairment. Br J Psychiatry 136: 256–269, 1980.
107. Jagust, WJ, Friedland, RP, and Budinger, TF: Positron emission tomography differentiates normal pressure hydrocephalus from Alzheimer's disease. J Neurol Neurosurg Psychiatr 48:1091–1096, 1985.
108. Jagust, WJ, Budinger, TF, and Reed, BR: The diagnosis of dementia with single photon emission computed tomography. Arch Neurol 44:259–262, 1987.
109. Joachim, CL, Morris, JH, and Selkoe, DJ: Clinically diagnosed Alzheimer's disease: Autopsy results in 150 cases. Ann Neurol 24:50–56, 1988.
110. Johnson, KA, Mueller, ST, Walshe, M, English, RJ, and Holman, BL: Cerebral perfusion imaging in Alzheimer's disease. Arch Neurol 44:165–168, 1987.
111. Kamo, H, McGeer, PL, Harrop, R, McGeer, EG, Caine, DB, Martin, WRW, and Pate, BD: Positron emission tomography and histopathology in Pick's disease. Neurology 37:439–445, 1987.
112. Kinkel, WR, Jacobs, L, Polachini, I, Bates, V, and Heffner, RR: Subcortical arteriosclerotic encephalopathy (Binswanger's disease). Arch Neurol 42: 951–959, 1985.
113. Knopman, DS, Christensen, KJ, Schut, LS, and Ngo, T: Neuropsychometric and computed tomographic findings in Pick's disease (abstr). Neurology (Suppl 1)38:228, 1988.
114. Koto, A. Rosenberg, G, Zingesser, LH, Horoupian, D, and Katzman, R: Syndrome of normal pressure hydrocephalus: Possible relation to hypertensive and arteriosclerotic vasculopathy. J Neurol Neurosurg Psychiatr 40:73–79, 1977.
115. Kuhl, DE, Metter, EJ, and Riege, WH: Patterns of local cerebral glucose utilization determined in Parkinson's disease by the [^{18}F]fluorodeoxyglucose method. Ann Neurol 15:419–424, 1984.
116. Kuhl, DE, Metter, EJ, Riege, WH, and Phelps, ME: Effects of human aging on patterns of local cerebral glucose utilization determined by the [18F]fluorodeoxyglucose method. J Cereb Blood Flow Metab 2:163–171, 1982.
117. Kuhl, DE, Metter, EJ, Benson, F, Ashford, JW, Riege, WH, Fujikawa, DG, Markham, CH, Mazziotta, JC, Maltese A, and Dorsey, DA: Similarities of cerebral glucose metabolism in Alzheimer's and Parkinson's dementia. J Cereb Blood Flow Metabol (Suppl 1)5:S169–170, 1985.
118. Kuhl, DE, Small, GW, Riege, WH, Fuji-

kawa, EJ, Metter, EJ, Benson, DF, Ashford, JW, Mazziotta, JC, Maltese, A, and Dorsey, DA: Cerebral metabolic patterns before the diagnosis of probable Alzheimer's disease (abstr). J Cereb Blood Flow Metabol (Suppl)7:S406, 1987.

119. Larson, EB, Reifler, BV, Sumi, SM, Canfield, CG, and Chinn, NM: Diagnostic tests in the evaluation of dementia: A prospective study of 200 elderly outpatients. Arch Intern Med 146:1917–1922, 1986.

120. Lebrun-Grandie, P, Baron, J, Soussaline, F, Loch, H, Sastre, J, and Bousser, M: Coupling between regional blood flow and oxygen utilization in the normal human brain. Arch Neurol 40:230–236, 1983.

121. LeMay, M: CT changes in dementing diseases: A review. AJNR 7:841–853, 1986.

122. LeMay, M and Hochberg, FH: Ventricular differences between hydrostatic hydrocephalus and hydrocephalus ex vacuo by computed tomography. Neuroradiology 17:191–195, 1979.

123. LeMay, M, Stafford, JL, Sandor, T, Albert, M, Haykal, H, and Samani, A: Statistical assessment of perceptual CT scan ratings in patients with Alzheimer type dementia. J Comput Assist Tomogr 10(5):802–809, 1986.

124. Lenzi, GL, Frackowiak, RS, Jones, T, Heather, JD, Lammertsma, AA, Rhodes, CG, and Pozzilli, C: $CMRO_2$ and CBF by the oxygen-15 inhalation technique. Results in normal volunteers and cerebrovascular patients. Eur Neurol 20:285–290, 1981.

125. Levasseur, M, Setter, G, Pappata, S, Laplane, D, Tran Dinh, Dubois, B, Baulac, M, and Baron, JC: Abnormal frontal cortex glucose utilization (CMRglu) in behaviorally impaired subjects with bilateral pallidal lesions (BPL): A PET study (abstr). Neurology (Suppl 1) 38:397, 1988.

126. Liston, EH and La Rue, A: Clinical differentiation of primary degenerative and multi-infarct dementia: A critical review of the evidence. Part II: Pathological Studies. Biol Psychiatry 18(12): 1467–1484, 1983.

127. Loeb, C, and Gandolfo, C: Diagnostic evaluation of degenerative and vascular dementia. Stroke (14(3):399–401, 1983.

128. Loewenstein, D, Yoshii, F, Barker, WW, Apicella, A, Emran, A, Chang, JY, and Duara, R: Predominant left hemisphere metabolic dysfunction in dementia. Arch Neurol 46:146–152, 1989.

129. Lotz, PR, Ballinger, WE, Jr, and Quisling, RG: Subcortical arteriosclerotic encephalopathy: CT spectrum and pathologic correlation. AJNR 7:817–822, 1986.

130. Maher, ER, and Lees, AJ: The clinical features and natural history of the Steele-Richardson-Olszewski syndrome (progressive supranuclear palsy). Neurology 36:1005–1008, 1986.

131. Manon-Espaillat, R, Lanska, D, Ruff, RL, and Marsaryk, T: Magnetic resonance imaging in progressive supranuclear palsy: Decreased signal intensity in the basal ganglia (abstr). Neurology (Suppl 1):38:192, 1988.

132. Marshall, VG, Bradley, WG Jr, Marshall, CE, Bhoopat, T, and Rhodes, RH: Deep white matter infarction: Correlation of MR imaging and histopathologic findings. Radiology 167:517–522, 1988.

133. Martin, WRW, Palmer, MR, Peppard, RF, and Caine, DB: Quantitation of presynaptic dopaminergic function with positron emission tomography (abstr.) Neurology (Suppl 1)39:163, 1989.

134. Mayeaux, R and Stern, Y: Intellectual dysfunction and dementia in Parkinson disease. In Mayeaux, R and Rosen, WG (eds): The Dementias. Raven Press, New York, 1983, pp 211–227.

135. Mayeaux, R, Stern, Y, and Spanton, S: Heterogeneity in dementia of the Alzheimer type: Evidence of subgroups. Neurology 35:453–461, 1985.

136. McGeachie, RE, Fleming, JO, Sharer, LR, and Hyman, RA: Diagnosis of Pick's disease by computed tomography. J Comput Assist Tomogr 3(1):113–115, 1979.

137. McGeer, PL, Kamo, H, McGeer, EG, Martin, WRW, Pate, BD, and Li, DKB:

Comparison of PET, MRI and CT with pathology in a proven case of Alzheimer's disease. Neurology 36:1569–1574, 1986.
138. McGeer, PL, Kamo, H, Harrop, R, Li, DKB, Tuokko, H, McGeer, EG, Adam, MJ, Ammann, W, Beattie, BL, Caine, DB, Martin, WRW, Pate, BD, Rogers, JG, Ruth, TJ, Sayre, CI, and Stoessel, AJ: Positron emission tomography in patients with clinically diagnosed Alzheimer's disease. Can Med Assoc J 134:597–607, 1986.
139. McKhann, G, Drachman, D, Folstein, M, Katzman, R, Price, D, and Stadlan, EM: Clinical diagnosis of Alzheimer's disease: report of the NINCDS-ADRDA work group under the auspices of department of health and human services task force on Alzheimer's disease. Neurology 34:939–944, 1984.
140. Melamed, E, Lavy, S, Bentin, S, Cooper, G, and Rinot, Y: Reduction in regional cerebral blood flow during normal aging in man. Stroke 11:31–35, 1980.
141. Meyer, JS, Sakai, F, Naritomi, H, and Grant, P: Normal and abnormal patterns of cerebrovascular reserve tested by ^{133}Xe inhalation. Arch Neurol 35: 350–359, 1978.
142. Miller, JD, deLeon, MJ, Ferris, SH, Kluger, A, George, AE, Reisberg, B, Sachs, SJ, and Wolff, AP: Abnormal temporal lobe response in Alzheimer's disease during cognitive processing as measured by ^{11}C-2-deoxy-D-glucose and PET. J Cereb Blood Flow Metabol 7:248–251, 1987.
143. Molsa, PK, Paljarvi, Rinne JO, Rinne, UK, and Sako, E: Validity of clinical diagnosis in dementia: A prospective clinicopathological study. J Neurol Neurosurg Psychiatr 48:1085–1090, 1985.
144. Morris, JC, Cole, M, Banker, BQ, and Wright, D: Hereditary dysphasic dementia and the Pick-Alzheimer spectrum. Ann Neurol 16:455–466, 1984.
145. Moss, MB, Albert, MS, Butters, N, and Payne, M: Differential patterns of memory loss among patients with Alzheimer's disease, Huntington's disease, and alcoholic Korsakoff's syndrome. Arch Neurol 43:239–246, 1983.
146. Munoz-Garcia, D, and Ludwin, K: Classic and generalized variations of Pick's disease: A clincopathological, ultrastructural, and immunocytochemical comparative study. Ann Neurol 16:467–480, 1984.
147. Naeser, MA, Alexander, MP, Helm-Estabrooks, N, Levine, HL, Laughlin, SA, and Geschwind, N: Aphasia with predominantly subcortical lesion sites. Arch Neurol 39:2–14, 1982.
148. Nahmias, C, Garnett, ES, Firnau, G, and Lang, A: Striatal dopamine distribution in parkinsonian patients during life. J Neurol Sci 69:223–230, 1985.
149. Naritomi, H, Meyer, JS, Sakai, F, Yamaguchi, F, and Shaw, T: Effects of advancing age on regional cerebral blood flow. Studies in normal subjects and subjects with risk factors for atherothrombotic stroke. Arch Neurol 36:410–416, 1979.
150. Neary, D, Snowden, JS, Shields, RA, Burjan, AWI, Northern, B, MacDermott, N, Prescott, MC, and Testa, HJ: Single photon emission tomography using ^{99m}Tc-HM-PAO in the investigation of dementia. J Neurol Neurosurg Psychiatr 50:1101–1109, 1987.
151. O'Brien, MD: Vascular dementia is underdiagnosed. Arch Neurol 45:797–798, 1988.
152. Office of Technology Assessment, US Congress. 07A-BA-323. Losing a million minds: Confronting the tragedy of Alzheimer's disease and other dementias. US Govt Printing Office, Washington, DC, April 1987.
153. Pantano, P, Baron, J, Lebrun-Grandie, P, Duquesnoy, N, Bousser, M, and Comar, D: Regional cerebral blood flow and oxygen consumption in human aging. Stroke 15:635–641, 1984.
154. Pastakia, B, Polinsky, R, Di Chiro, G. Simmons, JT, Brown, R, and Wener, L: Multiple system atrophy (Shy-Drager syndrome): MR imaging. Radiology 159:499–502, 1986.
155. Pawlik, G, Heiss, WD, Beil, C, Wienhard, K, Herholz, K, and Wagner, R: PET demonstrates differential age dependence, asymmetry and response to various stimuli of regional brain glucose metabolism in healthy volunteers

(abstr). J Cereb Blood Flow Metabol (Suppl 1) 7:S376, 1987.

156. Perani, D, Di Piero, V, Vallar, G, Cappa, S, Messa, C, Bottini, G, Berti, A, Passafiume, D, Scarlato, G, Gerundini, P, Lenzi, GL, and Fazio, F: Technetium-99m HM-PAO-SPECT study of regional cerebral perfusion in early Alzheimer's disease. J Nucl Med 29:1507–1514, 1988.
157. Perlmutter, JS and Raichle, ME: Regional blood flow in hemiparkinsonism. Neurology 35:1127–1134, 1985.
158. Perlmutter, JS, Kilbourn, MR, Raichle, ME, and Welch, MJ: Positron emission tomographic demonstration of upregulation of radioligand-receptor binding in human MPTP-induced parkinsonism (abstr). J Cereb Blood Flow Metabol (Suppl 1)7:S371, 1987.
159. Perlmutter, JS, Powers, WJ, Herscovitch, P, Fox, PT, and Raichle, ME: Regional asymmetries of cerebral blood flow, blood volume, and oxygen utilization and extraction in normal subjects. J Cereb Blood Flow Metabol 7:64–67, 1987.
160. Perry, RH: Recent advances in neuropathology. Br Med Bull 42(1):34–41, 1986.
161. Petersen, RC, Mokri, B, and Laws, R, Jr: Surgical treatment of idiopathic hydrocephalus in elderly patients. Neurology 35:307–311, 1985.
162. Podreka, I, Suess, E, Goldenberg, G, Steiner, M, Brucke, T, Muller, C, Lang, W, Neirinckx, RD, and Deecke, L: Initial experience with Technetium-99m HM-PAO brain SPECT. J Nucl Med 28:1657–1666, 1987.
163. Quinn, NP, Rossor, MN, and Marsden, CD: Dementia and Parkinson's disease: Pathological and neurochemical considerations. Br Med Bull 42(1):86–90, 1986.
164. Radue, EW, du Boulay, GH, Harrison, MJG, and Thomas, DJ: Comparison of angiographic and CT findings between patients with multi-infarct dementia and those with dementia due to primary neuronal degeneration. Neuroradiology 16:113–115, 1978.
165. Reisberg, B, Borenstein, J, Salob, SP, Ferris, SH, Franssen, E, and Georgotas, A: Behavioral symptoms in Alzheimer's disease: Phenomenology and treatment. J Clin Psychiatry (Suppl) 48:9–15, 1987.
166. Rinne, UK, Laihinen, A, Rinne, JO, Nagren, K, Bergman, J, and Ruotsalainen, U: Positron emission tomography (PET) demonstrates dopamine receptor supersensitivity in the striatum of patients with early Parkinson's disease (abstr). Neurology (Suppl 1)39:273, 1989.
167. Risberg, J: Regional cerebral blood flow measurements by ^{133}Xe-inhalation: Methodology and applications in neuropsychology and psychiatry. Brain Lang 9:9–34, 1980.
168. Roberts, MA, and Caird, FI: Computerized tomography and intellectual impairment in the elderly. J Neurol Neurosurg Psychiatr 39:986–989, 1976
169. Roman, GC: Senile dementia of the Binswanger type: A vascular form of dementia in the elderly. JAMA 258(13): 1782–1788, 1987.
170. Rosen, WG, Terry, RD, Fuld, PA, Katzman, R, and Peck, A: Pathological verification of ischemic score in differentiation of dementias. Ann Neurol 7: 486–488, 1980.
171. Rosenberg, GA, Kornfeld, M, Stovring, J, and Bicknell, JM: Subcortical arteriosclerotic encephalopathy (Binswanger): Computerized tomography. Neurology 29:1102–1106, 1979.
172. Salibi, NA, Lourie, GL, and Lourie, H: A variant of normal-pressure hydrocephalus simulating Pick's disease on computerized tomography. J Neurosurg 59:902–904, 1983.
173. Schlageter NL, Carson, RE, and Rapoport, SI: Examination of blood-brain barrier permeability in dementia of the Alzheimer type with [^{68}Ga]EDTA and positron emission tomography. J Cereb Blood Flow Metabol 67:1–8, 1987.
174. Schlageter, NL, Horwitz, B, Creasey, H, Carson, R, Duara, R, Berg, GW, and Rapoport, SI: Relation of measured brain glucose utilization and cerebral atrophy in man. J Neurol Neurosurg Psychiatr 50:779–785, 1987.
175. Schneider, E, Fisher, PA, Jacobi, P, Becker, H, and Hacker, H: The signifi-

cance of cerebral atrophy for the symptomotology of Parkinson's disease. J Neurol Sci 42:187–197, 1979.

176. Schoenberg, BS, Kokmen, E, and Okazaki, H: Alzheimer's disease and other dementing illnesses in a defined United States population: Incidence rates and clinical features. Ann Neurol 22:724–729, 1987.

177. Schwartz, M, Creasey, H, Grady, CL, DeLeo, JM, Frederickson, HA, Cutler, NR, and Rapoport, SL: Computed tomographic analysis of brain morphometrics in 30 healthy men aged 21 to 81 years. Ann Neurol 17:146–157, 1985.

178. Shapiro, MB, Ball, MJ, Grady, CL, Haxby, JV, Kaye, JA, and Rapoport, SI: Dementia in Down's syndrome: Cerebral glucose utilization, neuropsychological assessment and neuropathology. Neurology 38:938–942, 1988.

179. Sharp, P, Gemmell, H, Cherryman, G, Besson, J, Crawford, J, and Smith, F: Application of Iodine-123-labeled Isopropylamphetamine imaging to the study of dementia. J Nucl Med 27:761–768, 1986.

180. Shibayama, H, Kitoh, J, Marui, Y, Kobayashi, H, Iwase, S, and Kayukawa, Y: An unusual case of Pick's disease. Acta Neuropathol 59:79–87, 1983.

181. Sjögren, T, Sjögren, H, and Lindgren, A: Morbus Alzheimer and morbus Pick: Genetic, clinical and pathoanatomic study. Acta Psychiatr Scand (Suppl) 82:1–152, 1952.

182. Smith, JS and Kiloh, LG: The investigation of dementia: Results in 200 consecutive admissions. Lancet 1:824–827, 1981.

183. Soininen, H, Puranen, M, and Riekkinen, PJ: Computed tomography findings in senile dementia and normal aging. J Neurol Neurosurg Psychiatr 45:50–54, 1982.

184. Sroka, H, Elizan, TS, Yahr, MD, Burger, A, and Mendoza, MR: Organic mental syndrome and confusion states in Parkinson's disease: Relationship to computerized tomographic signs of cerebral atrophy. Arch Neurol 28:339–342, 1981.

185. Stein, SC and Langfitt, TW: Normal-pressure hydrocephalus. Predicting the results of cerebrospinal fluid shunting. J Neurosurg 41:463–470, 1974.

186. Steiner, A, Gomori, JM, and Melamed, E: Features of brain atrophy in Parkinson's disease. Neuroradiology 27:158–160, 1985.

187. Steingart, A, Hachinski, V, Lau, C, Fox, A, Diaz, F, Cape, R, Lee, D, Initari, D, and Merskey, H: Cognitive and neurologic findings in subjects with diffuse white matter lucencies on computed tomographic scan (leuko-araiosis). Arch Neurol 44:32–35, 1987.

188. Symon, L and Dorsch, NWC: Use of long-term intracranial pressure measurement to assess hydrocephalic patients prior to shunt surgery. J Neurosurg 42:258–273, 1975.

189. Sze, G, DeArmand, SJ, Brant-Zawadzki, M, Davis, RL, Norman, D, and Newton, TH: Foci of MRI signal (pseudolesions) anterior to the frontal horns: Histological correlations of normal findings. AJR 147:331–337, 1986.

190. Thal LJ, Grundman M, and Klanber MR: Dementia: Characteristics of a referral population and factors associated with progression. Neurology 38:1083–1090, 1988.

191. Tomlinson, RB, Blessed, G, and Roth, M: Observations on brains of demented old people. J Neurol Sci 53:413–421, 1970.

192. Valentine, AR, Moseley, IF, and Kendall, BE: White matter abnormalities in cerebral atrophy: Clinicoradiological correlations. J Neurol Neurosurg Psychiatr 43:139–142, 1980.

193. Vassilouthis, J: The syndrome of normal-pressure hydrocephalus. J Neurosurg 61:1501–1509, 1985.

194. Wade, JPH, Mirsen, TR, Hachinski, VC, Fisman, M, Lau, C, and Merskey, H: The clinical diagnosis of Alzheimer's disease. Arch Neurol 44:24–29, 1987.

195. Wechsler, AF, Verity, MA, Rosenschein, S, Fried, I, and Scheibel, AB: Pick's disease: A clinical, computed tomographic, and histologic study with golgi impregnation observations. Arch Neurol 39:287–290, 1982.

196. Weinberger, DR, Gibson, RE, Coppola, R, Jones, DE, Berman, KF, Braun, AR,

Zeeberg, B, Sunderland, T, and Reba, RC: ^{123}IodoQNB SPECT in Alzheimer's and Pick's disease (abstr). Neurology (Suppl 1):39;165, 1989.

197. Whitehouse, PJ: The concept of subcortical and cortical dementia: Another look. Ann Neurol 19:1–6, 1986.

198. Wilson, RS, Fox, JH, Huckman, MS, Bacon, LD, and Lobick, JJ: Computed tomography in dementia. Neurology 32:1054–1057, 1982.

199. Wolfson, LI, Leenders, KL, Brown, LL, and Jones, T: Alterations of regional cerebral blood flow and oxygen metabolism in Parkinson's disease. Neurology 35:1399–1405, 1985.

200. Wong, DF, Wagner, HN Jr, Dannals, RF, Links, JM, Frost, JJ, Ravert, HT, Wilson, AA, Rosenbaum AE, Gjedde, A,. Douglass, KH, Petronis, JD, Folstein, MF, Toung, JKT, Burns, D, and Kuhar MJ: Effects of age on dopamine and serotonin receptors measured by positron emission tomography in the living human brain. Science 226:1393–1396, 1984.

201. Wu, S, Schenkenbert, T. Wing, SD, and Osborn, AG: Cognitive correlates of diffuse cerebral atrophy determined by computed tomography. Neurology 31: 1180–1184, 1981.

202. Yamada, F, Fukuda, S, Samelima, H, Yoshii, N, and Kudo, T: Significance of pathognomonic features of normal-pressure hydrocephalus. Neuroradiology 16:212–213, 1978.

203. Yerby, MS, Sundsten, JW, Larson, EB, Wu, SA, and Sumi, SM: A new method of measuring brain atrophy: The effect of aging in its application for diagnosing dementia. Neurology 35:1316–1320, 1985.

204. Yoshii, F, Barker, WW, Chang, JY, Loewenstein, D, Apicella, A, Smith, D, Boothe, T, Ginsberg, MD, Pascal, S, and Duara, R: Sensitivity of cerebral glucose metabolism to age, gender, brain volume, brain atrophy, and cerebrovascular risk factors. J Cereb Blood Flow Metabol 8:654–661, 1988.

205. Zatz, LM, Jernigan, TL, and Ahumada, AJ: Changes on computed cranial tomography with aging: Intracranial fluid volume. AJNR 3:1–11, 1982.

206. Zatz, LM, Jernigan, TL, and Ahumada, AJ: White matter changes in cerebral computed tomography related to aging. J Comput Assist Tomogr 6 (1):19–23, 1982.

207. Zimmerman, RD, Fleming, CA, Lee, BCP, Saint-Louis, LA, and Deck, MDF: Periventricular hyperintensity as seen by magnetic resonance. AJR 146:443–450, 1986.

Chapter 10

MAGNETIC RESONANCE IMAGING OF ADULT WHITE MATTER DISEASE

Burton P. Drayer, M.D.

PATHOANATOMY
MRI STUDIES
DIFFERENTIAL DIAGNOSIS

With the advent of high-resolution, cross-sectional imaging over the past decade, powerful approaches have become available for the diagnosis of demyelinating diseases. These imaging methods are safe, relatively noninvasive, and able to provide detailed anatomic information of even submillimeter structures. Information obtained by x-ray computed tomography (CT) or magnetic resonance imaging (MRI) is thus an in vivo representation of gross pathology. Precise pathoanatomic studies in living patients have the additional advantage of permitting repeated examinations during the various stages of lesion development and of providing dynamic information concerning blood-brain barrier (BBB) integrity. Because of the exquisite sensitivity of MRI (even compared with x-ray CT) for the detection of white matter disease, the results of the MRI study will need to be integrated into the diagnostic paradigm used to detect, prognose, and evaluate therapeutic response in demyelinating diseases. One must be aware, however, that information derived from MRI, if not used in careful conjunction with clinical data, could complicate rather than assist in patient care.

At present, there are no systematic evaluations of patients with demyelinating disease using either PET or SPECT. Hence, this chapter will focus on the use of x-ray CT and MRI in these disorders.

PATHOANATOMY

Multiple Sclerosis (MS) and Variants

Pathologic studies of MS have elucidated various paradoxes that are reflected in imaging studies. Most importantly, the clinical localization of an active lesion does not necessarily correspond to the site of demyelination detected by x-ray CT, MRI, or at autopsy.[2,6,24,29,38] The detection of a subacute or chronic focus of demyelination is often associated with a gross loss of brain substance, along with enlarged ventricles and cortical sulci.[2,6] MS is a disease of the oligodendroglia-myelin complex, and the irregular, sharply outlined plaques are scattered in a fairly symmetric fashion throughout the white matter. These lesions are often perpendicular to the body of the lateral ventricles following a perivenular distribution ("Dawson's fingers").[1,2] Approximately 5% of the lesions in MS may be found in gray matter.[29] Certain plaques are extremely difficult to detect on gross inspection because they are small or have incomplete demyelination ("shadow plaques").[2]

The distribution of lesions in MS can be arbitrarily divided into four anatomic locales: (1) the optic nerves, chiasm, and tracts; (2) the cerebral white matter; (3) the brainstem and cerebellum; and (4) the spinal cord. Prototype lesions are best delineated in myelinated brain substance in close relationship to the ependymal lining of the ventricular system, the cerebral and cerebellar white matter, and the cortical and basal ganglia gray matter adjacent to the pial surface.[10,20,29] The typical perivenular distribution of MS lesions involves ependymal venules, cerebral medullary venules, and pial venules. On histopathologic inspection, phagocytic macrophages are prominent in acute and subacute MS lesions.[44] The lesions contain myelin debris and globules of sudanophilic lipid (such as triglycerides and cholesterol esters).[1,2] Intracellular and extracellular neutral fats at the border of the lesion coincide with lesion activity. The oldest portion of the MS lesion is generally gliotic (fibrillary gliosis), without the sudanophilic lipid material.[1,2] Macrophages may destroy myelin rather than merely act as secondary scavengers.[44] Another important pathologic feature of MS is the disruption of the BBB during the acute and subacute phases of the disease.[9,38] Many authors have suggested that abnormal enhancement on the x-ray CT or MR study correlates with disease exacerbation and that high-dose steroid infusion may decrease the degree of CT enhancement in MS lesions.[32,36,39,46,48,49] Unfortunately, clinical experience suggests that some lesions in remission may enhance, whereas many active, exacerbating lesions may not enhance.

A variety of MS subgroups have been described in addition to the common *Charcot type*.[2] An acute, nonremitting, more destructive and rapidly progressive form of MS, the *Marburg type*, has been described in younger adults and may be impossible to distinguish from acute disseminated encephalomyelitis (ADEM) when there is sparing of the optic nerves and posterior columns. *Balo's concentric sclerosis* is also acute, rapidly progressive, and consists of demyelinated areas that are separated by bands of preserved myelin and have a concentric appearance. *Devic's type* of MS involves the spinal cord and optic nerves, with focal areas of necrosis and often prominent cord swelling.

Acute disseminated encephalomyelitis (ADEM) is an acute, monophasic, often postviral or postvaccination immune-mediated, white matter disease often associated with excellent clinical recovery or mild symptomatology. An inflammatory infiltrate follows a perivenular course with surrounding demyelination.[2] The white matter changes may become confluent along the venular course but do not become globular as in MS. An experimental animal model, experimental allergic encephalomyelitis (EAE), closely mimics this clinical disorder. Hurst's *hemorrhagic leukoencephalitis* is a more severe demyelinating disorder, with petechial hemorrhages in the cerebral white matter and corpus callosum, severe edema, necrotic venous walls, and predominantly perivascular hemorrhagic tissue destruction.

Microangiopathic Leukoencephalopathy

In hypertensive patients, arterioles show hyaline degeneration (lipohyalinosis), fibrinoid necrosis, and microatheroma in <200-μm vessels (arteriolar sclerosis).[27] Arteriolar sclerosis may result in a spectrum of abnormalities ranging from état criblé (dilated perivascular spaces) to frank infarction.[5,17,18] In order to better understand the pathologic basis of the term "lacune" (small infarction), Poirier (42) divided these findings into three groups:

1. Type I, with small, often multiple areas of infarction (état lacunaire);
2. Type II, with cystic scars and hemosiderin-laden macrophages that are the residua of small hemorrhages; and
3. Type III, with dilated perivascular spaces (état criblé) but no frank infarction or definite clinical sequelae. These findings are most commonly seen in the hypertensive and elderly population and likely predispose them to more severe ischemic change in a clinical setting of systemic hypotension or hypoxia.[17,18]

Arteriolar sclerosis can be further categorized in the following clinicopathologic scheme:

État criblé is commonly seen in the white matter and basal ganglia in the elderly population and consists of multiple dilated perivascular (Virchow-Robin) spaces with a narrow border of fibrillary gliosis and a central normal or slightly fibrotic vessel (artery or capillary).[3,4,23] The surrounding tissue is intact or displays mild perivascular demyelination (*atrophic perivascular demyelination*).[35] Somewhat more extensive associated changes may occur in the cerebral white matter, capsular and basal ganglia region, and pons, particularly in the elderly. These parenchymal alterations generally consist of gliosis, myelin pallor, and demyelination, presumably secondary to the chronic ischemia that accompanies arteriolar narrowing.[4,35]

État lacunaire (lacunar state) consists of small cavities (lacunes) with a diameter of less than 20 mm. According to Fisher,[28] lacunes are associated with hypertension in 90% of cases. Such cavities are the result of small, deep infarcts. Small hemorrhages are also common, as suggested by the finding of hemosiderin-laden macrophages around the cavities. The lesion occasionally appears as a smooth cyst with a vessel in the center that could be created by parenchymal atrophy due to spiraled elongations of the vessel and pulsatile trauma to the surrounding brain with concurrent elevated blood pressure.[28] Lacunes are typically present in the basal ganglia and basis pontis, sparing the cerebral and cerebellar cortex.[26,28] There is a frequent relationship (35%) of putaminal and thalamic hemorrhage with lacunar disease. A striking correlation between lacunes and hypertension is widely accepted, whereas lacunes do not seem to be related to cerebral embolism or diabetes.[13]

Encephalitis subcorticalis chronica progressiva (subcortical arteriolosclerotic encephalopathy; Binswanger's disease; microangiopathic leukoencephalopathy).[7,12,16,18,31,34,40] This condition, noted in both hypertensive and normotensive patients, is characterized by diffuse or patchy degeneration of white matter that largely spares the subcortical arcuate fibers. The white matter abnormalities consist of interspersed discrete foci of coagulative necrosis within extensive, generalized, often sheetlike demyelination. The corpus callosum is frequently reduced in thickness, with relative preservation of the cerebral cortex. Histologically, arteriolar sclerosis (hyalinization) of long penetrating arterioles is usually present, as well as loss of myelin and axons, widespread gliosis, invasion by macrophages, and demarcated foci of myelin destruction in the white matter.[21,30,41] Although the focal lesions can be attributed to an ischemic factor, the diffuse component of white matter degeneration is poorly understood. One theory suggests that this alteration is a late effect of cerebral edema induced by prior hypertensive encephalopathy. Another theory proposes that progressive chronic ischemia is produced by arteriolosclerosis with the additional contribution of systemic factors (hypoxia, anemia, hypercoagulability, and/or hypotension).

Hypertensive patients may be more susceptible to ischemia because of an inability to compensate for a decrease in blood pressure, probably due to structural alterations of arterioles with a decreased capacity for vasodilatation. Overly aggressive institution of antihypertensive therapy may result in further ischemia because of the impaired vasoregulation. Ischemic damage secondary to hypoperfusion (as in hypotension, cardiac dysfunction) results in infarction at the boundary zones of the major cerebral vessels. Areas of the brain such as deep cerebral white matter that are supplied by narrowed and tortuous arterioles are further susceptible to episodes of hypoperfusion. This pertains not only to hypertensive subjects but also to normotensive elderly individuals who frequently present with ischemic, generally asymptomatic changes in the deep white matter at the boundaries of the major cerebral arteries.

De Reuck[15] described the pathogenesis of periventricular white matter lesions in arterial boundary zones. He described three types of periventricular arterial supply:

1. Ventriculopetal striate and medullary perforating end-arteries,
2. Ventriculopetal end-branches of the perforating arteries that terminate in a ventriculofugal course from 3 to 10 mm from the ventricular border,
3. Ventriculofugal arteries from the choroidal arteries of the lateral and third ventricles, and three periventricular white matter boundary zones:

1. Anterior corpus callosum and pons,
2. Deep white matter adjacent to the atrium and occipital horn of the lateral ventricle, and
3. Deep white matter adjacent to the frontal horn, anterior temporal horn, and body of the lateral ventricles.

These boundary zones are particularly susceptible to the decreased regional cerebral blood flow that occurs with acute cardiac insufficiency, hypotension, respiratory arrest, or vascular occlusion, and the effects are highlighted by the presence of arteriolar narrowing as seen with hypertension and aging.

Six areas of the brain (Table 10–1) are particularly susceptible to ischemic events in the presence of arteriolar disease (microangiopathy).[17,18] These regions have in common a blood supply by way of small, perforating end-arteries without a protective collateral supply. The superficial cerebral white matter and arcuate U-fibers are generally spared even in the presence of arteriolar disease due to the dual vascular supply from the medullary arteries and the leptomeningeal arteries (Duvernoy type 5 branches).

Table 10–1 BRAIN AREAS SUSCEPTIBLE TO ISCHEMIA RESULTING FROM MICROANGIOPATHY

Region	*Arterial Supply*
Deep cerebral white matter	Medullary arteries
Caudate, anterior limb of internal capsule	Recurrent artery of Heubner (medial lenticulostriates) branch of anterior cerebral artery
Putamen, globus pallidus, internal capsule	Lenticulostriate branches of middle cerebral artery
Thalamus	Thalamogeniculate branches of posterior cerebral artery
Posterior limb of internal capsule, posterior portion of globus pallidus	Anterior choroidal branches of internal carotid artery
Pons	Perforating branches of basilar artery

MRI STUDIES

Technique

The important role of proton MRI in the diagnosis of MS and other white-matter disorders is now well established. A spin echo (SE) pulse sequence with a long repetition time (TR) and echo delay (TE) ("T_2-weighted," SE 2800/90) and flow compensation (gradient moment nulling) provides the greatest sensitivity for detecting lesions (see Chapter 2). On "intermediate" images (SE 2800/30), the lesions (increased signal intensity) are often better detected as multiple bright foci on a background of an isointense ventricular system. These lesions may be obscured on the SE 2800/90 images because the intensity of both cerebrospinal fluid and lesion is bright.

"T_1-weighted images" (SE 600/20) are less sensitive than T_2 images but assure greater diagnostic specificity because the T_1 images distinguish subacute blood (hyperintense) from demyelination (hypointense). Multiplanar, multiecho gradient refocused (MPGR) images may also be acquired (TR 500 ms, TE 15/35, flip angle 20°) and are particularly valuable for detecting high-signal-intensity demyelinating lesions in the spinal cord and low-signal-intensity hemorrhagic lesions in the brain. Hypointensity on the MPGR images (caused, for example, by hemosiderin-laden macrophages) is a useful finding in excluding the diagnosis of MS and in delineating a common mimicking disease, cavernous malformation.[45]

Multiple Sclerosis

Young and colleagues[50] first compared intravenously enhanced CT scanning with 0.17 resistive MRI using inversion recovery pulse sequences in 10 patients with definite MS. They reported 3 lesions in the supraventricular white matter by x-ray CT and 9 by MRI, 16 periventricular white matter lesions by x-ray CT and 84 by MRI, and no brainstem lesions by x-ray CT and 38 by MRI. In another report on 10 patients,[37] x-ray CT was positive in 7 and MRI was positive in all 10. Thirteen lesions were seen on intravenously enhanced x-ray CT scanning; 158 lesions were noted on MRI. In this limited group of patients, T_2-weighted spin echo pulse sequences (SE 1500/56) were more sensitive than T_1-weighted pulse sequences. Other studies have confirmed the sensitivity of T_2-weighted MRI for detection of demyelination in MS. The excellent sensitivity of MRI for defining MS lesions and the superiority of T_2 images have been confirmed in subsequent studies.[24,41,47]

Drayer and coworkers[21] studied 47 patients with definite MS using T_2- (SE 2500/80), intermediate- (SE 2500/40), and T_1-weighted (SE 500/25) pulse sequences with a high-field-strength (1.5 T) MRI system. Areas of increased signal intensity on the T_2-weighted images were present in 43 of 47 patients. The T_2-weighted pulse sequence was strikingly more sensitive than the T_1-weighted images. Most lesions were in a *periventricular* location, and the intermediate (SE 2500/40) images were particularly valuable in delineating these increased-signal-intensity abnormalities from the adjacent ventricles. Other common sites for lesions included the more peripheral cerebral white matter, corpus callosum, middle cerebellar peduncle, brainstem, and internal capsule. The prolonged T_2 relaxation time in MS lesions may be attributed to neutral fats, albumin, edema, and/or astrocytic gliosis, whereas the central prolonged T_1 may be related to the chronic fibrillary gliosis in the inactive central portion of the plaque.

The common periventricular signal hyperintensities denoting MS plaques have a "jumpy-bumpy" appearance and are present adjacent to the frontal, temporal, and occipital horns as well as the body of the lateral ventricles (Fig. 10–1). Lesions are often perpendicular to the body of the lateral ventricles fol-

Figure 10–1. Multiple sclerosis (MS), in a 40-year-old female. Parts (*A*), (*C*), and (*E*) are through the basal ganglia and thalamus, whereas (*B*), (*D*), and (*F*) are at the level of the body of the lateral ventricle. In (*A*) and (*B*), multiple areas of signal hyperintensity are seen in the cerebral white matter and capsular region, due to MS plaques. Signal hypointensity in the thalamus and striatum, as often seen secondary to severe white-matter disease, suggests abnormal iron accumulation (T_2-weighted image, SE 2800/90). In (*C*) and (*D*), signal hyperintensity is better delineated throughout the cerebral white matter and capsular region because the CSF is isointense (mixed weighting, SE 2800/30). In (*E*) and (*F*) (T_1-weighted, SE 600/20), the white-matter abnormalities are not as well defined. Subtle hyperintensity in the parieto-occipital region is probably secondary to abnormal barrier permeability to albumin.

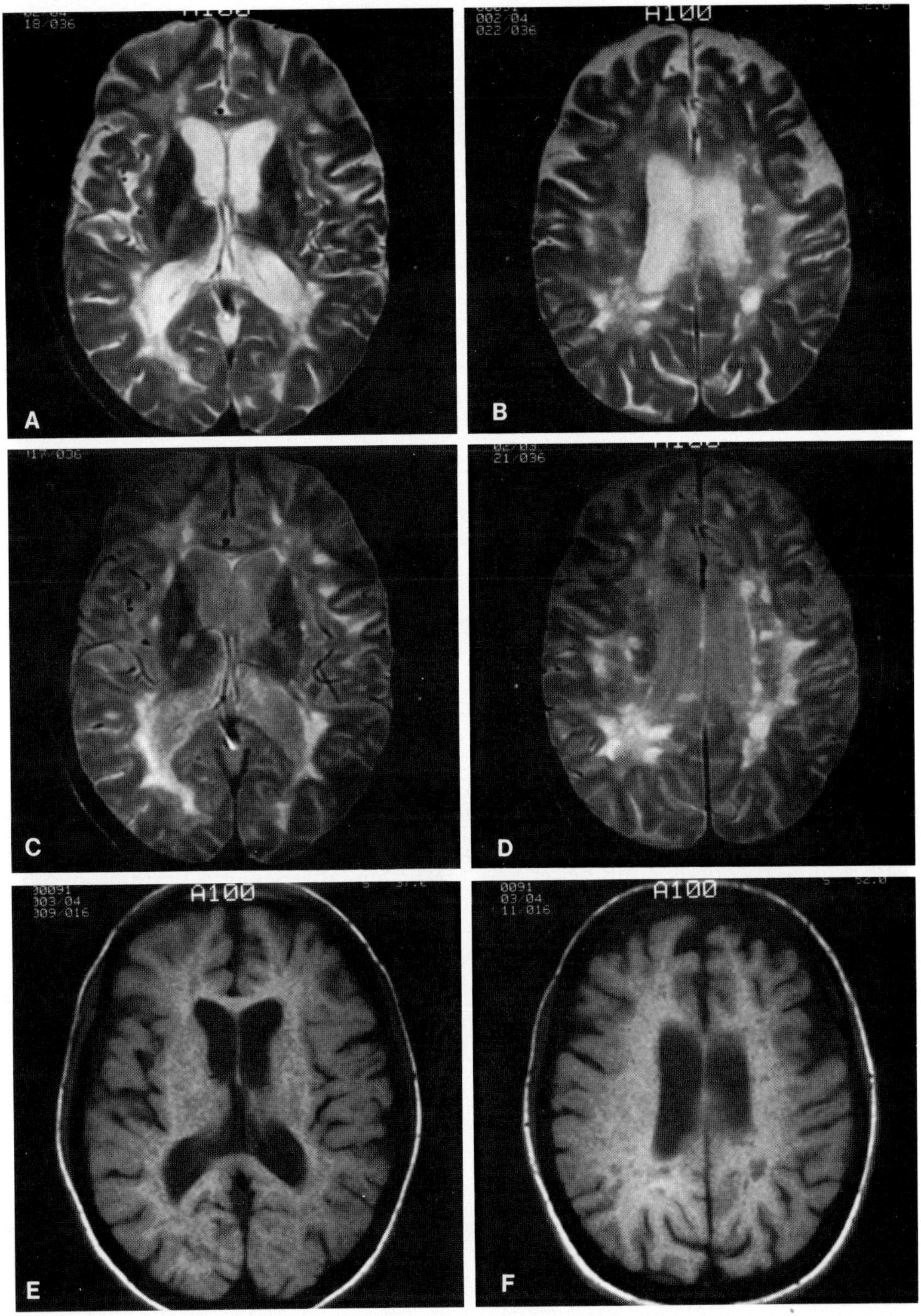
A
B
C
D
E
F

lowing a perivenular course ("Dawson's fingers"). Signal hyperintensities on T_2 images in the cerebellar peduncles are generally easy to detect because of their large size (Fig. 10–2). Brainstem lesions are more difficult to delineate on MRI studies than they are on gross pathologic inspection ("shadow plaques") (Fig. 10–3). Spinal cord lesions also are clearly visualized using MRI (Fig. 10–4). A spinal cord lesion, particularly without cord expansion in a young adult, should suggest MS. Further confirmation can be obtained with a brain MRI (although not always positive), visual evoked response study, and/or lumbar puncture. An isolated spinal cord MS plaque occurs in less than 5% of most study populations. It should be noted that MS is a disease of the oligodendroglia-vasculomyelin complex rather than of the white matter; therefore a small percentage of lesions may be found in the cortex and basal ganglia.

After the intravenous infusion of the paramagnetic contrast medium gadolinium Gd-DTPA (see Chapter 2), a variable degree of enhancement (as with x-ray CT) is sometimes noted with MRI.[32,39] Enhancement is best seen on T_1-weighted images as a focus of increased signal intensity. Abnormal enhancement denotes a disruption of the BBB and is, therefore, often better defined on a delayed, as opposed to an immediate, postinfusion T_1-weighted study. Further analyses are needed to determine whether abnormal enhancement (barrier permeability) correlates with lesion exacerbation or remission.[39] Rarely, a rim of increased signal intensity is seen surrounding larger, more prominent areas of decreased signal intensity on the nonenhanced T_1-weighted MRI study (see Fig. 10–1 *C–F*). This unusual finding may represent a prominently increased accumulation of protein (e.g., albumin) related to disruption of the BBB.

On high-field-strength MRI, Drayer and associates[21] noted decreased signal intensity (decreased T_2) on the SE 2500/90 images in the putamen and thalamus of MS patients (Fig. 10–1). Conversely, an age-matched group of normal individuals consistently showed a dominance of decreased signal intensity in the globus pallidus caused by the normal accumulation of iron.[22] The decreased signal intensity in the thalamus and putamen was only seen with severe involvement of the white matter and may reflect an abnormal accumulation of iron or other trace metals, although the mechanism is unclear. Mechanistic possibilities include oligodendroglial dysfunction in MS (iron is stored in oligodendroglia and astrocytes), abnormal BBB permeability to iron, decreased oxidative phosphorylation, and/or resultant iron accumulation from decreased metabolic demands in a critical sensory relay nucleus (thalamus). Of interest is a neuropathologic report of increased iron deposition adjacent to MS plaques.[14] This same finding has been observed using the Perls' stain for ferric iron on postmortem examination of patients with severe MS and multiple foci of abnormal blue (ferric iron) staining in MS plaques.[19] Of additional interest is that the most common histocompatibility loci of MS and hemochromatosis are the same.[14]

In summary, MRI is an extremely sensitive technique for the diagnosis of MS. The absence of a brain or spinal cord lesion on MRI is extremely unusual in this disease. A negative study should immediately call into question the accuracy of the diagnosis and set into motion a search for mimicking disorders. The absence of MRI findings suggesting MS should probably exclude an individual from a carefully controlled therapeutic trial.

Ischemic (Microangiopathic) Leukoencephalopathy

MRI is extremely sensitive in the detection of even subtle microvascular changes as reflected by signal hyperintensities on T_2-weighted images in the cerebral white matter and basal ganglia

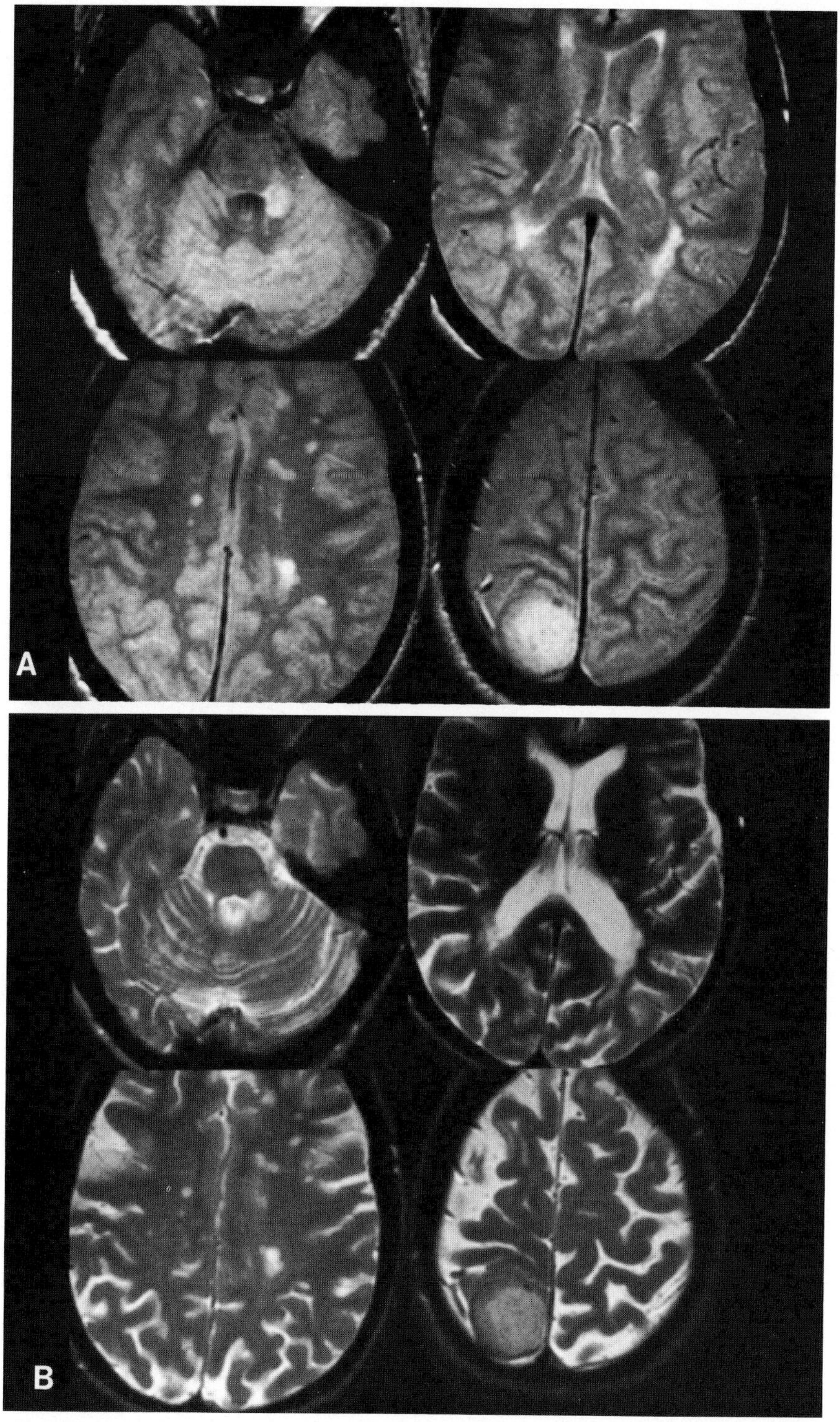

Figure 10–2. Multiple sclerosis in a 49-year-old female, with multiple-year history of remitting and exacerbating neurologic symptoms and optic neuritis. (*A*) (Mixed weighting, SE 2800/30) Multiple periventricular hyperintensities with a left middle cerebellar peduncle lesion typical of MS. A large, though clinically incidental, posterior parasagittal extra-axial mass is also shown. (*B*) (T_2-weighting, SE 2800/90) The MS lesions are not as clearly defined, but the signal characteristic (decreased signal intensity as compared to SE 2800/30 images) of the parasagittal mass is characteristic of a fibroblastic or transitional cell meningioma.

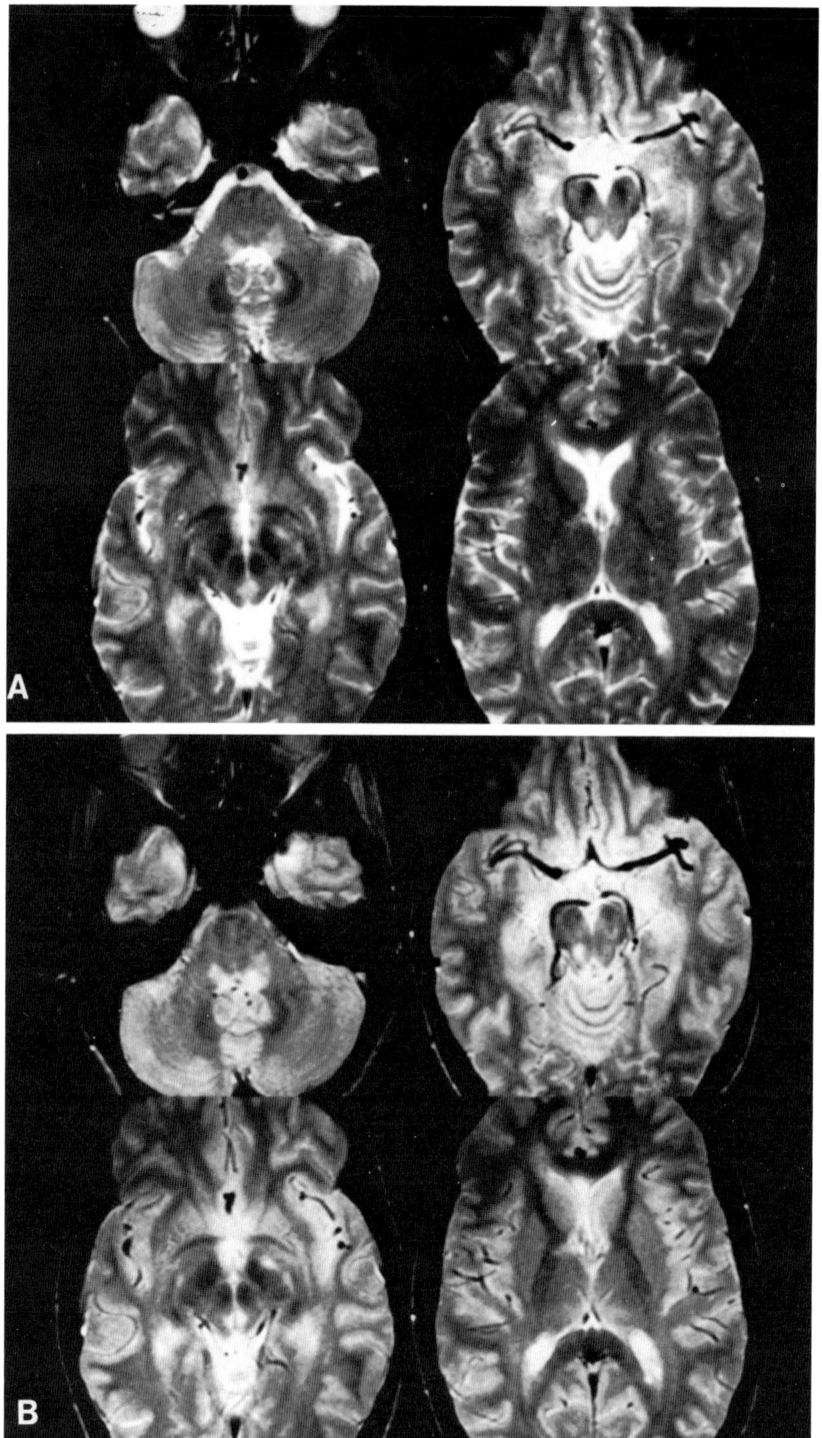

Figure 10–3. Multiple sclerosis (34-year-old female). (*A*) T_2-weighted MRI (SE 2800/90) shows abnormal increased signal intensity in the posterior midbrain tegmentum, middle cerebellar peduncles, and genu of the corpus callosum. (*B*) With mixed weighting (SE 2800/30), the MS plaques seen on the T_2 images are affirmed and more easily visualized.

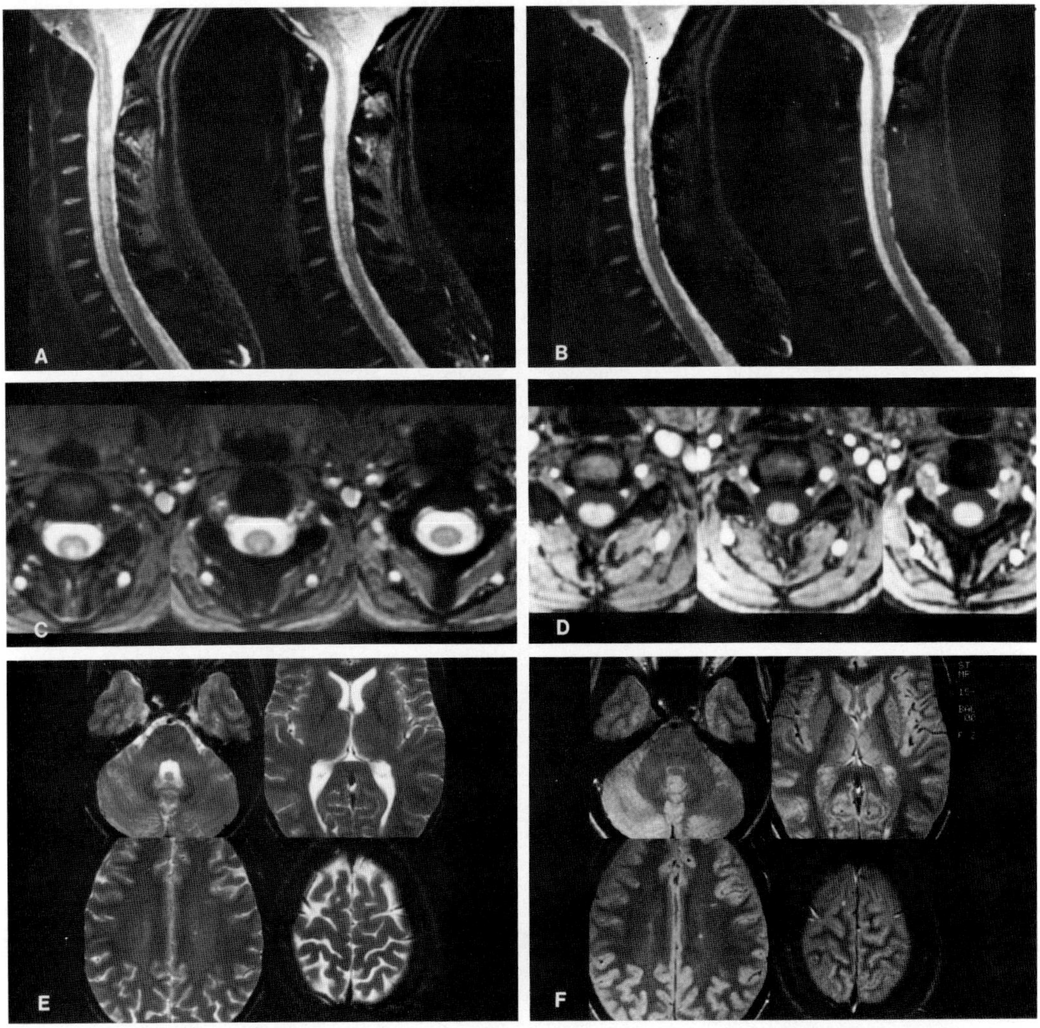

Figure 10–4. Multiple sclerosis (27-year-old female). (*A*) Gradient echo (GE 500/15/20°) shows a single spinal cord MS plaque at the C2-C3 level. (*B*) At GE 500/35/20°, greater T_2 weighting accentuates the cord lesion. The cervical cord is not enlarged and the cerebellar tonsils are in normal position. (*C*) At GE 500/20/20°, axial images also define the signal hyperintensity and absence of enlargement of the cord. (*D*) GE 50/13/45°—although these 1.5-mm-thick axial images acquired using a 3DFT acquisition mode provide elegant anatomic depiction of the spinal cord, neural foramen, bony anatomy, and vascular structures (white), they do not delineate the MS plaque, because of T_1 weighting. (*E*) T_2-weighted (SE 2800/90) brain images show only a few subtle hyperintensities (MS plaques) in the cerebral white matter. (*F*) Mixed-weighted (SE 2800/30) images better define the subtle periventricular and more peripheral right frontal MS plaques.

region (Fig. 10–5, Tables 10–2, 10–3). This exquisite sensitivity has added increasing complexity to the interpretation of MR images, particularly in the elderly.[17,18] Multiple punctate or more confluent foci of signal hyperintensity are commonly noted in the deep cerebral white matter and basal ganglia regions on T_2-weighted images even in patients without a focal or associated neurologic deficit. These are often called subcortical hyperintensities (SCHs) or, facetiously, unidentified bright objects (UBOs); and the pathologic substrate of these lesions is an important issue in MRI. Awad and

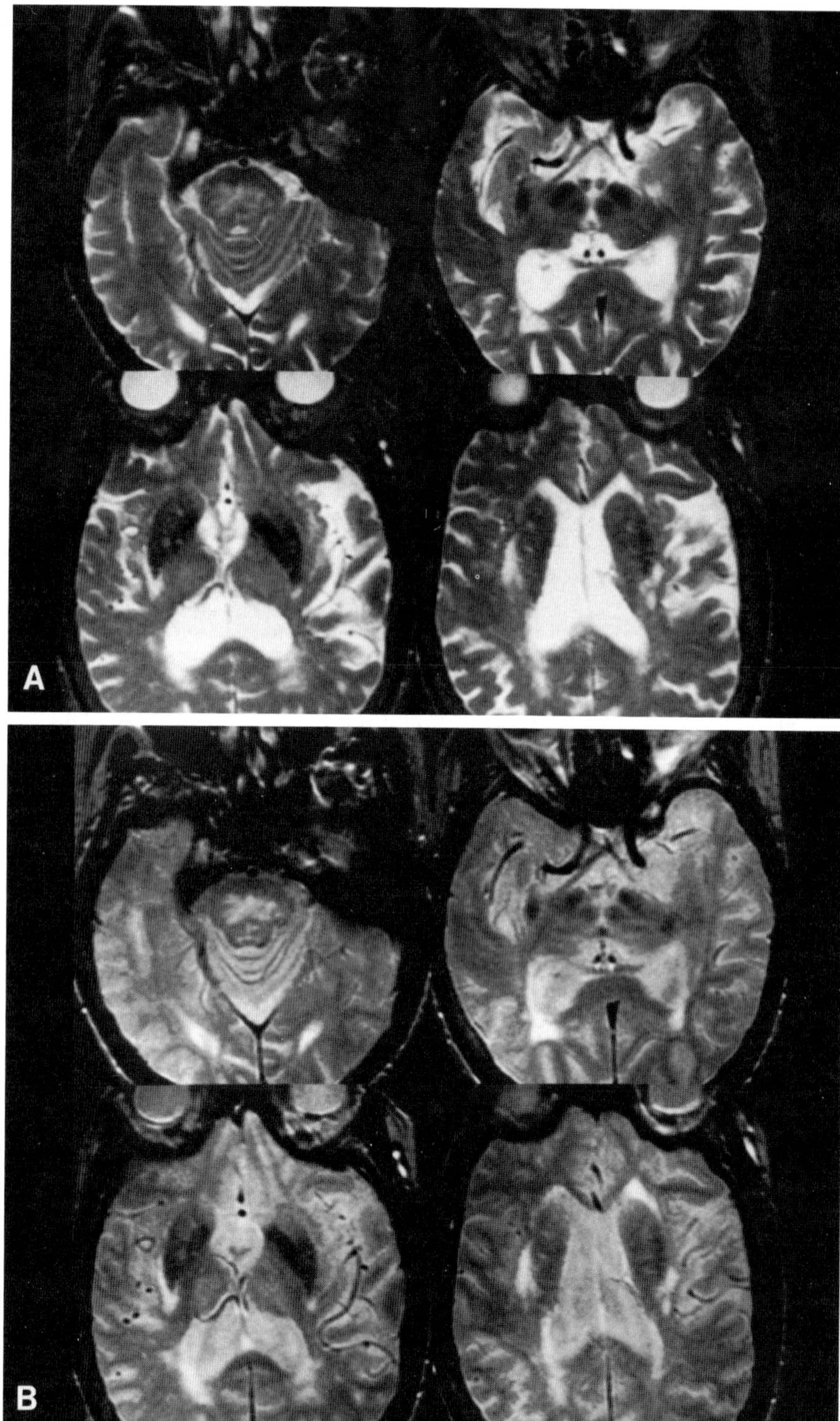

Figure 10–5. Hypertensive arteriolar disease (84-year-old hypertensive female). (*A*) T_2-weighted (SE 2800/90) MRI shows abnormal, confluent signal hyperintensities in the periventricular cerebral white matter, capsules, and pons in the distribution of noncollateralizing, perforating arteries. (*B*) Using mixed weighting (SE 2800/30), the extensive white matter and pontine alterations are more readily detected. This constellation of lesions is most commonly associated with hypoperfusion, hypertension, and/or aging.

Table 10–2 MRI FINDINGS IN CONDITIONS ASSOCIATED WITH HYPOPERFUSION

	Signal Weighting		
	T_1*	I†	T_2‡
État criblé (dilated perivascular spaces)	↓	—	↑
Demyelination: Myelin pallor	—	↑	↑
Isomorphic gliosis	—	↑	↑
Lacunar infarction	↓	↑	↑
Microangiopathic leukoencephalopathy	↓	↑	↑

*T_1-Short TR, short TE
†I = Intermediate weighting (long TR, short TE)
‡T_2 = Long TR, long TE

colleagues,[3,4] using clinical and post-mortem MRI-neuropathologic correlations, believed these SCHs represented a marker of cerebrovascular disease. They described dilated perivascular spaces secondary to arteriolar tortuosity (état criblé), gliosis, demyelination and infarction as having a similar appearance of SCH because of increased tissue water. Another group[35] felt that these hyperintensities were predominantly related to atrophic perivascular demyelination often found in the proximity of dilated perivascular spaces.

All investigators agree that SCHs increase in number with aging.[4,8,17] The most common underlying disorder associated with SCHs is hypertension, although other vascular risk factors and/or episodes of hypoperfusion (e.g., hypoxia, hypotension) may play an important role. The spectrum of arteriolar disorders and their MRI correlates are summarized in Table 10–2. Deep white matter and basal ganglia infarction may also be seen with carotid occlusive disease (Fig. 10–6). These MRI findings likely correlate with white matter x-ray CT changes described by Hachinski and coworkers[32b] as leuko-araiosis.

Table 10–3 RISK FACTORS FOR HYPOPERFUSIONAL WHITE MATTER HYPERINTENSITIES ON T_2 MRI STUDIES

In rank order of importance:
A. Hypertension
B. Aging
C. Hypotension
   Hypoxia
   Cardiac dysfunction
D. Arteritis
   Migraine
E. Diabetes mellitus?

The most severe form of diffuse arteriolar disease, with relatively symmetric, confluent, and extensive hyperintensities throughout the cerebral white matter, represents microangiopathic leukoencephalopathy of the Binswanger type (BML).[18] There is frequent sparing of the arcuate subcortical U-fibers, interspersed foci of cavitation (hypointensity on T_1 images as well as striking hyperintensity on T_2 images), multifocal hyperintensities in the basal ganglia, and enlargement of cortical sulci. These extensive changes may be seen in individuals without neurologic dysfunction, a confusing dilemma often encountered in routine clinical practice. In addition, a clinically dementing illness in a patient with even extensive SCHs does not confirm the diagnosis of a vascular dementia (see Chapter 9). In one study,[11] white matter changes (myelin pallor, fibrohyaline arteriosclerosis, partial loss of axons and myelin sheaths, and mild reactive astrocytosis) were found in 30 of 48 autopsies in patients with Alzheimer's disease (AD). These alterations correlated best with hypoperfusion and cardiac dysfunction (32 of 48 patients) rather than with hypertension (1 of 48 patients). An MRI study[25] confirmed the presence of white matter abnormalities in AD.

In summary, the *absence* of multiple white matter abnormalities in the atrophic brain of a demented individual strongly favors the diagnosis of a primary degenerative dementia (e.g., AD) but the *presence* of these changes does not confirm vascular dementia. A significant percentage of the population, particularly over age 65, may have signal hyperintensities on T_2-weighted images without neurologic deficit.

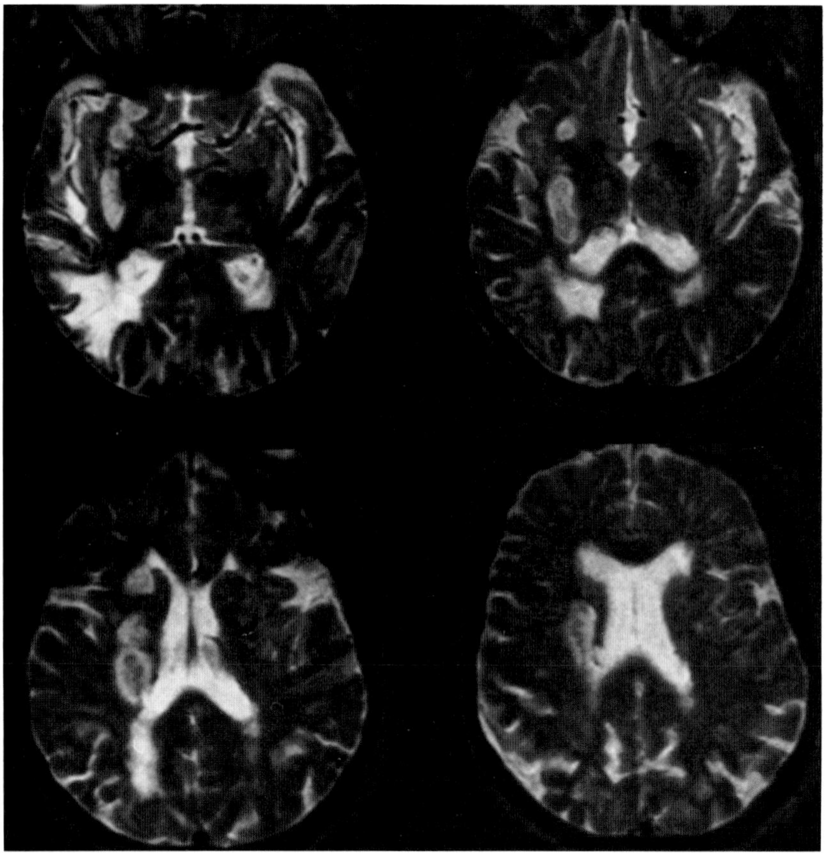

Figure 10–6. Boundary zone infarction (76-year-old female). T_2-weighted images (SE 2800/90) define a basal ganglia–capsular infarction in the distribution of the lenticulostriate branches of the right middle cerebral artery, and a parieto-occipital white-matter infarction in the boundary zone between the right middle and posterior cerebral arteries, secondary to occlusion of the right middle cerebral artery (absence of signal void). Unilateral boundary-zone infarction predominantly involves the deep white matter and is most often caused by ipsilateral carotid or middle cerebral stenosis or occlusion.

DIFFERENTIAL DIAGNOSIS*

It is practical from an imaging standpoint to separate disorders that predominantly involve the white matter into three groups:

1. Multiple sclerosis and closely associated *demyelinating (myelinoclastic)* disorders in which a secondary insult, possibly immune-related, affects normally developed myelin or, more precisely, the oligodendroglia-myelin-vascular complex.

2. *Leukoencephalopathic* disorders involving a toxic, metabolic, infectious, or ischemic insult to normal myelin, as seen with radiation injury (Fig. 10–7), ischemic microangiopathy, acquired immune deficiency syndrome (AIDS), chemotherapy, nutritional deficiency, and central pontine and extrapontine myelinolysis.

3. *Dysmyelinating (leukodystrophic)* disorders in which there is a primary metabolic abnormality in myelin synthesis or turnover, as seen with metachromatic leukodystrophy (MLD), Alexander's disease (Fig. 10–8), and sudanophilic leukodystrophies (e.g., Pelizaeus Merzbacher Type 1–6;

*Tables 10–4, 10–5

Table 10–4 PERIVENTRICULAR INCREASED WHITE MATTER MRI SIGNAL: DIFFERENTIAL DIAGNOSIS

A. Younger patient (age <50 yr)
   1. Multiple sclerosis
   2. Increased Virchow-Robin perivascular spaces
   3. Systemic lupus erythematosus (SLE)
   4. AIDS
      a. Primary HIV encephalitis
      b. Toxoplasmosis
      c. PML
      d. Lymphoma

B. Older patient (age >50 yr)
   1. Infarcts
      a. Tend to be relatively symmetric
      b. Spares the corpus callosum
      c. Spares the subcortical U-fibers
      d. +/− contiguous with ependyma
      e. +/− confluent lesions (i.e., with one another)
   2. Multiple sclerosis (10% of cases in patients age >50 yr)
      a. Can affect corpus callosum
      b. Can affect subcortical U-fibers
      c. +/− discrete, separate lesions; globular or linear perpendicular ("Dawson's fingers"), periventricular lesions.
      d. +/− not contiguous with ependyma
      e. Involves middle cerebellar peduncle
   3. Arteritis
      a. Peripheral > periventricular white matter involvement
      b. Multifocal, asymmetric

Table 10–5 DIFFERENTIAL DIAGNOSIS OF WHITE MATTER DISEASE DETERMINED WITH NEUROIMAGING

	Typical Onset	*Clinical Setting*	*White Matter Anatomic Predilection*	*Abnormal Enhancement (BBB)*
		I. Demyelinating (Myelinoclastic)		
A. Multiple sclerosis	Adult	Remissions Exacerbations Multifocal Abn VER/CSF+	Periventricular white matter Middle cerebellar peduncle Optic nerves Spinal cord	Yes (suggests lesion activity)
B. Acute Disseminated encephalomyelitis	All	Postviral Postvaccination (Animal model: EAE)	Multifocal, scattered, perivenular. Spares optic nerves, posterior columns (if acute hemorrage→Hurst hemorrhagic leuko-encephalopathy)	Yes

(*Continued*)

Table 10–5—*Continued*

	Typical Onset	*Clinical Setting*	*White Matter Anatomic Predilection*	*Abnormal Enhancement (BBB)*
		II. Leukoencephalopathy		
A. Central pontine myelinolysis (CPM)	Adult	Sodium swings Ethanolism Nutritional	Pons Extrapontine (capsule, cerebral white matter)	No
B. Marchiafava-Bignami	Adult	Italian wine ? CPM variant	Corpus callosum	No
C. Progressive multifocal leuko-encepha-lopathy	Adult	Immune sup-pression Lymphoma	Cerebral white matter, often asymmetric AIDS: gray = white	Yes
D. Radiation injury	All	>6 mo post-radiation If necrosis, difficult to distinguish from tumor	Diffuse (in radiation port) Disseminated necrotizing leukoencepha-lopathy (DNL): metho-trexate + radiation	Yes (if necrosis)
E. Microangiopathic leukoencepha-lopathy	Elderly	Hypertension Arteriolopathy Hypoperfusion (Hypoxia/ hypotension)	Distribution of deep, noncol-lateralizing perforating arteries (e.g., medullary, striate, pontine): Cerebral white matter Pons/thalamus Basal ganglia/ capsule	No
F. HIV Encephalitis	Adult	AIDS; dementia	Multifocal cerebral white matter and capsule	No
		III. Dysmyelinating (Leukodystrophy)		
A. Adrenoleuko-dystrophy	Child	Familial Male	Parietal/occipital white Splenium	Yes
B. Metachromatic	Child	↓Aryl Sulf A Abnormal NCV	Diffuse cerebral white	No
C. Alexander's (Canavan's)	Child	Large head	Diffuse cerebral white	No
D. Sudanophilic (e.g., Pelizaeus Merzbacher)	Child	Slows deteri-oration of function	Diffuse cere-bral white	No
F. Navajo neuropathy (Leukodystrophy)	Child	Familial Navajo Indians	Cerebellar white	No

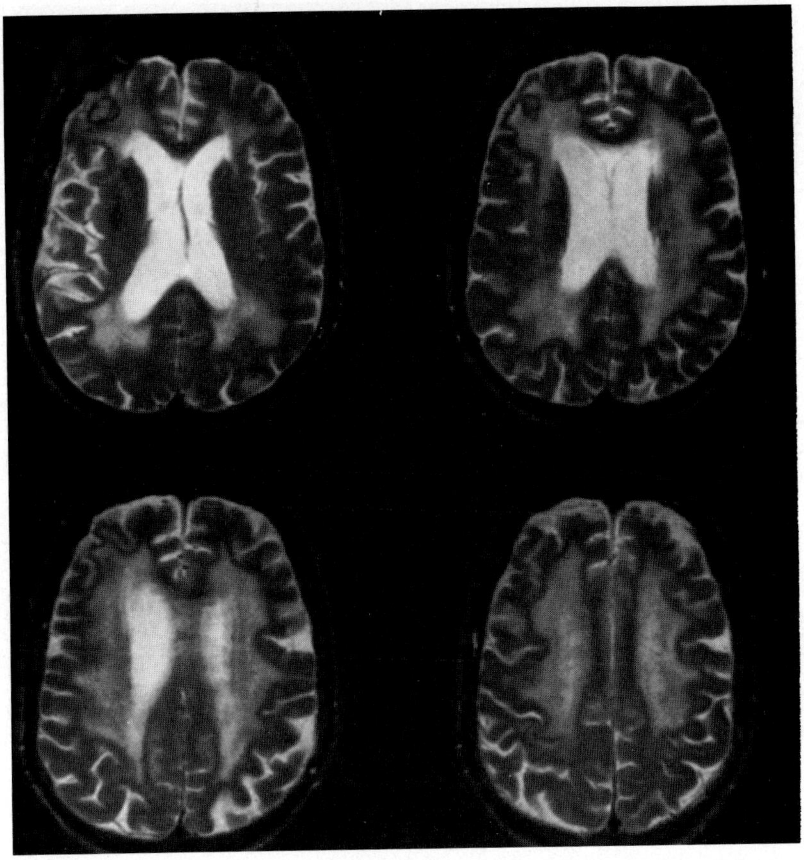

Figure 10–7. Radiation injury (76-year-old male). Extensive sheetlike signal hyperintensity involving the cerebral white matter symmetrically and bilaterally on T_2-weighted images (SE 2800/90). Radiation therapy for metastatic disease was performed 10 months prior to the MRI. Note the small hemorrhagic metastasis in the anterolateral frontal lobe at the gray-white junction.

Type 4 is adult variant) (see Chapter 12).

Although each of these disorders generally causes an abnormally increased signal intensity in the white matter on intermediate and T_2-weighted images, knowledge of patient age, clinical presentation, and anatomic predilection of lesions in the different pathologic entities will greatly improve the diagnostic specificity of MRI (see Table 10–5). For example, the leukodystrophies exhibit diffuse, extensive, symmetric, and confluent signal hyperintensity on T_2 images in younger individuals with a progressive deterioration in neurologic function. Because BBB disruption is not a prominent feature of the leukodystrophies, the introduction of Gd-DTPA to the clinical practice of MRI should not only improve the capability for determining MS plaque activity but also should improve diagnostic specificity. The BBB is intact in all the dysmyelinating disorders except adrenoleukodystrophy.[33] The barrier is also intact in ischemic white matter disorders, thus distinguishing SCHs from subtle metastatic foci with vasogenic edema.

Human immune deficiency virus (HIV) encephalitis has become a common cause of demyelination in the appropriate population. The usual clinical presentation involves a progressive dementing illness. White matter lesions are often initially small with enlargement and confluence noted on serial interval studies; cortical atrophy is al-

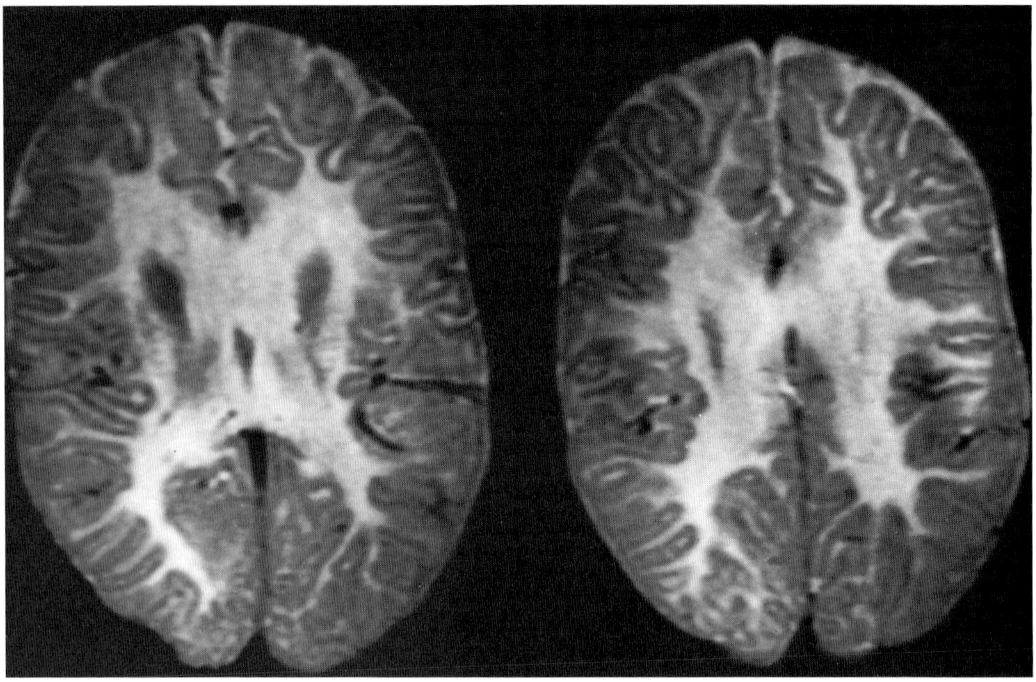

Figure 10–8. Alexander's disease (3-year-old male). Extensive, confluent, symmetrical increased signal intensity on T_2-weighted images (SE 2800/90) involves almost the entire cerebral white matter, except for partial sparing of the subcortical arcuate "U" fibers, characteristic of a dysmyelinating disorder.

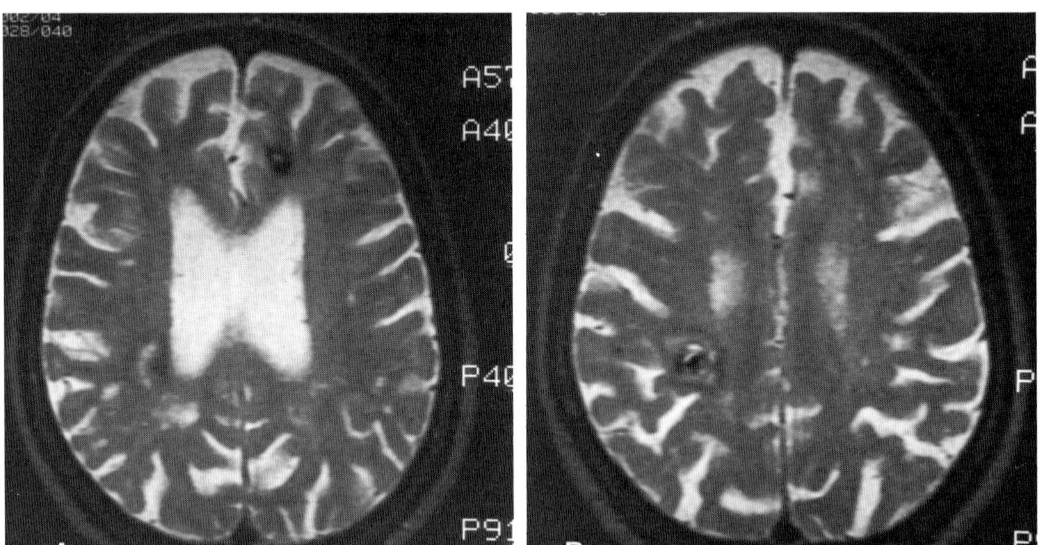

Figure 10–9. Cavernous malformations (28-year-old female). Abnormal signal hypointensities are noted in the frontal and parietal white matter, characteristic of hemosiderin-laden macrophages on these T_2-weighted (SE 2800/90) images. Punctate hyperintensities suggesting ischemia also are present. The multiplicity of hypointense lesions without surrounding edema and remitting neurologic symptoms (at times mimicking MS) strongly suggest familial cavernous malformation.

most always present.[43] The white matter abnormalities with HIV cannot be definitively distinguished by MRI from alterations noted with cytomegalovirus (CMV) encephalitis or progressive multifocal leukoencephalopathy (PML). Primary central nervous system lymphoma and toxoplasma encephalitis usually do not cause differential diagnostic difficulty, as they will generally enhance with Gd-DTPA.

SUMMARY

MRI has become the initial diagnostic imaging procedure of choice to evaluate individuals with clinically suspected MS. Due to the exquisite sensitivity of MRI for the detection of white matter lesions, the absence of an abnormality on the MR study makes the diagnosis of any white matter disease extremely unlikely. MRI thus becomes an exceptionally valuable noninvasive technique for screening the much larger group of patients with clinical features (e.g., optic neuritis, paresthesia, weakness, ataxia) that raise the suspicion of MS.

Various authors have suggested that MRI is too sensitive and nonspecific; experience in our institution suggests this is not true. If the interpreter has a good working knowledge of MRI principles as well as of the pathologic features and dominant distribution of white matter lesions, a diagnosis can generally be made with a high degree of accuracy. Other diseases that may mimic MS clinically (e.g., Chiari I malformation, cavernous malformation [Fig. 10–9], spinocerebellar degenerations) are clearly defined using MRI (see Chapter 11). In addition, improved sensitivity will ultimately improve specificity (e.g., a single large white matter lesion on x-ray CT may represent glioma rather than demyelination, while the MRI demonstration of multiple additional lesions will strongly favor the diagnosis of demyelination).

Perhaps the most exciting feature of MRI is that it permits the noninvasive and repeated study of patients with white matter disease and should provide a sophisticated characterization of the temporal course of demyelination and, potentially, even of the response of brain white matter to therapeutic interventions.

REFERENCES

1. Adams CWM: Pathology of multiple sclerosis: Progression of the lesion. Br Med Bull 33:15–20, 1977.
2. Allen, IV: Demyelinating diseases. In Adams, JH, Corsellis, JAN, and Duchen, LW (eds): Greenfield's Neuropathology. John Wiley & Sons, New York, 1984, pp 338–384.
3. Awad, IA, Spetzler, RF, Hodak, JA, Johnson, PC, and Awad, CA: Incidental lesions noted on magnetic resonance imaging of the brain: Prevalence and clinical significance in various age groups. Neurosurgery 20:222–227, 1987.
4. Awad, IA, Johnson, PC, Spetzler, RF, and Hodak, JA: Incidental subcortical lesions identified on magnetic resonance imaging in the elderly. II. Postmortem pathological correlations. Stroke 17:1090–1097, 1986.
5. Bamford, JM and Warlow, CP: Evolution and testing of the lacunar hypothesis. Stroke 19(9):1074–1082, 1988.
6. Barrett L, Drayer B, and Shin, C: High-resolution computed tomography in multiple sclerosis. Ann Neurol 17:33–38, 1985.
7. Binswanger, O: Die Abgrenzung der algemeinen progressiven Paralyse (Referat, erstattet auf der Jahresversammlung des Vereins Deutscher Irrenarzte zu Dresden am 20 Sept., Berl Klin Wochschr 31:1103–1105, 1137–1139, 1180–1186, 1894.
8. Brant-Zawadzki, M, Fein, G, Van Dyke, C, et al: MR imaging of the aging brain: Patchy white-matter lesions and dementia. AJNR 6:675–682, 1985.
9. Broman, T: Blood-brain barrier damage in multiple sclerosis: Supravital test-observations. Acta Neurol Scand 40(Suppl 10):21–24, 1964.
10. Brownell, B and Hughes, JT: The distri-

bution of plaques in the cerebrum in multiple sclerosis. J Neurol Neurosurg Psychiatr 25:315–320, 1962.
11. Brun A and Englund, E: A white matter disorder in dementia of the Alzheimer type: A Pathoanatomical study. Ann Neurol 19:253–262, 1986.
12. Caplan, LR and Schoene, WC: Clinical features of subcortical arteriosclerotic encephalopathy (Binswanger disease). Neurology 28:1206–1215, 1978.
13. Cole, FM and Yates, P: Comparative incidence of cerebrovascular lesions in normotensive and hypertensive patients. Neurology 18:255–259, 1968.
14. Craelius, W, Migdal, MW, Luessenhop, CP, et al: Iron deposits surrounding multiple sclerosis plaques. Arch Pathol Lab Med 106:397–399, 1982.
15. De Reuck, J: The human periventricular arterial blood supply and its anatomy of cerebral infarctions. Eur Neurol 5:321–334, 1971.
16. De Reuck, J, Crevits, L, DeCoster, W, et al: Pathogenesis of Binswanger chronic progressive subcortical encephalopathy. Neurology 30:920–928, 1980.
17. Drayer, BP: Imaging of the aging brain. Part I. Normal findings. Radiology 166:785–796, 1988.
18. Drayer, BP: Imaging of the aging brain. Part II. Pathologic conditions. Radiology 166:797–806, 1988.
19. Drayer, BP: Magnetic resonance imaging of multiple sclerosis. BNI Quarterly 3:65–73, 1987.
20. Drayer, BP and Barrett, L: Magnetic resonance imaging and CT scanning in multiple sclerosis. Ann NY Acad Sci 436:294–314, 1984
21. Drayer, B, Burger, P, Hurwitz, B, Dawson, D, and Cain, J: Reduced signal intensity on MR images of thalamus and putamen in multiple sclerosis: Increased iron content? AJNR 8:413–419, 1987.
22. Drayer, BP, Burger, P, Darwin, R, Riederer, S, Herfkens, R, and Johnson, GA: Magnetic resonance imaging of brain iron. AJNR 7:373–380, 1986; and AJR 147:103–110, 1986.
23. Durand-Fardel, M: Mémoire sur une altération particuliére de la substance cérébrale. Gaz Med Paris 10:23–38, 1842.
24. Edwards, MK, Farlow, MR, Stevens, JC: Multiple sclerosis: MRI and clinical correlation. AJR 147:571–574, 1986.
25. Fazekas, F, Chawluk, JB, Alavi, A, et al: MR signal abnormalities at 1.5 T in Alzheimer's dementia and normal aging. AJNR 8:421–426, 1987.
26. Fisher, CM: Lacunar strokes and infarcts: A review. Neurology 32:871–876, 1982.
27. Fisher, CM: Arterial lesions underlying lacunes. Acta Neuropathol 12:1–15, 1969.
28. Fisher, CM: Lacunes—Small, deep cerebral infarcts. Neurology 15:774–784, 1965.
29. Fog, T: The topography of plaques in multiple sclerosis with special reference to cerebral plaques. Acta Neurol Scand (Suppl 15)41:1–161, 1965.
30. George, AE, de Leon, MJ, Kalnin, A, et al: Leukoencephalopathy in normal and pathologic aging. II. MRI of brain lucencies. AJNR 7:567–570, 1986.
31. Goto, K, Ishii, N, and Fukasawa, H: Diffuse white-matter disease in the geriatric population. Radiology 141:687–695, 1981.
32. Grossman, RI, Gonzalez-Scarano, F, Atlas, SW, et al: Multiple sclerosis: Gadolinium enhancement in MR imaging. Radiology 161:721–725, 1986.
32b. Hachinski, VC, Potter, P, and Merskey, H: Leuko-araiosis. Arch Neurol 44:21–23, 1987.
33. Heinz, ER, Drayer, BP, Haenggelli, CA, Painter, MJ, and Crumrine, P: CT scanning in white matter disease. Radiology 130:371–378, 1979.
34. Kinkel, WR, Jacobs, L, and Polachini, I: Subcortical arteriosclerotic encephalopathy (Binswanger's disease): Computed tomographic, nuclear magnetic resonance, and clinical correlations. Arch Neurol 42:951–959, 1985.
35. Kirkpatrick, JB and Heyman, LA: White-matter lesions in MR imaging of clinically healthy brains of elderly subjects: Possible pathologic basis. Radiology 162:509–511, 1987.
36. Lebow, S, Anderson, DC, Mastri, A, and Larson, D: Acute multiple sclerosis with contrast enhancing plaques. Arch Neurol (Chicago) 35:435–439, 1978.

37. Lukes, SA, Crooks, LE, Aminoff, MJ, et al: Nuclear magnetic resonance imaging in multiple sclerosis. Ann Neurol 13:592–601, 1983.
38. McDonald, WI: Pathophysiology in multiple sclerosis. Brain 97:179–196, 1974.
39. Miller, DH, Rudge, P, Johnson, G, et al: Serial gadolinium enhanced magnetic resonance imaging in multiple sclerosis. Brain 111:927–939, 1988.
40. Olzewski, J: Subcortical arteriosclerotic encephalopathy: Review of the literature on the so-called Binswanger's disease and presentation of two cases. World Neurol 3:359–375, 1962.
41. Ormerod, IEC, Miller, DH, McDonald, WI, Du Boulay, EPGH, Rudge, P, Kendall, BE, Moseley, IF, Johnson, G, Tofts, PS, Halliday, AM, Bronstein, AM, Scaravilli, F, Harding, AE, Barnes, D, and Zilkha, KJ: The role of NMR imaging in the assessment of multiple sclerosis and isolated neurological lesions: A quantitative study. Brain 110:1579–1616, 1987.
42. Poirier, J and Derouesné, C: Le concept de lacune cérébrale de 1838 à nous jours. Rev Neurol (Paris) 141:3–17, 1985.
43. Post, MJD, Tate, LG, Quencer, RM, Hensley, GT, Berger, JR, Sheremata, WA, and Maul, G: CT, MR, and pathology in HIV encephalitis and meningitis. AJNR 9:469–476, 1988.
44. Prineas JW and Wright, RG: Macrophages, lymphocytes, and plasma cells in the perivascular compartment in chronic multiple sclerosis. Laboratory Investigation 38:409–421, 1978.
45. Rigamonti, D, Hadley, MN, Drayer, B, Johnson, PC, Hoenig-Rigamonti, K, Knight, T, and Spetzler, RF: Cerebral cavernous malformations: Incidence and familial occurrence. N Engl J Med 319(6):125–130, 1988.
46. Sears, ES, Tindall, RSA, and Zarnow, H: Active multiple sclerosis: Enhanced computerized tomographic imaging of lesions and the effect of corticosteroids. Arch Neurol 35:426–434, 1978.
47. Sheldon, JJ, Siddharthan, R, Tobias, J, et al: MR imaging of multiple sclerosis: Comparison with clinical and CT examinations in 74 patients. AJNR 6:683–690, 1985.
48. Troiano, R, Hafstein, M, Ruderman, M, Dowling, P, and Cook, S: Effect of high-dose intravenous steroid administration on contrast-enhancing computed tomographic scan lesions in multiple sclerosis. Ann Neurol, 15:257–263, 1984.
49. Viñuela, FV, Fox, AJ, Debrun, GM, Feasby, TE, and Ebers, GC: New perspectives in computed tomography of multiple sclerosis. AJR 139:123–127, 1982.
50. Young, IR, Hall, AS, Pallis, CA, et al: Nuclear magnetic resonance imaging of the brain in multiple sclerosis. Lancet 2:1063–1066, 1981.

Chapter 11

CEREBELLAR DISORDERS

Sid Gilman, M.D., and Stephen S. Gebarski, M.D.

DEGENERATIVE DISEASES
DEMYELINATIVE DISEASE
CEREBELLAR ANOMALIES
VASCULAR DISEASE
CEREBELLAR ABSCESS
ALCOHOLIC CEREBELLAR DEGENERATION
NEOPLASMS

Imaging studies provide important information in the clinical and laboratory evaluation of patients with disorders of cerebellar function. Imaging procedures should be undertaken only after a careful history, physical examination, and neurologic examination have indicated the possibility of a disorder of the cerebellum and brainstem. The symptoms suggesting cerebellar or brainstem disease observed most frequently consist of headache, gait difficulty, clumsiness of limb movements, nausea, vomiting, and various complaints that are often termed "dizziness."[29] The symptom of dizziness from lesions of the posterior fossa usually consists of a sense of lightheadedness, but some patients experience true vertigo.[29,58] The signs of cerebellar disease consist of disorders of stance and gait; titubation; rotated or tilted postures of the head; oculomotor disorders, including gaze-paretic nystagmus, rebound nystagmus, square wave jerks, periodic alternating nystagmus, ocular dysmetria, and optokinetic nystagmus; limb hypotonia; ataxic dysarthria; dysmetria; dysdiadochokinesis and dysrhythmokinesis; ataxia; tremor; abnormal check and rebound; and limb weakness.[29]

In this chapter, we describe the common cerebellar disorders, discuss their usual modes of presentation, and then evaluate the utility of imaging studies in the evaluation of these conditions. Heretofore, pneumoencephalography was the only means of directly imaging structures in the posterior fossa. This technique was extremely uncomfortable to the patient and involved substantial risks to patients with mass lesions in this location. X-ray computed tomography (CT) has almost completely replaced pneumoencephalography and has become the single most commonly used imaging study for disease of the posterior fossa. With modern techniques, the beam hardening and scatter artifact limitations of x-ray CT in the posterior fossa can be diminished (see Chapter 1). These artifacts cannot be completely eliminated, however, and the inherent risk of ionizing radiation must be taken into account. Magnetic resonance imaging (MRI) is, in most cases, superior to x-ray CT in imaging the posterior fossa. Where it is easily available, MRI often replaces x-ray CT as the primary imaging modality to evaluate subacute and chronic posterior fossa diseases. The principal shortcomings of MRI (see Chapter 2), besides lack of availability, are:

1. Generally longer image acquisition time than CT, leading to motion artifact with uncooperative patients;

2. Ferromagnetic limitations where structures that are influenced by high magnetic fields, such as cerebral aneurysm clips, indwelling pacemakers, and neurostimulators and their leads, may be displaced or have current induced along them, with injury of tissue;

3. Insensitivity for certain diseases such as acute hemorrhages, meningiomas, and subtle changes in cortical bone; and

4. Patient intolerance of the procedure.

The most common absolute contraindications to MR are cardiac pacemakers and cerebral aneurysm clips. Magnetically switched pacemakers may malfunction if placed within the magnetic field, and certain types of aneurysm clips may move in a dangerous fashion.

Ancillary imaging modalities in posterior fossa disorders include angiography, positron emission tomography (PET; see Chapter 3), and single photon emission computed tomography (SPECT; see Chapter 4). Angiography is presently used as the initial imaging evaluation only in certain vascular diseases, usually atherosclerotic arterial occlusive disease. Even then, most patients will have already undergone x-ray CT. More often, angiography is called upon to demonstrate the detailed vascular morphology and vascular dynamics of lesions thought to have a significant vascular component. PET has been used to study adult-onset cerebellar degenerations (olivopontocerebellar atrophy,)[30,54,85] Friedreich's ataxia,[31] alcoholic cerebellar degeneration,[32] and paraneoplastic cerebellar degeneration.[4] Attenuation correction is needed for PET studies, and for structures of the posterior fossa it may be accomplished with either transmission scans or with the standard ellipse method[30] (see Chapter 3). SPECT has not been used in systematic studies of cerebellar disorders.

DEGENERATIVE DISEASES

The diagnosis of a degenerative disease of the cerebellum usually ensues when a patient develops progressive gait difficulty or limb ataxia with nystagmus in the absence of signs of a space-taking posterior fossa lesion. In most cases, the diagnosis of a degenerative disease is made after the exclusion of other disorders, including demyelinative disease, anomalies, vascular disease, infections, toxic metabolic diseases, paraneoplastic processes, and neoplasms. The presence of a positive family history is often helpful in the diagnosis of a degenerative disease. Imaging studies can be very helpful in the evaluation of patients with degenerative disease. The two most common diseases are olivopontocerebellar atrophy and Friedreich's ataxia.

Olivopontocerebellar Atrophy (OPCA)

OPCA is a progressive neurologic disorder characterized by neuronal degeneration in the cerebellar cortex, inferior olives, and pons.[20,21,29,40] The disease has been termed Menzel's hereditary ataxia if a clearly defined heritable pattern is established. Both autosomal recessive and autosomal dominant modes of transmission have been reported.[29,40] The disease also occurs sporadically and is then generally simply called "OPCA." Two other related adult-onset idiopathic degenerative diseases involve the cerebellum. One is hereditary cerebellar olivary degeneration of Holmes.[35,44,106] The other is sporadic parenchymatous cerebellar cortical atrophy,[35,40,61] also known as late cortical cerebellar atrophy (LCCA). These four types of cerebellar degeneration are difficult to distinguish clinically, making the distinctive characteristics in imaging studies important. Generally speaking, imaging studies can help separate Menzel and sporadic OPCA from Holmes and LCCA but cannot further differentiate among them.

OPCA is characterized clinically by a progressive cerebellar ataxia, which usually begins with a disorder of gait and an ataxic dysarthria. Later there is the progressive development of incoordination of all of the limbs. Most patients present only with symptoms of cerebellar involvement. A number of other features have been described, including pigmentary retinal degeneration; ophthalmoplegia; optic atrophy; dementia; extrapyramidal disturbances, including rigidity, chorea, and athetosis; and amyotrophy of the limbs or tongue.[29] In some cases, OPCA includes a widespread multisystem atrophy, which involves the Shy-Drager syndrome, with a combination of autonomic insufficiency, cerebellar ataxia, and extrapyramidal symptoms.

Imaging studies in OPCA commonly show diminished volume of the structures in the posterior fossa. There is often atrophy of the cerebellar folia and smallness of the brainstem, with enlargement of the fourth ventricle and of the cisterna magna. Pneumoencephalographic information on OPCA was confusing, with reports of a wide range of affected regions and degrees of atrophy. X-ray CT studies have provided more consistent data. Sporadic OPCA and Menzel ataxia demonstrate disproportionate, and often marked, atrophy of the basis pontis, whereas this region is relatively spared in LCCA and Holmes type. All four of these degenerative disorders usually demonstrate more marked atrophy of the cerebellum than of the cerebrum.[6,14,17,109] Ordinarily, the cerebellar wasting is greater in the hemispheres than in the vermis; both cerebral and vermian involvement appear later in the course of the disease.[14]

Although x-ray CT is quite effective in the evaluation of degenerative cerebellar diseases, MRI is even better.[27,71] MRI permits sensitive, relatively artifact-free images of the basis pontis and inferior olivary nuclei. A major advantage is the availability of sagittal-plane images without a change of the patient's physical position (Fig. 11–1). This makes pontine morphology easy to evaluate and reduces scalar errors in volume estimation imposed by a poorly controlled angle of image acquisition. More importantly, MRI provides a sensitive means of evaluation for diseases that may mimic the clinical presentation of OPCA (Fig. 11–2). If one of these four degenerative diseases is present, MRI should show the expected distribution of atrophy without signal aberration or mass. Signal aberration, usually hyperintense (white) areas in the white matter, and less so in the gray matter, would suggest other etiologies, commonly ischemic sequelae or multiple sclerosis. However, MRI may fail to identify these four degenerative disorders early in their course when the expected pattern of atrophy has not yet developed. In such cases, PET becomes especially valuable.

PET studies of patients with OPCA have been carried out with [^{18}F]2-fluoro-2-deoxy-D-glucose (^{18}F-FDG) to examine local cerebral metabolic rates for glucose (LCMRGlc).[30,54,85] These studies reveal significant hypometabolism in the cerebellar hemispheres, cerebellar vermis, and brainstem in comparison with normal control subjects (Fig. 11–3).[30] Cerebral blood flow is reduced in these regions as well.[32b] In most of these cases, x-ray CT reveals some degree of atrophy in the cerebellum. A significant relationship occurs between the degree of atrophy and the reduction in LCMRGlc in the cerebellum and the brainstem.[30] Nevertheless, some patients have minimal atrophy and substantially reduced LCMRGlc, suggesting the atrophy does not fully account for the finding of hypometabolism. LCMRGlc is within normal limits for the thalamus, basal ganglia, and cerebral cortex.

In further PET studies of LCMRGlc in patients with OPCA, the severity of ataxic and spastic dysarthria was compared with LCMRGlc. Perceptual analysis was used to examine the speech disorders, and rating scales were devised to quantitate the degree of ataxia and spasticity in the speech of each patient. A significant inverse correlation was found between the severity of ataxia in speech and the LCMRGlc within the

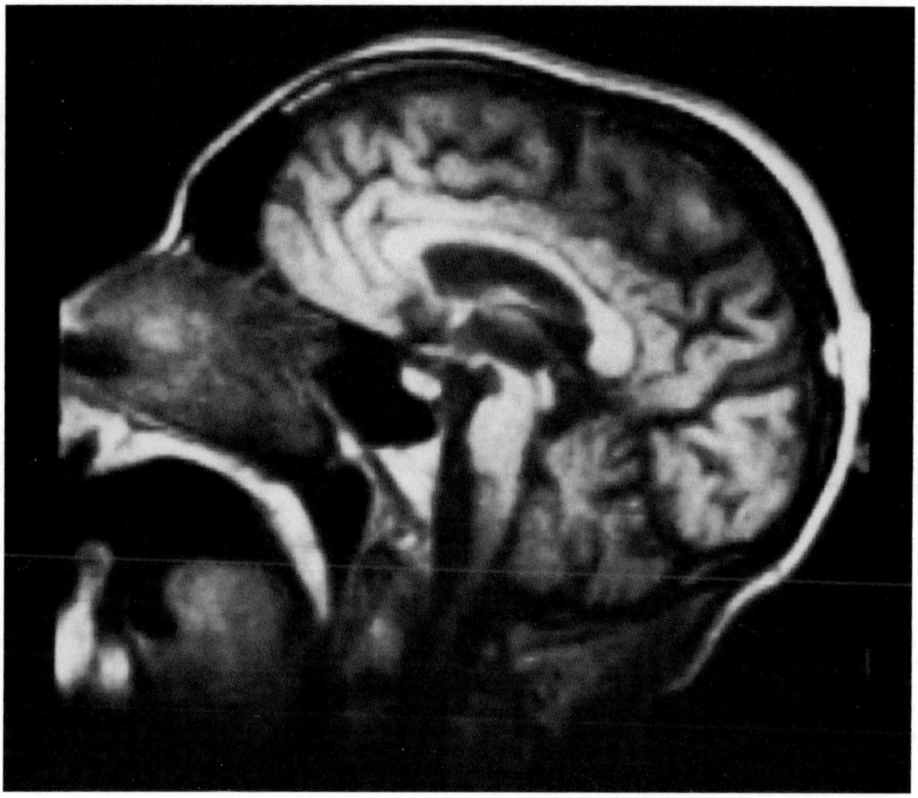

Figure 11–1. Olivopontocerebellar atrophy. Sagittal MRI. This plane is the most dependable for evaluation of basis pontis and vermian atrophy, which are marked in this young man.

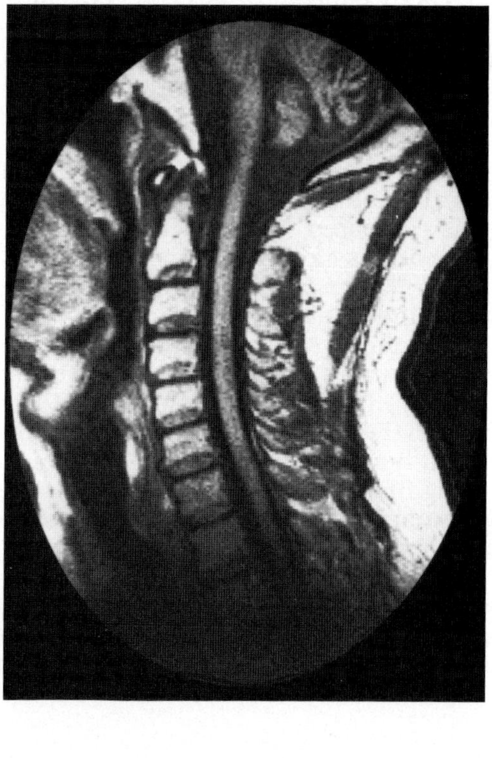

Figure 11–2. Olivopontocerebellar atrophy. This sagittal cervical spinal cord MR image, taken with a specialized cervical spine coil in a patient with OPCA, shows not only the atrophy of the cerebellar vermis and basis pontis, but also the normal size of the cervical spinal cord. This sequence is useful if Friedreich's ataxia is suspected; in Friedreich's ataxia, vermian and spinal cord atrophy may be present but the basis pontis is usually normal in size.

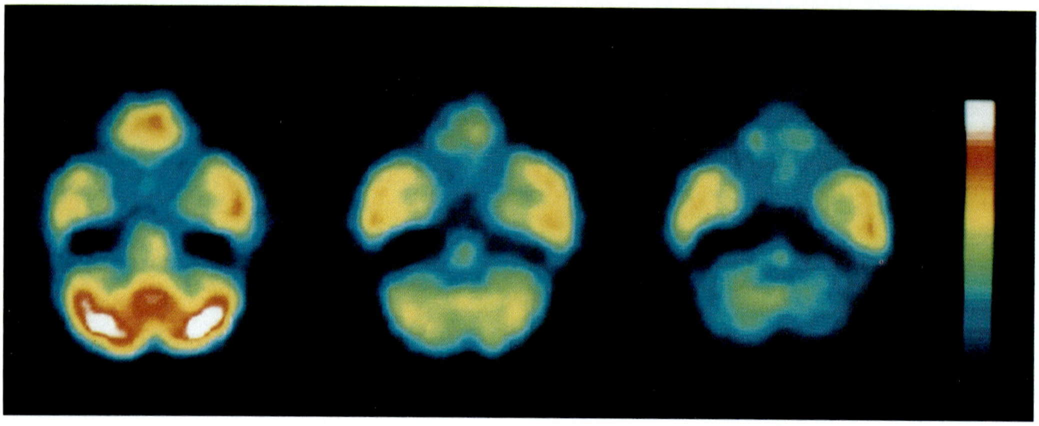

Figure 11–3. Olivopontocerebellar atrophy. PET scans showing cerebral glucose utilization as detected with ^{18}F-FDG. The scans show a horizontal section at the level of the cerebellum and the base of the temporal and frontal lobes. The color bar indicates glucose utilization rates in mg per 100 g per min extending from 0.0 to 7.7. (*Left*) Female control subject, aged 64 years. Note that the glucose utilization rates are slightly higher in the cerebellum than in the temporal lobes. (*Center*) Female patient with OPCA, aged 61 years. The patient has moderately severe ataxia of speech and limb motor function. Note the moderate degree of hypometabolism in the cerebellar vermis, cerebellar hemispheres, and brainstem. (*Right*) Female patient with OPCA, aged 59 years. The patient has a severe degree of ataxia of speech and limb motor function. Note the marked degree of hypometabolism in the cerebellar vermis, cerebellar hemispheres, and brainstem. (From Kluin, et al,[54] with permission.)

cerebellar vermis, cerebellar hemispheres, and brainstem, but not within the thalamus.[54] No significant correlation was found between the severity of spasticity in speech and LCMRGlc in any of these structures, however. These findings support the view that the severity of ataxia in speech in OPCA patients is related to the functional activity of the cerebellum and its connections in the brainstem.[54]

In additional studies, the severity of cranial and somatic motor dysfunction was compared with LCMRGlc and the degree of tissue atrophy in patients with OPCA.[85] A scale was devised to measure the degree of ataxia in the neurologic examinations. A significant correlation was found between the severity of motor impairment and LCMRGlc within the cerebellar vermis, both cerebellar hemispheres, and the brainstem. A significant but weaker relationship was noted between the degree of tissue atrophy in these regions and clinical severity. A partial correlation analysis revealed that LCMRGlc, not the amount of atrophy, is the more important correlate of motor dysfunction in OPCA.

Recently, PET has been utilized to determine the density of GABA/benzodiazepine receptors in the cerebellum of patients with OPCA.[32a] Antecedent autoradiographic studies of postmortem cerebral tissue from patients with OPCA demonstrated a decrease of both glutamatergic[2a,60a] and GABAergic[2a] neurotransmitter receptors. Preliminary investigations utilizing [^{11}C] flumazenil and PET revealed decreased binding to GABA/benzodiazepine receptors in the cerebellum of patients with OPCA compared to normal control subjects.[32a] These studies indicate that, utilizing PET with new ligands specific for certain neurotransmitters and neurotransmitter receptors, it may be possible to characterize the biochemical disorders in patients with OPCA. This characterization may help to classify the cerebellar degenerations more fully and to devise strategies for treatment.

Friedreich's Ataxia (FA)

FA is a chronic progressive neurologic disorder that is inherited as an autosomal recessive trait.[29,40,97] The onset is usually before puberty, with progressive muscle weakness and ataxia of gait. As these symptoms worsen, other symptoms and signs appear, including limb ataxia; scoliosis; pes cavus; loss of position, vibration, and light touch sensations of the limbs; loss of the deep tendon reflexes; and the appearance of extensor plantar responses. Cardiomyopathy occurs in essentially all patients with FA and usually accounts for death by middle age. Dysarthria usually occurs early in the disease. Muscle atrophy and degeneration of the optic nerves may be late effects. Diabetes mellitus is found in a substantial percentage of patients with FA.

The principal neuropathologic abnormalities in FA involve degeneration in the peripheral sensory nerves, the dorsal root ganglia, and the dorsal roots.[77,78,103] Degeneration also occurs within the spinal cord, affecting posterior columns, the lateral corticospinal tracts, and the dorsal and ventral spinocerebellar tracts. There is loss of cells in Clarke's column and in the substantia gelatinosa. The cerebellum and brainstem commonly show little or no change, but occasionally there is volume loss in the pons and medulla, as well as patchy atrophy of Purkinje cells. Many cases show degeneration of neurons in the dentate nuclei. Degenerative changes also may occur in the reticular and vestibular nuclei of the brainstem.

As expected from the histopathology, x-ray CT and MRI findings in the posterior fossa may not be helpful in FA. Up to one third of the patients, sometimes even those patients with longstanding disease, have a normal cerebellum and brainstem on x-ray CT.[82] Many patterns of cerebellar and, at times, cerebral atrophy have been reported in FA but no uniformly distinctive pattern has emerged.[14,17,82] When x-ray CT is abnormal in FA, it usually demonstrates more marked rostral vermian atrophy with relative sparing of the cerebellar hemispheres. As a rule, the more marked the clinical impairment, the more marked the cerebellar atrophy.[14]

Recently, PET scanning with ^{18}F-FDG was carried out in 22 patients with FA, and the results were compared with the scans of 23 normal control subjects.[31] There was a significant increase of LCMRGlc in the patient with FA in the cerebral cortex, caudate nucleus, and lenticular nucleus, but not in the thalamus, cerebellar vermis, cerebellar hemispheres or brainstem. The patients with FA were divided into two groups, ambulatory and nonambulatory, to study the correlation between severity of disease and LCMRGlc. The results showed that LCMRGlc was significantly increased in the ambulatory group compared with the normal controls in the cerebral cortex, caudate nucleus, lenticular nucleus, thalamus, cerebellar vermis, cerebellar hemispheres, and mesencephalon, but not in the pons (Fig. 11–4). LCMRGlc was significantly increased in the nonambulatory patient with FA compared with the normal controls in the caudate nucleus and lenticular nucleus, but not in the other structures. LCMRGlc was significantly increased in the ambulatory FA patients in comparison with the nonambulatory FA patients in the thalamus, cerebellar vermis, cerebellar hemispheres, mesencephalon, and pons, but not in the cerebral cortex or basal ganglia (Fig. 11–5).

The results of PET studies in FA revealed evidence of widespread cerebral glucose hypermetabolism in the central nervous system of patients with FA who are still ambulatory in comparison with normal control subjects. Increased glucose metabolism was also found in nonambulatory patients with FA, but only within the basal ganglia. These results suggest that glucose metabolic rate is increased throughout the central nervous system early in the disease and decreases as the disease progresses. The increased metabolism may reflect a fundamental biochemical defect in FA relating to carbohydrate metabolism. The decline in metabolic rate with disease progression may be due to loss of neurons and synaptic terminals.

Because spinal cord atrophy is the most marked morphologic abnormality in FA, a safe and simple means of imag-

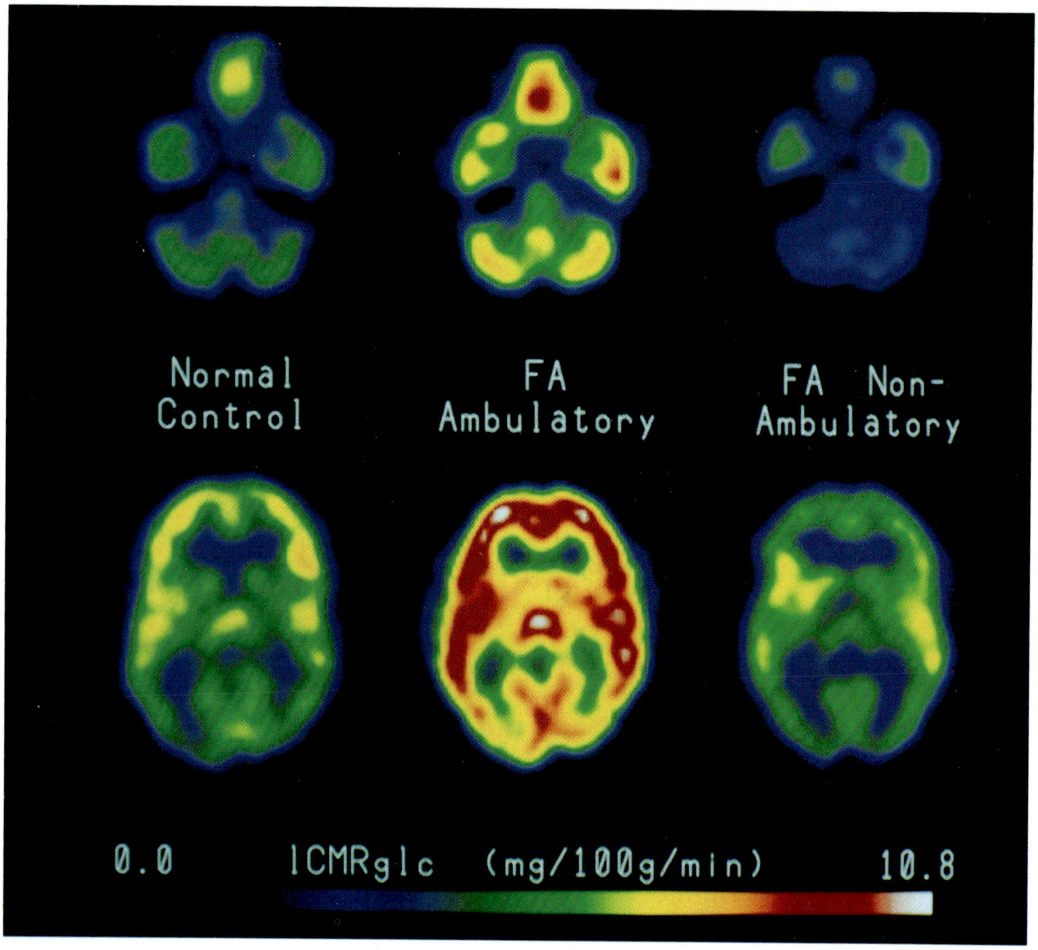

Figure 11–4. PET scans showing cerebral glucose utilization studied with ^{18}F-FDG. The upper 3 scans show horizontal sections at the level of the cerebellum and the base of the temporal and frontal lobes. The lower 3 scans show the level of the basal ganglia and thalamus. The color bar indicates the rate of glucose utilization. The upper and lower scans on the left are from a normal control female aged 24 years. The upper and lower scans in the middle are from a woman with Friedreich's ataxia, aged 25, who remains ambulatory. The upper and lower scans on the right are from a woman with Friedreich's ataxia, aged 29, who is nonambulatory. There is glucose hypermetabolism in the ambulatory patient with Friedreich's ataxia compared with the control subject and the nonambulatory patient. (From Gilman et al,[31] pp. 750–757, with permission).

ing both the brain and spinal medullary substance would be ideal. X-ray CT without intrathecal contrast material is relatively insensitive in the estimation of spinal cord size, however, and myelography or even more simple intrathecal contrast instillation for x-ray CT are invasive procedures and thus usually are not indicated (see Chapter 1).

MRI, unlike x-ray CT, can image both the brain and spinal cord without the addition of contrast material. Hence, when FA is suspected, MRI is the study of choice and should include examination of at least the cervical spinal cord as well as the brain. Because of the variation in size of the normal spinal cord, only the more marked cases of atrophy can be dependably identified. Despite this limitation, useful imaging information can be obtained.[82] Although imaging cannot separate other spinal cord–dominant atrophic processes, such as hereditary spastic ataxia, from FA, the age at clinical presentation and systems involved allow differentiation.

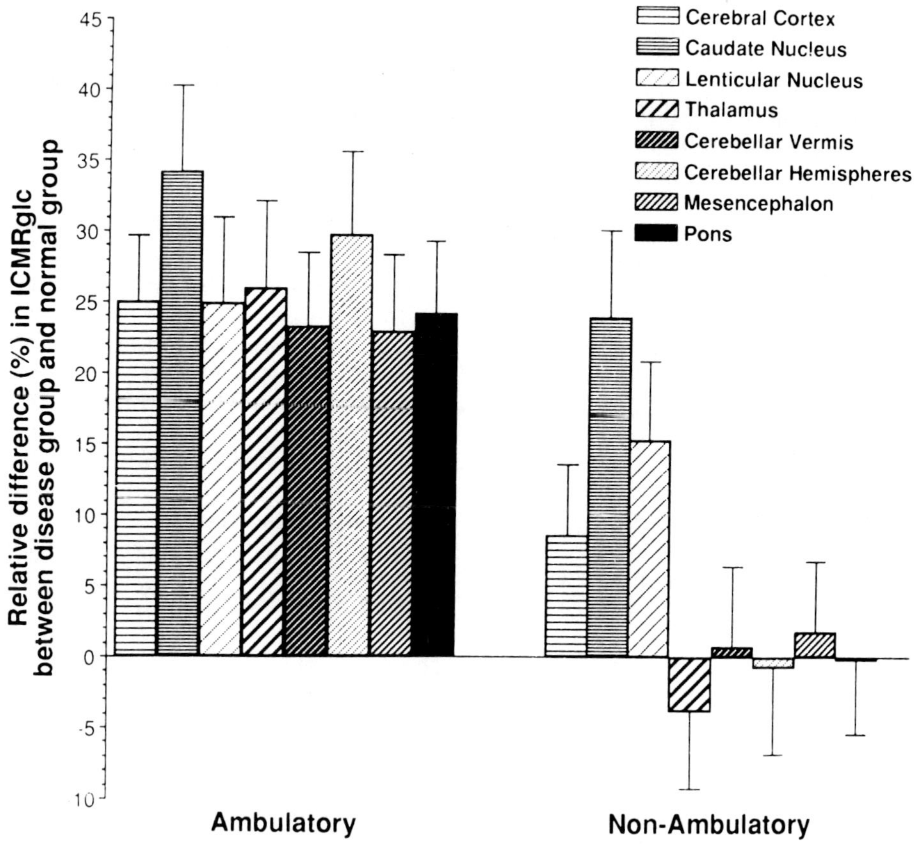

Figure 11–5. Mean local cerebral metabolic rate for glucose (LCMRGlc), relative to the levels in normal controls, for patients with Friedreich's ataxia. Error bars represent the standard error of the mean. (From Gilman et al,[31] pp. 750–757, with permission.)

Paraneoplastic Cerebellar Degeneration

Cerebellar degeneration can occur as a result of neoplasms occurring outside the central nervous system.[7,41] Anti-Purkinje cell antibodies have been detected in this condition, leading to the speculation that it may be an autoimmune disorder.[15,36,37,46] Cerebellar deficits usually evolve over days or months and the progression of symptoms may stop as abruptly as they began, but the deficits are largely irreversible. The causative neoplasms in adults include lung, breast, uterine, and ovarian carcinomas. In children, neuroblastoma is the neoplasm frequently associated with cerebellar degeneration. The clinical effects of paraneoplastic cerebellar degeneration are similar to those resulting from infectious or neoplastic diseases of the cerebellum, and include ataxia of gait and speech, titubation, limb dysmetria, hyporeflexia, opsoclonus, and myoclonus. Sensory disturbance also may occur, as well as progressive external ophthalmoplegia and muscle atrophy.

Neuropathologic examination in patients with paraneoplastic cerebellar degeneration usually reveals widespread loss of Purkinje cells, thinning of the molecular layer, and depletion of the granular layer. Most often, the dentate and olivary nuclei are normal. There is often demyelination of the superior cerebellar peduncles. The diagnosis of paraneoplastic cerebellar degeneration is assisted by the finding of anti–Purkinje cell antibodies in the serum.[36] Testing for these antibodies can be performed at several institutions in the United States, including Memorial Hospital in New York City, the Mayo Clinic, the University of Utah in Salt Lake City, and the University of Oregon in Portland.

Imaging studies in the early phase of this disease usually show no abnormality. With time, however, atrophy appears and x-ray CT will show a diffusely decreased volume for the cerebellum in a nonspecific pattern.[86] MRI assists somewhat, providing more artifact-free evaluation of cerebellar atrophy and greater sensitivity in the detection of brain metastases[33] (Fig. 11–6).

To date, only a limited number of patients with paraneoplastic cerebellar degeneration have been studied with PET and ^{18}F-FDG.[4] These patients had widespread hypometabolism throughout the central nervous system (Fig. 11–7). There was metabolic coupling between the cerebellum, cuneus, posterior temporal, lateral frontal, and paracentral cortex, possibly because of loss of cerebellar efferents to thalamus and forebrain structures.

DEMYELINATIVE DISEASE

Multiple sclerosis (MS) commonly affects the cerebellum, cerebellar pathways, and the brainstem.[65] Patients with MS, however, only rarely have signs limited to the cerebellum and its systems.[29,65] Although usually characterized by exacerbations and remission, at times MS presents as a progressive neurologic disorder.

Patients with MS commonly develop ataxia, spasticity, visual loss, sensory disturbance, and urinary dysfunction. Cerebellar disorders are uncommon at the onset of the disease, but by the time a neurologist is consulted, signs of

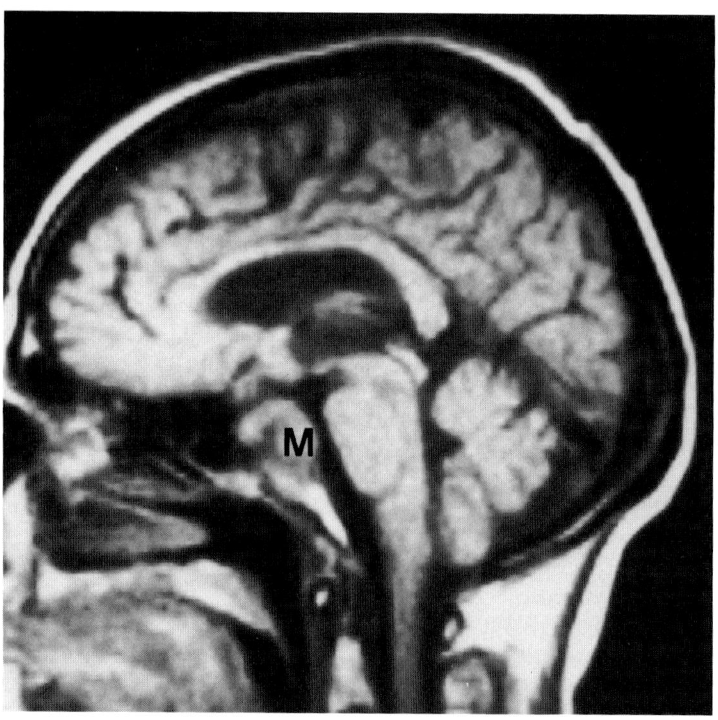

Figure 11–6. Paraneoplastic cerebellar degeneration. This sagittal MR image shows slight cerebellar atrophy, but dramatically demonstrates a clival metastasis from bronchogenic carcinoma (*M*).

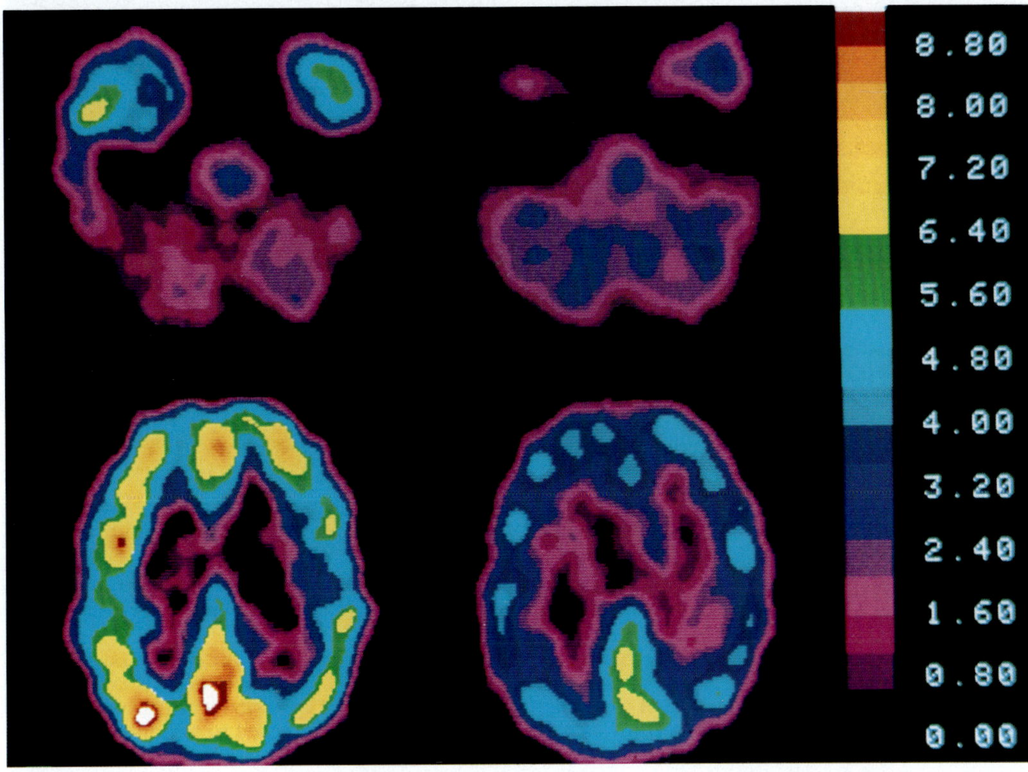

Figure 11–7. Paraneoplastic cerebellar degeneration. PET scans showing cerebral glucose utilization as detected with ^{18}F-FDG. The scans show horizontal sections at the level of the cerebellum (*upper pair*) and frontoparietal cortex (*lower pair*) from two patients with paraneoplastic cerebellar degeneration. The color bar indicates glucose utilization rates in mg per 100 g per min. In the patient whose scans are shown on the left, hypometabolism is restricted to the brainstem and cerebellum. In the patient whose scans are shown on the right, the cerebral cortex is hypometabolic as well. (From Anderson, et al,[4] pp. 533–540, with permission).

cerebellar disease are frequent.[65] In patients with established disease, cerebellar deficits are common; in Kurtzke's[56] series, 84% of patients had these signs. Cerebellar gait disturbances occur commonly in association with truncal ataxia, limb tremors, titubation, nystagmus, and dysarthria.

Diagnostic evaluation of patients suspected of having MS is assisted by cerebrospinal fluid (CSF) analysis and by somatosensory, auditory, and visual evoked potentials. Routine brain x-ray CT demonstrates abnormalities in roughly 50% or less of patients with MS,[42,106] whereas high doses of intravenous iodinated contrast material may demonstrate abnormalities in up to 70% of these patients.[96,106] X-ray CT abnormalities usually include small periependymal low-attenuation lesions with variable contrast enhancement. The rare presentation of MS as a mass lesion or "pseudotumor" is easily imaged on x-ray CT. Unfortunately, there are no distinctive x-ray CT imaging characteristics to separate this from other solitary mass lesions.

Compared with x-ray CT, MRI has much greater sensitivity in the detection of MS by imaging[23,24] (Fig. 11–8; see also Chapter 10). When early and established cases are considered together, sensitivity exceeds 90%. MRI and analysis of CSF for oligoclonal bands are the most cost-effective corro-

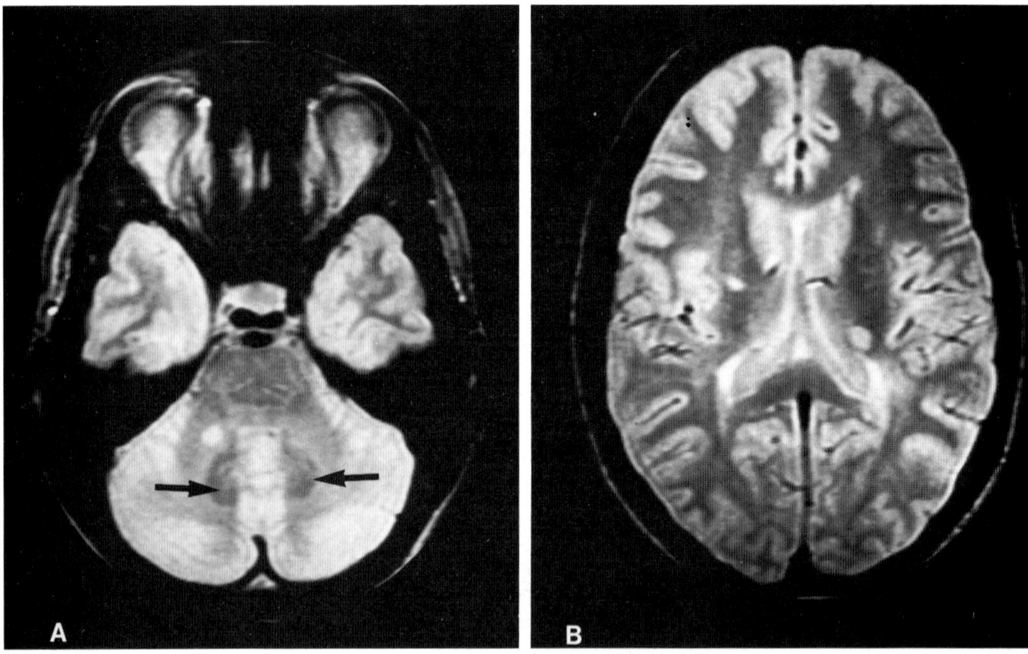

Figure 11–8. (*A,B*) Multiple sclerosis. Axial T_2-weighted MR images showing the classic nodular and punctate high-signal (white) periependymal lesions of multiple sclerosis. The lower-signal (dark) central structures indicated by the arrows on (*A*) represent the dentate nuclei. The lower signal is due in part to iron deposition. Iron deposition in certain parts of the brain may be increased in patients with MS.

borative investigations.[24] There is good correspondence between the number and size of lesions and the topography expected to be involved by clinical examination,[24,97] making MRI a useful tool for following the course of established MS.

Only a few patients with MS have been studied with PET.[9] The studies included measurement of regional oxygen utilization, oxygen extraction, blood flow, and blood volume. Cerebral oxygen utilization and blood flow were reduced significantly in cerebral gray and white matter in MS patients as compared with normal controls. Oxygen consumption in the cerebellum, however, was no different in MS patients than in controls. It is unclear why the cerebellum was spared in this study, since MS frequently involves cerebellar white matter.

CEREBELLAR ANOMALIES

The most common cerebellar anomalies are the Chiari malformations, the Dandy-Walker malformation, and von Hippel-Lindau disease.

Chiari Malformations

There are four types of Chiari malformations.[29] In *type I*, also called the adult Chiari malformation, the cerebellar tonsils are herniated into the foramen magnum and may extend into the cervical canal (Fig. 11–9). Other associated features include hydrocephalus, syringomyelia, syringobulbia, and an imperforate foramen of Magendie. The symptoms evolve slowly and include disorders of gaze, dysarthria, headache, dizziness, blurred vision, vomiting, and

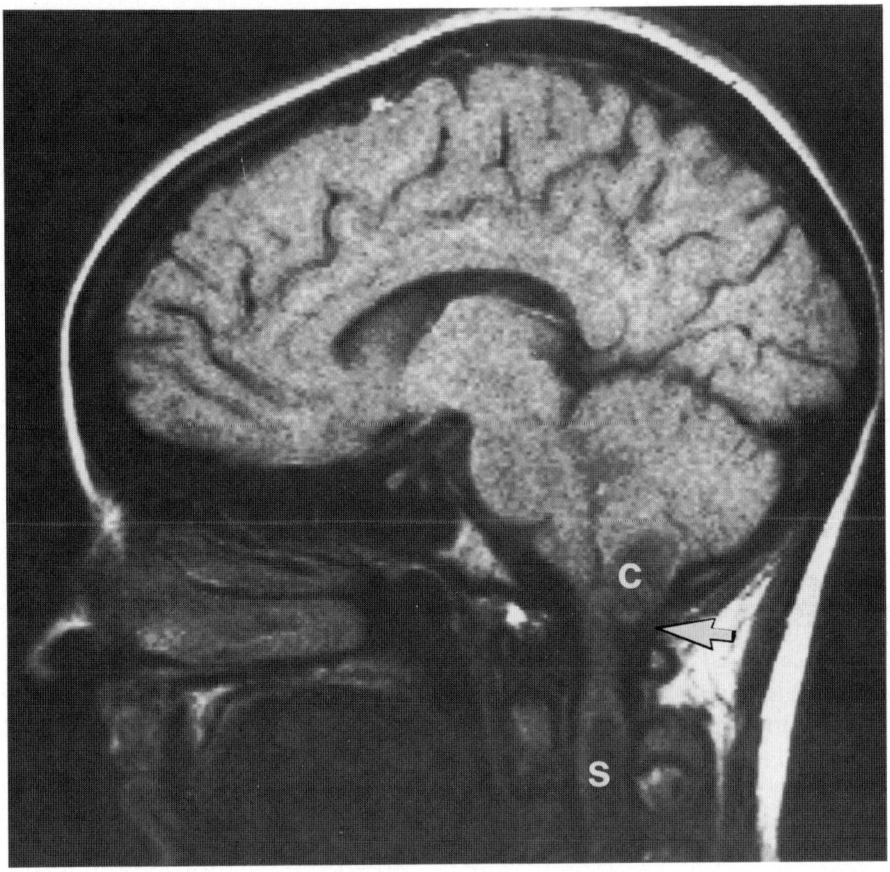

Figure 11–9. Chiari I malformation. A sagittal MRI in this severe Chiari I malformation demonstrates not only the cerebellar tonsillar ectopia (*arrow*) extending nearly as far caudal as the superior aspect of the ring of C-1, but also easily demonstrates associated cysts of the spinal cord (S) and cerebellum (C). Images of the intra-axial and spinal medullary cysts would be extremely difficult to obtain with any other modality. Clearly, MRI would assist surgical planning in such a case.

vertigo. Headaches occurring frequently and lasting less than a few minutes can occur with this malformation. All of the symptoms may be improved by decompression of the posterior fossa.

Type II Chiari malformation, also known as the Arnold-Chiari malformation, involves both the cerebellum and the brainstem. There is caudal displacement of the medulla oblongata, often with an S-shaped deformity of the cervicomedullary junction. The brainstem is placed low, so that the lower cranial nerves must course upward through the foramen magnum before exiting the skull. The cerebellar vermis extends to or below the foramen magnum. Hydrocephalus often develops. The posterior fossa is small, the tentorium is low, and spina bifida often is present in association with a myelomeningocele and hydrocephalus. The conus medullaris usually is low in the spinal canal and there is little or no filum terminale between the end of the cord and its attachment to the sacrum. This anomaly is called a tethered cord. In some patients there may be basilar impression of the skull, malformation of the cervical spine, mesencephalic spur formation, malformation of the falx cerebri, fenestration of the septum pellucidum, enlarged intrathalamic connection, and hydromyelia. Other abnormalities can include stenosis of the aqueduct of Sylvius, microgyria, intraventricular heterotopias, hypoplasia of the tentorium cerebelli, and dilation of the foramen of Monro.

In the *type III* Chiari malformation, there is a disturbance in the formation of both the hindbrain and the occipital bone. The cerebellum is small and positioned abnormally about a kinked brainstem. The medulla oblongata is flattened and appears to have remained split in development.

Type IV Chiari malformation is no longer considered to be a distinct entity. This malformation consists of cerebellar hypoplasia or dysgenesis.

The diagnosis of a Chiari malformation often becomes apparent at birth when a child presents with myelomeningocele. In many patients, however, there is no evidence of a Chiari malformation until adulthood. Then the patient may develop headaches, ataxia of gait, nystagmus, dysphagia, limb weakness, impaired sensation, and spasticity. Down-beat nystagmus is a common presenting sign.

Imaging studies greatly assist in the diagnosis of the Chiari malformations. Overall, routine axial x-ray CT is a relatively poor technique for imaging these malformations. Associated supratentorial abnormalities, most often aqueductal-level obstructive hydrocephalus, can be discerned in type II and III malformations. In type II malformation the findings in the posterior fossa include enlargement of the foramen magnum, tight "packing" of the posterior fossa with brain substance, pointed or "beaked" quadrigeminal plate and cistern, upward herniation of a distorted vermis through a wide tentorial incisura, and low-lying fourth ventricle.[72–74] More specialized high-resolution x-ray CT can provide detailed images of small regions of interest with artifact suppression. These studies can demonstrate tonsillar and vermian ectopia, and encystation of the fourth ventricle or syringobulbia. Such images can be reformatted to provide sagittal images for better visualization of the topographic relationships of all portions of the lesion. Intrathecal contrast material helps outline these structures; before MRI became available, intrathecal contrast with x-ray CT was an important method of defining intra-axial cyst formation. Myelography without x-ray CT will demonstrate the tonsillar ectopia but is not otherwise very useful. The morbidity of myelography increases with the amount of contrast material directed intracranially. Angiography will show distortion of the vascular tree from the ectopia, especially of the tonsillohemispheric branches of the posterior inferior cerebellar arteries, but is now rarely performed for this indication.

MRI has supplanted all of the above imaging modalities in the initial evaluation and follow-up of Chiari malformations. MRI easily provides sagittal images to delineate the interrelationships of all portions of the malformation (see Fig. 11–9). It permits resolution of intra-axial cyst formation in the brainstem and spinal cord as well as of vascular distortion without the addition of contrast material of any type. Effective planning for decompressive surgery results from clear delineation of the degree of cerebellar ectopia, distortion of the rostral cervical spinal canal, associated encystation of the fourth ventricle, hydromyelia or syrinx formation, and the extent of distortion of the vasculature. Follow-up of these heretofore difficult-to-image lesions is thus markedly simplified with MRI.

The high sensitivity of MRI in the craniocervical region has demonstrated that many normal people have slight degrees of asymptomatic tonsillar ectopia. MRI evidence for distortion of the structures in this region, especially if signal aberration is superimposed, when coupled with clinical evidence for dysfunction, would suggest that decompressive surgery may be needed. Without these findings, however, it would seem reasonable to assume that normal variation includes protrusion of 3 mm or less of nondistorted cerebellar tonsillar material below the foramen magnum.[1]

Dandy-Walker Syndrome

Dandy-Walker syndrome is a cystic malformation in the posterior fossa consisting of a hypoplastic cerebellar vermis, high placement of the tentorium cerebelli, enlargement of the posterior fossa, and elevation of the transverse sinuses.[29] These are the major features; other common abnormalities include hydrocephalus, agenesis of the corpus callosum, atresia of the foramina of Luschka and Magendi, neuronal and glial heterotopias, agenesis of the cerebellar flocculi and tonsils, and gyral anomalies of the cerebrum. Associated disorders include renal malformation and polydactyly. A substantial percentage of patients with the Dandy-Walker malformation are stillborn or die shortly after birth with progressive hydrocephalus. Clinical signs of the malformation usually appear in infancy with progressive hydrocephalus, a feeding disturbance, nausea and vomiting. The symptoms and signs at onset in older children and adults include ocular palsies, visual loss, hearing disorder, gait instability, and nystagmus. In many patients the Dandy-Walker malformation may present with a gradual onset of quadriparesis of spastic type without signs of cerebellar disturbance. In some the malformation may be asymptomatic throughout life.

Imaging studies are key to the diagnosis of the Dandy-Walker syndrome. Skull x-rays occasionally show elevation of the transverse sinus grooves and thinning of occipital bone with enlargement of the occipital region of the calvarium. X-ray CT demonstrates a nearly central CSF collection that cannot be completely separated from the fourth ventricle (Fig. 11 – 10). This finding helps to differentiate the Dandy-Walker syndrome from patients with simply a large cisterna magna. In the Dandy-Walker syndrome, little or no vermis is visible, depending on the degree of hypoplasia in the particular patient. Secondary elevation of the transverse sinuses and tentorium can be discerned. Severe cases invariably have aqueductal-level obstructive hydrocephalus and, many times, the associated abnormalities mentioned above. As with the Chiari malformation, there appears to be a spectrum of morphologic and clinical involvement in the Dandy-Walker syndrome. The most mildly affected cases show only "prominent valleculae" secondary to minimal vermian hypoplasia.[38,63]

Again, as with the Chiari malformation, MRI has supplanted all other imaging modalities in evaluation of the Dandy-Walker malformation. The above-described findings are more easily seen with MRI, and the easily obtained sagittal images provide much better topographic relationships.

Von Hippel-Lindau Disease

Von Hippel-Lindau disease is the association of cerebellar hemangioblastomas with retinal angiomas and visceral cysts or tumors.[29] It is a hereditary disorder transmitted as an autosomal dominant trait with variable penetrance. Commonly, patients with this condition develop visual disorders from retinal tumors which may be the presenting complaint, or the initial presentation may be symptoms from cerebellar or brainstem dysfunction, including headache, vertigo, and vomiting.[45,68] Cysts and angiomas may affect the adrenal glands, pancreas, liver, epididymis, kidney, and other abdominal organs. Pheochromocytomas develop in some families and renal cell carcinomas may occur later in life.

Imaging studies that are helpful in this diagnosis include arteriography, x-ray CT, and MRI. Arteriography may reveal the hemangioblastoma as well as other angiomatous tumors. Routine brain x-ray CT affords good delineation

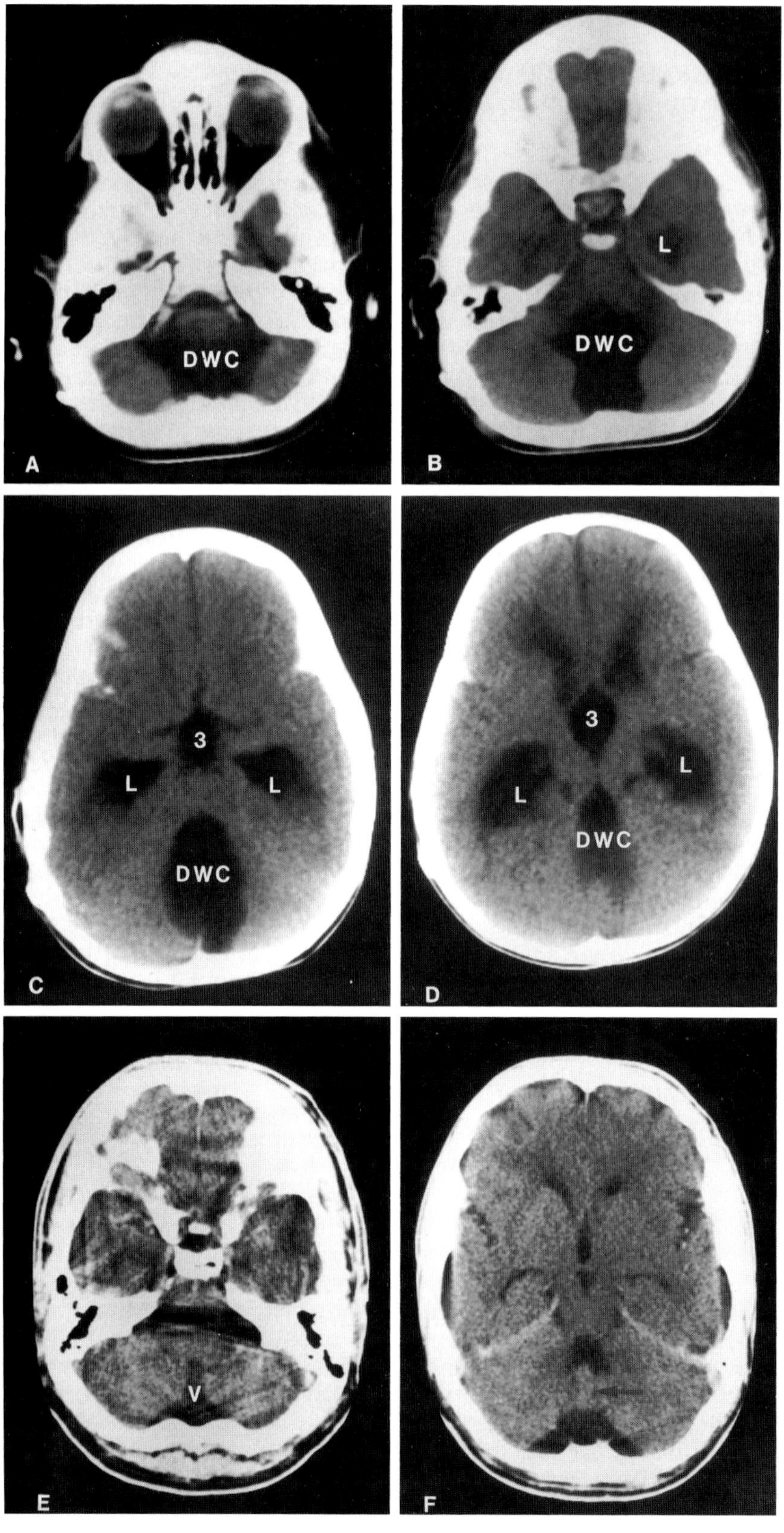
DWC
A
L
DWC
B
3
L
L
DWC
C
3
L
L
DWC
D
V
E
F

of moderate-to-large hemangioblastomas and their attendant cysts. However, small lesions and extension of the cysts into the spinal cord can be missed with x-ray CT.[83]

MRI provides more sensitivity than x-ray CT in detecting all of the hemangioblastomas as well as their arterial supply and venous drainage, and without the addition of contrast material (Fig. 11–11). It also reveals the exact relationships of the solid and cystic portions of the lesion, and improves topographic understanding with easily obtained sagittal and coronal images. Thus, it provides the most accurate data for surgical planning.[91] If acute hemorrhage is suspected, an x-ray CT scan should be obtained first, since MRI may be less sensitive in this situation. Both abdominal x-ray CT and MRI are useful in evaluation of the visceral components of this syndrome.[91]

Angiography is used as a confirmatory or preoperative examination. Angiography usually demonstrates intense hypervascularity in the nidus of the lesion, with dilated feeding arteries and draining veins. A mass effect may be seen if the cyst is large enough to compress neighboring structures.

VASCULAR DISEASE

Transient Ischemic Attacks

A transient ischemic attack involving the brainstem and cerebellum results from diminished flow through the vertebrobasilar arterial system.[11] The attack consists of an episode of focal neurologic disorder with abrupt onset and resolution within 24 hours. The common symptoms include vertigo, deafness, syncope, transient blurring of vision, and unsteadiness of gait.[75] Other common symptoms include double vision, ataxia of the limbs, and even bilateral limb weakness or sensory deficits. Dysphagia, bilateral visual field disturbances, and tinnitus are less common.[12] Occipital headache often accompanies these signs and symptoms, so that a distinction between complicated migraine and vertebrobasilar insufficiency can be difficult. The risk factors for transient ischemic attacks in the posterior circulation include hypertension, diabetes, cigarette smoking, and hypercholesterolemia.

X-ray CT is the best choice for imaging acute ischemic brain injury,[102] although the artifacts caused by beam hardening can make small lesions difficult to identify (see Fig. 1–9*A*). While MRI is more sensitive in locating lesions of this type, small acute hemorrhages may be missed (see Chapter 7, p. 183). Such hemorrhages usually radically change the management of these lesions with respect to anticoagulation. In many patients, however, the symptoms are subacute or chronic, and in these cases, MRI is clearly superior to x-ray CT.[52] Brainstem and cerebellar ischemic changes usually can be seen as regions of increased intensity that may be remarkably symmetric on the two sides. There may be clearly demarcated focal loss of brain substance, suggesting older completed infarcts. Subacute lesions usually will show low signal on T_1-weighted images and high signal on T_2-weighted images, as well as mass effect (see Chapter 2, p. 40).[89] Gadolinium helps considerably in finding small, subacute lesions.

Angiography, usually with selective intra-arterial injections and film-

Figure 11–10. (*A–D*) Dandy-Walker malformation. Four serial, contiguous 10 mm axial x-ray CT sections show severe vermian hypoplasia. The large CSF attenuation space (DWC) represents the Dandy-Walker cyst. As in most cases, obstructive hydrocephalus has occurred, as indicated by dilation of the third (3) and lateral (L) ventricles. Prominent cisterna magna. Two serial 5 mm axial sections (*E–F*) show a prominent cisterna magna and a large vallecula (V). As opposed to the Dandy-Walker malformation, however, the fourth ventricle can be clearly separated from the cisterna magna by the vermis (*arrow*).

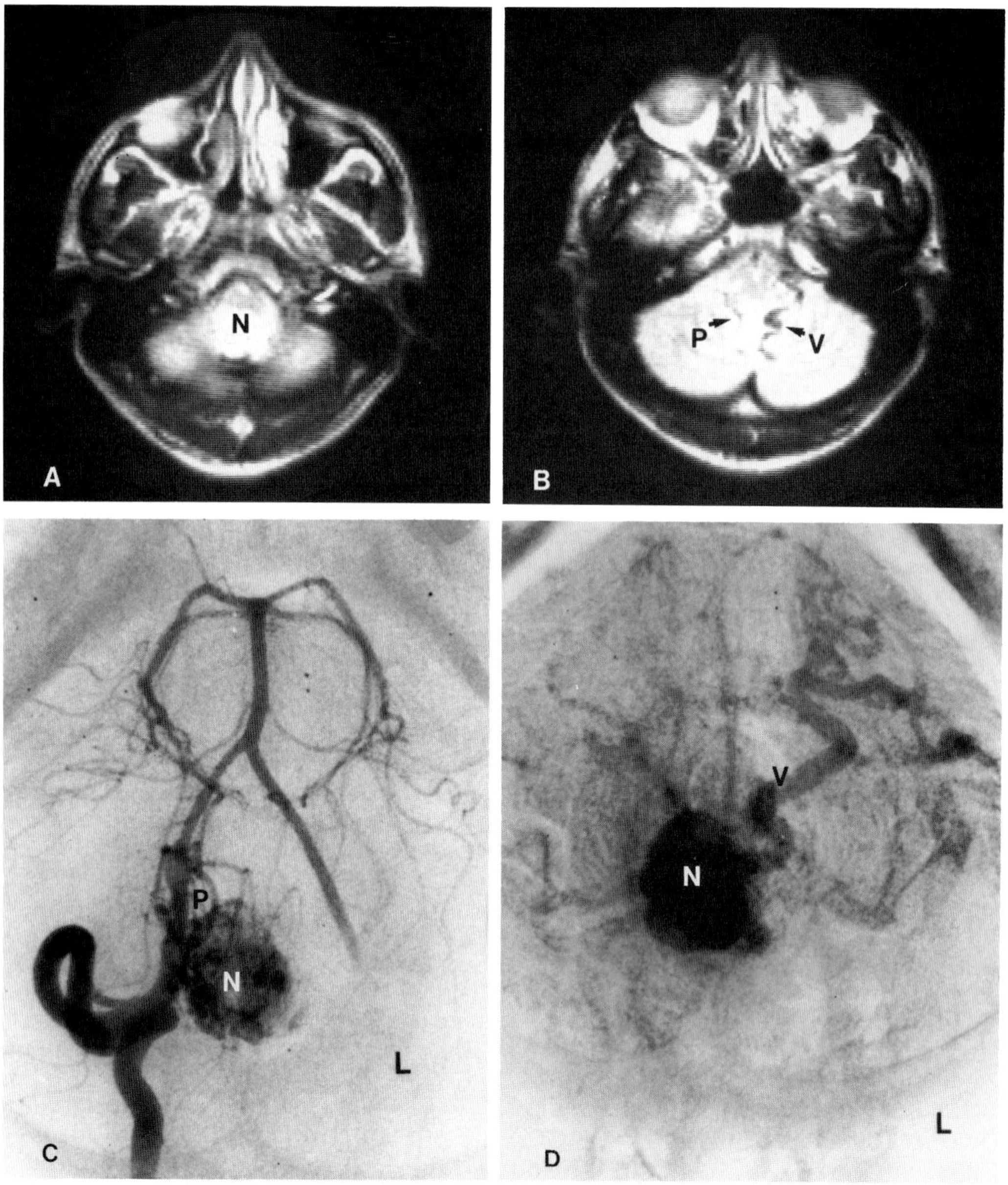

Figure 11–11. Von Hippel-Lindau syndrome—cerebellar hemangioblastoma. (*A,B*) Axial MR images show a high-signal nidus (N), enlarged posterior inferior cerebellar artery (P) feeding the nidus, and a dilated lateral recess vein (V) draining the nidus. The correspondence between these MR images and subtraction-technique submental vertex vertebral arteriography (*C,D*) is dramatic.

screen images for fine detail, can be used in these patients to define the dominant region of occlusive disease and permit planning of management.[11,43] Because proximal lesions are generally more common than distal lesions, angiography must include arch aortography as well as head and neck imaging.[28] Angiography usually is performed with the neck in a neutral position and not rotated. It is useful to change the position of the neck, particularly in rotation, if clinical evidence for positional change is present (e.g., symptom onset with rotation or a decrease in upper extremity pulses with neck rotation). Filming in flexed, extended, or rotated positions is termed "dynamic" or "stress" angiography and can be helpful, although it is performed infrequently.

Cerebellar Infarction

Infarction within the cerebellum usually results from thrombosis of a branch of the vertebrobasilar artery,[13,99] most commonly stemming from arteriosclerosis. Cerebellar infarction rarely results from emboli migrating into the vertebrobasilar system from the heart or from complicated migraine, trauma, and infections. The most frequent site of infarction is in the posterior inferior half of a single cerebellar hemisphere, because of lesions of the posterior inferior cerebellar artery[19,59] (Fig. 11–12).

The presenting complaints with cerebellar infarction consist of difficulty with standing or walking, nausea and vomiting, dizziness or vertigo, slowed speech, and clumsiness of limb movements.[58] Headache characteristically occurs in this condition and is either in the frontal or occipital region.[59] Mentation may be impaired early in the course, probably because of increased intracranial pressure. With progression of the symptoms, most patients develop disturbances of extraocular movements, including a sixth-nerve palsy or a gaze palsy. Gaze-evoked nystagmus also occurs commonly. Facial weakness may occur, but usually other cranial nerves are spared unless brainstem structures are directly infarcted.[59]

Hydrocephalus develops in a substantial number of patients with cerebellar infarction, and impaired cognition occurs in about half of those with hydrocephalus.[34,100] Hydrocephalus results from tonsillar herniation with obstruction of CSF flow at the level of the fourth ventricle. Transtentorial herniation of the cerebellum may result in compression of the posterior cerebral artery and cause impaired vision or cortical blindness from occipital lobe ischemia.[29]

Imaging studies have been discussed in the preceding section. Small infarctions can be managed with careful observation, but extensive infarctions require exploration of the posterior fossa and resection of necrotic cerebellar tissue.[19,59] Although the mortality rate approaches 80% in patients with extensive infarction untreated surgically if the patient becomes stuporous or comatose, this figure is around 50% if the patient is treated surgically before obtundation occurs.[34] The prognosis of cerebellar infarction depends upon the degree of involvement of the cerebellum.[51] In rapidly progressive cases, the infarcted cerebellum becomes edematous and soon exceeds the volume of the posterior fossa. Tonsillar herniation results and cardiorespiratory failure occurs. Death from brainstem compression is frequently an outcome in these cases.[51]

Cerebellar Hemorrhage

Hypertension is the most common cause of cerebellar hemorrhage.[84] Other etiologies include anticoagulation therapy, intrinsic coagulation defects, vascular malformations, neoplasms, infection, and trauma.[8,49]

Clinically, differentiation of cerebellar hemorrhage from cerebellar infarction is difficult. Headache occurs more commonly with hemorrhage, but may occur with infarction as well.[59,99] The sudden onset of an occipital headache with vomiting, dizziness, and gait difficulty is most characteristic of hemorrhage, particularly in a hypertensive person.[79] Gait or truncal ataxia occurs more frequently than limb ataxia, but both may be present. If a hemorrhage involves one cerebellar hemisphere, dysmetria of the ipsilateral limbs may occur. Gaze palsies and facial palsies are common.[79] Difficulty with conjugate gaze often occurs and usually is ipsilateral to the side of the hemorrhage, most

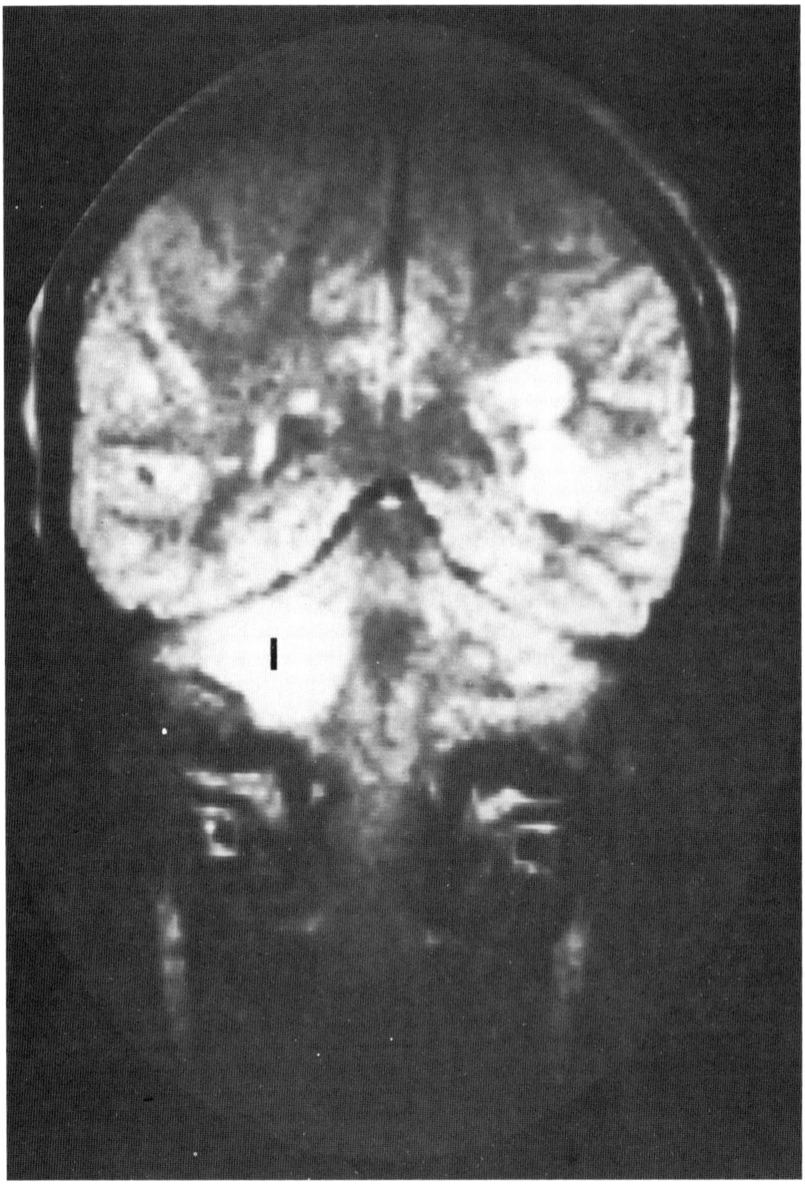

Figure 11–12. Cerebellar infarction. Coronal T_2-weighted MR image shows large high-signal (white) infarct in the right cerebellar hemisphere (I). Similar but smaller signal aberrations are seen about the lateral ventricles above the tentorium, consistent with chronic ischemic white-matter injuries.

likely resulting from brainstem compression. A sixth-nerve palsy may occur on the side of the hemorrhage. In some patients there is a gaze preference to the side opposite the cerebellar hemorrhage. Frequently, patients with cerebellar hemorrhage will be in coma at the time of their initial hospital admission.[67] These patients usually have complete ophthalmoplegia. In patients who are still awake after a cerebellar hemorrhage, the common signs are miotic pupils, gaze-evoked horizontal nystagmus, decreased corneal reflexes, neck stiffness, dysarthria, and vertigo.[67,79] Forced deviation of the eyes or head toward the unaffected side is observed in many patients with hemorrhage into a cerebellar hemisphere. Ocular bobbing occurs rarely.

X-ray CT provided a major advance in the diagnosis of cerebellar hemorrhage. The high attenuation of acutely extravasated blood compared with brain allows rapid recognition (Fig. 11–13). X-ray CT is also useful in following the course of the hemorrhage over time. As discussed under ischemic disease, MR is not the best imaging modality in cases of suspected acute hemorrhage, because subtle lesions of this type can be missed (see Chapter 7). Some patients with cerebellar hemorrhage should be taken from x-ray CT to arteriography in order to identify the bleeding site. Although not generally indicated for all intraparenchymal cerebellar hemorrhages, meticulous magnification film-screen selective arteriography is essential if a vascular malformation or an aneurysm is suspected. An arteriogram is usually elected if hemorrhagic ischemic injury is suspected clinically.

MRI becomes useful, although secondary, if x-ray CT and angiography fail to define the etiology of the hemorrhage or if more data are needed on the topographic relationships of a known lesion such as a vascular malformation.[55]

Aneurysms

Aneurysms of the posterior fossa usually occur at the bifurcation of the basilar artery into the posterior cerebral arteries, or along the basilar artery itself (see Fig. 7–6). The initial manifestation may consist of a subarachnoid hemorrhage; in this case, the patient often will

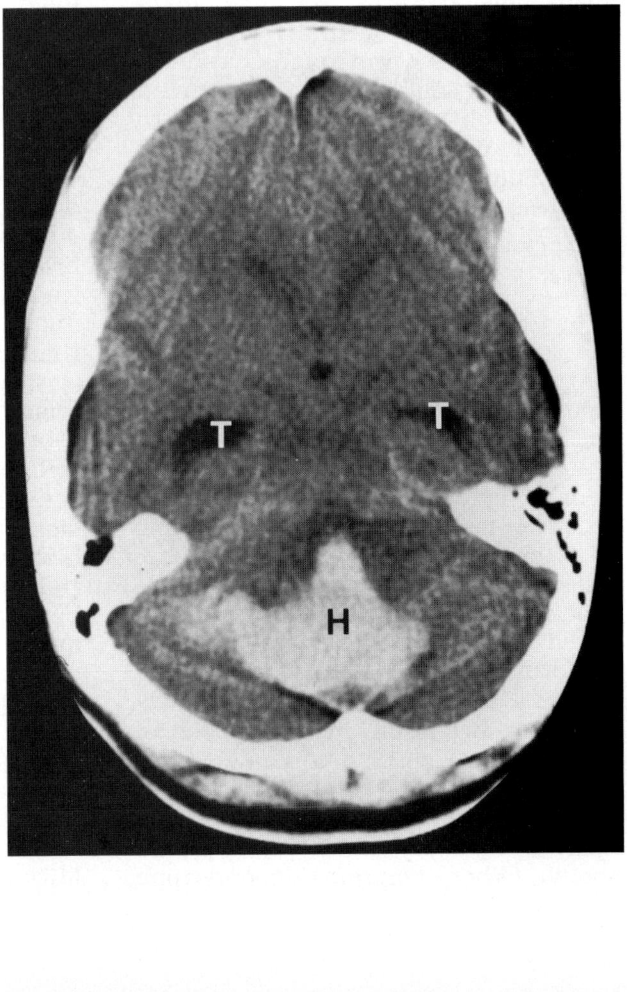

Figure 11–13. Cerebellar hemorrhage. Axial x-ray CT demonstrates massive intraventricular and intraparenchymal cerebellar hemorrhage (H), with marked local mass effect obliterating the basilar cistern and causing early obstructive hydrocephalus, indicated by dilation of the temporal horns of the lateral ventricles (T). The etiology of this hemorrhage was a vascular malformation.

lose consciousness or become confused following complaints of a severe headache. Nausea, vomiting, and photophobia also may occur. The occurrence of ataxia and dysarthria accompanying headache, nausea, and vomiting give a clue to the origin of the aneurysm. Aneurysms of the vertebral artery may cause bleeding into or compression of the cerebellum.[47] Through progressive enlargement, aneurysms of the cerebellar branch arteries near the take-off from the basilar artery may produce a cerebellopontine-angle syndrome with impaired hearing, facial weakness, and limb ataxia on the side of the lesion. Rarely, an aneurysm of the anterior inferior cerebellar artery will produce symptoms suggestive of a cerebellopontine-angle mass.[47]

X-ray CT and MRI will demonstrate only the larger aneurysms, and thus angiography is required if this diagnosis is suspected. Angiography for detection of aneurysms requires selective intra-arterial injections, usually with film-screen technique and magnification for high detail. Oblique views and cross-compression technique are frequently needed to delineate completely the circle of Willis and to separate overlapping arteries.

Arteriovenous Malformations

Arteriovenous malformations may occur within or around the cerebellum and usually present clinically with an acute hemorrhage[60] or with progressive signs of cerebellar dysfunction. Cerebellar hemorrhage is the most common initial cause of symptoms. When a cerebellar hemorrhage occurs, it usually is difficult to determine whether it has resulted from a bleeding arteriovenous malformation, an aneurysm, an angioma, a hemangioblastoma, or a venous malformation in the posterior fossa. Patients with hemorrhage from a vascular malformation usually present with headache, dizziness, nausea, vomiting, diplopia, dysarthria, and photophobia. Other symptoms depend upon the degree of involvement of additional posterior fossa structures. The course may be slowly progressive, sudden in onset, or intermittent.

X-ray CT without and with intravenous contrast enhancement usually will reveal the larger vascular malformations.[50] Typical findings in a posterior fossa vascular malformation would include acute mixed intraparenchymal and subarachnoid hemorrhage, perhaps with an intraventricular component. Most of the hemorrhage is usually in the posterior fossa, but there may be a substantial amount of blood above the tentorium by the time the patient is imaged. A fair proportion of patients will present without acute hemorrhage, as discussed above. Whether or not there is acute hemorrhage, intravenous contrast administration usually reveals serpiginous structures representing the site of moderate-to-large arteriovenous-type vascular malformations with dilated feeding arteries and draining veins. In the acute case, arteriography usually is performed immediately following x-ray CT. The details of arteriography are the same as discussed above. If there is no acute hemorrhage, x-ray CT may show focal ex-vacuo change in and about the vascular malformation, suggesting antecedent hemorrhage and brain injury. There also may be a distinctive calcification pattern in and about the vascular malformation and at times in the injured brain adjacent to it.

Although x-ray CT is useful in the imaging of subacute and chronic presentations of vascular malformations, MRI excels in this task with its greater sensitivity in detecting intra-axial lesions and its ability to delineate flowing blood without additional contrast material[55] (Fig. 11 – 14).[7–3,7–4] MRI may also be employed in acute lesions if x-ray CT and angiography do not demonstrate a source of bleeding or if precise topographic relationships are needed to plan treatment. Even if MRI strongly suggests a vascular malformation, however, angiography is required to plan therapy. The usual appearance of a racemose arteriovenous malformation on MRI is that of a tangle of low-intensity

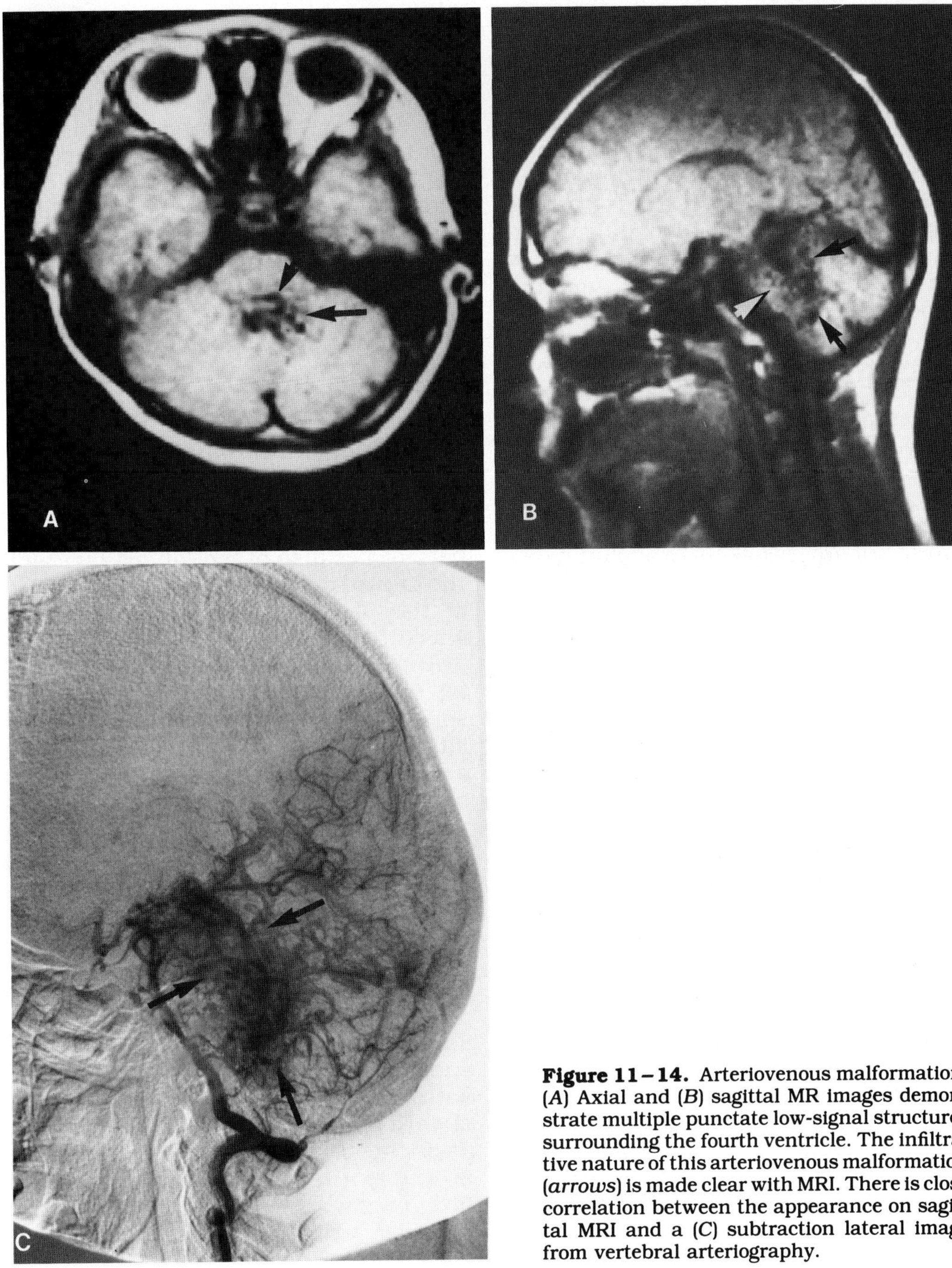

Figure 11–14. Arteriovenous malformation. (*A*) Axial and (*B*) sagittal MR images demonstrate multiple punctate low-signal structures surrounding the fourth ventricle. The infiltrative nature of this arteriovenous malformation (*arrows*) is made clear with MRI. There is close correlation between the appearance on sagittal MRI and a (*C*) subtraction lateral image from vertebral arteriography.

(black) serpiginous structures, perhaps with a well-defined nidus, associated with dilated supplying arteries and draining veins. There may or may not be mass effect and/or edema, depending upon how irritating the lesion is and whether or not previous brain injury from local hemorrhage has occurred. The perisylvian region is an especially common site of involvement by these lesions.

Telangiectatic vascular malformations, perhaps the most common type in the posterior fossa, may defy all attempts to localize them regardless of the imaging modalities employed, because they often infiltrate about the pia of the brainstem and exhibit contrast-transit characteristics nearly identical to those of normal arteries and veins in this region. This area is also difficult to study with angiography because it is surrounded by dense bone, making subtraction artifacts more common. Fortunately, the racemose high-flow arteriovenous malformations, which may be the type that most frequently hemorrhages, are relatively easy to image with x-ray CT, MRI, and angiography. Venous angiomas and cavernous angiomas, not uncommon in the posterior fossa, can be slightly more difficult to image but are less likely to hemorrhage.

CEREBELLAR ABSCESS

Abscesses in the posterior fossa usually develop from infection within or adjacent to the central nervous system; only a small percentage of cerebellar abscesses result from infection at a remote site.[5,22] Retrograde septic thrombophlebitis is a common cause for the spread of infection into the cerebellum.[90] The lung and heart are the most likely sources of bacterial infection when a source in close proximity to the nervous system is not apparent.[90]

The clinical symptoms of cerebellar abscess usually involve the manifestations of increased intracranial pressure rather than cerebellar dysfunction.[22,70] The most frequent presenting complaint is headache,[69] but with time, deficits occur in cranial nerve functions and in the state of alertness.[70] Papilledema occurs commonly,[69] along with facial weakness, hearing loss, and dysconjugate gaze.

Imaging studies are the diagnostic procedures of choice when cerebellar abscesses are suspected. Lumbar puncture is contraindicated because of the chance of herniation, and because the findings with lumbar puncture often are misleading.[70,90] X-ray CT is helpful in diagnosis, particularly if a ring of pathologic contrast enhancement can be seen about a lower-attenuation (generally necrotic) center (Fig. 11 – 15). Contributory findings are local edema, ventricular and/or subarachnoid enhancement suggesting brain inflammation, and, rarely, low attenuation in adjacent dural venous sinuses, suggesting thrombophlebitis. The "ring-lesion" imaging characteristics of abscess are not pathognomonic, however. They can be seen in neoplasms (both primary and metastatic), in stroke, and in maturing hemorrhage, but the combination of clinical findings and x-ray CT often is diagnostic.

MRI shows similar findings but generally is not employed in the acutely ill patient because of motion artifact and the hazard of placing such a patient out of the physician's reach, even for a short interval.

Angiography is only rarely performed for the evaluation of abscess. It is reserved for cases in which dural venous sinus involvement is suspected but not adequately proved by clinical, x-ray CT, or MRI studies.

ALCOHOLIC CEREBELLAR DEGENERATION

Cerebellar degeneration from alcoholism can develop over an interval of days, weeks, or months. It may evolve slowly and insidiously, rapidly with subsequent stabilization, or erratically with episodic exacerbations.[104] Frequently the disorder of gait seen with alcoholic cerebellar degeneration improves as the patient becomes detoxified under treatment. In many patients, however, a substantial disorder of gait persists after detoxification.

The principal clinical findings in patients with alcoholic cerebellar degeneration are a disturbance of gait and of truncal stability with little or no impairment of speech, oculomotor function, or coordinated movements of the upper limbs. Only a small percentage of pa-

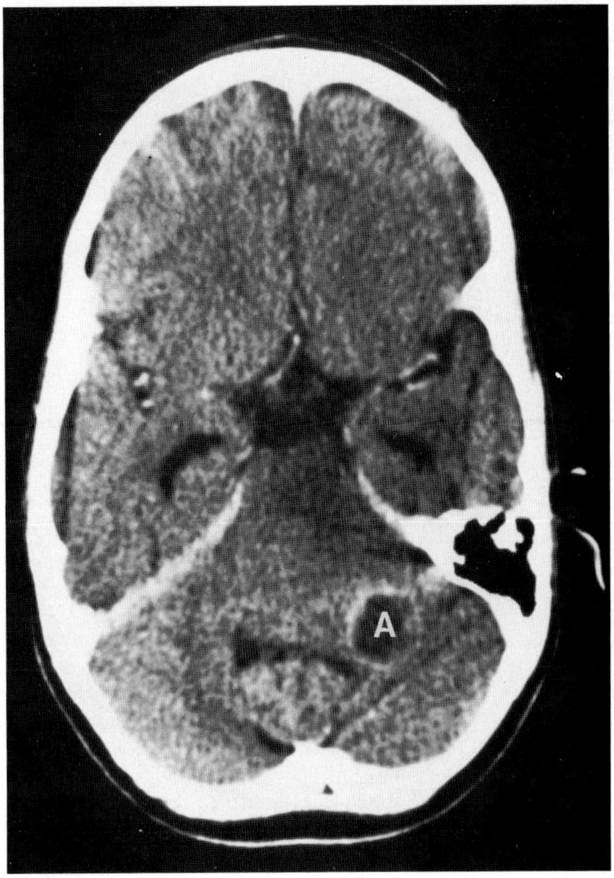

Figure 11–15. Cerebellar abscess. Contrast-enhanced axial x-ray CT scan shows the classic imaging characteristics of abscess (A): a thin rim of pathologic contrast enhancement surrounding a necrotic, low-attenuation center. This CT scan also demonstrates low attenuation in the brainstem caused by local inflammation.

tients develop a tremor of the head or limbs. The condition is thought to result from nutritional deficiency rather than from the direct effects of alcohol.

The pathologic changes in the cerebellum with alcoholic cerebellar degeneration are indistinguishable from those occurring with Wernicke's syndrome.[2,104] There is atrophy in all layers of the cerebellum in the anterior and superior portion of the vermis.[104] Purkinje cells are decreased to absent in this region, and neuronal loss may be prominent also in the dentate and inferior olivary nuclei.[104] The cerebellar hemispheres are involved much less than is the vermis.

X-ray CT in alcoholic cerebellar degeneration demonstrates atrophy of both the cerebral hemispheres and the cerebellar vermis (Fig. 11–16); the cerebellar hemispheres are somewhat spared. Perhaps the most notable differentiating feature of alcoholic cerebellar degeneration is the relatively early involvement of the cerebral hemispheres, especially the frontal lobes, compared with other types of cerebellar degenerations.[14] In patients with the appropriate clinical findings, x-ray CT is helpful in making the diagnosis. MRI offers better resolution of the structures of interest but may be degraded if patient cooperation is poor and, as noted above, is less widely available than x-ray CT. In many patients it can be difficult to differentiate alcoholic cerebellar degeneration from other progressive cerebellar degenerations such as olivopontocerebellar atrophy. Metabolic scanning with PET seems likely to be helpful.

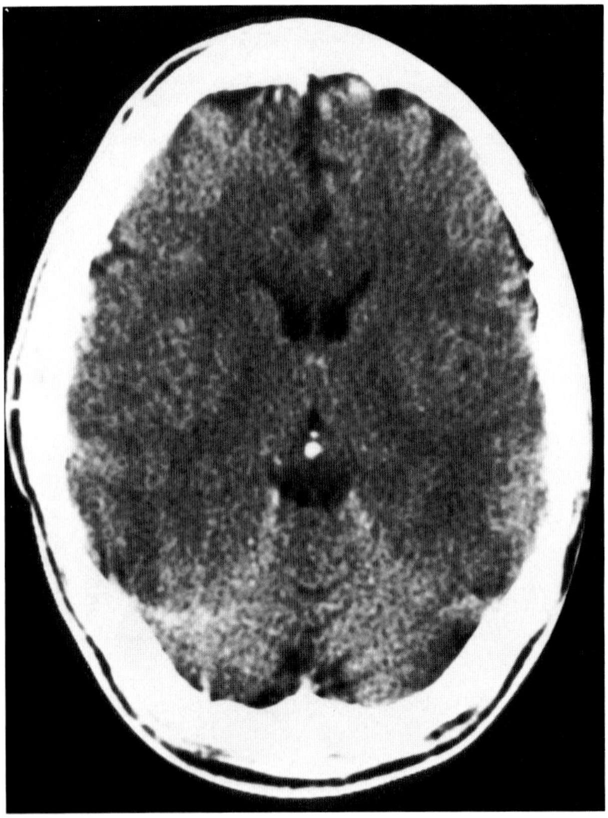

Figure 11–16. Alcoholic cerebellar degeneration. Contrast-enhanced axial x-ray CT demonstrates atrophy of the cerebellar vermis and frontal lobe cortex with relative sparing of the cerebellar hemispheres in this 25-year-old alcoholic man.

In a recent study utilizing PET, LCMRglc was studied using ^{18}F-FDG in 14 chronically alcohol dependent patients and 8 normal control subjects.[32] Nine of the 14 alcohol dependent patients had clinical signs of alcoholic cerebellar degeneration and the remaining 5 patients did not. All 9 patients with clinical signs of cerebellar degeneration had significantly decreased LCMRGlc in the superior cerebellar vermis in comparison with the normal controls (Fig. 11–17). The 5 patients without clinical signs of cerebellar degeneration did not show decreased LCMRGlc in the cerebellum. All 14 chronically alcohol dependent patients had diminished LCMRGlc bilaterally in the medial frontal area of the cerebral cortex in comparison with the normal control subjects. The degree of atrophy found in x-ray CT scans was significantly correlated with the LCMRGlc in the medial frontal area of the cerebral cortex, but not in the cerebellum. The findings indicate that hypometabolism in the superior cerebellar vermis is closely related to clinical symptoms in patients with alcoholic cerebellar degeneration and does not occur in alcohol dependent patients unless they show clinical signs of cerebellar degeneration. Hypometabolism in the medial frontal cortex, along with atrophy in this region, appears to be a frequent finding in chronically alcohol dependent patients with or without alcoholic cerebellar degeneration.

NEOPLASMS

Signs and Symptoms of Cerebellar Tumors

The intraparenchymal tumors most commonly affecting the cerebellum and adjacent structures are medulloblas-

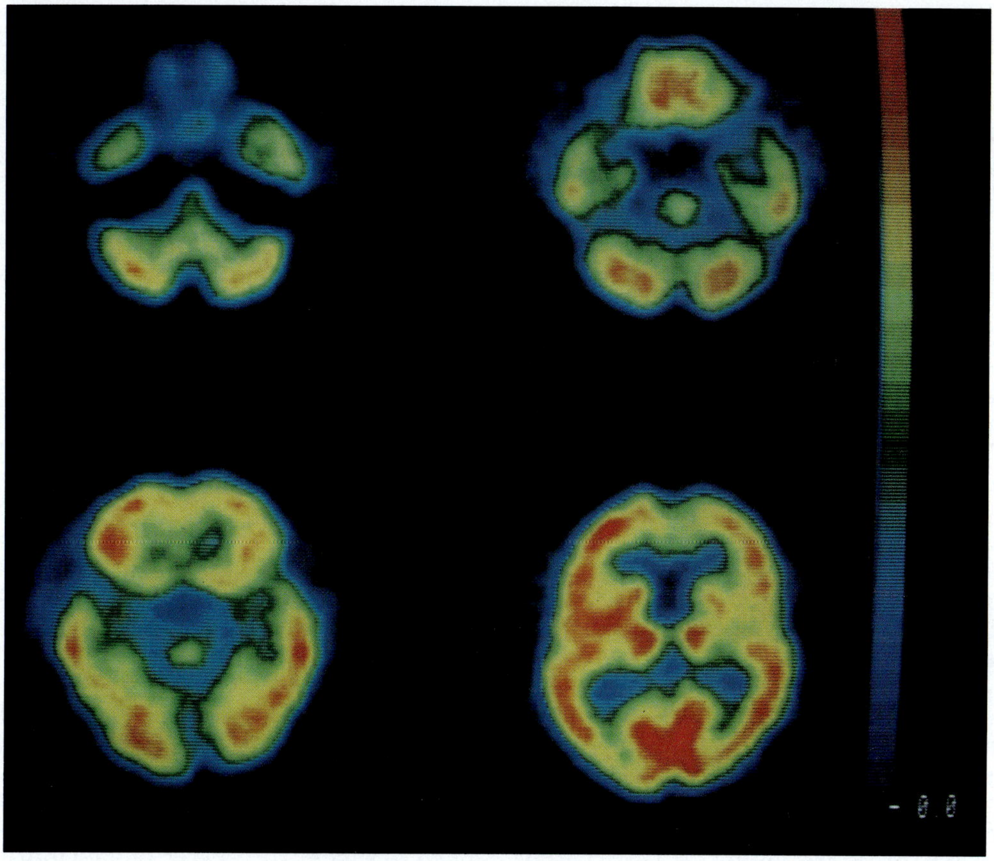

Figure 11–17. Alcoholic cerebellar degeneration. PET scans showing cerebral glucose utilization as detected with ^{18}F-FDG. The scans show horizontal sections at the level of the cerebellum (*upper left*), a slightly higher level of the cerebellum (*upper right*), the highest level that still shows the cerebellum (*lower left*), and the level of the basal ganglia and thalamus (*lower right*). The scans were taken from a 55-year-old man with alcoholic cerebellar degeneration. Note the hypometabolism of the cerebellar vermis. The lower two scans also show hypometabolism of the frontal lobes. The color bar indicates glucose utilization rates in mg per 100 g per min extending from 0.0 to 10.5.

tomas, astrocytomas, metastatic tumors, and ependymomas.[3,48,57,61] Other related neoplasms occurring in the posterior fossa are angioreticulomas, sarcomas, and other forms of glioma. Lymphomas, neuroblastomas, and gangliocytomas may occur in the cerebellum but are rare.[81,93,107] Hemangiomas and hemangioblastomas occur with intermediate frequency.[98] The incidence of the different types of cerebellar tumors varies with age and cell type. Metastatic tumors in the posterior fossa are found most commonly in middle age, whereas astrocytomas and medulloblastomas appear most frequently in childhood (see Chapters 6 and 12).

Patients with cerebellar neoplasms frequently present with signs of neurologic dysfunction early in life. About one third of patients with cerebellar tumors develop symptoms and signs of their neoplasms within the first 10 years of life.[3] Twenty-five percent of the patients have symptoms that begin less than 2 months before the time they come to medical attention; one fourth have complaints extending more than 6 months. The duration of the history is longer with astrocytomas than with medulloblastomas or ependymomas. The most frequent presenting symptoms with cerebellar tumor are headache and difficulty with standing and walking.[3] Infants, however, may present with restlessness, irritability, or lethargy;[48] hydrocephalus manifested by an enlarging head may be an initial presentation, along with head tilt, neck stiffness, and vomiting.[48]

The neurologic signs occurring with cerebellar tumor consist of papilledema, nystagmus, limb hypotonia, and ataxia. Papilledema occurs at the time of the initial diagnosis in about three fourths of all patients with cerebellar neoplasms. Optic nerve atrophy may occur if the papilledema is chronic.[29] A cerebellar neoplasm should be suspected when a patient presents with frontal or occipital headaches associated with nausea, vomiting, unsteady gait, and clumsiness.[25] Associated signs include unilateral limb ataxia, diplopia, rebound nystagmus, titubation, pendular deep tendon reflexes, dysarthria, and kinetic tremors.[29]

A frequent problem in the diagnosis of cerebellar neoplasms is that the lesion may produce few localizing signs. Often the only presenting signs will be those resulting from an increase in intracranial pressure owing to ventricular obstruction.[66]

Intra-axial Cerebellar Tumors

The evaluation of intra-axial posterior fossa neoplasms with imaging usually begins with x-ray CT, generally performed after the infusion of intravenous contrast material. Large lesions are immediately apparent and there are relatively distinct topographic and imaging characteristics for each type of neoplasm. If there is suspicion of calcification or hemorrhage, a noncontrast x-ray CT should also be obtained. Small lesions, especially those of the medulla oblongata or pons, and subtle infiltrative lesions with little mass effect can be missed with x-ray CT, however (Fig. 11 – 18*A*). Before MRI, cisternography with intrathecal myelographic contrast material was employed to avoid beam hardening artifacts and to study the outlines of the brainstem more effectively.

At the present time, mainly because of the greater accessibility of x-ray CT, MRI usually follows CT in the evaluation of these lesions. While MRI is consistently helpful in these cases, it is especially important if x-ray CT is negative and the clinical presentation is worrisome. MRI is also important if more detail regarding precise topographic relationships of a mass seen on x-ray CT are needed (Fig. 11 – 18*B*). MRI not only defines the external relationships of the mass, but also delineates the amount of intra-axial infiltration with far more sensitivity than does x-ray CT.[39] Many cerebellar lesions also will be studied with MRI for the same reasons. If surgery is being considered for any lesion that is thought to be a posterior fossa neoplasm, an MRI scan should be obtained if it is available.

With high-quality x-ray CT, and especially now with MRI, angiography is less frequently performed in the basic evaluation of posterior fossa neoplasms. Angiography now is most frequently used to assess the degree of vascularity of the lesion and to evaluate the vascular topographic relationships in lesions with a marked vascular component as suggested on x-ray CT, MRI, or both. Although angiographic mass effect can be used to localize lesions, this procedure is known to be insensitive and is no longer important, since x-ray CT and MRI are far more effective methods.

X-ray CT has been a great asset in the diagnosis of patients with suspected brain tumors. Posterior fossa neoplasms usually show low or high attenuation of x-rays in comparison with adjacent brain tissue, and thus good resolution may be obtained without additional invasive procedures (Table 11 – 1). Moreover, intravenous injection of contrast material may cause tumors isodense with the cerebellum to appear more dense after injection.

The modes of therapy available for cerebellar neoplasms are surgery, irradiation, and chemotherapy. Surgical decompression allows tissue to be ob-

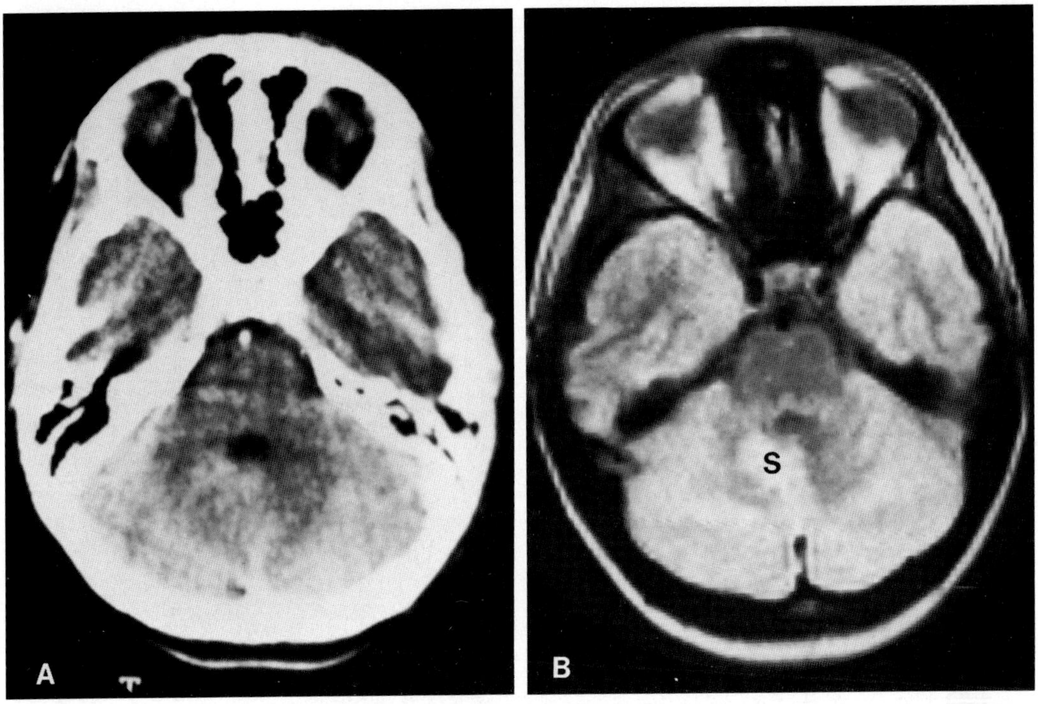

Figure 11–18. Primitive neuroectodermal tumor. (*A*) Intravenous-contrast-enhanced axial CT scan shows subtle pathologic contrast enhancement about the right lateral recess of the fourth ventricle. (*B*) Axial MR image at the same level definitively demonstrates signal abberration (S) and subtle mass effect, as well as the infiltrative character of this lesion. At surgery, the histopathology demonstrated a primitive neuroectodermal neoplasm.

tained for histopathologic examination. Some brain tumors are highly sensitive to radiation therapy, particularly some medulloblastomas. X-ray CT and MRI offer simple and safe methods to follow the course of the neoplasm with time and treatment.

Metastatic Disease of the Cerebellum

This is the most common tumor in the posterior fossa of the adult, usually occurring after the third to fourth decade of life.[29] Solitary lesions occur more often than multiple tumors.[64,92] Twenty-five percent of solitary metastases in the brain occur in the cerebellum.[64] The sources of the most common metastatic tumors are the lung, breast, gastrointestinal tract, skin, and kidney. Bronchogenic carcinoma is the most frequent source of metastases in all patients, but breast carcinoma is responsible for many cerebellar tumors in women.

X-ray CT is generally the first imaging study performed and, as discussed above, usually is sufficient. MRI is commonly reserved for clinically suspicious but CT-negative cases, or for situations in which more precise knowledge of topographic relationships is needed for treatment planning. Angiography is employed, if at all, usually only as a preoperative evaluation.

Extraparenchymal Tumors

Meningiomas may arise within the posterior fossa and usually cause cerebellar dysfunction from pressure rather than as a result of invasion. Menin-

Table 11–1 FREQUENT IMAGING CHARACTERISTICS OF COMMON POSTERIOR FOSSA MASSES

			MRI*	
Lesion Type	***Location***	***X-ray CT****	***T_1-weighted***	***T_2-weighted***
I. Adults				
A. Metastatic neoplasm (most common types are carcinoma of the lung and breast)	Entire posterior fossa contents including bone, meninges, and parenchyma. Most often seen in cerebellar parenchyma.	Variable appearance, but usually one of two types: 1. *Target lesion.* Central core of high attenuation after contrast infusion with surrounding low-attenuation vasogenic edema. 2. *Ring lesion.* Concentric ring of low-attenuation edema surrounding moderate-attenuation "active" neoplasm with a central low-attenuation core of necrosis.	Center moderate intensity if target lesion, very low intensity if ring lesion. Both with surrounding low-intensity edema.	Entire lesion is usually high-signal but somewhat heterogeneous.
B. Schwannoma	Usually eighth-nerve neoplasms centered about the internal acoustic canal in cerebellopontine-angle cistern.	Moderate increase to isoattenuation before contrast. Prominent high attenuation after administration of contrast material. Can be heterogeneous, but usually very discrete lesions.	Usually isointense, mass effect if large enough. Sensitivity markedly increased with IV gadolinium-DTPA; lesion becomes hyperintense.	Usually hyperintense and easily seen.
C. Meningioma	Tentorium or anterior portions of cerebello pontine-angle cistern. Rarely, if ever, extends into internal acoustic canal.	Slightly high attenuation before contrast, usually with prominent pathologic contrast enhancement. The lesion usually has a broad base upon a meningeal surface and is quite homogeneous in appearance.	Isointense. Hyperintense after IV gadolinium-DTPA. (Meningioma may be missed on MRI unless IV gadolinium-DTPA administered.)	Isointense. Large lesions will show mass effect. Some show high-intensity surrounding edema.

D. Abscess	Meningeal-based or parenchyma. This has become an uncommon lesion.	"Ring lesion." Usually has a thinner rim of contrast enhancement than metastatic neoplasm.	Similar to metastatic neoplasm but usually has thinner-walled rim.	
II. Children				
A. Medulloblastoma	Central cerebellar parenchyma, many times remarkably symmetric.	Bulky, mainly homogeneous iso- to moderate–attenuation mass before contrast. Prominent homogeneous pathologic contrast enhancement. Usually presents with obstructive hydrocephalus.	Mainly homogeneous. Moderate to low intensity.	Mainly homogeneous. Very high intensity.
B. Ependymoma	Fourth ventricle	Bulky inhomogeneous moderate- to low-attenuation lesion before contrast. Moderate, somewhat less marked, inhomogeneous pathologic contrast enhancement	Like medulloblastoma but usually more inhomogeneous.	
C. Astrocytoma (usually pilocytic)	Cerebellar hemisphere	Thin-walled, discrete "cystic" lesion with pathologic contrast enhancement of the cyst wall.	Moderate intensity, thin-walled "cystic" lesion with low-intensity center.	Homogeneous high-intensity mass.

*All imaging characteristics compared with surrounding normal brain; i.e., "isointense" means isointense compared with brain.

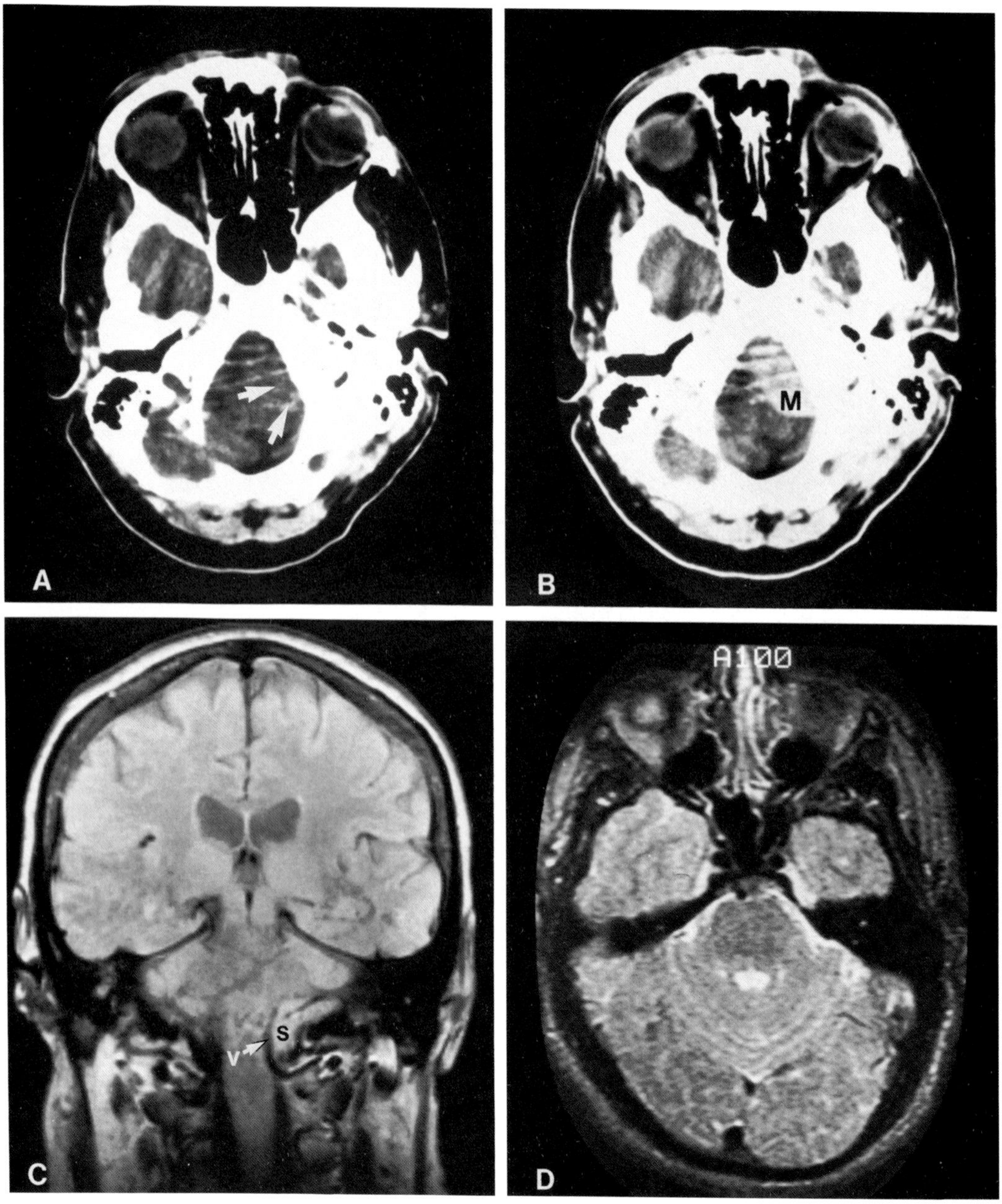

Figure 11–19. Foramen magnum meningioma. Axial x-ray CT (*A*) before and (*B*) after infusion of intravenous contrast material shows the typical imaging characteristics of meningioma, with subtle high attenuation in the lesion before contrast (*arrows*) and bright pathologic enhancement after contrast infusion (M). As usual, this neoplasm has a broad base along the inner table of the skull. (*C*) A coronal MR image rather dramatically shows the mass effect upon the vertebral artery (V), but demonstrates only slightly increased signal within the large mass (S). Intravenous infusion of paramagnetic contrast material would make this lesion far brighter. Without use of such material, meningiomas can be completely MR occult (see Fig. 1–16). Tentorial meningioma. (*D*) Axial T_2-weighted and (*E*) T_1-weighted MRI scans show no convincing lesion. (*F*) Axial and (*G*) coronal T_1-weighted MRI scans immediately following intravenous infusion of gadolinium-DTPA demonstrate the dramatic enhancement typical of meningiomas. The (*G*) coronal image shows that the meningeal surface involved is the tentorium and not that of the cerebellopontine angle. The ease of acquisition of multiple orthogonal planes makes MRI superior to x-ray CT in providing topographic definition of lesions.

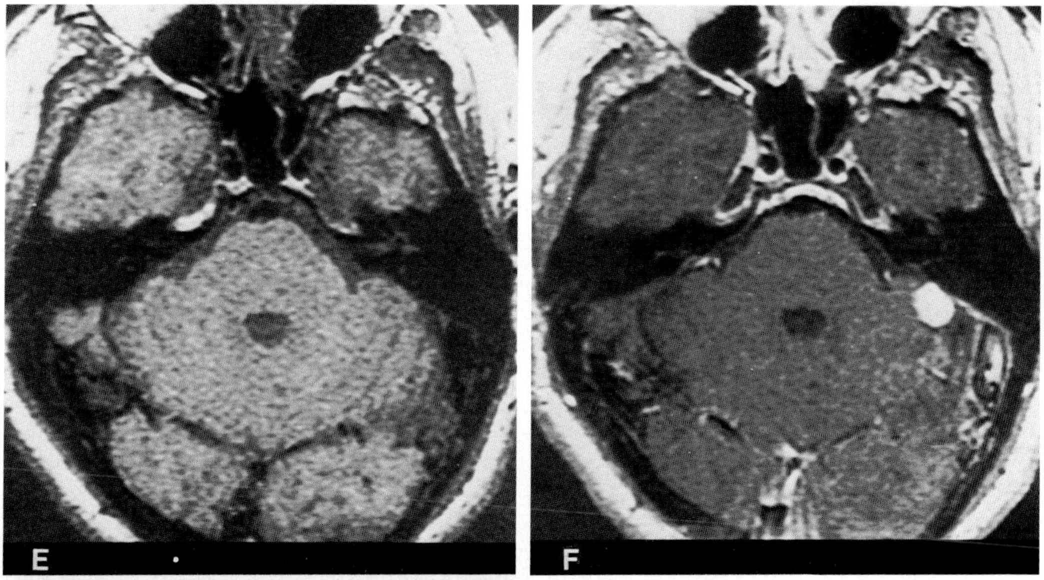

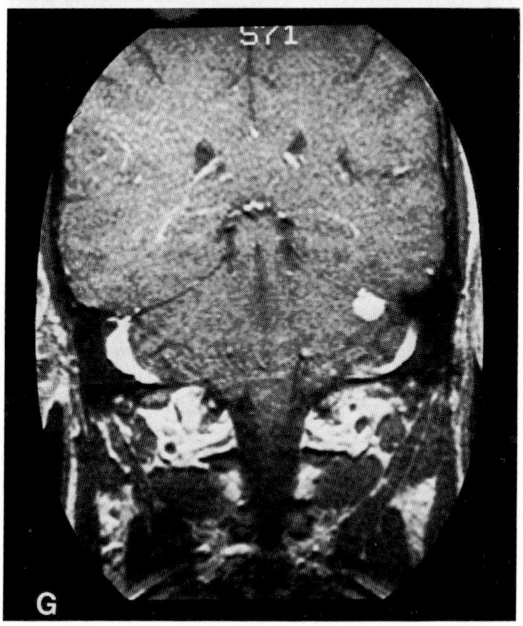

Figure 11–19. *Continued.*

giomas of the posterior fossa occur primarily in adults, and are infrequent, representing less than 10% of all intracranial meningiomas.[88] Meningiomas commonly affect the clivus, the cerebellopontine angle, and the squamous portion of occipital bone.

Meningiomas usually produce only chronic headache as a major symptom. Unless the tumor appears in the cerebellopontine angle, the mass may be very large before the patient receives medical attention. Often papilledema owing to early obstructive hydrocephalus is an early sign.[29] When cerebellar dysfunction occurs, it usually results from compression of a portion of the cerebellum.

X-ray CT without and with intravenous contrast material provides high sensitivity and specificity in the detection of most meningiomas, with a predictive accuracy approaching 90%.[87] The classic appearance is that of a mass with slightly increased attenuation before contrast material is administered, and then prominent contrast enhancement (Fig. 11–19). The mass usually has a broad extra-axial base and most commonly is found about the cerebellopontine angle cistern, tentorium, or foramen magnum. Fourth-ventricular meningiomas are uncommon. Lesions with these imaging characteristics and topography are nearly pathognomonic for meningioma. With high-resolution x-ray CT, even subtle lesions in difficult areas, such as the foramen magnum, can be delineated.[108] Once a meningioma is suggested by clinical and x-ray CT findings and surgical therapy is indicated, arteriography must follow. The arteriographic characteristics are also nearly pathognomonic if a prominent meningeal arterial supply is delineated. In posterior fossa meningiomas, this arterial supply is usually from the posterior meningeal artery or the meningohypophyseal trunk.[101] There is variable brain parenchymal supply, almost directly proportional to the degree of brain invasion. Some meningiomas, especially the en plaque type, can be missed by angiography.

MRI will locate meningiomas, but overall, has a lower sensitivity than does x-ray CT for this lesion,[110] because the MR signal characteristics of meningiomas are often identical to those of brain.[94] Subtle degrees of cortical bone induction or scalloping, frequently seen in meningiomas, are also difficult to assess with MRI. With MR intravenous contrast material, these recommendations are likely to change and MRI will become extremely sensitive in the detection of meningiomas.[94,110]

Treatment of meningiomas of the posterior fossa is surgical. A cure is possible with complete resection of benign tumors.

Cerebellopontine-Angle Schwannoma

Tumors of the cerebellopontine angle usually arise from Schwann cells of the eighth nerve and are termed "acoustic neuromas" or "acoustic schwannomas."[29] Many other tumors may develop in the cerebellopontine angle, including meningiomas, ependymomas, lipomas, hemangiomas, arteriovenous malformations, metastatic tumors, and choroid plexus papillomas. Giant aneurysms of branches of the vertebral artery also may be difficult to distinguish from cerebellopontine-angle tumors.

Acoustic neuromas occur often in patients with von Recklinghausen's neurofibromatosis. Bilateral acoustic neuromas in childhood are essentially diagnostic of neurofibromatosis.

Patients with unilateral acoustic neuromas usually have unilateral hearing loss and tinnitus. A small percentage will have dysphagia, and a very few will have symptoms of corticospinal tract disturbance. Vertigo and ataxia of gait may develop as the tumor expands into the cerebellum, but the signs usually are limited to slight dysmetria or kinetic tremor on one side of the body.

Imaging studies are helpful diagnostically (Figs. 11–20, 11–21; also see Fig. 1–13). Skull x-rays alone may provide good evidence of a cerebellopontine-angle mass. Eighth-nerve schwannomas will cause enlargement of the internal auditory canal. Air contrast studies have been used in the past but now are seldom employed. Routine brain x-ray CT, after intravenous contrast material, will demonstrate most lesions 2 cm or larger. The classic appearance is that of a pathologically enhancing mass lesion extending directly into a widened internal acoustic canal. Meningiomas may simulate this shape and attenuation exactly, but almost never extend into the internal acoustic canal as perfectly as do schwannomas. High-resolution x-ray CT, especially with small region-of-interest scanning,

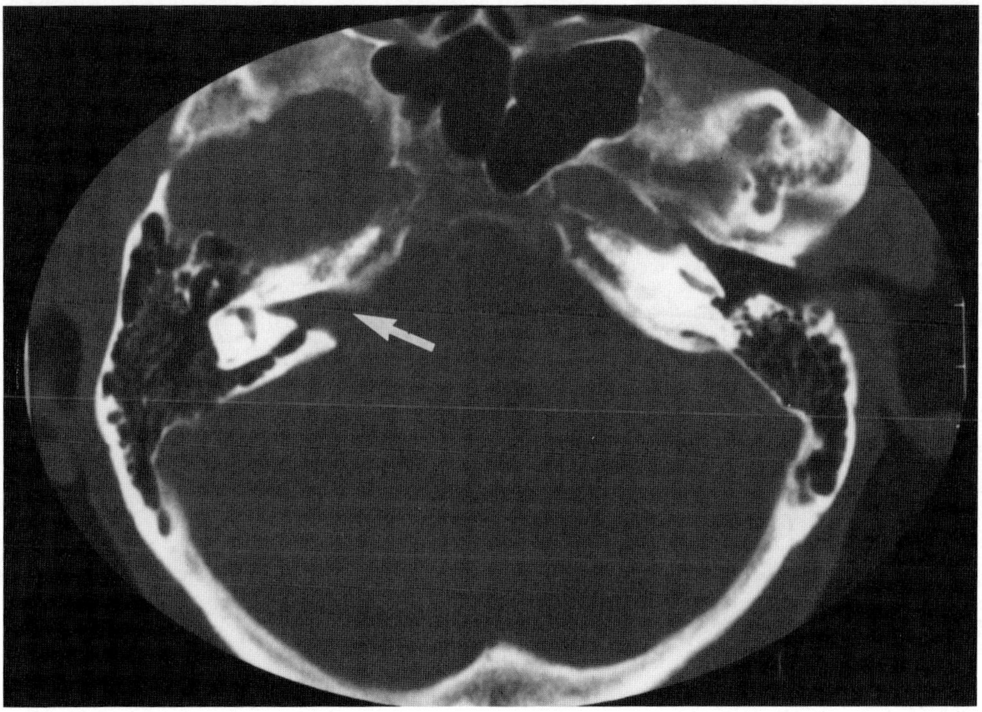

Figure 11–20. Eighth-nerve schwannoma (acoustic neuroma). Axial-targeted bone-algorithm x-ray CT nicely demonstrates widening of the internal acoustic canal (*arrow*) caused by the direct pressure effects from the schwannoma.

will locate nearly all of these lesions if there is any extracanalicular extension.[18,80] X-ray CT with intrathecal contrast material, be it iodinated contrast agents or gas, will further increase the sensitivity and allow detection of intracanalicular lesions.[18] These studies are unpleasant for the patient, however, usually causing headache and nausea.

MRI (see Fig. 11–21*B,C*) affords sensitivity nearly equal to that of high-resolution intrathecal contrast-enhanced x-ray CT,[76] with little or no discomfort. Now that MR intravascular contrast material has become available for general clinical use, MRI sensitivity should increase even further.[16] If the clinical picture is distinctive, many physicians omit x-ray CT and use MRI as the initial imaging in eighth-nerve schwannomas. This plan is not wise if lesions elsewhere in the temporal bone are suspected, however, since MR sensitivity in these other lesions is poorer than that of x-ray CT.[26]

Treatment of most cerebellopontine-angle tumors involves surgical intervention. A substantial number of these tumors can be removed completely.

SUMMARY

Imaging studies have greatly contributed to the diagnosis and management

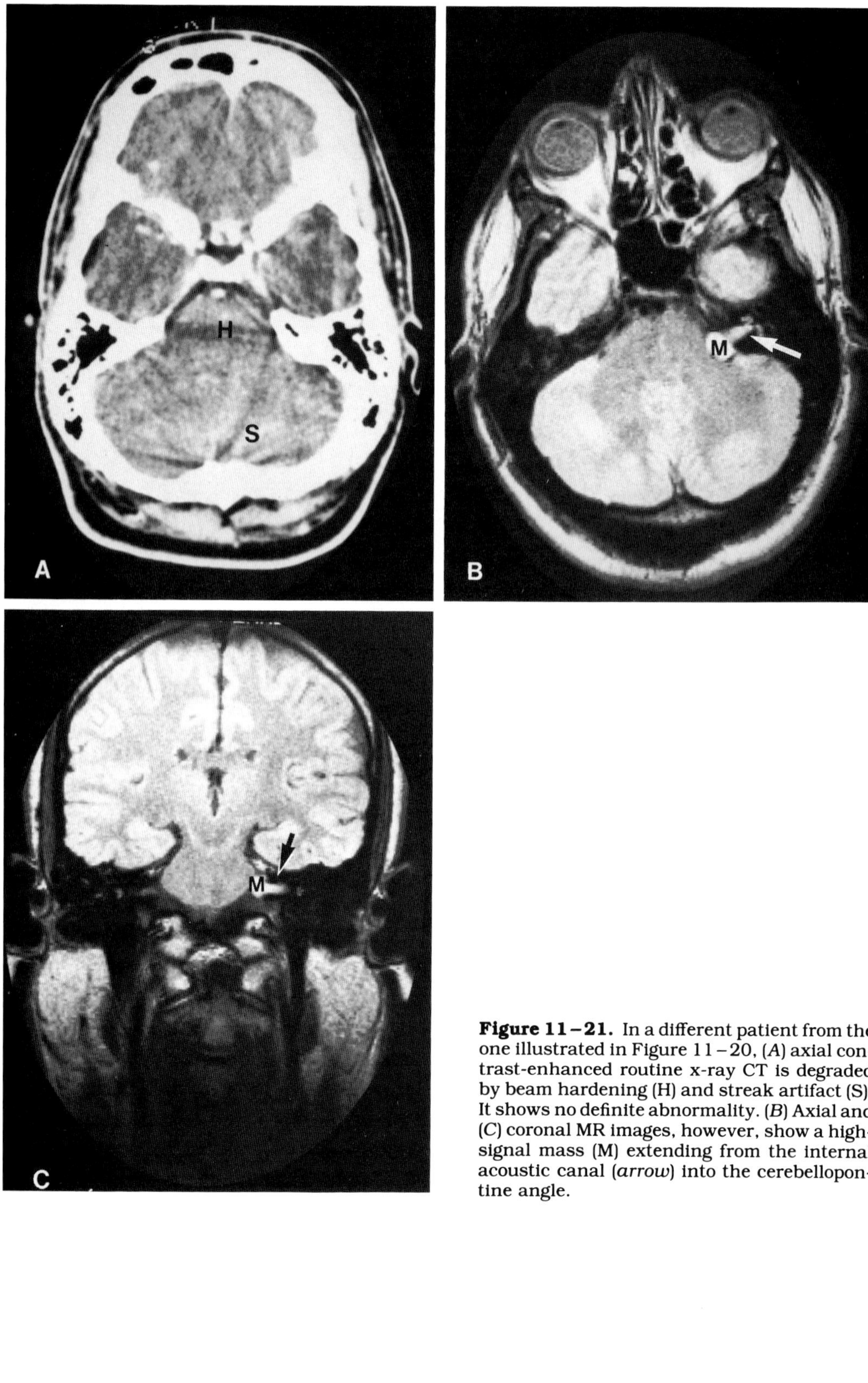

Figure 11–21. In a different patient from the one illustrated in Figure 11–20, (*A*) axial contrast-enhanced routine x-ray CT is degraded by beam hardening (H) and streak artifact (S). It shows no definite abnormality. (*B*) Axial and (*C*) coronal MR images, however, show a high-signal mass (M) extending from the internal acoustic canal (*arrow*) into the cerebellopontine angle.

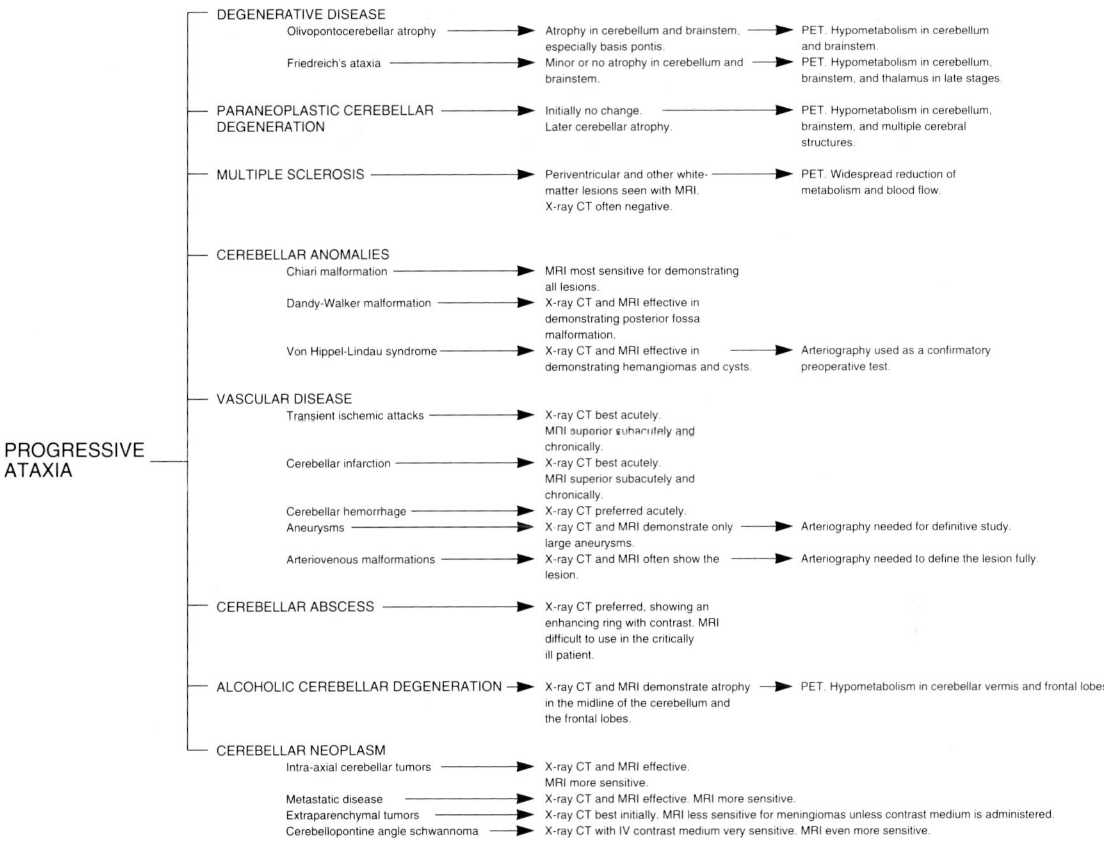

Figure 11–22. Imaging methods in the differential diagnosis of cerebellar ataxia in the adult. By clinical evaluation and laboratory tests, rule out medication effects (for example, phenytoin [Dilantin]), thyroid disease, vitamin B_{12} deficiency, vitamin E deficiency, collagen vascular disease, peripheral neuropathy, tertiary syphilis, chronic renal or hepatic disease, and chronic meningoencephalitis, as from cryptococcosis, sarcoid, tuberculosis, or AIDS. With the appropriate clinical findings, consider the possibilities shown.

of cerebellar disorders. Although x-ray CT studies are limited by artifacts, CT remains the most versatile and widely available imaging study for diseases of the posterior fossa. MRI is generally superior to x-ray CT in imaging this region of the nervous system, but its availability is relatively limited. Functional studies such as single photon emission computed tomography (SPECT) and positron emission tomography (PET) have just begun to be used to explore disorders of the posterior fossa. Figure 11–22 presents a summary of imaging methods in the differential diagnosis of cerebellar ataxia in the adult.

REFERENCES

1. Aboulezz, AO, Sartor, K, Geyer, CA, and Gado, MH: Position of cerebellar tonsils in the normal population and in patients with Chiari malformation: Quantitative approach with MR imaging. J. Comput Assist Tomogr 9:1033–1036, 1985.
2. Adams, RD and Victor, M: Principles of Neurology, ed 3. McGraw-Hill, New York, 1985.
2a. Albin, RL and Gilman, S: Autoradiographic localization of inhibitory and excitatory amino acid neurotransmitter receptors in human normal and olivo-

pontocerebellar atrophy cerebellar cortex. Brain Res 522:37–45, 1990.
3. Amici, R, Avanzini, G, and Pacini, L: Cerebellar tumors. Monographs in Neural Sciences, Vol 4. Karger, Basel, 1976.
4. Anderson, NE, Posner, JB, Sidtis, JJ, Moeller, JR, Strother, SC, Dhawan, V, and Rottenberg, DA: The metabolic anatomy of paraneoplastic cerebellar degeneration. Ann Neurol 23:533–540, 1988.
5. Beller, AJ, Sahar, A, and Praiss, I: Brain abscess: Review of 89 cases over a period of 30 years. J Neurol Neurosurg Psychiatr 36:757–768, 1973.
6. Bianco, F, Bozzao, L, Colonnese, C, and Fantozzi, L: The value of computerized tomography in the diagnosis of cerebellar atrophy. Ital J Neurol Sci 1:65–68, 1983.
7. Brain, WR and Wilkinson M: Subacute cerebellar degeneration in patients with carcinoma. In Brain, WR and Norris FH (eds): The Remote Effects of Cancer on the Nervous System. Grune & Stratton, New York, 1965, pp 17–23.
8. Brennan, R and Berglund, R: Acute cerebellar hemorrhage: Analysis of clinical findings and outcome in 12 cases. Neurology 27:527–532, 1977.
9. Brooks, DJ, Leenders, KL, Head, G, Marshall, J, Legg, NJ, and Jones, T: Studies on regional cerebral oxygen utilization and cognitive function in multiple sclerosis. J Neurol Neurosurg Psychiatr 47:1182–1191, 1984.
10. Caplan, LR: Vertebrobasilar occlusive disease. In Barnett, JHM, Mohr, JP, Stein, BM, and Yatsu, F (eds): Stroke. Pathophysiology, Diagnosis, and Management, Vol. 1 Churchill-Livingstone, Edinburgh, 1986, pp 549–619.
11. Caplan, LR and Rosenbaum, A: Role of cerebral angiography in vertebrobasilar occlusive disease. J Neurol Neurosurg Psychiatr 38:601–612, 1975.
12. Cartlidge, NE, Whisnant, JP, and Elveback, LR: Carotid and vertebral-basilar transient cerebral ischemic attacks. A community study, Rochester, Minnesota. Mayo Clin Proc 52:117–120, 1977.
13. Castaigne, P, Lhermitte, F, Gautier, JC, Escourolle, R, Derouesne, C, Der-Agopian, P, and Popa, C: Arterial occlusions in the vertebrobasilar system. A study of 44 patients with postmortem data. Brain 96:133–154, 1973.
14. Claus, D and Aschoff, JC: Cranial computerized tomography in spinocerebellar atrophies. NYAS 374:831–838, 1981.
15. Cunningham, J, Graus, F, Anderson, N, and Posner, JB: Partial characterization of the Purkinje cell antigens in paraneoplastic cerebellar degeneration. Neurology 36:1163–1168, 1986.
16. Curati, WL, Graif, M, Kingsley, DPE, Niendorf, HP, and Young, RI: Acoustic neuromas: Gd-DTPA enhancement in MR imaging. Radiology 158:447–451, 1986.
17. Diener, HC, Muller, A, Thron, A, Poremba, M, Dichgans, J, and Rapp, H: Correlation of clinical signs with CT findings in patients with cerebellar disease. J Neurol 233:5–12, 1986.
18. Dubois, PL, Drayer, B, Bank, WO, Deeb, ZL, and Rosenbaum, AE: An evaluation of current diagnostic radiologic modalities in the investigation of acoustic neurilemmomas. Radiology 126: 173–179, 1978.
19. Duncan, GW, Parker, SW, and Fisher, CM: Acute cerebellar infarction in the PICA territory. Arch Neurol 32:364–368, 1975.
20. Eadie, MJ: Olivo-ponto-cerebellar atrophy (Dejerine-Thomas type). In Vinken, PJ and Bruyn, GW (eds): Handbook of Clinical Neurology. North-Holland, Amsterdam, 1975, pp. 415–431.
21. Eadie, MJ: Olivo-ponto-cerebellar atrophy (Menzel type). In Vinken, PJ and Bruyn, GW (eds): Handbook of Clinical Neurology. North-Holland, Amsterdam, 1975, pp. 433–449.
22. Gardner-Thorpe, C and Al-Mufti, ST: Metastatic cerebellar abscess producing nerve deafness. J Neurol Neurosurg Psychiatr 32:360–361, 1969.
23. Gebarski, SS, Allen, R, and Stiennon-Gebarski, KM: Magnetic resonance imaging of white matter diseases excluding multiple sclerosis (MS) and ischemic leukoencephalopathy (IL). AJNR 6:468, 1985.
24. Gebarski, SS, Gabrielsen, TO, Gil-

man, S, Knake, JE, Latack, JT, and Aisen, AM: The initial diagnosis of multiple sclerosis: Clinical impact of magnetic resonance imaging. Ann Neurol 17:469–474, 1985.

25. Geissinger, JD and Bucy, PC: Astrocytomas of the cerebellum in children. Arch Neurol 24:125–135, 1971.
26. Gentry, LR, Jacoby, CG, Turski, PA, Houston, LW, Strother, CM, and Sackett, JF: Cerebellopontine angle-petromastoid mass lesions: Comparative study of diagnosis with MR imaging and CT. Radiology 162:513–520, 1987.
27. Gerke, KF, and Gebarski, SS: Magnetic resonance imaging of olivopontocerebellar degeneration. AJR 144:428, 1985.
28. Gerke, KF, Gebarski, SS, Chandler, WF, and Phillips, TW: External carotid-vertebral artery anastomosis for vertebrobasilar insufficiency. AJNR 6:33–37, 1985.
29. Gilman, S, Bloedel, JR, and Lechtenberg, R: Disorders of the Cerebellum. FA Davis, Philadelphia, 1981.
30. Gilman, S, Markel, DS, Koeppe, RA, Junck, L, Kluin, KJ, Gebarski, SS, and Hichwa, RD: Cerebellar and brainstem hypometabolism in olivopontocerebellar atrophy detected with positron emission tomography. Ann Neurol 23:223–230, 1988.
31. Gilman, S, Junck, L, Markel, DS, Koeppe, RA, and Kluin, KJ: Cerebral glucose hypermetabolism in Friedreich's ataxia detected with positron emission tomography. Ann Neurol 28:750–757, 1990.
32. Gilman, S, Adams, K, Koeppe, RA, and Berent, S, Kluin, K, Modell, JG, Kroll, P, and Brunberg, IA: Cerebellar and frontal hypometabolism in alcoholic cerebellar degeneration studied with positron tomography. Ann Neurol 28:775–785, 1990.

32a. Gilman, S, Holthoff, V, Koeppe, RA, Frey, KA, Junck, L, Kluin, KJ, and Brunberg, J: Decreased cerebellar GABA/benzodiazepine receptor binding in OPCA studied with [^{11}C] flumazenil and PET. J Cereb Blood Flow Metab (in press) 1991.

32b. Gilman, S, Koeppe, RA, Markel, DS, Junck, L, Kluin, KJ: Relationship between cerebral blood flow and glucose metabolic rate in olivopontocerebellar atrophy studied with positron emission tomography. Neurology 41:225, 1991 (abstract).

33. Graif, M, Bydder, GM, Steiner, RE, Niendorf, FP, and Thomas, MH: Contrast-enhanced MR imaging of malignant brain tumors. AJNR 6:855–862, 1985.
34. Greenberg, J, Skubick, D, and Shenkin, H: Acute hydrocephalus in cerebellar infarct and hemorrhage. Neurology 29:409–413, 1979.
35. Greenfield, JG: The spino-cerebellar degenerations. Blackwell Scientific Publications, Oxford, 1954.
36. Greenlee, JE and Brashear, HR: Antibodies to cerebellar Purkinje cells in patients with paraneoplastic cerebellar degeneration and ovarian carcinoma. Ann Neurol 14:609–613, 1983.
37. Greenlee, JE, Brashear, HR, and Herndon, RM: Immunoperoxidase labeling of rat brain sections with sera from patients with paraneoplastic cerebellar degeneration and systemic neoplasia. J Neuropathol Exp Neurol 47: 561–571, 1988.
38. Groenhout, CM, Gooskens, RH, Veiga-Pires, JA, Ramos, L, Willemse J, and van Nieuwenhuizen, O: Value of sagittal sonography and direct sagittal CT of the Dandy-Walker syndrome. AJNR 5: 476–477, 1984.
39. Han, JS, Bonstelle, CT, Kaufman, B, Benson, JE, Alfidi, RJ, Clampitt, M, Van Dyke, C, and Huss RG: Magnetic resonance imaging in the evaluation of the brainstem. Radiology 150:705–712, 1984.
40. Harding, AE: The hereditary ataxias and related disorders. Churchill-Livingstone, Edinburgh, 1984.
41. Henson, RA and Urich, H: Cancer and the nervous system. The Neurological Complications of Systemic Malignant Diseases. Oxford, Blackwell Scientific Publications, 1982.
42. Hershey, LA, Gado, MH, and Trotter, JL: Computerized tomography in the diagnostic evaluation of multiple sclerosis. Ann Neurol 5:32–39, 1979.
43. Hinshaw, DB Jr, Thompson, JR, Hasso, AN, and Casselman, ES: Infarc-

tions of the brainstem and cerebellum: A correlation of computed tomography and angiography. Radiology 137:105–112, 1980.

44. Holmes, G: A form of familial degeneration of the cerebellum. Brain 30:466–489, 1907.
45. Horton, WA, Wong, V, and Eldridge, R: Von Hippel-Lindau disease. Clinical and pathological manifestations in nine families with 50 affected members. Arch Intern Med 136:769–777, 1976.
46. Jaeckle, KA, Graus, F, Houghton, A, Cardon-Cardo, C, Nielsen, SL, and Posner, JB: Autoimmune response of patients with paraneoplastic cerebellar degeneration to a Purkinje cell cytoplasmic protein antigen. Ann Neurol 18:592–600, 1985.
47. Johnson, JH and Kline, DG: Anterior inferior cerebellar artery aneurysms. J Neurosurg 48:455–460, 1978.
48. Kageyama, N, Takakura, K, Epstein, F, Hoffman, JH, and Schut, L: Intracranial tumors in infancy and childhood. Basic research, diagnosis and treatment. In Homburger, F (ed): Progress in Experimental Tumor Research, Vol. 30. Karger, Basel, 1987.
49. Kase, CS and Caplan, LR: Parenchymatous posterior fossa hemorrhage in stroke. In Barnett, HJM, Mohr, JP, Stein, B, and Yatsu, F (eds): Stroke: Pathophysiology, Diagnosis and Management. Churchill-Livingstone, Edinburgh, 1985, pp. 621–641.
50. Kelly, JJ Jr, Mellinger, JF, and Sundt, TM Jr: Intracranial arteriovenous malformations in childhood. Ann Neurol 3:338–343, 1978.
51. Khan, M, Polyzoidis, KS, Adegbite, AB, and McQueen, JD: Massive cerebellar infarction: "Conservative" management. Stroke 14:745–751, 1983.
52. Kircheff, II: Arteriosclerotic ischemic cerebrovascular disease. Radiology 162:101–109, 1987.
53. Kistler, JP, Buonanno, FS, DeWitt, LD, Davis, KR, Brady, TJ, and Fisher, CM: Vertebral-basilar posterior cerebral territory stroke: Delineation by proton nuclear magnetic resonance imaging. Stroke 15:417–426, 1984.
54. Kluin, KJ, Gilman, S, Markel, DS, Koeppe, RA, Rosenthal, G, and Junck, L: Speech disorders in olivopontocerebellar atrophy correlate with positron emission tomography findings. Ann Neurol 23:547–554, 1988.
55. Kucharczyk, W, Lemme-Pleghos, L, Uske, A, Brant-Zawadski, M, Dooms, G, and Norman, D: Intracranial vascular malformations: MR and CT imaging. Radiology 156:383–389, 1985.
56. Kurtzke, JF: Clinical manifestations of multiple sclerosis. In Vinkin, PJ and Bruyn, GW (eds): Handbook of Clinical Neurology, North-Holland, Amsterdam, 1970, pp 161–216.
57. Laws, ER Jr, Bergstralb, EJ, and Taylor, WF: Cerebellar astrocytoma in children. In Homburger, F (ed): Progress in Experimental Tumor Research, Vol 30. Karger, Basel, 1987, pp 122–127.
58. Lechtenberg, R and Gilman, S: Speech disorders in cerebellar disease. Ann Neurol 3:285–290, 1978.
59. Lehrich, JR, Winkler, GF, and Ojemann, RG: Cerebellar infarction with brainstem compression: Diagnosis and surgical treatment. Arch Neurol 22: 490–498,1970.
60. Lusins, J and Sencer, W: Posterior fossa vascular malformations. Long-term follow-up. NY State J Med 76: 416–420, 1976.

60a. Makowiecz, RL, Albin, RL, Cha, J-H-J, Young, AB, and Gilman, S: Two types of quisqualate receptors are decreased in human olivopontocerebellar atrophy cerebellar cortex. Brain Res 523:309–312, 1990.

61. Marie, P, Foix, C, and Alajouanine, T: De l'atrophie cérébelleuse tardive à prédominance corticale. Rev Neurol 38:849–1082, 1922.
62. Marsh, WR and Laws, ER Jr: Intracranial ependynomas. In Homburger F (ed): Progress in Experimental Tumor Research, Vol 30. Karger, Basel, 1987, pp 175–180.
63. Masdeu, JC, Dobben, GD, and Azar-Jia, B: Dandy-Walker syndrome studied by computed tomography and pneumoencephalography. Radiology 147:109–114, 1983.
64. Masucci, EF: Posterior fossa metastases simulating primary tumors. Acta Neurol Scand 42:589–603, 1966.
65. Matthews, WB, Acheson, ED, Batche-

lor, JR, and Weller, RO: McAlpine's Multiple Sclerosis. Churchill-Livingstone, Edinburgh, 1985.

66. Maurice-Williams, RS: Mechanism of production of gait unsteadiness by tumors of the posterior fossa. J Neurol Neurosurg Psychiatr 38:143–148, 1975.
67. McKissock, W, Richardson, W, and Walsh, L: Spontaneous cerebellar hemorrhage. Brain 83:1–9, 1960.
68. Miller, RG, Porter, RJ, Nielsen, SL, and Hosobuchi, H: Von Hippel-Lindau's disease. Can J Neurol Sci 3:29–33, 1976.
69. Morgan, H and Wood, MW: Cerebellar abscesses: A review of seventeen cases. Surg Neurol 3:93–96, 1975.
70. Morgan, H, Wood, MW, and Murphey, F: Experience with 88 consecutive cases of brain abscess. J Neurosurg 38:698–704, 1973.
71. Nabatame, H, Fukuyama, H, Akiguchi, I, Kaneyama, M, Nishimura, K, and Nakano, Y: Spinocerebellar degeneration: Qualitative and quantitative MR analysis of atrophy. JCAT 12:298–303, 1988.
72. Naidich, TP, Pudlowski, RM, Naidich, JB, Gornish, M, and Rodriguez, FJ: Computed tomographic signs of the Chiari II malformation part I: Skull and dural partitions. Radiology 134:64–71, 1980.
73. Naidich, TP, Pudlowski, RM, and Naidich, JB: Computed tomographic signs of the Chiari II malformation part II: Midbrain and cerebellum. Radiology 134:391–398, 1980.
74. Naidich, TP, Pudlowski, RM, and Naidich, JB: Computed tomographic signs of the Chiari II malformation part III: Ventricles and cisterns. Radiology 134:657–663, 1980.
75. Naritomi, H, Sakai, F, and Meyer, JS: Pathogenesis of transient ischemic attacks within the vertebrobasilar arterial system. Arch Neurol 36:121–128, 1979.
76. New, PFJ, Bachow, TB, Wismer, GL, Rosen, BR, and Brady, TJ: MR imaging of the acoustic nerves and small acoustic neuromas at 0.6 T. AJR 144:1021–1026, 1985.
77. Oppenheimer, DR: Brain lesions in Friedreich's ataxia. Can J Neurol Sci 6:173–176, 1979.
78. Oppenheimer, DR: Diseases of the basal ganglia, cerebellum and motor neurons. In Adams, JH, Corsellis, JAN, and Duchens, LW (eds): Greenfield's Neuropathology, ed 4. John Wiley & Sons, New York, 1984, pp 699–747.
79. Ott, KH, Kase, CS, Ojemann, RG, and Mohr, JP: Cerebellar hemorrhage: Diagnosis and treatment. A review of 56 cases. Arch Neurol 31:160–167, 1974.
80. Pinto, RS, Kricheff, II, Bergeron, RT, and Cohen, N: Small acoustic neuromas: Detection by high resolution gas CT cisternography. AJR 139:129–132, 1982.
81. Pritchett, PS and King, TI: Dysplastic gangliocytoma of the cerebellum: An ultrastructural study. Acta Neuropathol (Berlin) 42:1–5, 1978.
82. Ramos, A, Quintana, F, Diez, C, Leno, C, and Berciano, J: CT findings in spinocerebellar degeneration. AJNR 8:635–640, 1987.
83. Rebner, M and Gebarski, SS: Magnetic resonance imaging of spinal cord hemangioblastoma. AJNR 6:287–289, 1985.
84. Richardson, AE: Spontaneous cerebellar hemorrhage. In Vinken, P and Bruyn, GW (eds): Handbook of Clinical Neurology. North-Holland, Amsterdam, 1972, pp 54–67.
85. Rosenthal, G, Gilman, S, Koeppe, RA, Kluin, KJ, Markel, DS, Junck, L, and Gebarski SS: Motor dysfunction in olivopontocerebellar atrophy is related to cerebral metabolic rate studied with positron emission tomography. Ann Neurol 24:414–419, 1988.
86. Rothman, SLG and Glanz, S: Cerebellar atrophy: The differential diagnosis by computerized tomography. Neuroradiology 16:123–136, 1978.
87. Russell, EJ, George, AE, Kricheff, II, and Budzilovich, G: Atypical computed tomographic features of intracranial meningioma. Radiology 135:673–682, 1980.
88. Salamon, GM, Combalbert, A, Raybaud, C, and Gonzalez, J: An angiographic study of meningiomas of the posterior fossa. J Neurosurg 35:731–741, 1971.

89. Salomon, A, Yeates, AE, Burger, PC, and Heinz, ER: Subcortical arteriosclerotic encephalopathy: Brain stem findings with MR imaging. Radiology 165:625–629, 1987.
90. Samson, DS and Clark, K: A current review of brain abscess. Am J Med 54:201–210, 1973.
91. Sato, Y, Waziri, M, Smith, W, Frey, E, Yuh, WTC, Hanson, J, and Franken, EA. Von Hippel-Lindau disease: MR imaging. Radiology 166:241–246, 1988.
92. Sharr, MM and Garfield, JS: Management of intracranial metastases. Br Med J 1:1535–1537, 1978.
93. Shin, W, Laufer, H, Lee, Y, Aftalion, B, Hirano, A, and Zimmerman, HM: Fine structure of a cerebellar neuroblastoma. Acta Neuropathol (Berlin) 42:11–13, 1978.
94. Spagnoli, MV, Goldberg, HI, Grossman, RI, Bilaniuk, LT, Gomori, JM, Hackney, DB, and Zimmerman, RA: Intracranial meningiomas: High-field MR imaging. Radiology 161:369–375, 1986.
95. Spiegel, SM, Vinuela, F, Fox, AJ, and Pelz, DM: CT of multiple sclerosis: Reassessment of delayed scanning with high doses of contrast material. AJNR 6: 533–536, 1985.
96. Stevens, JC, Farlow, MR, Edwards, MK, and Yu, P: Magnetic resonance imaging, clinical correlation in 64 patients with multiple sclerosis. Arch Neurol 43:1145–1148, 1986.
97. Stumpf, DA: The inherited ataxias. Neurol Clin North Am 2:47–57, 1985.
98. Sundbarg, G, Brun, A, Efsing, HO, and Lundberg, N: Non-neoplastic expanding lesions of the vermis cerebelli. J Neurosurg 37:55–64, 1972.
99. Sypert, G and Alvord, E: Cerebellar infarction: A clinicopathological study. Arch Neurol 32:357–363, 1975.
100. Taneda, M, Ozaki, K, Wakayama, A, Yogi, K, Kaneda, H, and Irino T: Cerebellar infarction with obstructive hydrocephalus. J Neurosurg 57:83–91, 1982.
101. Taveras, JM and Wood, EH: Diagnostic Neuroradiology, ed 2. Williams & Wilkins, Baltimore, 1976.
102. Tsai, FY, Teal, JS, Heishima, GB, Zee, CS, Grinnell, VS, Mehringer, CM, and Segall, HD: Computed tomography in acute posterior fossa infarcts. AJNR 3:149–156, 1982.
103. Tyrer, JH: Friedreich's ataxia. In Vinken, P and Bruyn, GW (eds.) North-Holland, Amsterdam, 1975, pp 319–364. Handbook of Clinical Neurology.
104. Victor, M, Adams, RD, and Mancall, EL: A restricted form of cerebellar cortical degeneration occurring in alcoholic patients. Arch Neurol 1:579–688, 1959.
105. Vinuela, FV, Fox, AJ, Debrun, GM, Feasby, TE, and Ebers, GC: New perspectives in computed tomography of multiple sclerosis. AJR 139:123–127, 1982.
106. Weber, FP and Greenfield, JG: Cerebello-olivary degeneration: An example of heredofamilial incidence. Brain 65:220–231, 1942.
107. White, BE and Rothfleisch, S: Primary cerebellar lymphoma: A case report. Neurology 18:582–586, 1968.
108. Williams, AL, Haughton, VM: Cranial Computed Tomography: A Comprehensive Text. CV Mosby, St. Louis, 1985.
109. Yamamoto, H, Yasuhiko, A, Takatoshi, W, Yoshitaka, H, Yasushi, M, and Sobue, I. Evaluation of supra- and infratentorial brain atrophy by computerized tomography in spinocerebellar degeneration. Jap J Med 25:238–245, 1986.
110. Zimmerman, RD, Fleming, CA, Saint-Louis, LA, Lee, BCP, Manning, JJ, and Deck, DF: Magnetic resonance imaging of meningiomas. AJNR 6:149–157, 1985.

Chapter 12

PEDIATRIC DISORDERS

Harry T. Chugani, M.D., and
Rosalind B. Dietrich, MB, ChB

NORMAL BRAIN DEVELOPMENT
BRAIN MALFORMATIONS
HYPOXIC-ISCHEMIC ENCEPHALOPATHY IN THE NEWBORN
CHILDHOOD EPILEPSY
METABOLIC DISEASES
PRACTICAL CONSIDERATIONS

The recent availability of new and sophisticated imaging modalities has made it possible for the first time to study noninvasively both the structure and function of the pediatric brain. The high-resolution multiplanar images obtained by x-ray computed tomography (x-ray CT) and magnetic resonance imaging (MRI) show an in vivo representation of both the normal anatomic changes and the pathologic processes that occur during childhood. Positron emission tomography (PET) and single photon emission CT (SPECT) imaging, on the other hand, are able to demonstrate both the diffuse and local functional changes occurring within the brain. Used appropriately and in combination with clinical information, these imaging modalities not only offer the opportunity to detect and differentiate the different disease entities that occur in this age range but also may give us additional insight into disease etiology and evolution over time.

NORMAL BRAIN DEVELOPMENT

During intrauterine and extrauterine development, the brain undergoes the sequential anatomic, functional, and organizational changes necessary to support the complex adaptive behavior of a fully mature normal individual. A clear understanding of these normal maturational changes is essential in comprehending and elucidating the mechanisms involved in the myriad of conditions resulting in abnormal brain development. Indeed, a recent study of the prenatal and perinatal factors associated with brain disorders[53] concluded that our understanding of normal developmental processes is still very limited. One important reason for this lack of knowledge has been the paucity of suitable techniques available for the in vivo study of many sequential changes occurring in the nervous system during its development. The recent availability of new neuroimaging modalities, has aroused great interest in applying these techniques to the study of human brain development. Before we describe the data that have been generated in this area with the neuroimaging approach, we will present a brief account of the development of the central nervous system. More detailed descriptions can be found in the many excellent reviews.[12,30]

The nervous system originates from the ectodermal layer of the embryonic disc with the initial formation of the neural plate, neural tube, and neural crest. Following closure of the neural tube and formation of the telencephalic vesicles, neuronal migration occurs. This is an organized process involving neuronal and glial stem cells that originate in the ventricular and subventricular portions of the telencephalon. Neuronal migration, guided by an organized system of radial glial fibers, follows in a radial centrifugal manner from the periventricular regions to the site of future neocortex. In the human fetus, neuronal migration takes place between 7 and 16 weeks of gestational age. As a rule, cells that migrate later will ultimately be situated in a more peripheral cortical layer than cells that migrate earlier. Following migration, the neurons differentiate into subtypes depending upon their location and layer.

Ample evidence now exists both in humans[67,68,128] and in other species[43,44,95,119,126] that during development, the brain produces a vast excess of neurons, synapses, and dendritic spines. The overproduction of neurons and their synaptic contacts is biologically advantageous in reducing the genetic load that would otherwise be required for specifically programming the enormous numbers of synaptic contacts in the nervous system.[21,71] Subsequently, many neurons die, and there is a regression of dendritic spines and synapses.[29] This form of cell death occurs early in development, by 2 years of age in humans, but the loss of synaptic elements is a more protracted process that continues well into the second decade of life.[67,68]

The biologic rules governing regression of neuroanatomic elements are poorly understood but these phenomena are believed to account, at least in part, for nervous-system plasticity.[44] The concept that there are mechanisms that act to retain those pathways in which patterns of external stimuli induce activity and eliminate potential connections not so activated has been termed "functional validation" by Jacobson[71] and "selective stabilization" by Changeux and coworkers.[21] This process would account for the contribution of early experience of the developing individual toward the final neuroanatomic composition and neurophysiologic representation within the nervous system.

In order to accommodate and organize the large number of cells and their processes, the formation of cerebral convolutions typical of advanced mammals enables the total surface area of the brain to be greatly increased without the impracticality of an excessively large brain. This process in humans follows the formation of the cerebral hemispheres, which has occurred by about 31 days' gestation. Subsequently, the first sulcus to become apparent is the lateral (sylvian) sulcus, which is evident during the third month of gestation. Secondary and tertiary sulci develop during the final months of the prenatal period.

Myelination is a process that greatly enhances the functional efficiency of neurons by increasing the speed of conduction. Although it is apparent in some brain structures as early as the third month of fetal life, much of the process of myelination occurs after birth, continuing into the second decade of life.[64,152] Furthermore, there is evidence to suggest that the myelin sheaths undergo remodeling throughout life.[51]

Structural Imaging

High-quality images of the living brain, demonstrating good anatomic detail, were obtained for the first time following the advent of the cross-sectional imaging modalities, x-ray CT and MRI.* Because of direct multiplanar

*References 9,17,35,64,74,98,120,127.

imaging capabilities and superior tissue-contrast differentiation, MRI has proved to be the modality of choice for demonstrating the normal structural changes occurring in the developing brain during maturation, and for demonstrating both normal and abnormal acquisition of myelin.[9,35,64,74,98]

MRI demonstrates effectively the transition of the developing preterm brain from the presence of a relatively smooth cortex with no or few convolutions to that of an extensively and compactly infolded cortex seen in the normal term infant.[101,102,109] McArdle and associates[101,102] (Fig. 12–1) have documented and defined the sequential MRI appearances of the developing brain at different ages. An increasingly complex arrangement of sulci and gyri is seen with increasing maturity. The exact age of premature neonates can thus be determined in vivo using these data. This work also establishes the normal range of widths of the extracerebral CSF spaces and lateral ventricles in this patient population.[102]

The process of myelination has been well documented pathologically in small numbers of infant brains,[13,32,40,90,94,152] most recently in a larger series of cases.[18] Until recently, however, myelination could not be studied in vivo or sequentially in the same child. Because myelination is a dynamic process starting in some sites during intrauterine life and continuing after birth, it can be an extremely useful index of

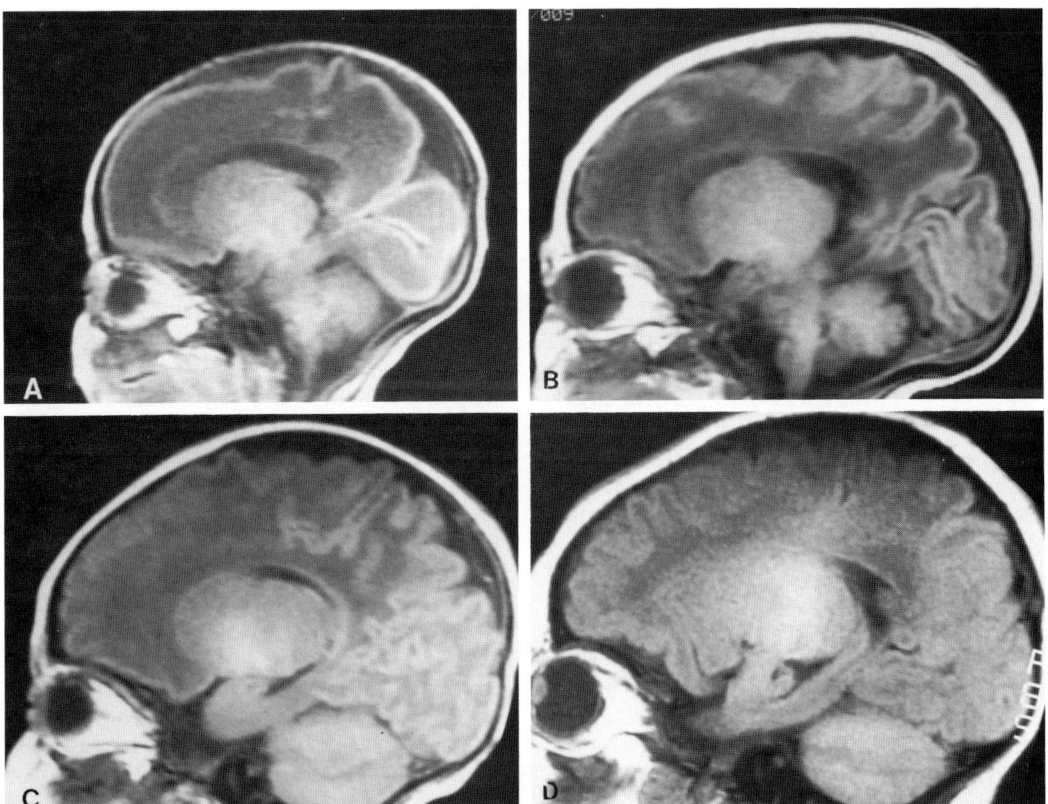

Figure 12–1. Anatomy of the premature brain. Sequential images obtained after 31, 35, 38, and 44 weeks of gestation. Saggital T_1-weighted (SE 600/32) images demonstrate an increasingly complex development of the sulci and gyri over the cerebral hemispheres as brain development progresses. (Images courtesy of Craig B. McArdle, Houston, TX.)

brain maturation during infancy. This is particularly true in the first two years, when changes occur most rapidly. Because MRI is highly sensitive to the differences in water and lipid content of gray and white matter, it offers a unique opportunity to study white matter maturation in vivo both sequentially and relative to a known standard. Care has to be taken, however, in the interpretation of myelination changes on images obtained on different magnetic field strength scanners and with different pulse sequence parameters.[115] To visualize the myelin present within the white matter of the brain, T_2-weighted spin echo or heavily T_1-weighted (either IR or short-TR, short-TE spin echo) pulse sequences should be obtained, since these maximize inherent tissue-contrast differentiation (see Chapter 2).

GRAY-WHITE MATTER DIFFERENTIATION

T_2-weighted spin echo pulse sequences can distinguish between gray and white matter in infants and demonstrate early progression of myelination. This MRI-sensitive gray-white differentiation is primarily due to differences in the water content of the gray and white matter at different ages.[92,120] During the first year of life, the water content of the infant brain decreases rapidly, from 88% at birth to 82% at 6 months of age.[40,120] There is then a continued steady decrease in water content until 2 years of age, followed by a plateau thereafter.

Although developmentally normal children show a spectrum of relative intensities of gray and white matter, their gray-white matter patterns fall into three distinct groups: infantile, isointense, and early adult.[35] At birth and generally for the first 8 months, the infantile pattern shows reversal of the normal adult pattern seen on T_2-weighted images; that is, in neonates white matter has a more intense signal than gray matter (Figs. 12–2, 12–3). Children aged 8–12 months demonstrate the transient isointense phase, with poor differentiation of gray and white matter (Fig. 12–4). The early adult pattern, where gray matter has higher signal intensity than white matter, is seen in all normal children over 12 months (Fig. 12–5) and may be seen as early as 10 months of age. The transient isointense pattern is rarely seen throughout the entire brain at one time. Patients more frequently show an infantile-isointense pattern or an adult-isointense pattern. In some children, all three patterns may be seen concomitantly. When a transition from one pattern to another is seen in the brain of the same child, the more immature pattern is consistently present in the areas of later myelination.

MYELINATION

As myelin is deposited, the lipid and protein content of the brain increase. These changes occur concomitantly with the aforementioned water loss, possibly because of the relatively hydrophobic nature of myelin. On T_2-weighted sequences, as the process of myelination progresses, the previously nonmyelinated, high-intensity, infantile white matter develops lower signal intensity on T_2-weighted sequences following established patterns.[9,35,64] At birth some myelin is already present supratentorially in the thalamus and infratentorially in the inferior cerebellar peduncles (see Fig. 12–2). In children over 1 month of age, myelin can be seen in the region of the posterior limb of the internal capsule (see Fig. 12–3). As myelination continues, areas of lower signal intensity are also identified sequentially in the optic radiations (see Fig. 12–3), in the anterior limb of the internal capsule and radiations to the precentral gyrus (6 months), in the parietal and frontal white matter (8 months) (see Fig. 12–4), and in the white matter of the temporal lobes (1 year) (see Fig. 12–5C). After 1 year of age, the portion of myelinated central white matter increases progressively as myelination extends more peripherally and causes

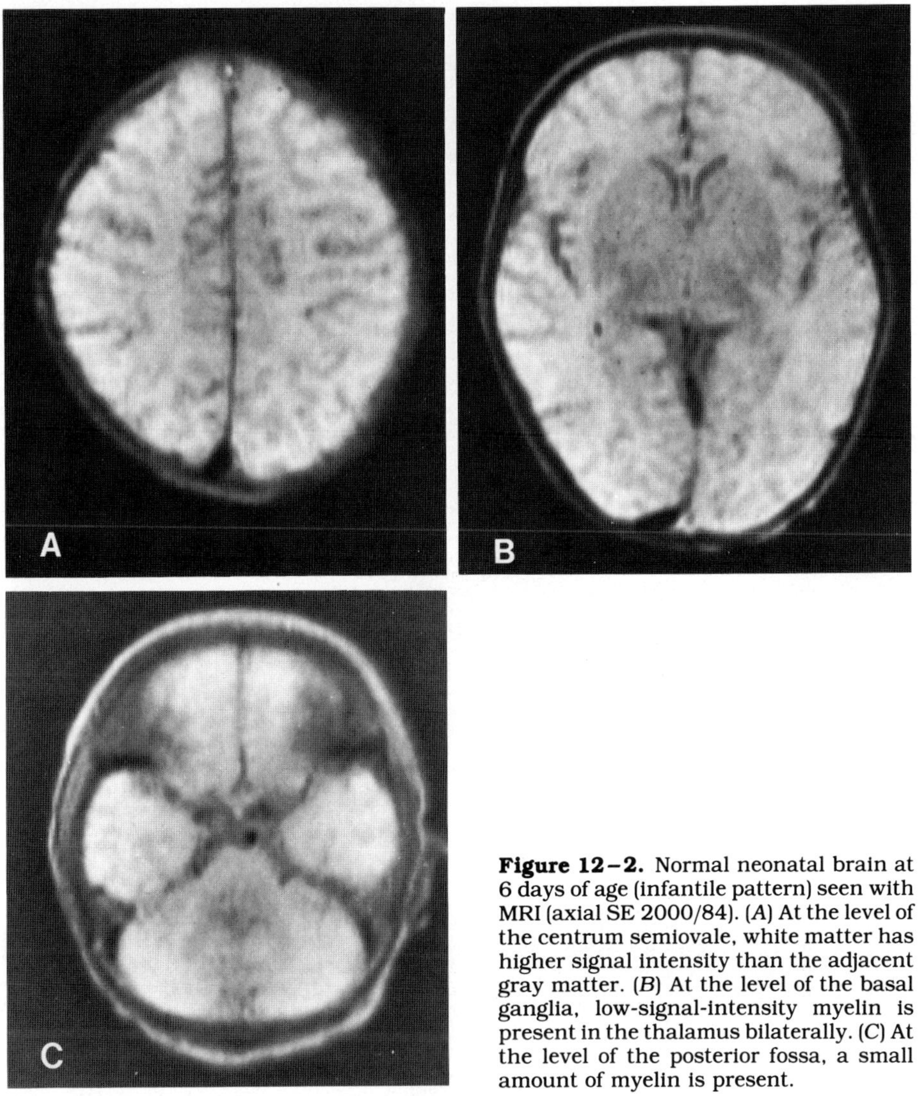

Figure 12–2. Normal neonatal brain at 6 days of age (infantile pattern) seen with MRI (axial SE 2000/84). (*A*) At the level of the centrum semiovale, white matter has higher signal intensity than the adjacent gray matter. (*B*) At the level of the basal ganglia, low-signal-intensity myelin is present in the thalamus bilaterally. (*C*) At the level of the posterior fossa, a small amount of myelin is present.

finer branching of the myelinated subcortical fibers and increased differentiation of the signal intensity of the gray and white matter. These changes are summarized in Table 12–1.

On inversion recovery images, areas of the white matter already myelinated have high signal intensity compared with adjacent nonmyelinated areas[74] (Fig. 12–6). The progression of myelination seen on inversion recovery sequences parallels that seen on spin echo sequences. Although the presence of myelin in any specific tract may be seen earlier on T_1-weighted images, the timing of the deposition of myelin as seen on T_2-weighted sequences better correlates with that seen on autopsy sections stained for myelin.[9] In children with clinical developmental delay, MRI often shows the same sequential appearance of myelin deposition, but demonstrates both a delay in the development of myelin in the white matter and

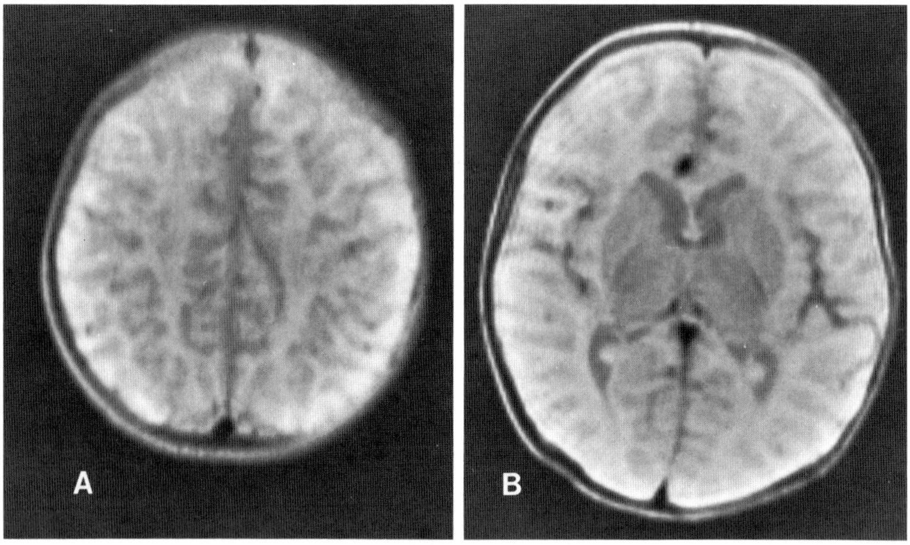

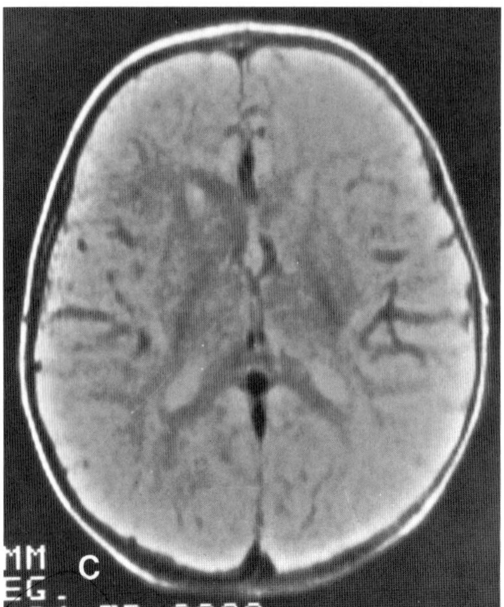

Figure 12–3. Normal neonatal brain at 3 months of age (infantile pattern) seen with MRI (axial SE 2000/84). (*A*) At the level of the centrum semiovale, the white matter still maintains high-signal intensity compared to the adjacent gray matter. (*B*) At the level of the basal ganglia, myelin is now present in the region of the posterior limb of the internal capsule and is beginning to be deposited in the white matter of the occipital lobe. (*C*) At the level of the posterior fossa, more myelin is present than was seen at 6 days (Fig. 12–2*C*).

in the transition from one gray-white matter differentiation pattern to another[35] (Fig.12–7).

Functional Imaging

Before the development of PET and SPECT, local functional maturation of the human brain could not be studied adequately in vivo. Global cerebral blood flow (CBF) and oxygen utilization, however, could be measured in the developing brain with the Kety-Schmidt method.[82,85] Using a modification of this technique, Kennedy and Sokoloff[82] demonstrated that the average global CBF in nine normal children (age 3–11 years) was approximately 1.8 times that of normal young adults. Similarly,

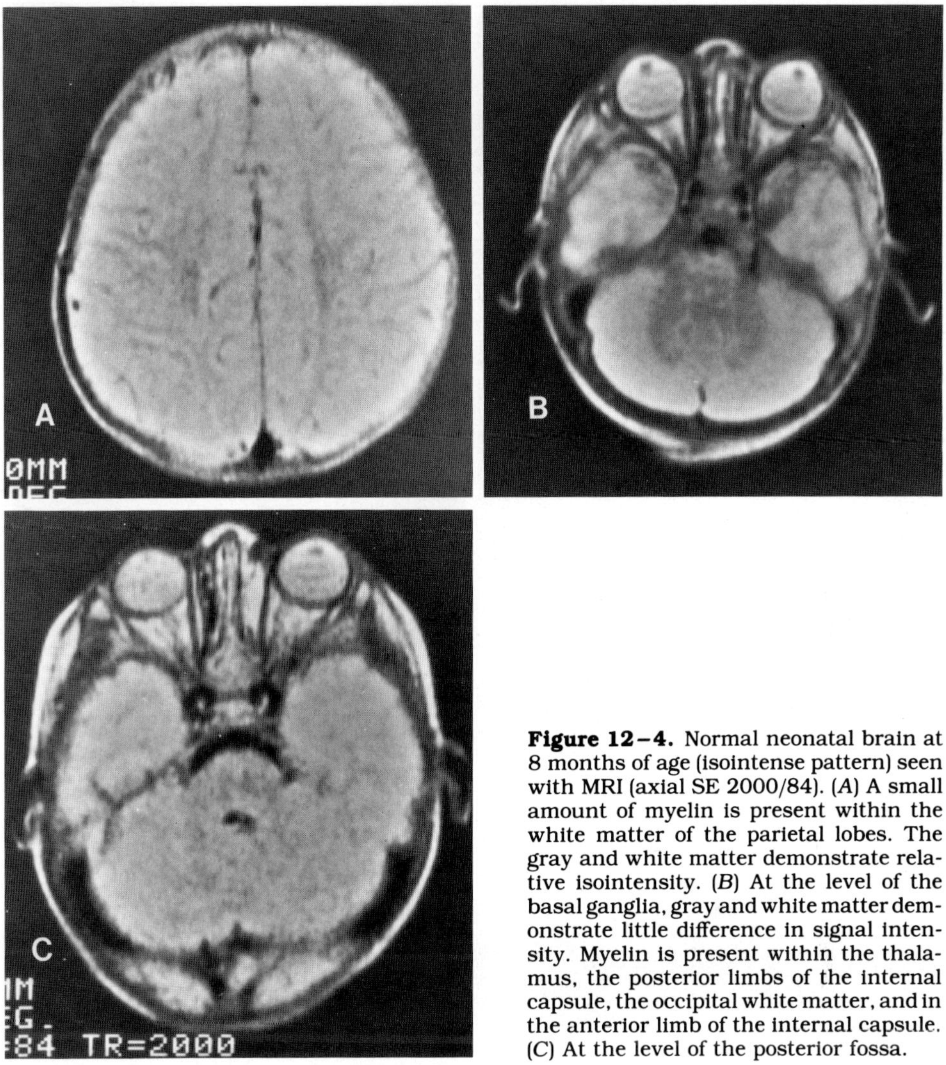

Figure 12–4. Normal neonatal brain at 8 months of age (isointense pattern) seen with MRI (axial SE 2000/84). (*A*) A small amount of myelin is present within the white matter of the parietal lobes. The gray and white matter demonstrate relative isointensity. (*B*) At the level of the basal ganglia, gray and white matter demonstrate little difference in signal intensity. Myelin is present within the thalamus, the posterior limbs of the internal capsule, the occipital white matter, and in the anterior limb of the internal capsule. (*C*) At the level of the posterior fossa.

average cerebral oxygen utilization was approximately 1.3 times higher in children than in adults.

Although PET and SPECT are ideally suited for studying local functional changes in the brain during normal development, such studies in entirely normal children cannot be performed because of ethical considerations, including radiation exposure, venipuncture and blood sampling. The usual dose of fluorodeoxyglucose (FDG) for children is 0.143 mCi/kg, approximately 25% lower than that used in adults (see Chapter 3, Table 3–5). With this dose, the whole body radiation exposure is about 300 m rad (0.003 Gy). Peak exposure is to the bladder and is 2 rad (0.02 Gy). The dose to the brain is about 500 m rad (0.005 Gy). At UCLA, children less than 2 years of age are intravenously administered 0.45% saline solution (10 ml/kg over 2 hours) beginning 15 minutes after FDG injection. At 40, 100, and 160 minutes, urination is stimulated in infants by Credé's

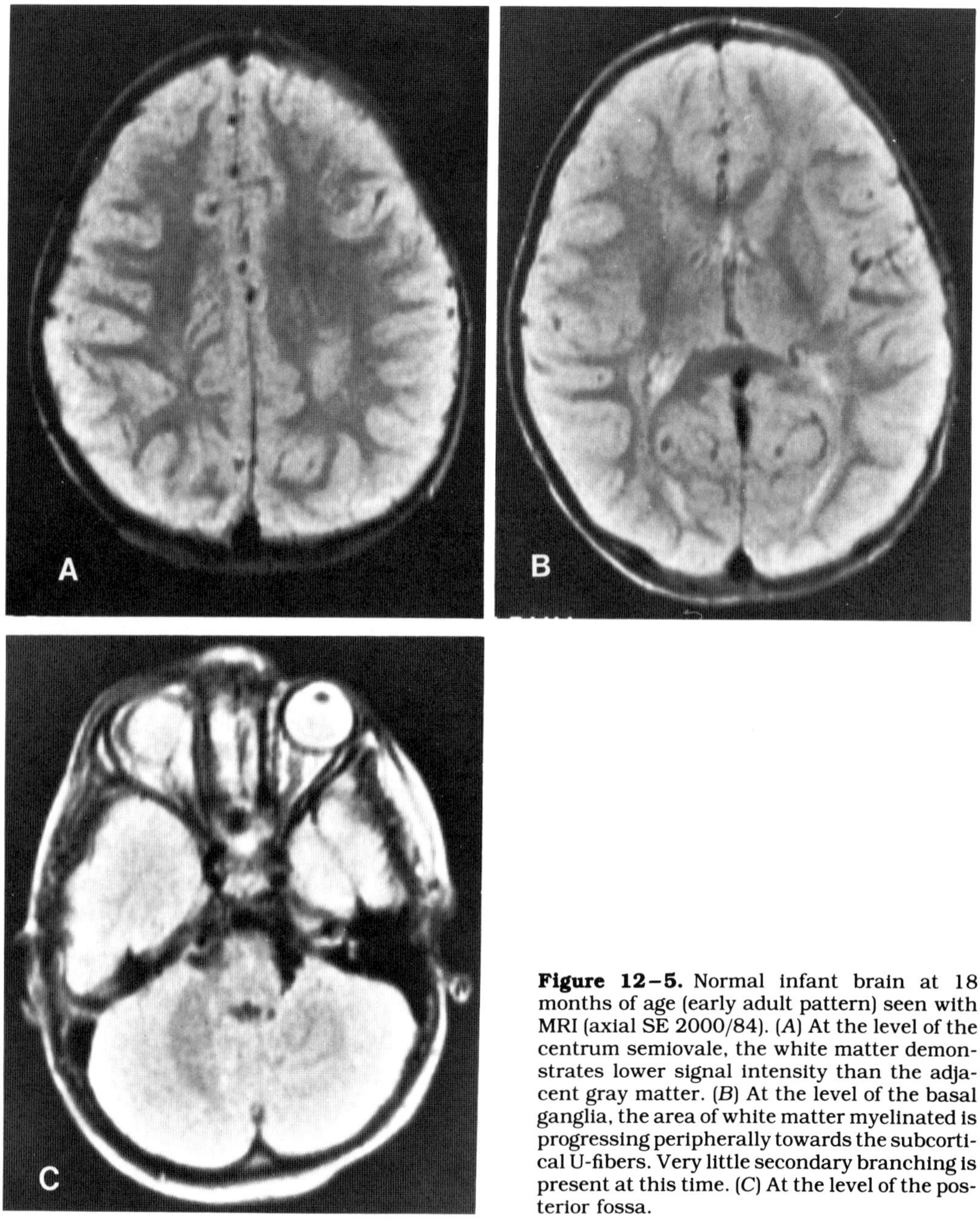

Figure 12–5. Normal infant brain at 18 months of age (early adult pattern) seen with MRI (axial SE 2000/84). (*A*) At the level of the centrum semiovale, the white matter demonstrates lower signal intensity than the adjacent gray matter. (*B*) At the level of the basal ganglia, the area of white matter myelinated is progressing peripherally towards the subcortical U-fibers. Very little secondary branching is present at this time. (*C*) At the level of the posterior fossa.

method. Older children are encouraged to urinate immediately following the FDG uptake period. Although these maneuvers are effective in reducing bladder and total body radiation exposure, the study of normal children with PET is still not justifiable. Therefore, normative data have to be acquired indirectly using a variety of strategies. One strategy[23,25] is to select retrospectively from all the children who have undergone PET a subgroup who had either experienced transient neurologic events that did not significantly interfere with

Table 12–1 NORMAL WHITE MATTER MATURATION MILESTONES

Age	*Site of Myelin*	*Gray-White Pattern**
Birth	Thalamus, cerebellar peduncles	Infantile
1 mo	Posterior limb internal capsule	Infantile
3 mo	Optic radiations	Infantile
6 mo	Radiations to precentral gyrus	Infantile
8 mo	Parietal and frontal white matter	Isointense
1 yr	Temporal white matter	Early adult
2 yr	Further branching of subcortical fibers	Early adult

*Gray-white pattern on spin echo T_2-weighted axial images (SE 2000/84). *Infantile:* White matter hyperintense compared with gray matter. *Isointense:* White and gray matter isointense. *Early adult:* White matter hypointense compared to gray matter.

neurologic development, or in whom neurologic disease was eventually ruled out. The children comprising this subgroup are reasonably representative of normal children, enabling investigators to characterize normal maturational changes of local cerebral metabolic rates for glucose (LCMRGlc) during development.[23,25]

One such analysis included 29 infants and children of various ages ranging from 5 days to 15 years, and consisting of 16 males and 13 females. In this population, LCMRGlc in the first month of postnatal life was highest in sensorimotor cortex, thalamus, brainstem, and cerebellar vermis, all of which are relatively old structures on

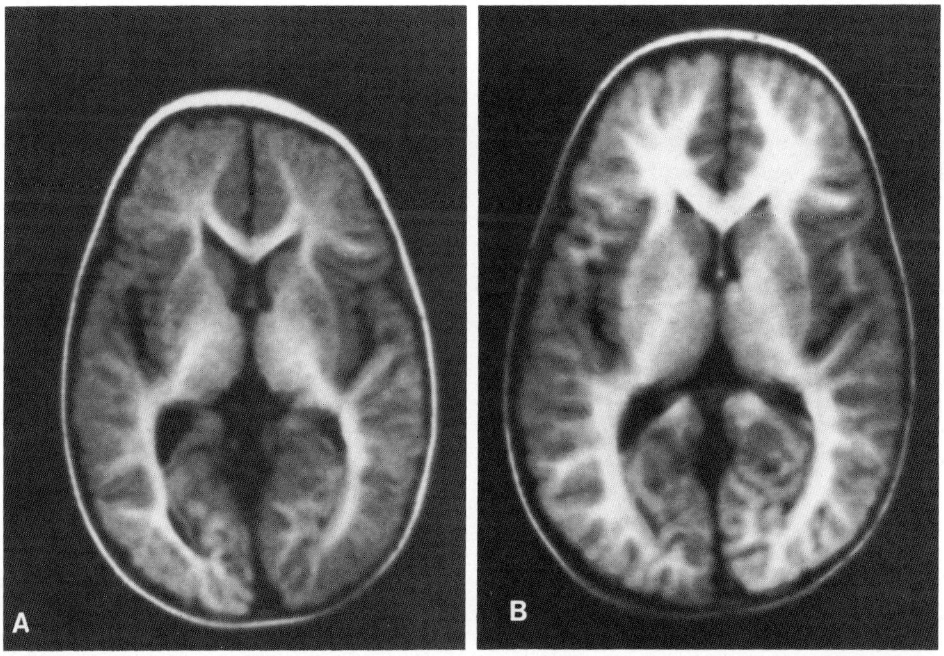

Figure 12–6. Normal progression of myelination on inversion recovery sequences (axial IR 1800/60/44). (*A*) A 10-month-old child. Myelinated areas are seen as high-signal intensity on this sequence. (*B*) Same child at 39 months of age. The areas of myelinated white matter now extend more peripherally to the subcortical U-fibers. (Images courtesy of Graeme Bydder, Hammersmith Hospital, London.)

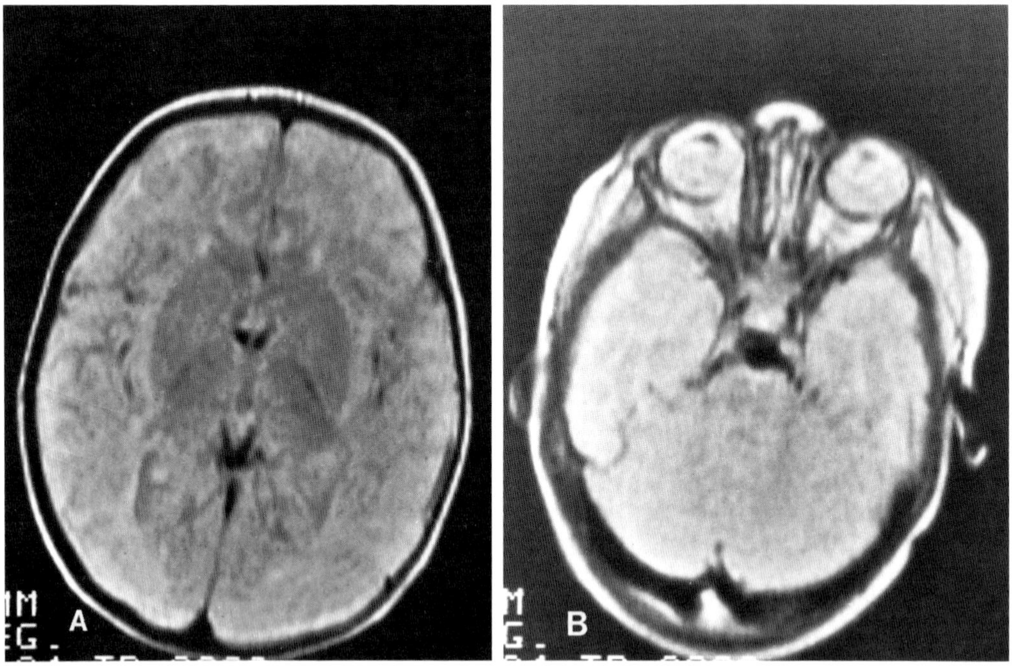

Figure 12–7. Delayed myelination in an 18-month-old girl with clinical developmental delay (axial SE 2000/84). (*A*) At the level of the basal ganglia, the gray and white matter demonstrate a transition pattern between an infantile and isointense pattern. Myelin is seen to be present within the posterior limb of the internal capsule and in the optic radiations, consistent with a normal child of 4 to 6 months of age. (*B*) At the level of the posterior fossa, the gray-white matter differentiation pattern demonstrates the infantile pattern, with white matter having higher signal intensity than gray. Only a small amount of myelin has been laid down in the posterior fossa.

the phylogenic scale (Figs. 12–8, 12–9*D*). During the second and third months, LCMRGlc increased in the basal ganglia, parietal, temporal, and primary visual cortices, and in the cerebellar hemispheres. The frontal cortex, however, lagged behind the other cortical regions in its glucose metabolic development (Fig. 12–8*C,D*). By approximately 8 months, the frontal and various association cortical regions also became metabolically active (Fig. 12–8*E,F*). Within the frontal cortex, the lateral and inferior portions were the first to show a maturational rise in LCMRGlc. The last area of the brain to display an increase in LCMRGlc was the dorsal prefrontal cortex, which is the most recent area of the frontal lobe to undergo extensive differentiation on the phylogenic scale. The detailed temporal sequence in which structures become metabolically mature[23,25], therefore, supports the statement that "ontogeny recapitulates phylogeny." By 1 year of age, the anatomic pattern of LCMRGlc resembles that of the young healthy adult (Fig. 12–8*G,H*).

Quantitative analysis of LCMRGlc in various gray matter structures from birth to adulthood in the 29 control children and in 7 young healthy adults revealed the following: LCMRGlc was lower at birth (13–25 μmol/minute per 100 g among various anatomic structures) than in adults, rapidly rose to reach adult values (19–33 μmol/minute per 100 g) by age 2 years, and continued to rise until age 3–4 years, when LCMRGlc in most gray matter regions reached values of 49–65 μmol/minute per 100 g. These high rates (in excess of adult values) were maintained until about age 9–10 years, when they began

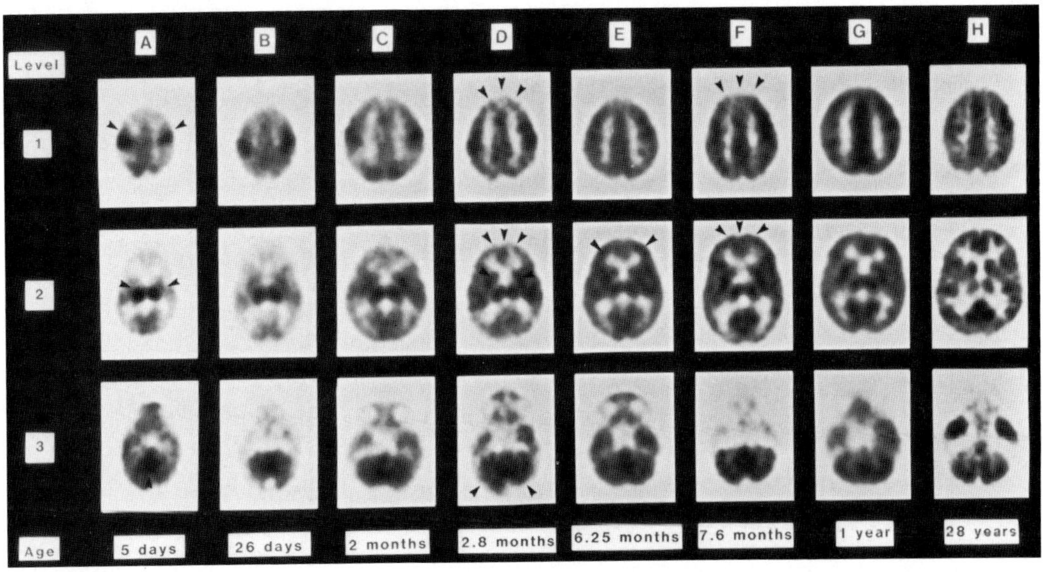

Figure 12–8. FDG-PET images illustrating developmental changes in glucose metabolism (LCMRGlc) in the normal human infant with increasing age, as compared to that of the adult (image sizes not on the same scale). Gray scale is proportional to LCMRGlc, with black being highest. In each image, the anterior portion of the brain is at the top of the image. (*A*) In the 5-day-old infant, LCMRGlc is highest in sensorimotor cortex, thalamus, cerebellar vermis (*arrows*), and brainstem (*not shown*). (*B, C, D*) LCMRGlc gradually increases in parietal, temporal, and calcarine cortices, basal ganglia, and cerebellar cortex (*arrows*), particularly during the second and third months. (*E*) By approximately 6 months, LCMRGlc increases first in the lateral prefrontal regions of the frontal cortex. (*F*) By approximately 8 months, LCMRGlc also increases in the medial aspects of the frontal cortex (*arrows*), as well as in the dorsolateral occipital cortex. (*G,H*) By 1 year, the LCMRGlc pattern resembles that of adults.

to decline, reaching adult values by the latter part of the second decade (see Fig. 12–9).

The distribution of LCMRGlc depicted by PET in the neonate is consistent with infant behavior at this age, which is, in general, mediated by subcortical brain structures. Furthermore, intrinsic brainstem reflexes (e.g., Moro, root, grasp reflexes) are present. Subsequently, the gradual suppression of intrinsic brainstem reflexes and the transition to "mature" EEG patterns during the second and third months also correspond to the process of "encephalization" reflected in the pattern of cerebral metabolism revealed by PET. An important behavioral hallmark of this age is the ability of the infant to engage in visuo-spatial and visuo-sensorimotor integration; for example, the infant is now able to track visually and to reach out for objects of interest.[149] The increase of LCMRGlc in frontal and association cortical regions during the seventh and eighth months is consistent with the emergence of higher cortical function and increasing cognitive development during this period.[79] These patterns of functional maturation support the notion proposed by Kennedy and colleagues[83] that, in general, there is a relationship between a metabolic increase within a neuroanatomic structure and the emergence of corresponding behavior.

The finding of higher LCMRGlc in children compared with adults is consistent with the excessive numbers of dendritic processes and synapses in childhood, since these elements account for most of the glucose utilized.[78,99,116] Therefore, the large surface area of an excessive number of processes might lead to high resting glucose metabolic rates for mainte-

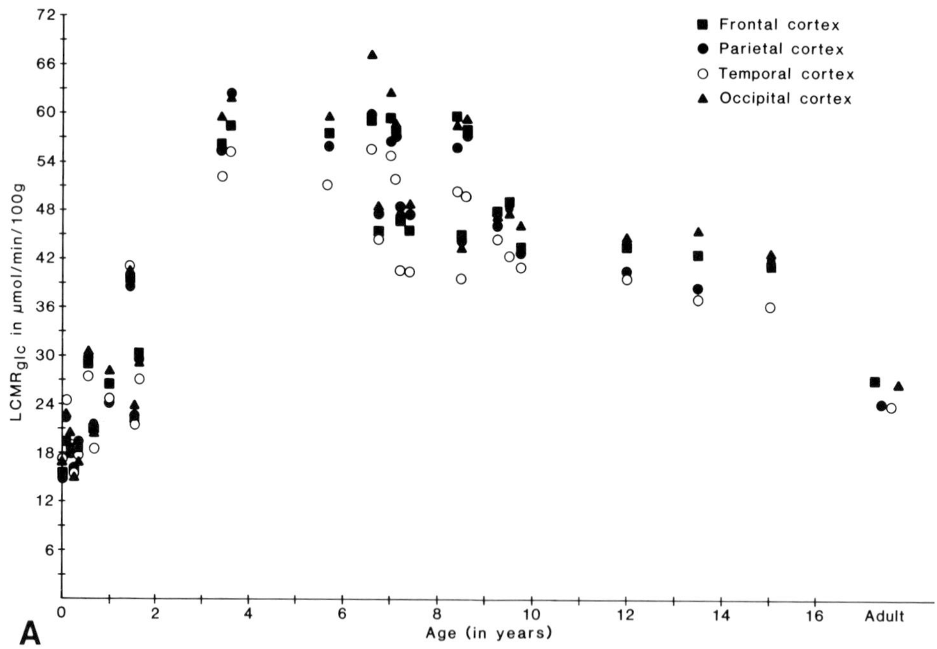

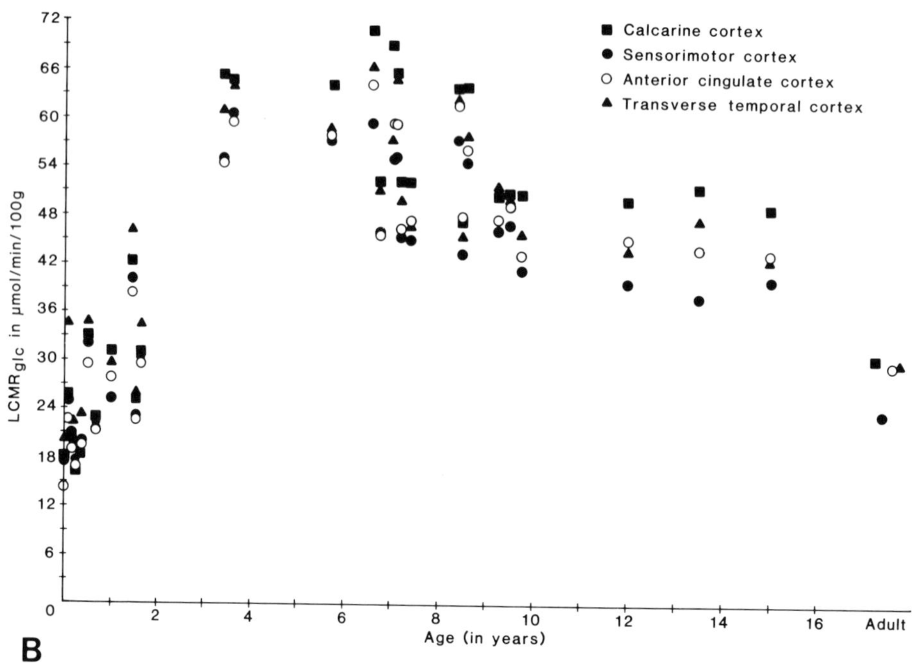

Figure 12–9. Absolute values of LCMRGlc for selected brain regions plotted as a function of age for 29 infants and children and 7 young adults. In the infants and children, points represent individual values of LCMRGlc; in adults, points are *mean* values from 7 subjects. (*A,B*) Selected regions of cerebral cortex.

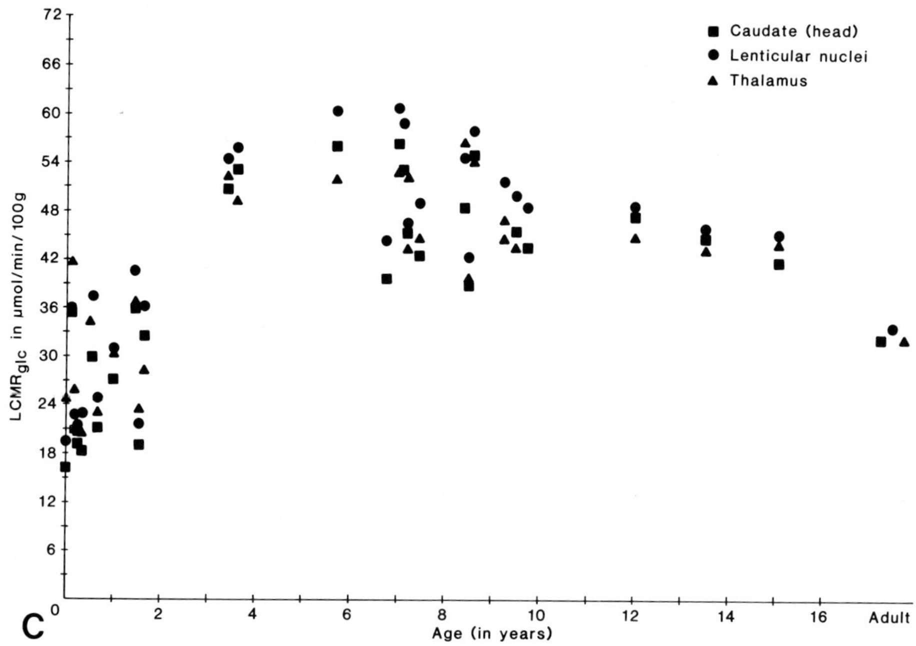

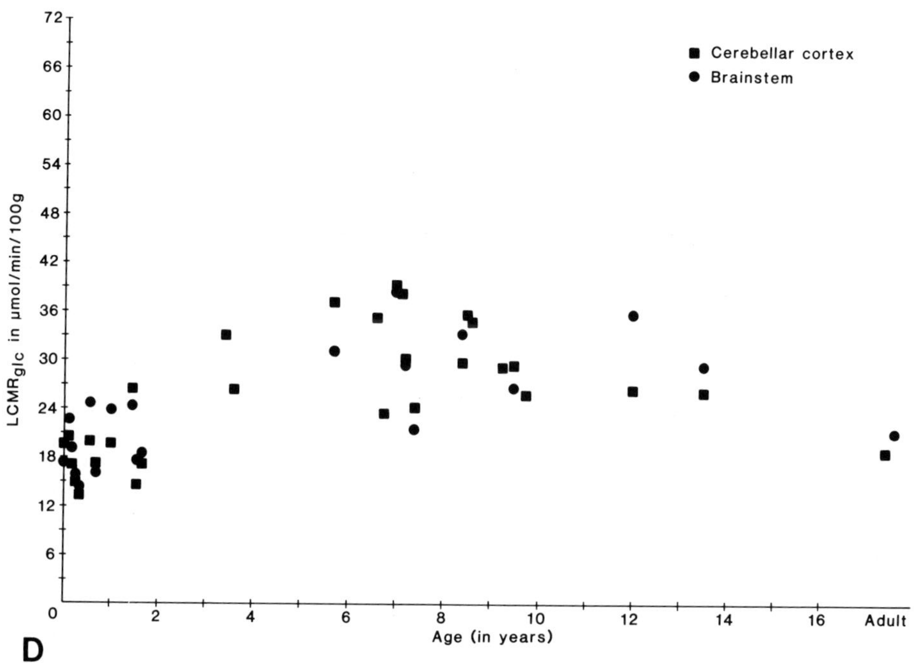

Figure 12–9. *Continued* (*C*) Basal ganglia and thalamus. (*D*) Cerebellar cortex and brainstem.

nance of membrane potentials. As the density of processes diminishes with age, LCMRGlc also decreases to approach adult levels.

A second cause for high LCMRGlc in the developing brain may be excessive metabolic expenditure by oligodendroglia during myelination, which, as indicated above, is another developmental process that proceeds into the second decade of life. Conversely, incomplete myelination of brain pathways may result in suboptimal conduction efficiency, thus requiring greater energy expenditure. The relative contributions of these possible mechanisms in accounting for the high LCMRGlc in the developing brain are unknown.

The measurement of LCMRGlc is only one parameter in the developing brain that can be studied with PET, and illustrates the potential wealth of information that can be obtained using this technique. In the foreseeable future, the mapping of ontogenetic changes in local protein synthesis, blood flow, and binding to various receptors will greatly enhance our understanding of normal brain development.

BRAIN MALFORMATIONS

Of all organ systems, the nervous system has the highest incidence of congenital malformations. With the development of high-resolution, multimodality neuroimaging techniques, the extent and type of brain malformations are increasingly being diagnosed antemortem rather than at autopsy. The advent of x-ray CT and MRI allowed visualization of cross-sectional anatomy of the brains of living children with congenital abnormalities. Because sequential studies can be obtained noninvasively, these modalities can give valuable information regarding the evolution of abnormalities. This is particularly important in the less severe anomalies, since children with such problems are rarely studied at autopsy. In this section, only supratentorial brain malformations are considered. Posterior fossa abnormalities are considered in Chapter 11.

Clinical/Pathophysiologic Background

Malformations of the brain include, among others, disturbances of neuronal migration (cerebral cortical dysgenesis), abnormal gyral formation, hypoplasia or agenesis of various structures, cyst formation, and dysraphic states. The presence of these different congenital anomalies is related to events occurring at various stages of brain development, which chronologically consist of dorsal induction, ventral induction, neuronal proliferation, neuronal migration, neuronal organization, and myelination. The more commonly encountered abnormalities that develop because of problems occurring at these stages are listed in Table 12–2.

Structural Imaging

Because MRI is able to image in multiple planes without the need to reposition the patient, it is an ideal modality for evaluating the structural anatomy of congenital anomalies.[60,92,122] Short-TR and short-TE sequences, with their superior resolution and shorter imaging times, are best for the depiction of displacement of structures and evaluation of the gyral-sulcal pattern and the size and shape of the ventricles and the extracerebral space, since on these sequences, the cerebrospinal fluid (CSF) has lower signal intensity than the adjacent gray and white matter. T_2-weighted sequences are useful to give additional information demonstrating associated abnormalities of meylination or the presence of hamartomatous lesions.

Functional Imaging

There have been very few functional neuroimaging studies of patients with

Table 12–2 CONGENITAL ANOMALIES ASSOCIATED WITH DIFFERENT STAGES OF BRAIN DEVELOPMENT

Developmental Process	*Gestational Time*	*Anomalies*
Dorsal induction	3–4 wk	Anencephaly Encephalocele Myelomeningocele Spinal dysraphism
Ventral induction	4–8 wk	Holoprosencephaly Septo-optic dysplasia
Neuronal proliferation	2–4 mo	Megalencephaly Micrencephaly vera
Neuronal migration	4–7 mo	Lissencephaly Pachygyria Polymicrogyria Schizencephaly Heterotopias

brain malformations. Details of those that have been studied are included in the appropriate subsection.

Cerebral Malformations

CLINICAL/ PATHOPHYSIOLOGICAL BACKGROUND AND STRUCTURAL IMAGING

Children with holoprosencephaly show a failure of normal development of the cerebral hemispheres, thalamus, and hypothalamus caused by a defect of cleavage. There is fusion of the lateral ventricles, which have failed to separate, and a lack of development of the interhemispheric fissure and falx.[54] In more severe forms (alobar prosencephaly) there is a large single ventricular cavity with a saucerlike rim of cerebral tissue anteriorly and a large dorsal cyst (Fig. 12–10*A*). In less severe forms (lobar prosencephaly), there is partial separation into cerebral lobes, but the frontal horns of the lateral ventricles are fused, although separate occipital horns are visible. The interhemispheric fissure and the falx are only partially developed and may be seen posteriorly. The roof of the single ventricle is indented downward in the midline (Fig. 12–10*B*). In lobar prosencephaly the interhemispheric fissure is usually present from the occiput to the anterior portion of the frontal lobes. There may be only a small portion of cortex fused just ahead of the anterior portion of the corpus callosum. The bodies of the lateral ventricles have a narrowed appearance, with fusion of the anterior horns.

Septo-optic dysplasia is a syndrome consisting of blindness, hypoplasia of the optic discs, and absence of the septum pellucidum. Patients with this condition frequently have hypopituitarism. X-ray CT and MRI studies show small optic nerves, absence of the septum, and enlargement of the chiasmatic cistern. The falx and interhemispheric fissure are normal[117] (Fig. 12–11).

Megalencephaly is a rare anomaly that develops because of abnormal neuronal proliferation. It may be unilateral or bilateral in distribution. Infants with this condition present with early seizures and severe encephalopathy (Fig. 12–12). Neuropathologic examination typically reveals a chaotic hyperplasia and hypertrophy of neuronal elements, resulting in an abundance of disorganized brain parenchyma. The x-ray CT and MRI findings in five children with this anomaly were recently described and show hemispheric hypertrophy with lateral ventricle dilatation, abnormal gyral patterns, and thickened cortex on the enlarged side.[80]

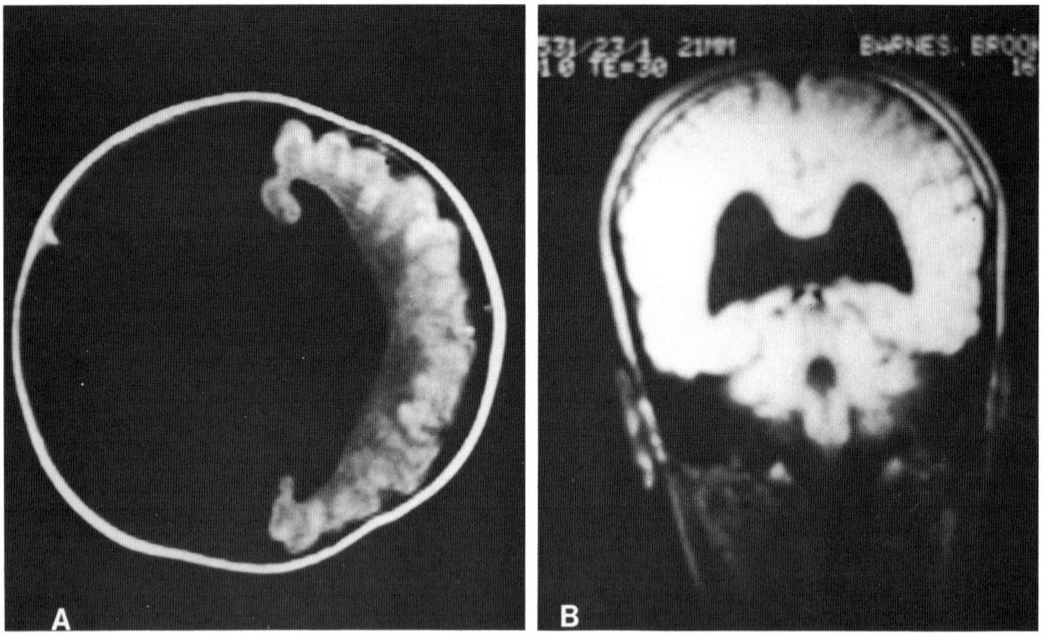

Figure 12–10. Holoprosencephaly. (*A*) Axial MRI (SE 1000/30). A saucerlike rim of cerebral tissue is seen anterior to a large dorsal cyst. (*B*) Coronal image (SE 1000/30). Indentation of the single ventricle is present. There is incomplete falx formation.

When abnormalities of migration occur, the cortex develops abnormal thickness and folding and becomes disorganized. Early disturbances in migration produce changes that are more severe and more nearly symmetric than do those occurring later.[155] In the more severe forms of migrational defects, MRI clearly defines the surface anatomy of the brain,[10,156] showing the paucity of gyri and sulci in such conditions as lissencephaly and pachygyria. In extreme cases, agyria (that is, complete lissencephaly) occurs, with complete absence of gyri (Fig. 12–13). Migrating neurons are unable to reach the superficial layers of the cortex, which are thickened, and the white matter becomes "reduced in size", changes that are seen even on T_2-weighted images. Normal gyral formation does not occur, so the surface of the brain remains smooth. In cases of pachygyria, T_1-weighted images show broad gyri separated by shallow sulci; the temporal and frontal lobes are hypoplastic and separated by shallow sylvian fissures. The lateral ventricles are moderately dilated. These children also have characteristic craniofacial dysmorphism, with a narrow forehead and hollow temporal fossae. Clinical signs and symptoms depend on the severity of the abnormality and include a lack of psychomotor development, microcephaly, hypotonia, and seizures.

In polymicrogyria, multiple small abnormal gyri, with either histologically incomplete or absent intervening sulci and lack of secondary branching, are present. These abnormal gyri may be seen by MRI[156] (Fig. 12–14).

In children with schizencephaly (Fig. 12–15), who have unilateral or bilateral clefts traversing the brain tissue, lined on either side by gray matter, imaging in multiple planes is necessary to define fully the extent of the anomalous anatomy. If images are performed only in one plane, the cleft may be entirely missed.[11]

MRI is particularly valuable in the demonstration of heterotopic gray matter. Gray matter heterotopias are collec-

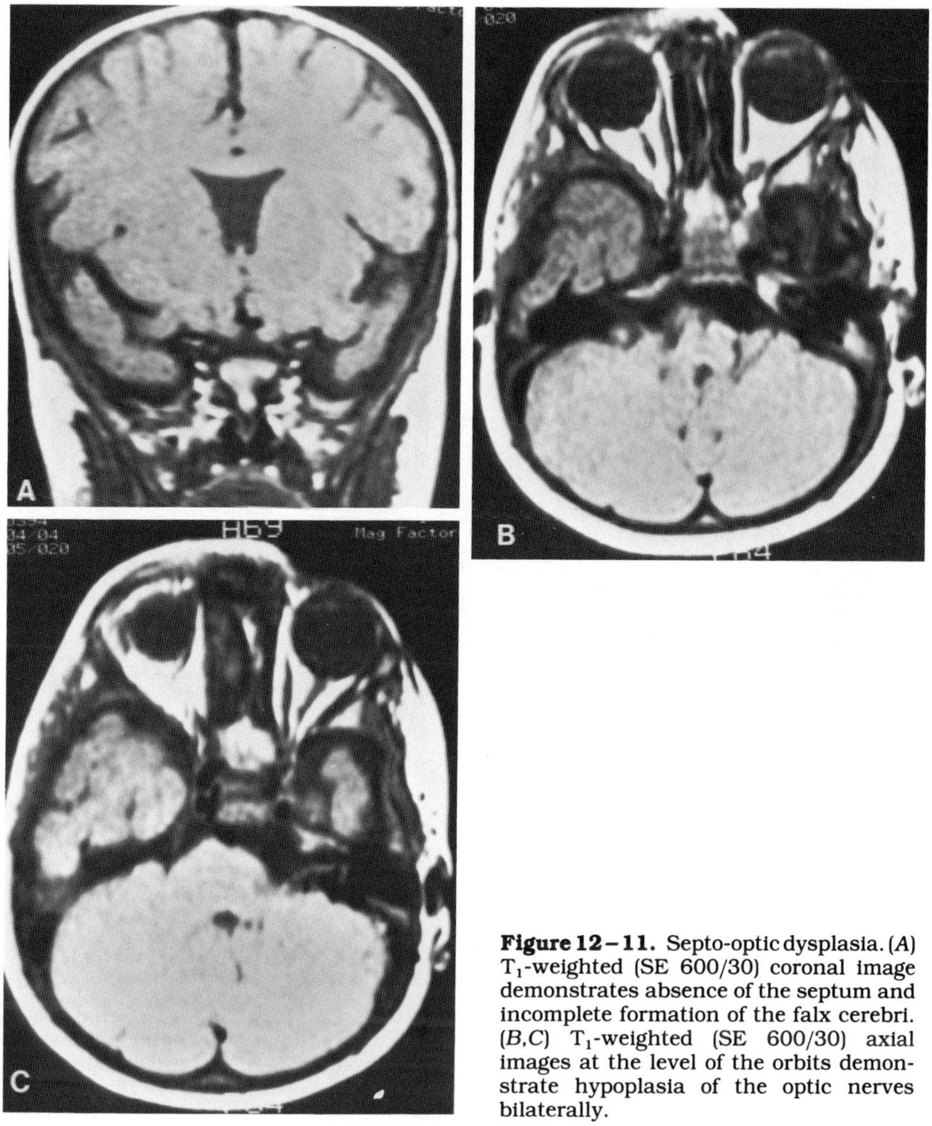

Figure 12–11. Septo-optic dysplasia. (*A*) T_1-weighted (SE 600/30) coronal image demonstrates absence of the septum and incomplete formation of the falx cerebri. (*B,C*) T_1-weighted (SE 600/30) axial images at the level of the orbits demonstrate hypoplasia of the optic nerves bilaterally.

tions of nerve cells that are in abnormal locations owing to their arrest along the migration pathway from the germinal matrix to the cortex. These areas have the same signal intensity as adjacent gray matter, no matter what MRI pulsing parameters are used. Those in a periventricular location can be seen on both MRI and x-ray CT as pseudomasses invaginating into the lateral ventricles. Only MRI, however, can identify the areas of heterotopic gray matter that are buried within the white matter of the brain. These are optimally seen on sequences with long TR values that show good gray-white matter differentiation (see Fig. 12–14).[7,33] Additional MRI images to show the pattern of myelination are often helpful in this group of patients, who frequently demonstrate delay in the myelination process.

Images in multiple planes also are useful in evaluating abnormalities of the corpus callosum and associated lesions.[5,81] In such patients, sagittal

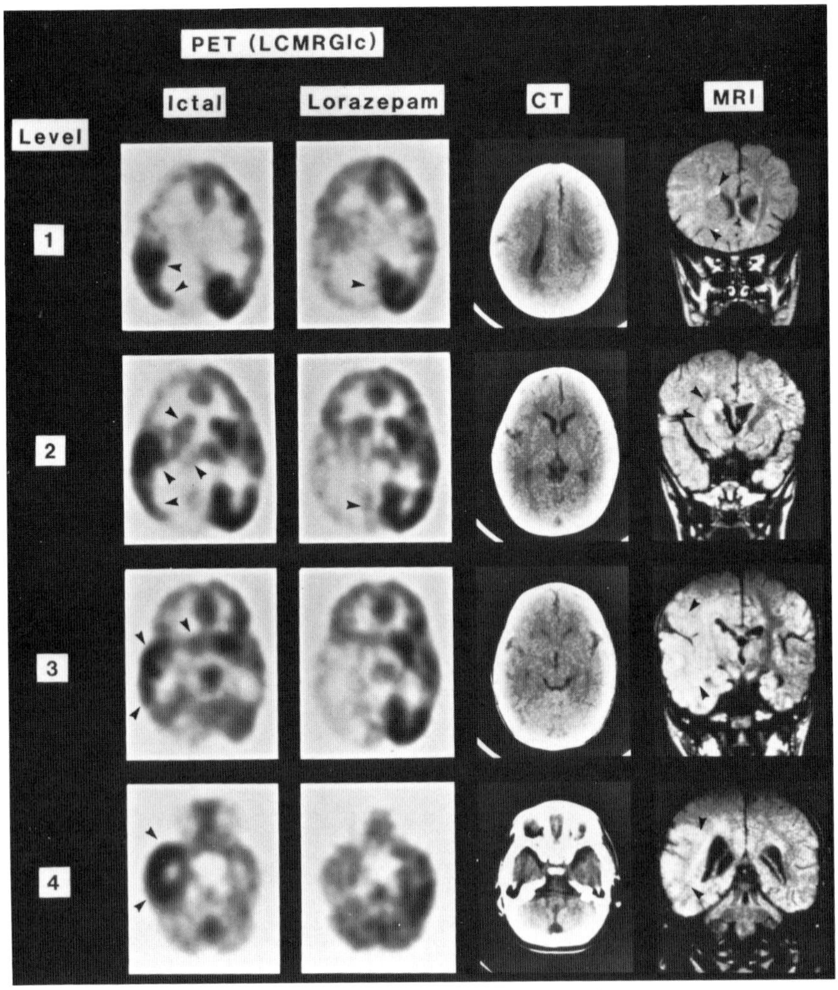

Figure 12–12. FDG-PET, x-ray CT, and MRI (SE 2000/40) images of an infant with intractable seizures beginning at 1 month of age. X-ray CT and MRI both revealed left hemimegalencephaly. MRI also showed dilated left lateral ventricle and increased signal intensity throughout the left cerebral hemisphere, particularly in the area of the caudate nucleus. Ictal PET depicted high LCMRGlc in the midbrain, right calcarine cortex, and left temporal and parietal regions, compared to the rest of the left hemisphere. Interictal PET (following 9.2 mg per kg lorazepam IV) revealed diffuse cortical and subcortical hypometabolism in the left cerebral hemisphere, and a relatively normal LCMRGlc pattern in the right hemisphere. EEG showed multifocal left-sided spikes and polyspike-wave activity. Thiopental infusion revealed a marked absence of drug-induced beta over the left hemisphere, with a normal response over the right. The patient underwent a left cerebral hemispherectomy, and has been seizure-free since. Neuropathologic examination of the excised hemisphere showed areas of disorganized cortex with scattered clusters of atypical astrocytes and scattered swollen neurons.

images will demonstrate total or partial absence of the corpus callosum; distortion of the cingulate gyrus; radiation of the midline sulci; and the presence of associated lesions such as lipomas, cysts or posterior fossa anomalies, including Dandy-Walker and Chiari malformations. Axial images show the characteristic appearance of the lateral ventricles, with dilatation of the occipital horns of the lateral ventricles and separation of the beaked anterior horns (Fig. 12–16). When partial absence of the corpus callosum occurs, it is usually

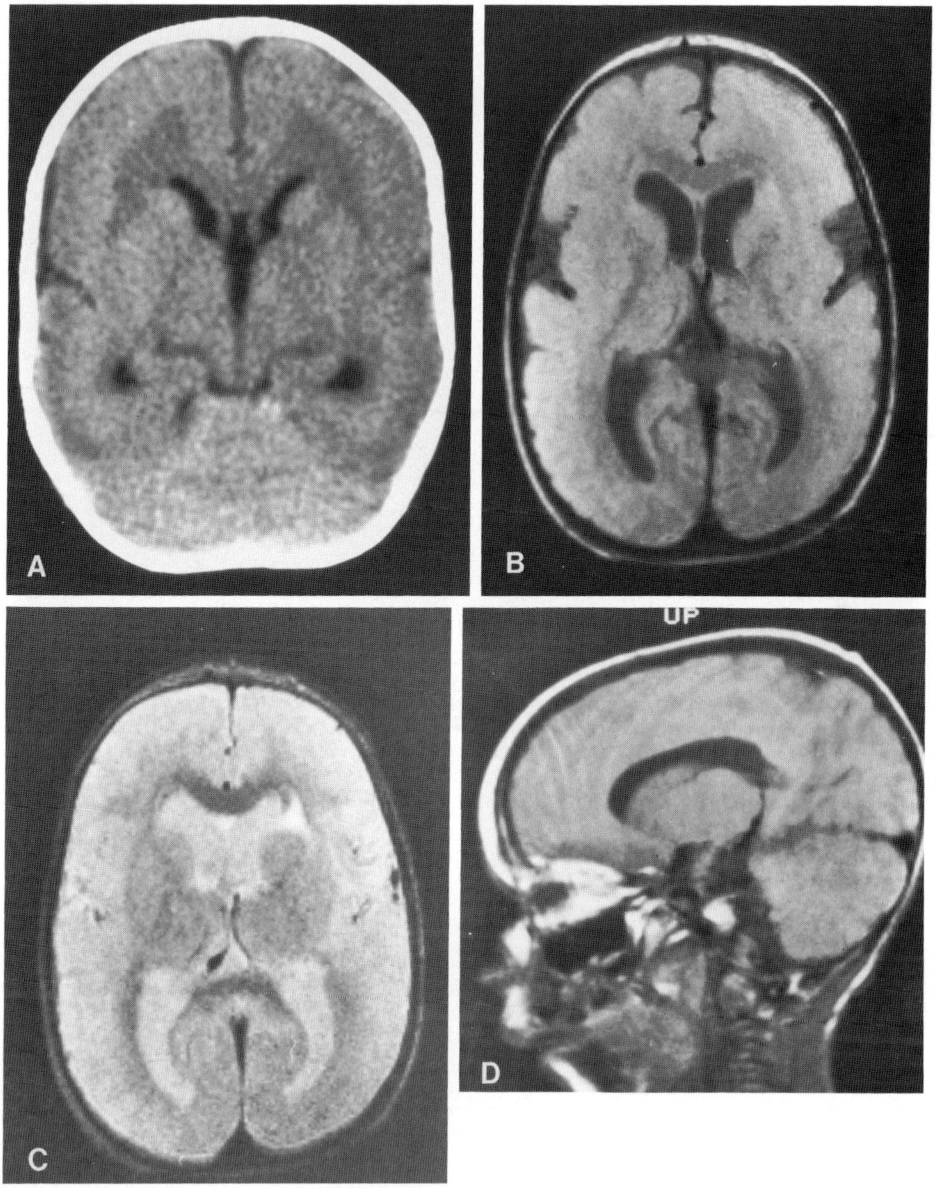

Figure 12–13. Lissencephaly. (*A*) Axial x-ray CT scan at the level of the basal ganglia demonstrates a thickened cortex and straight, obliquely oriented sylvian fissures. (*B*) Axial MRI (SE 600/30). There is a paucity of sulci and gyri along the surface of the cerebral hemispheres. Mild dilatation of the lateral ventricles is present. (*C*) Axial MRI (SE 3000/80). Thickened gray matter at the cortex is evident, with a paucity of white matter in the periventricular region. (*D*) Parasagittal MRI (SE 600/30). Note the absence of sulci and gyri along the surface of the cerebral hemispheres on this T_1-weighted sequence.

the posterior portion that is absent, since development occurs from anterior to posterior. Less frequently, as a result of early vascular insult, absence of the anterior portion of the corpus callosum may be seen.

FUNCTIONAL IMAGING

In a single patient with cortical heterotopia located in the deep right frontoparietal area, FDG-PET revealed LCMRGlc in this region to be identical to

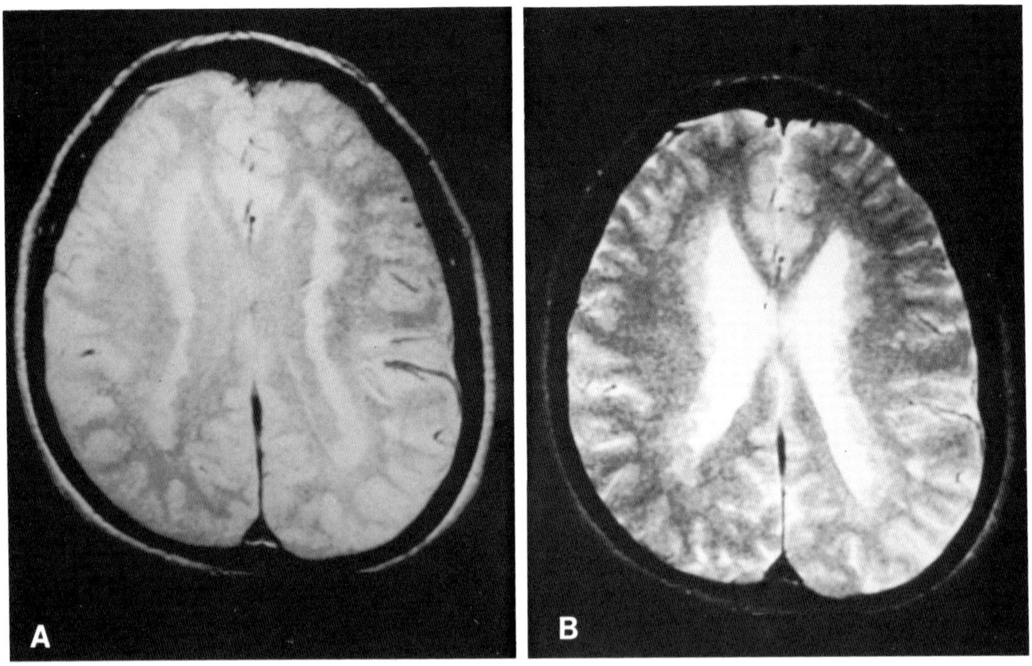

Figure 12–14. Polymicrogyria and heterotopic gray matter. (*A*) Axial MRI (SE 3000/40) and (*B*) axial MRI (SE 3000/80). Nodular masses of tissue seen bilaterally in periventricular regions demonstrate the same signal intensity as the adjacent gray matter and represent rests of heterotopic gray matter. The surface of the brain has shallow sulci and increased numbers of gyri, consistent with a diagnosis of polymicrogyria.

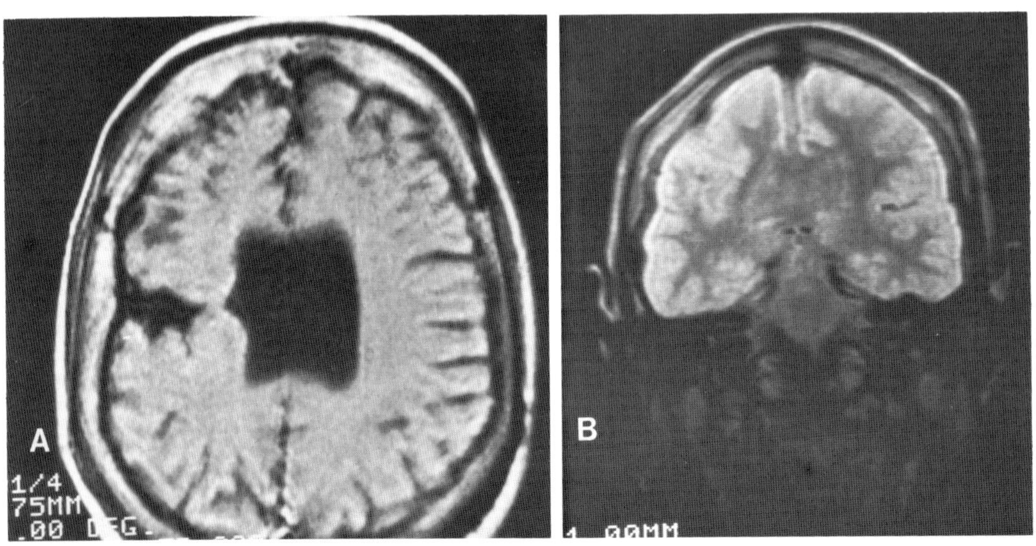

Figure 12–15. Schizencephaly. (*A*) Axial MRI (SE 800/28). A unilateral cleft is seen extending from the surface of the right parietal lobe, connecting with the right lateral ventricle. (*B*) Coronal MRI (SE 2000/84). On this T_2-weighted image, the gray matter is seen to extend along the lips of the cleft bilaterally.

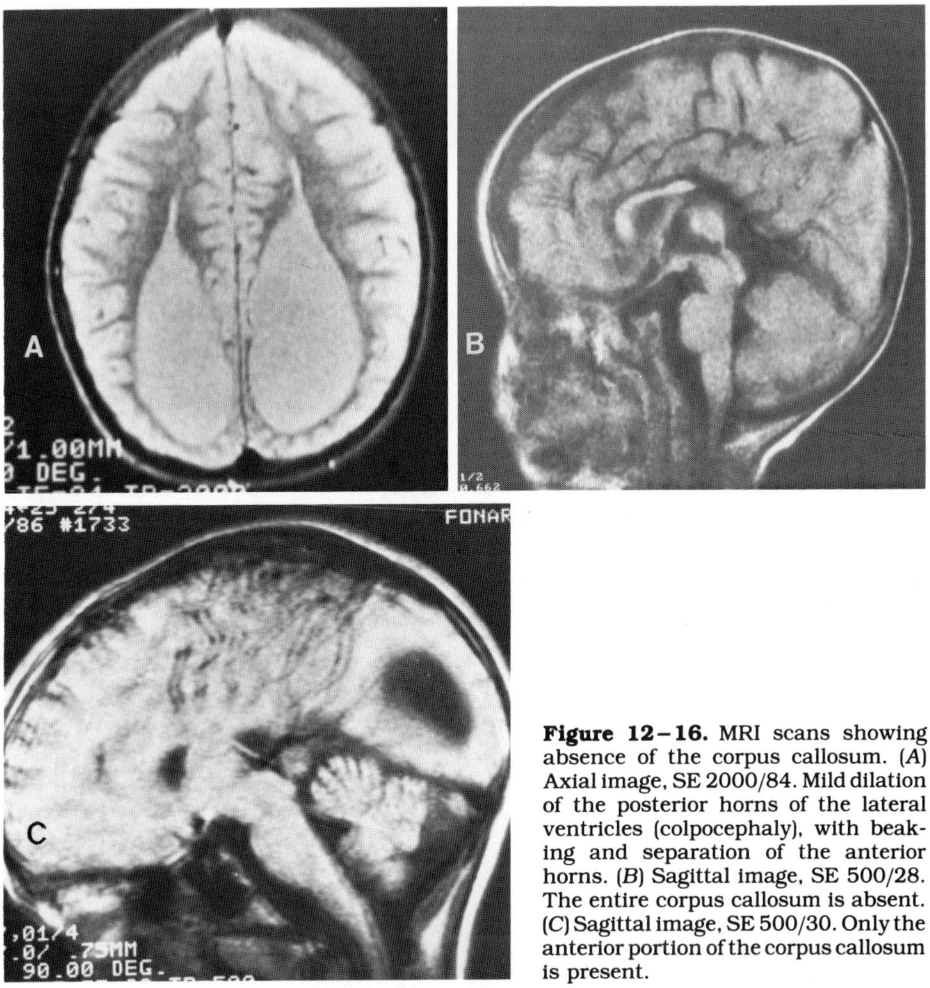

Figure 12–16. MRI scans showing absence of the corpus callosum. (*A*) Axial image, SE 2000/84. Mild dilation of the posterior horns of the lateral ventricles (colpocephaly), with beaking and separation of the anterior horns. (*B*) Sagittal image, SE 500/28. The entire corpus callosum is absent. (*C*) Sagittal image, SE 500/30. Only the anterior portion of the corpus callosum is present.

that of the contralateral frontoparietal cortex.[7] This patient suffered from psychomotor retardation and epilepsy. Although paroxysmal activity on the EEG was bilateral, it was most prominent over the right hemisphere.

In some centers, PET and SPECT have become an integral part of the evaluation of children, with intractable epilepsy being considered for surgical excision of the epileptic focus.[27,69] These techniques not only have successfully identified hamartomas and unilateral megalencephalic malformations (see Fig. 12–12) corresponding to the epileptic discharges, but also have demonstrated the functional integrity of brain regions outside the area of proposed surgical resection.[27]

Neuropathologic correlation of surgically resected epileptic tissue in children with intractable seizures has revealed that FDG-PET is a sensitive test capable of detecting cytoarchitectural disturbances, even when x-ray CT and MRI fail to show any abnormalities. Although the extent of surgical resection in children undergoing focal excision is usually determined with the guidance of intraoperative electrocorticography, the distribution of malformed (epileptic) tissue has, thus far, precisely matched that depicted by PET.[118]

Hamartomas and Arachnoid Cysts

Hamartoma of the tuber cinereum (Fig. 12–17) is a congenital malformation consisting of a tumorlike, ectopic mass of neuronal tissue. Children with this abnormality present with precocious isosexual puberty or neurologic symptoms such as seizures, intellectual impairment, and behavioral problems. X-ray CT and MRI typically reveal a mass in the region of the interpeduncular cistern that does not enhance after administration of contrast agents.[124] These lesions remain unchanged in size on consecutive studies. (Other types of tumors are described in Chapter 6.)

Arachnoid cysts develop when fluid is loculated within arachnoidal layers. They most frequently occur adjacent to the temporal horns, in the interhemispheric region, over the convexities, in the cerebellopontine angle, or in the suprasellar region. Both x-ray CT and MRI show the cysts to have thin walls and to contain fluid. The adjacent brain parenchyma is displaced inward and the adjacent calvarium may be eroded. Cysts situated adjacent to the ventricular system may cause hydrocephalus owing to obstruction of CSF flow.

Phakomatoses

Disorders of histiogenesis, or the phakomatoses, are hereditary developmental disorders characterized by disordered ectodermal cell proliferation, both in the nervous system and in the skin.

TUBEROUS SCLEROSIS

Tuberous sclerosis is a hereditary disease with dominant inheritance and variable expression. Fibrocellular nodules or tubers are present in the cerebral cortex and in the periventricular areas. Clinically, these patients are often mentally retarded and develop epilepsy. On examination they have de-

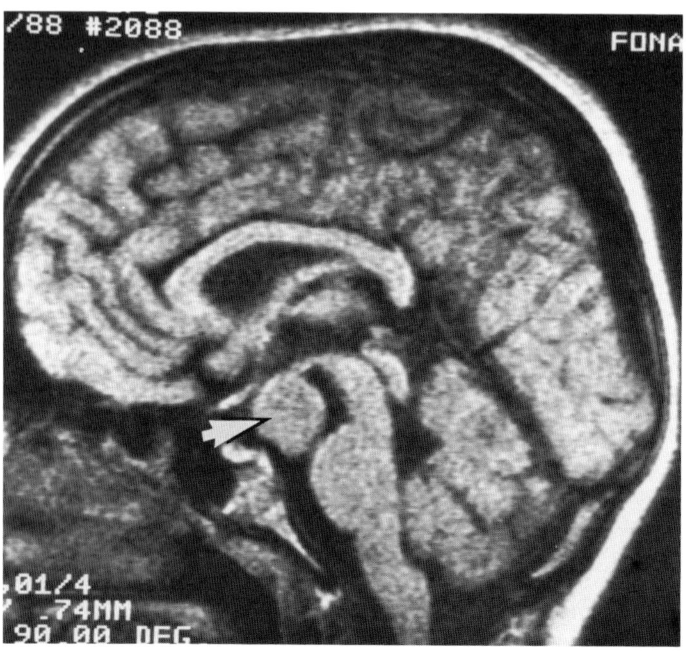

Figure 12–17. Hamartoma of the tuber cinerum. Sagittal MRI scan (SE 500/28). The isointense mass is seen in the suprasella region.

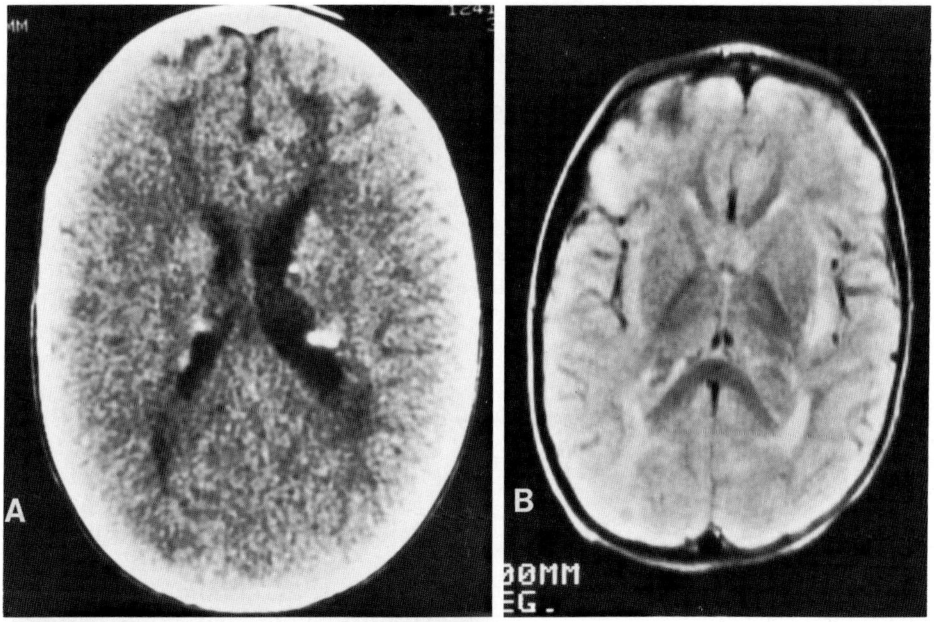

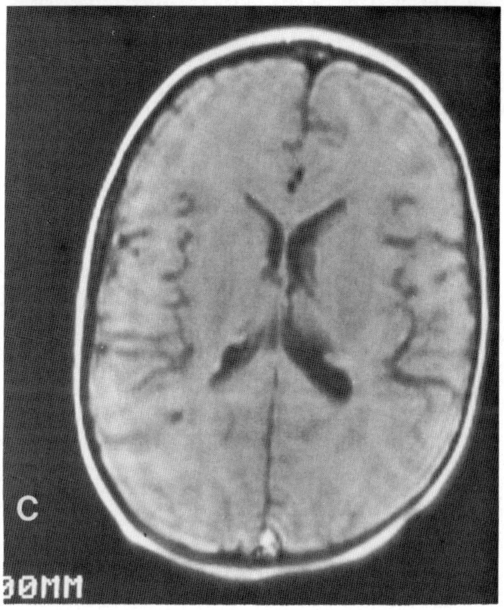

Figure 12–18. Tuberous sclerosis. (*A*) Axial x-ray CT scan demonstrates multiple periventricular calcifications. (*B*) Axial MRI scan (SE 2000/85). The high-intensity areas present in gray and white matter represent hamartomatous lesions. (*C*) Sagittal MRI scan (SE 800/30). Periventricular tubera are seen invaginating into the lateral ventricles.

pigmented nevi and sebaceous adenomas of the face. They may also have retinal phakomas, cardiac rhabdomyomas, and renal angiolipomas. Nodules may obstruct the foramen of Monro, leading to hydrocephalus, and may develop into subependymal giant-cell astrocytomas. On x-ray CT, tubers can be seen as calcified subependymal masses that do not enhance after contrast administration (Fig. 12–18). Enhancement is seen in lesions that have developed into giant-cell tumors. MRI shows the subependymal masses but is less sensitive in detecting calcification. Despite this, MRI is the study of choice for the evaluation of patients with possible tuberous sclerosis.[129,144] Because of its superior tissue-contrast differentiation, it allows identification of the plaques in the cortex and white matter that can not be well identified by x-ray CT (see Fig. 12–18). The MRI contrast agent gadolinium-DTPA (Gd-DTPA) should prove useful in the future to help identify developmental giant-cell tumors, which may occur in these patients.

NEUROFIBROMATOSIS

Neurofibromatosis is inherited in an autosomal dominant manner, occurring in 1/2500–1/3000 births. It has both peripheral and central nervous system manifestations. Peripherally, multiple, subcutaneous nerve-sheath tumors may be present.

Centrally, optic gliomas are frequently seen. Although these can be demonstrated by both x-ray CT and MRI, MRI better visualizes the intracanalicular portions of the optic nerves, and the optic chiasm. For demonstration of the optic nerves, T_1-weighted sequences should be used, owing to their superior anatomic resolution. T_2-weighted sequences are also needed, however, to demonstrate possible extension of the gliomas along the optic radiations. T_2-weighted sequences can show areas of high signal intensity within the white matter or basal ganglia regions. These areas are thought to represent hamartomatous lesions or areas of gliosis[86] (Fig. 12–19). In older children and adults, meningiomas and cranial nerve neurinomas, particularly of the acoustic nerve, are seen, but these are uncommon in younger children. Occasionally aqueductal stenosis occurs with secondary hydrocephalus detectable by x-ray CT and MRI.

The osseous dysplasia seen in some children with neurofibromatosis is unilateral involvement of the sphenoid bone. The bony changes present can be demonstrated both by x-ray CT and by MRI, but are better seen by the former.

STURGE-WEBER SYNDROME

Clinical/Pathophysiologic Background. The Sturge-Weber syndrome (SWS), in its classic form, consists of facial capillary hemangioma (port-wine stain) in the distribution of one or more divisions (usually the upper division) of the fifth cranial nerve, and ipsilateral leptomeningeal angiomatosis. The intracranial, extracerebral vascular malformation often leads to epilepsy, intracerebral calcification, and contralateral hemiparesis, hemiatrophy, and homonymous hemianopsia. Other features often associated with SWS are glaucoma and mental retardation.[1,106] The presence of facial capillary hemangioma with or without ipsilateral glaucoma does not necessarily imply SWS, a term that should be reserved for patients who also have cerebral involvement.[46]

Cerebral angiography in patients with SWS has demonstrated the variable presence of arterial thromboses, absence of cortical veins, aberrant cerebral venous drainage, and arteriovenous malformations, in addition to the characteristic leptomeningeal angioma commonly located in the posterior parietal distribution.[14,125] These findings, together with those from ^{99m}Tc-pertechnetate brain scanning studies,[87] have suggested that unilateral chronic cerebral ischemia may be at least partially accountable for ultimate cerebral calcification and cerebral cell death in SWS.[60]

Structural Imaging. Both x-ray CT and MRI can be used to define the extent of the cerebral angioma in SWS. The findings differ, depending on the age of the child at the time of scanning. Before 1-2 years of age, x-ray CT may show the affected hemisphere to be enlarged, with small arachnoid spaces and lateral ventricles. Post–contrast enhancement opacification of the angioma and adjacent hemisphere can be seen. There is ipsilateral enlargement of the choroid plexus. Alternatively, the arachnoid spaces and ipsilateral ven-

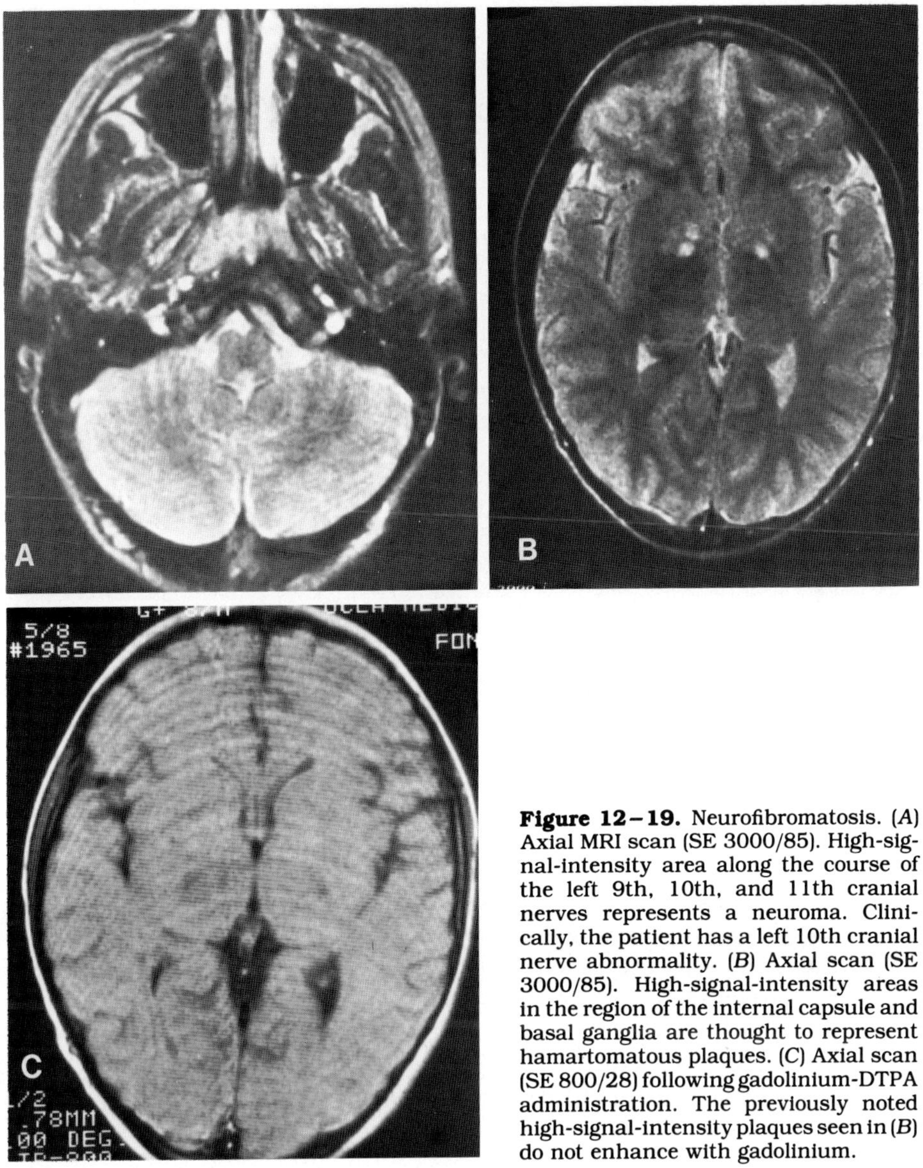

Figure 12–19. Neurofibromatosis. (*A*) Axial MRI scan (SE 3000/85). High-signal-intensity area along the course of the left 9th, 10th, and 11th cranial nerves represents a neuroma. Clinically, the patient has a left 10th cranial nerve abnormality. (*B*) Axial scan (SE 3000/85). High-signal-intensity areas in the region of the internal capsule and basal ganglia are thought to represent hamartomatous plaques. (*C*) Axial scan (SE 800/28) following gadolinium-DTPA administration. The previously noted high-signal-intensity plaques seen in (*B*) do not enhance with gadolinium.

tricle may appear enlarged, and contrast administration may enhance the involved cerebral convolutions.[46a,97a] Calcifications may be seen within the angioma. MR images obtained at this time reflect the x-ray CT findings. Two MRI studies of children less than 1 year of age with Sturge-Weber syndrome have been reported and demonstrate accelerated myelination of the involved hemisphere compared with the contralateral side.[72] These findings are thought to reflect the fact that the angiomas are richly vascularized in children under approximately 2 years of age. In older children the angioma is progressively excluded from the circulation. Large areas of calcification are seen and focal or generalized cerebral atrophy develops, probably secondary

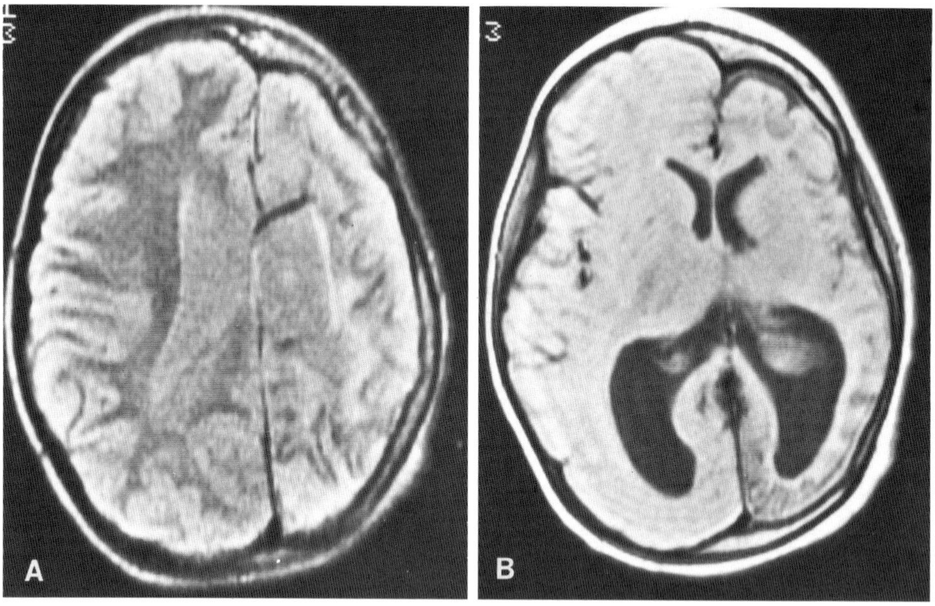

Figure 12–20. Sturge-Weber syndrome. (*A*) Axial MRI scan (SE 2000/84). Hemiatrophy of the left cerebral hemisphere with compensatory thickening of the calvarium on the ipsilateral side is identified. The lateral ventricles are enlarged bilaterally. The ribbonlike low-signal-intensity area along the sulci of the posterior parietal lobe is due to calcification. (*B*) On this T_1-weighted sequence (SE 800/28), the hemiatrophy and area of calcification are again seen. There is hypertrophy of the choroid plexus on the ipsilateral side.

to chronic ischemia and prolonged seizures (Fig. 12–20). In these older patients, both x-ray CT and MRI will show atrophy. X-ray CT better demonstrates the calcifications and MRI the vascular channels of the angioma.

Functional Imaging. In children and adults with advanced SWS, FDG-PET typically reveals widespread unilateral hypometabolism ipsilateral to the facial nevus (Fig. 12–21). In two infants less than 1 year of age with early-stage SWS, however, interictal PET revealed a pattern of widespread cerebral cortical *hyper*metabolism ipsilateral to the facial nevus (Fig. 12–22). In one of these infants, contralateral cerebellar hypermetabolism was also seen, presumably as a result of activation through crossed cerebellar connections. As the disease advanced, this infant became progressively hemiplegic, and PET, at age 3 years, revealed the typical pattern seen in older children: diffuse cerebral hypometabolism ipsilateral to the facial nevus.[28] Among six infants with the facial stigmata of SWS and no clinical evidence of neurologic involvement, five had normal PET studies of glucose metabolism, but one had hypometabolism in the right parieto-occipital region, highly suspicious for the SWS.[28]

Clinical/Pathophysiologic Correlations. The mechanisms causing increased LCMRGlc of the ipsilateral cerebral cortex and contralateral cerebellum in the young infant with newly diagnosed SWS are unclear, particularly because primary structural involvement of the cerebellum is not a feature of SWS.[2] Several possible explanations should, however, be considered. First, although the presence of epileptiform activity can result in increased LCMRGlc,[45] this is unlikely to have been the case in this interictal study because there was no evidence of seizure clinically or on EEG. Second, although anaerobic glucose metabolism, which is considerably less efficient in energy production than aerobic metab-

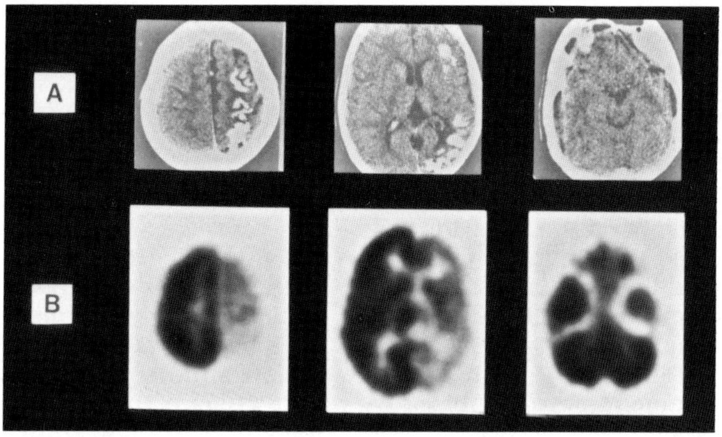

Figure 12–21. A 14-year-old girl with Sturge-Weber syndrome. Facial capillary hemangioma was present in the V1, V2, V3 distribution, neck, and shoulder. (*A*) X-ray CT showed cerebral hemiatrophy with diffuse calcification in the gyral patterns. (*B*) FDG-PET revealed severe diffuse hemispheric cortical and subcortical hypometabolism; LCMRGlc values for all regions in the right hemisphere and cerebellum were in the normal range for the patient's age.

olism, may have accounted for increased LCMRGlc in the affected cerebral hemisphere, it would not explain the increased LCMRGlc in the contralateral cerebellum, which is normally perfused in SWS.[2] Third, although accelerated myelination (see above) could account for increased LCMRGlc in the affected cerebral hemisphere, this mechanism, again, would not explain increased LCMRGlc of the contralateral cerebellum. Finally, the LCMRGlc patterns observed in this infant may be related to chronic ischemia in the affected hemisphere, causing pathways (such as the cortico-ponto-cerebellar cir-

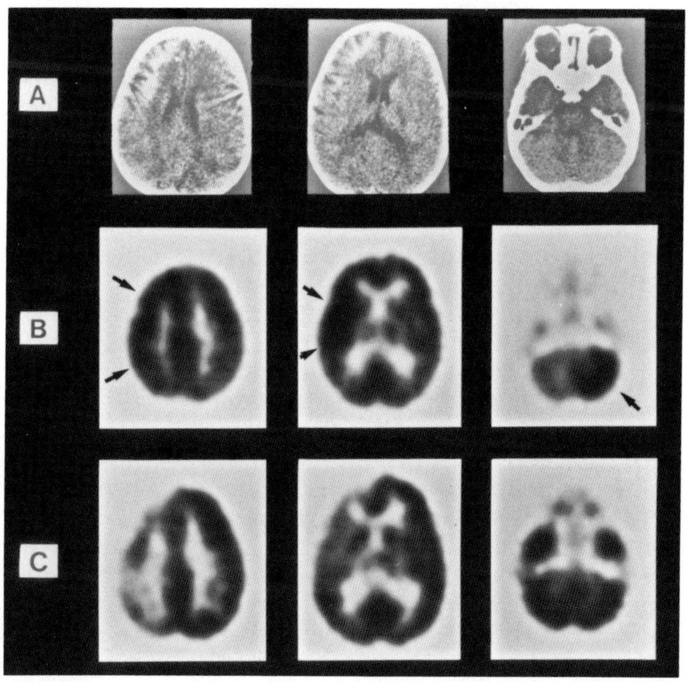

Figure 12–22. A 9-month-old infant with Sturge-Weber syndrome. Facial capillary hemangioma involved only the right ophthalmic trigeminal distribution. (*A*) X-ray CT showed early right frontal and parietal calcification (sparing the cerebellum). (*B*) FDG-PET revealed that LCMRGlc in the right hemisphere and left cerebellum exceeded control values for age (see Fig. 12–9). There was no clinical or EEG evidence of seizure during PET. (*C*) At age 3 years and 1 month, x-ray CT revealed further right hemispheric calcification, and PET showed diffuse right hemispheric hypometabolism, similar to that of the patient in Figure 12–21.

cuitry) to be episodically activated without necessarily producing a seizure.

Early diagnosis of SWS is important, since in some of these infants, cerebral hemispherectomy, if performed during the first year of life, can prevent an otherwise unremitting clinical deterioration.[63] Hemispherectomy performed after the age of 1 year in these patients is accompanied by less successful outcome with respect to intellectual function and residual motor and sensory deficit.[63] The role of PET in these patients is complementary to that of x-ray CT or MRI, which provide evidence of gross anatomic involvement, whereas PET is a sensitive tool that delineates the distribution and severity of functional impairment in specific brain regions early in the process of cerebral cell death. Together, these procedures may be used in the careful selection of suitable candidates for early hemispherectomy.[28] In addition, serial FDG-PET studies in patients with early SWS may provide important insight into the mechanisms of unilateral cerebral degeneration in this disease, and may be used as a sensitive index of disease progression when evaluating the benefits of potential medical therapies.

HYPOXIC-ISCHEMIC ENCEPHALOPATHY IN THE NEWBORN

Clinical/Pathophysiologic Background

In both preterm and term babies, hypoxic-ischemic encephalopathy from perinatal asphyxia can result in subsequent chronic neurologic disability such as cerebral palsy, mental retardation, and epilepsy.[130,147] The incidence of birth asphyxia resulting in permanent injury to the central nervous system is difficult to ascertain, but has been estimated to be 1%–5% of live births.[19,96] Epidemiologic studies, however, have suggested that perinatal asphyxia is a rare cause of cerebral palsy.[15,113] Although the incidence of intracranial (particularly intraventricular) hemorrhage is higher in preterm than in full-term infants,[147] the mortality from birth asphyxia is higher in full-term infants than in preterms.[96] Other factors significantly correlated with an adverse outcome include increasing severity of encephalopathy and the presence of intractable seizures.[49,133]

The acute management of infants with perinatal asphyxia includes the avoidance or treatment of cerebral edema to ensure adequate cerebral perfusion, suppression of seizures, and the correction of metabolic disturbances. Recently, animal studies of neonatal brain anoxia have shown that inhibition of excitatory neurotransmission in the acute phase of the insult is associated with an attenuation of cerebral edema[138] and neuronal necrosis.[137] Clinical trials in humans using this approach, however, have not yet been performed.

Structural Imaging

Ultrasonography is an important imaging modality in the newborn infant and is used in the neonatal nursery both as a screening tool for the possible presence of abnormalities and for serial imaging of visualized abnormalities. The appearances of neonatal pathology with this modality have been extensively described[50,132] and are beyond the scope of this chapter.

The uses of MRI in the evaluation of children who have had hemorrhagic and/or ischemic anoxic events have been reported recently.[36,74,76,103,104,123]

Children who have suffered anoxic-ischemic events in utero may demonstrate hemispheric defects or porencephalies. Porencephaly is a cystic malformation of the brain probably secondary to destruction and subsequent absorption of a portion of the brain parenchyma. This results in one or more cystic cavities that communicate with the ventricles and frequently with the subarachnoid space. Both x-ray CT and MRI can demonstrate these cystic cavities. Multiplanar T_1-weighted MR images are more likely to

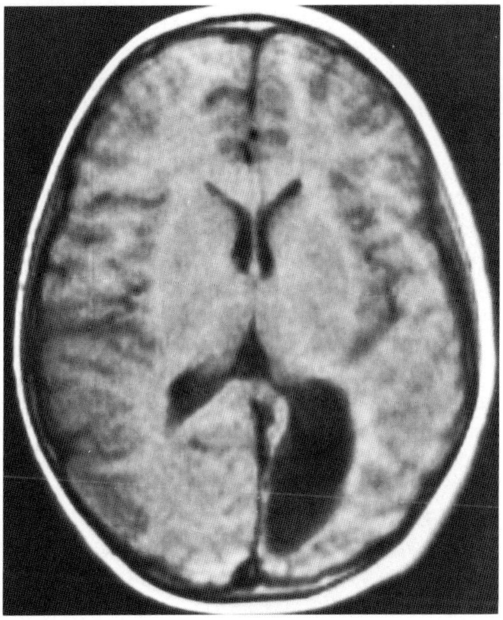

Figure 12–23. Porencephaly. Axial MRI scan (SE 800/28). Cystic cavity with the same signal intensity as CSF communicates with the posterior horn of the left lateral ventricle.

demonstrate communication of the cavity with the ventricular system than are axial CT images (Fig. 12–23). At times, however, it is not possible to differentiate porencephalic and arachnoid cysts with either modality.

Intraventricular and periventricular hemorrhage is a frequent and severe complication of prematurity. Bleeding usually occurs in the subependymal germinal matrix adjacent to the head of the caudate nucleus. The hemorrhage may rupture into the lateral ventricles and can be seen collecting in the occipital horns, fourth ventricle, and cisterna magna. Clots within the ventricular system may lead to obstruction of CSF flow. More severe cases have associated intraparenchymal hematomas. Ultrasound and x-ray CT are superior to MRI in detecting parenchymal hemorrhage in the first few days after its occurrence. After this time MRI is the single best modality for visualization of hemorrhage and is superior at all times for the identification of subdural or epidural hemorrhage[57,103,123] (Fig. 12–24). MR phase mapping techniques have been reported to improve the detection of small areas of hemorrhage in this patient population, but are not routinely used at this time, since most MRI scanners do not have the capability of obtaining these specialized images.[153]

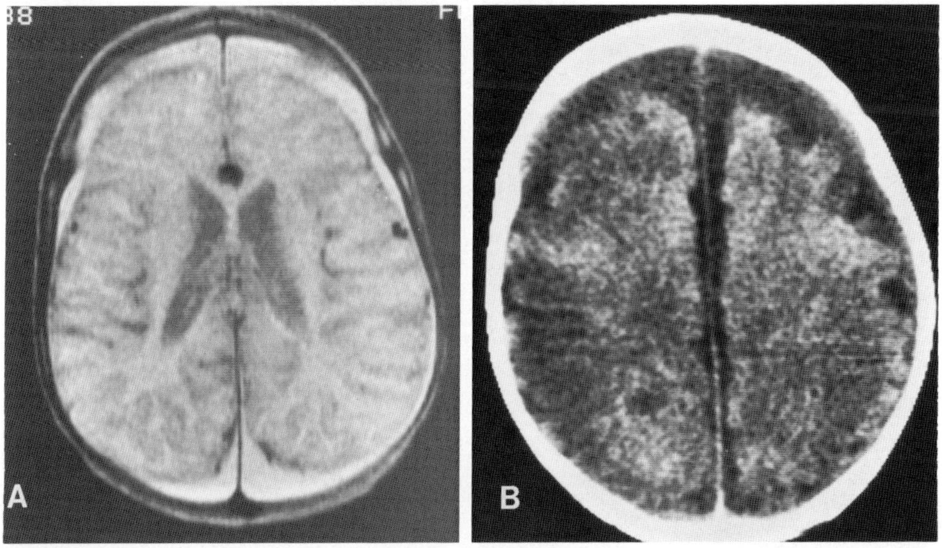

Figure 12–24. Bilateral subdural hematomas and brain infarction. (*A*) Axial MRI scan (SE 2000/84). Bilateral subdural fluid collections are identified peripherally. There is a subtle loss of the gray-white matter differentiation pattern in the left occipital region suggestive of an area of edema. (*B*) Axial x-ray CT scan demonstrates low-density areas in the parieto-occipital lobes bilaterally, consistent with a diagnosis of bilateral infarctions.

Periventricular leukomalacia may develop in premature infants with cardiorespiratory disturbances and, less commonly, in term births with congenital heart disease.[34,52,135,151] Ischemic areas develop in the watershed zones bordering the lateral ventricles, particularly around the foramen of Monro or along the course of the optic radiations.[34] In these regions ischemic necrosis is followed by development of gliosis. In more severe cases, loss of brain substance occurs. Radiographically, the borders of the dilated lateral ventricles demonstrate irregularity; in more severe cases, cystic areas may be seen in the periventricular white matter (Fig. 12–25).

In term infants, perinatal ischemic injury may lead to massive cerebral infarction. In the acute phase, this is usually manifested as diffuse cerebral edema. Both x-ray CT and MRI show compression of the lateral ventricles. X-ray CT shows the cerebral parenchyma to have diffuse edema compared with the adjacent nonischemic cerebellum and brainstem (Fig. 12–26). These findings also may be demonstrated by MRI. A case has been reported, however, in which the normal higher water content of the neonatal brain compared to that of the adult apparently masked a large acute infarction that was seen on later studies.[110] More localized areas of edema may also be difficult to detect using MRI (see Fig. 12–24).

Localized lesions in the brainstem and basal ganglia may result from prenatal or perinatal asphyxia or hypoxic-ischemic encephalopathy, and if large enough can be identified by imaging modalities. Delayed MRI studies in children with severe hypoxic ischemic episodes may show areas of gliosis in the basal ganglia regions and cortical areas. These areas may be associated with areas of low signal intensity in the basal ganglia and/or white matter that are thought to represent areas of iron

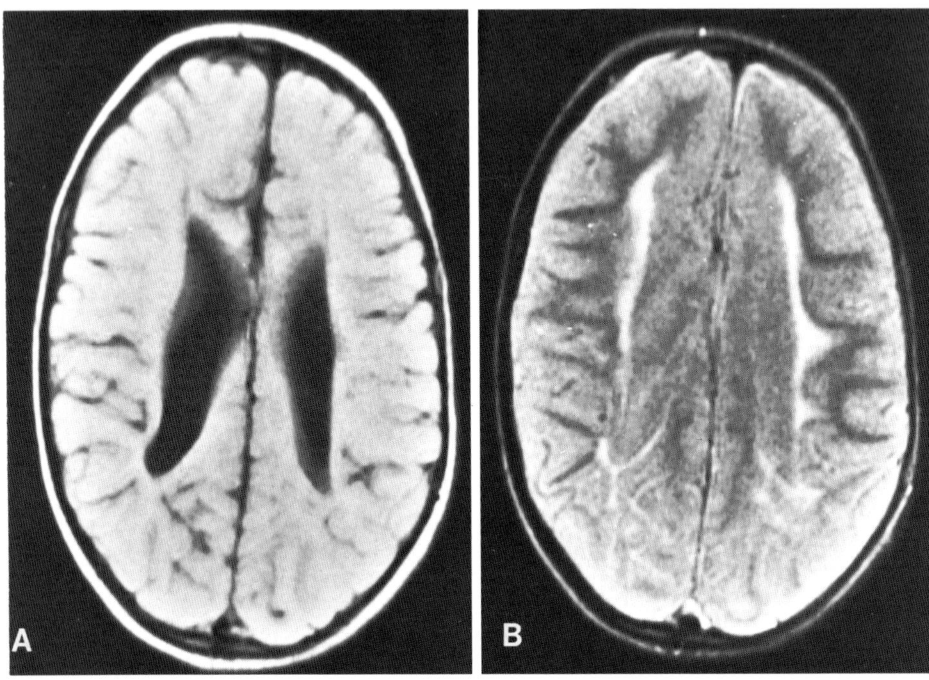

Figure 12–25. Periventricular leucomalacia. (*A*) Axial MRI scan (SE 800/30). The lateral ventricles have irregular borders. (*B*) On a T_2-weighted sequence (SE 2000/85), there is high-signal intensity bordering the irregularly shaped lateral ventricles.

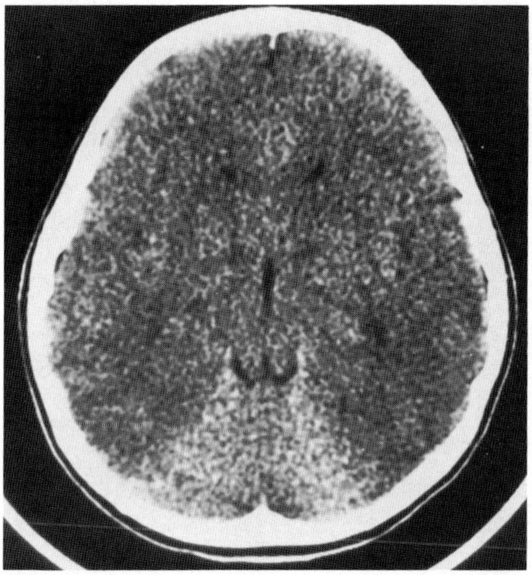

Figure 12–26. Cerebral edema. On this axial x-ray CT scan, diffuse low density is seen in the edematous cerebral hemispheres, contrasting with normal density of the cerebellum.

deposition. In some cases, calcification may also be present.[36]

Functional Imaging

Only a few studies have used PET or SPECT in the acutely asphyxiated newborn infant, partly because these infants are usually very ill and difficult to transport out of the intensive care nursery for prolonged periods.

In the very first PET measurement of glucose utilization in infants, Doyle and colleagues[11] demonstrated that the area of functional impairment (hypometabolism) in preterm infants with intraventricular hemorrhage extended beyond the regions shown on x-ray CT to be anatomically involved. Subsequent measurements of local cerebral blood flow with PET in preterm infants with intraventricular and intracerebral hemorrhage demonstrated that, in addition to a paucity of cerebral blood flow in the area of hemorrhagic involvement, blood flow throughout the affected cerebral hemisphere was markedly reduced.[145] It appeared, therefore, that in these premature infants, intracerebral hemorrhage is but one manifestation of a large ischemic infarct.

In full-term asphyxiated neonates, PET revealed that the most consistent abnormality of cerebral blood flow is a relative hypoperfusion to the parasagittal regions of the brain.[146] When studied later with FDG-PET, these children often show a pattern of LCMRGlc resembling that of a normal newborn. In other words, while brain structures that are relatively mature metabolically at birth are spared, the severe birth insult appears to halt the functional maturation of less metabolically mature brain regions (Fig. 11–27).

Recently, it was shown that following birth asphyxia, some infants may have cerebral blood flow rates of less than 10 ml/minute per 100 g and yet survive without apparent neurologic deficit.[3] The authors therefore cautioned against using blood flow criteria in establishing brain death in newborns.

Clinical/Pathophysiologic Correlations

In addition to the primary hypoxic-ischemic event in the newborn, a number of factors described in adult ischemic events during the recovery period may also play a role in causing further damage in neonates.[131] These factors include the failure to reperfuse ischemic areas after circulation has been restored (the "no-reflow phenomenon"); poor reactivity of the cerebral circulation, thus compromising oxygen delivery; and, possibly, other biochemical derangements. In order to provide effective therapeutic intervention, these and other factors must be identified and understood.

The PET studies of cerebral blood flow described above in both preterm and term infants appear to indicate an important role of impaired cerebral perfusion in causing brain damage.[145,146] In the preterm infants, a large cerebral infarct appears to be the primary event, suggesting that the intracranial hemorrhage is probably a secondary epiphen-

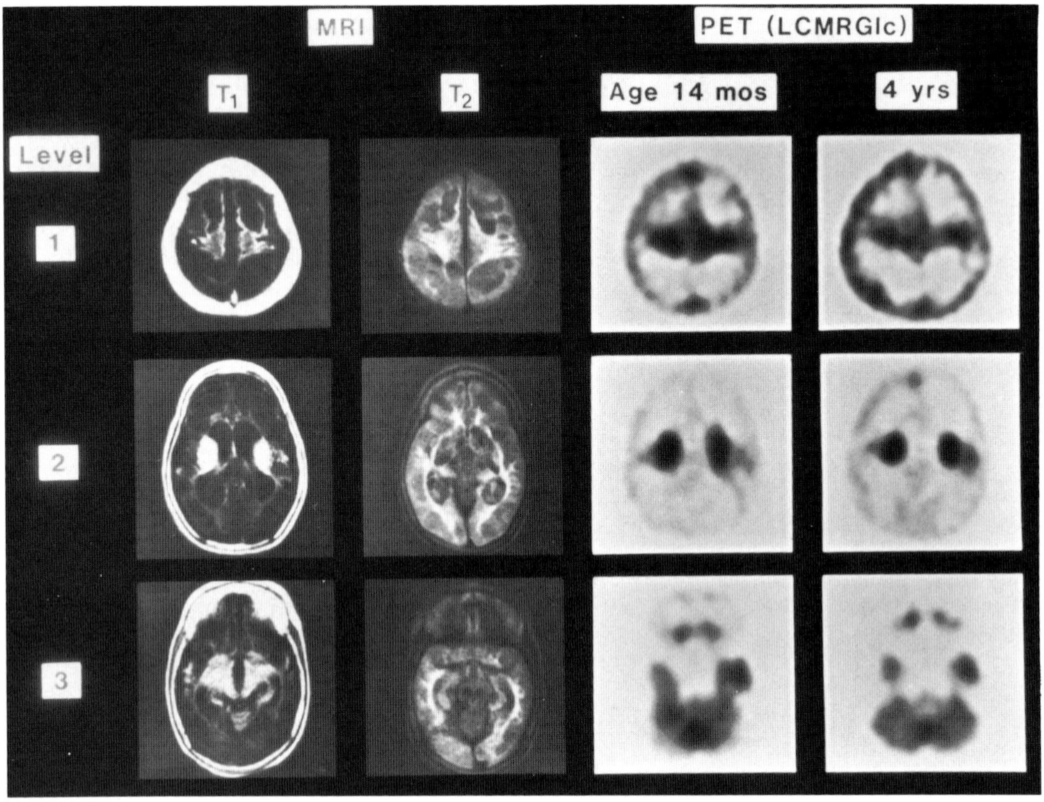

Figure 12–27. Profound psychomotor retardation following hypoxic-ischemic encephalopathy sustained at birth. Child is cortically blind, has no consistent auditory function, and suffers from seizures (for which she is given phenobarbital and valproic acid). Neurologic exam reveals generalized spasticity and persistence of primitive reflexes. MRI shows large areas of porencephaly, sparing portions of the sensorimotor cortex, thalamus, basal ganglia, brainstem, and cerebellum (particularly the vermis). FDG-PET at 14 months revealed a pattern of very low LCMRGlc throughout most of the cerebral cortex (~2 μmol per minute per 100 g), relative to higher (20–25 μmol per minute per 100 g) LCMRGlc in the thalamus and cerebellum, particularly the vermis.

omenon. In term infants, the pattern of cerebral blood flow impairment (to parasagittal brain areas) is suggestive of ischemic damage in cerebrovascular watershed areas, possibly as a result of systemic hypotension associated with perinatal asphyxia.

CHILDHOOD EPILEPSY

Epilepsy is one of the most common neurologic disorders of childhood. In this section we will primarily consider the more malignant or medically refractory forms of childhood epilepsy, since these are the types requiring alternate treatment approaches, and hence those in which new neuroimaging modalities are most widely applied. Because the partial epilepsies of childhood are similar to those occurring in adults, they are discussed in Chapter 5.

Lennox-Gastaut Syndrome

CLINICAL/PATHOPHYSIOLOGIC BACKGROUND

In 1939, Gibbs and colleagues[56] first used the term "petit mal variant" to describe the EEG pattern of a group of patients who differed both clinically and electrographically from patients with classical petit mal epilepsy. Subsequent descriptions led to the commonly used eponym "Lennox-Gastaut syndrome" to delineate a group of patients characterized by the triad of $1-2\frac{1}{2}$ Hz spike-wave pattern on EEG, some degree of intellectual impairment, and the presence of multiple seizure types, including various combinations of minor-motor, tonic-clonic, atypical absence, and partial seizures.[100]

Despite the presence of these common features, patients with Lennox-Gastaut syndrome are markedly heterogeneous with respect to etiologic factors, which may include prenatal and perinatal complications, structural abnormalities, metabolic disease, trauma, infection, and other causes.[120] Because the seizures in these patients are typically difficult to control with medical management, surgical treatment is frequently sought.

STRUCTURAL IMAGING

No study has yet been published that evaluates the ability of MRI to detect focal lesions in patients with Lennox-Gastaut syndrome. As with other types of epilepsy, MRI will probably prove to be slightly more sensitive than CT in detecting such abnormalities,[91,93,97] but still may demonstrate abnormal findings only in a small number of these patients.

In some patients with the Lennox-Gastaut syndrome, x-ray CT has identified focal lesions that have been amenable to successful surgical resection, leading to improved seizure control.[4,66] In general, however, x-ray CT scans in these patients are either normal or reveal diffuse cortical atrophy.

FUNCTIONAL IMAGING

Studies of cerebral glucose metabolism with FDG-PET in children with Lennox-Gastaut syndrome have resulted in a new classification based on metabolic anatomy. Four major metabolic subtypes have been identified (Fig. 12–28): unilateral focal hypometabolism, unilateral diffuse hypometabolism, bilateral diffuse hypometabolism, and normal pattern.[24,70,143] Unilateral focal hypometabolism in the temporal lobe had previously been reported in two adults with Lennox-Gastaut syndrome studied with PET.[58]

CLINICAL/PATHOPHYSIOGICAL CORRELATIONS

A number of patients with Lennox-Gastaut syndrome and unilateral focal hypometabolism on PET had corresponding focal epileptiform discharges on their EEGs in addition to the characteristic generalized slow spike-wave activity. X-ray CT and MRI may also show focal abnormalities such as calcification, or may be normal. These children should be further evaluated for focal resection of the epileptic focus if their seizures remain uncontrolled medically.[24]

The metabolic subtype with unilateral diffuse hypometabolism on PET often shows lateralized epileptiform discharges on EEG in addition to generalized $1-2\frac{1}{2}$ Hz spike-wave activity. If it can be demonstrated that all the seizures in these patients arise from one hemisphere, then corpus callosotomy or cerebral hemispherectomy may be considered as a means of seizure control.

Children with bilateral diffuse hypometabolism or with a normal pattern on PET would not be considered surgical candidates. Unfortunately, these groups contain the largest numbers of patients, and in one study,[143] these were the only metabolic patterns encountered. (That study contained a small number of patients, and those with focal findings on neurologic examination, x-ray CT, or EEG were excluded.) Nevertheless, new advances in neuroimaging hold great potential in the clinical management of the Lennox-Gastaut syndrome.

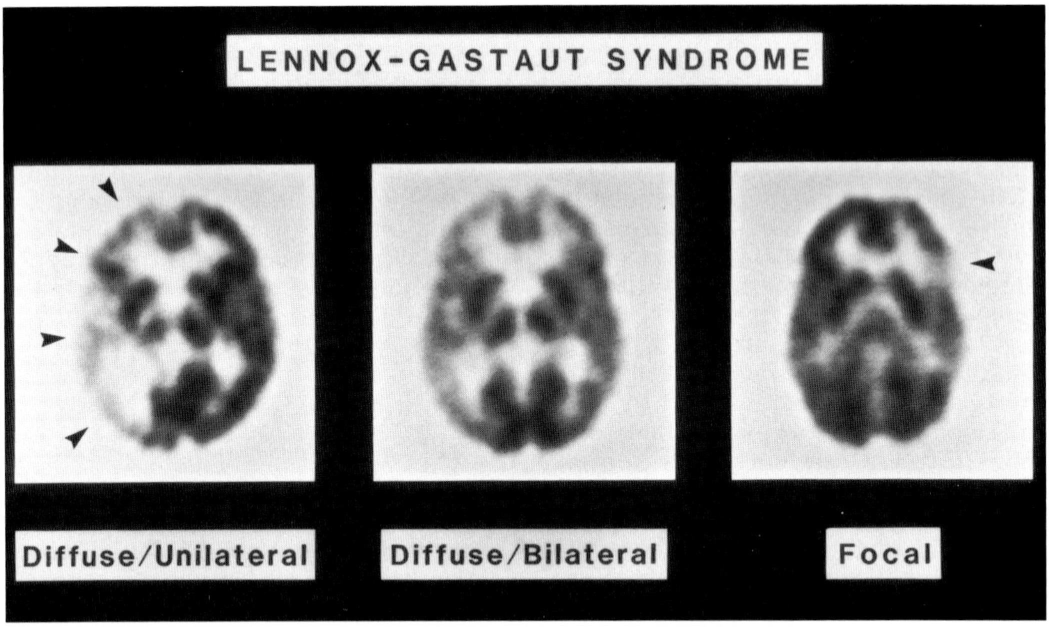

Figure 12–28. Three interictal abnormalities in the patterns of cerebral glucose utilization seen in children with Lennox-Gastaut syndrome, using FDG-PET. The child with left diffuse hypometabolism was an 8-year-old boy with normal x-ray CT and predominantly right tonic seizures, followed by transient right hemiparesis. Bilateral diffuse hypometabolism is illustrated in a 6-year-old whose CT scan demonstrated only diffuse cortical atrophy. X-ray CT of the 5-year-old boy with right posterior frontal hypometabolism revealed a small calcified lesion just lateral to the head of the right caudate nucleus, but not all patients with focal hypometabolism have a corresponding structural lesion on x-ray CT or MRI.

Infantile Spasms

CLINICAL/PATHOPHYSIOLOGIC BACKGROUND

Infantile spasms are characterized by brief flexion, extension, or mixed flexion and extension jerks of the muscles of the neck, trunk, or extremities. The disorder is age-specific, occurring typically in infants between 3 and 8 months of age.[73] Interictal EEG recordings in these infants usually reveal the pattern known as hypsarrhythmia, but during the ictal state, when clusters of spasms occur, a transient diffuse electrodecremental pattern is observed on the EEG. The etiology of infantile spasms is multifactorial, consisting of metabolic abnormalities, dysplastic or dysgenetic conditions, and a variety of prenatal, perinatal and postnatal insults. When an etiology is found, the spasms are referred to as symptomatic infantile spasms. In about 40% of patients, however, the cause is unknown; these infants are described as the cryptogenic group.[107] Although developmental delay and ultimately psychomotor retardation is the outcome in more than 90% of those with symptomatic spasms, the prognosis is far better for those in the cryptogenic group, provided treatment with ACTH or prednisone is initiated early.[107]

The hypsarrhythmic EEG pattern of patients with infantile spasms, as well as the spasms themselves, often (but not always) improve with steroid therapy rather than with conventional anticonvulsants. This suggests that infantile spasms are different from other seizure types. The lack of a topographic relationship between clinical manifestations of the spasms and EEG activity in these infants suggests that the spasms may involve subcortical regions predominantly, and hence may be more closely related to myoclonus or motor dyskinesias than to epilepsy.

STRUCTURAL IMAGING

For diagnostic and prognostic purposes, it is important to perform x-ray CT or MRI scans on all infants and children with infantile spasms. X-ray CT on 37 infants and children with infantile spasms revealed diffuse cerebral atrophy predominating in the frontotemporal regions in 30 cases.[55] Of five cases with subependymal calcification, all had tuberous sclerosis. A tumor of the basal ganglia was seen in one case. Agenesis of the corpus callosum was diagnosed in four cases. A more recent study[48] on 58 cases of infantile spasms revealed cerebral atrophy in 30 cases, calcification in 11 cases, agenesis of the corpus callosum in 3 cases, and other abnormalities in 4 cases. Normal x-ray CT scans were seen in 10 cases. Other structural abnormalities such as choroid plexus papilloma[16] and temporal lobe astrocytoma[108] have also been detected with x-ray CT. In both series,[48,55] infants and children with abnormal CT scans had a worse prognosis. There are no studies comparing x-ray CT and MRI in children with infantile spasms.

FUNCTIONAL IMAGING

FDG-PET studies in babies with cryptogenic infantile spasms have revealed a symmetric pattern in which LCMRGlc in subcortical structures such as the lenticular nuclei and brainstem are higher than in the cerebral cortex[22] (Fig. 12–29).

Babies with the symptomatic form of infantile spasms, in contrast, have additional foci of metabolic disturbances on FDG-PET that may not be visualized on x-ray CT. For example, in some infants with tuberous sclerosis, hypometabolic areas in the cerebral cortex believed to represent cortical tubers have been seen.[22] These foci of hypometabolism are similar to those demonstrated with FDG-PET in adults with tuberous sclerosis.[141] In a baby with infantile spasms who had been born prema-

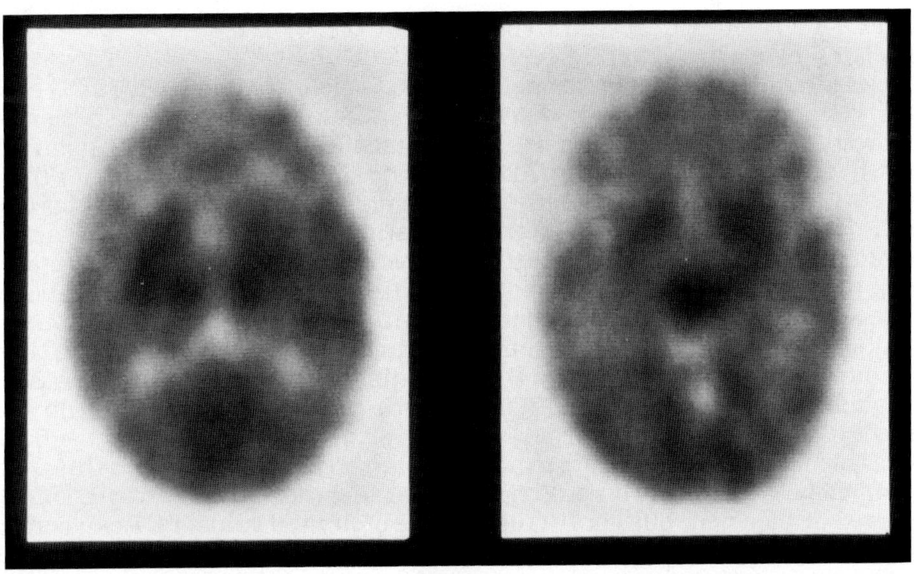

Figure 12–29. FDG-PET in a 5-month-old baby with cryptogenic infantile spasms and hypsarrhythmia. Therapy with ACTH had been instituted prior to the study, but several clusters of spasms occurred during the FDG-uptake period. Note the relatively high glucose metabolic rates in the lenticular nuclei and brainstem compared to that in the cerebral cortex.

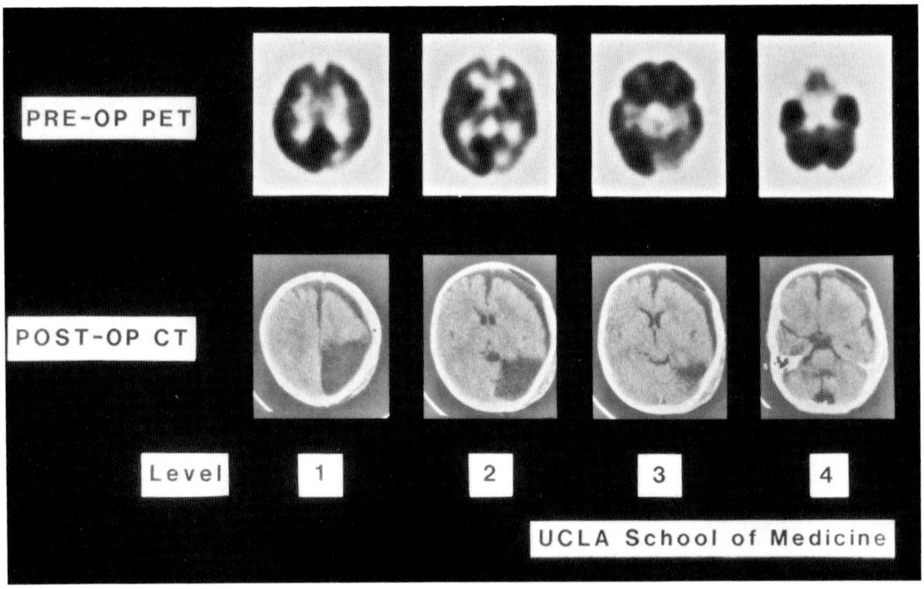

Figure 12–30. A 13-month-old girl who, following normal birth, developed seizures at 10 weeks of age. Seizures were uncontrolled and, at 6 months of age, infantile spasms developed. EEG-telemetry showed onset of seizures in right posterior temporal area. X-ray CT and MRI scans were normal. FDG-PET showed right occipitoparietal hypometabolism. Intraoperative corticography showed a right occipitoparietal focus, in agreement with PET; this focus was resected. Patient is seizure-free 2 years postoperatively and is developing normally, although a right hemianopsia is present. Pathology: hamartomatous malformation.

turely and suffered intracranial hemorrhage, PET revealed widespread hypometabolism extending well beyond structures identified as abnormal based on x-ray CT. Hamartomas in the cerebral cortex as a cause of infantile spasms have been detected with PET (Fig. 12–30) when not visualized by x-ray CT or MRI. Surgical removal of the hamartoma abolishes the infantile spasms, and results in normal subsequent development.[118] Finally, in an infant initially assigned to the cryptogenic group, PET revealed a focus in the hypothalamic region, where LCMRGlc exceeded that in all other brain regions. Because this focus of relative hypermetabolism was inaccessible, it could not be resected or biopsied, but ventriculoperitoneal shunt placement has successfully relieved the obstructive hydrocephalus, with improvement of symptoms in this infant.

CLINICAL/PATHOPHYSIOLOGIC CORRELATIONS

It is clear that PET with FDG can play a potentially useful role in patients with infantile spasms. It can assist in classifying these infants into either the cryptogenic or symptomatic subgroups, a distinction that is of clinical and prognostic relevance.[107] Furthermore, the pattern of relative hypermetabolism in lenticular nuclei and brainstem when compared to cortex in many of these infants (of both subgroups) is consistent with the notion that infantile spasms involve predominantly subcortical brain structures. Thus, in this paroxysmal disorder where x-ray CT and MRI are of limited value, PET can contribute not only to the clinical management of the patient, but also towards understanding the basic mechanisms involved in infantile spasms.

METABOLIC DISEASES

Clinical/Pathophysiologic Correlations

Included in this group of diseases are the disorders of amino acid metabolism; carbohydrate metabolism; the mucopolysaccharidoses; the mucolipidoses and disorders in glycoprotein metabolism; the organic acidurias; disorders of lipid, metal, and purine metabolism; and the peroxisomal disorders. Although many of these individual entities are rare, as a group they are widespread. Important advances have been made in recent years in the diagnosis and treatment of these diseases. A full description of each of these entities is beyond the scope of this chapter. The interested reader should consult a number of excellent reviews.[20,39,111,112]

Structural Imaging

The findings seen in metabolic disorders by both x-ray CT and MRI are relatively nonspecific. However, both modalities can often differentiate those subgroups of disease that predominantly involve the gray matter, the white matter, or the basal ganglia. In some instances a more exact diagnosis can be established based on the specific distribution of the abnormalities.

In the metabolic diseases that involve predominantly the gray matter (such as neuronal ceroid lipofuscinosis, Menke's disease, and Alper's disease), both the x-ray CT and MRI findings are nonspecific and usually show only progressive atrophy as the disease evolves.[61,62,89,134] Occasionally calcifications may be seen in the basal ganglia.[61]

In the leukodystrophies, however, as in adult white matter disorders, MRI has demonstrated unprecedented sensitivity in the detection and the demonstration of the extent of the abnormal areas of white matter.* Although demyelination or dysmyelination can be seen on x-ray CT the extent of involvement is more difficult to detect with this modality.[114] The changes in density seen on x-ray CT scans and in signal intensity seen on MR images in the areas of white matter abnormality are thought to be predominantly related to the increase in water content of these regions. MRI is extremely sensitive in demonstrating even small differences in water content of tissue. On x-ray CT scans areas of abnormal myelin and/or edema have lower density than adjacent tissue,[6,42,47,65,105,140,142] whereas on MR images the same areas demonstrate high signal intensity on T_2-weighted images, and low or isointensity on T_1-weighted images.[37,114]

In the majority of these disease entities (such as metachromatic leukodystropy, Pelizaeus-Merzbacher disease, and Krabbe's disease), the regions of high signal intensity on MRI are seen diffusely throughout the white matter[8,37,65,77,114,121,142] (Fig. 12–31).

In certain diseases within this group, a more characteristic distribution of the abnormal myelin may be seen. In MRI studies of some children with adrenoleukodystrophy, the white matter involvement is predominantly posterior in distribution, involving the occipital lobes first and progressing anteriorly with time[6,88] (Fig. 12–32). When an iodinated contrast agent or Gd-DTPA is administered to these patients, enhancement is seen only in the "leading edge," presumably where the disease process is active. By comparison, some children with Alexander's disease may demonstrate a predominantly anterior distribution of their disease[47,142] (Fig. 12–33).

In Leigh's disease, or subacute necrotizing encephalomyelopathy, x-ray CT findings consist of symmetric areas of low density in the basal ganglia, brainstem, and cerebellum. Atrophy and white matter involvement may also be present. On MRI, the same areas of involvement show high signal intensity on T_2-weighted images and low signal

*References 31, 59, 75, 88, 114, 136, 139, 154.

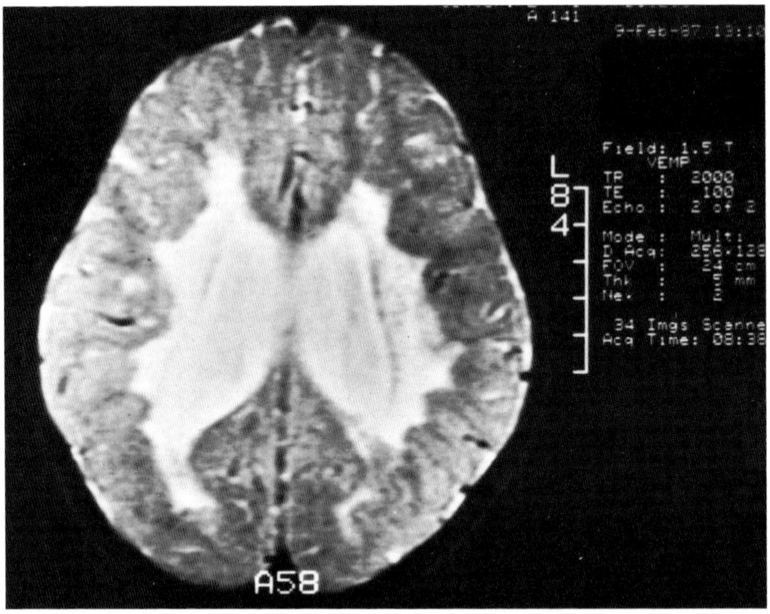

Figure 12–31. Metachromatic leukodystrophy. Axial MRI scan (SE 3000/90). High signal intensity is present in the periventricular white matter, in association with atrophy.

intensity on T_1-weighted images[31,59,137] (Fig. 12–34).

In children with mucopolysaccharidoses who demonstrate central nervous system involvement, x-ray CT and MRI again demonstrate nonspecific patterns of cerebral involvement.[75,150] Hydrocephalus, atlantoaxial subluxation, and dural thickening also may be seen.

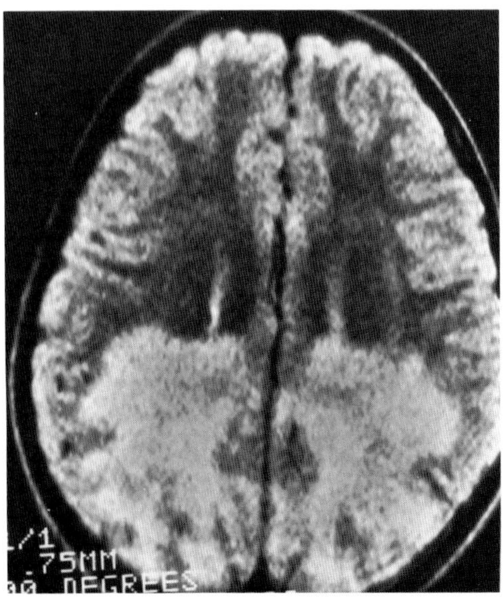

Figure 12–32. Adrenoleukodystrophy. Axial MRI scan (SE 2000/84) reveals areas of abnormal white matter that show high signal intensity in the occipitoparietal lobes.

Clinical/Pathophysiologic Correlations

In general, structural imaging in patients with metabolic disorders seldom allows a specific diagnosis to be made. This is not unexpected, since a multitude of biochemical defects affecting the central nervous system all can lead to similar gross degenerative changes. In some cases, however, (for example, the leukodystrophies), the distribution of abnormalities can be quite revealing, as discussed above. Even so, recent studies have shown that the severity of the disease process as graded by MRI does not correlate well with the clinical severity of disease.[38]

The biochemical errors that are known can potentially be studied with PET or SPECT as more specific radiolabeled probes become available. Some

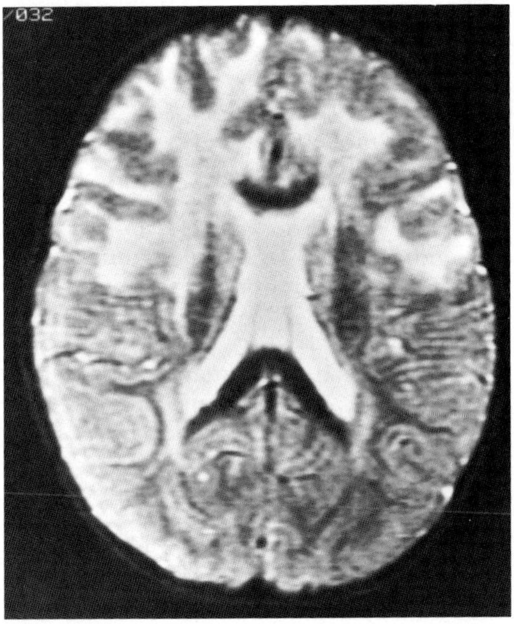

Figure 12–33. Alexander's disease. Axial MRI scan (SE 2000/85). The abnormal white matter is predominantly anterior in distribution.

tracers, such as ^{11}C-pyruvate, have already been synthesized and theoretically should be useful in the study of pyruvate and lactate metabolic disorders.

PRACTICAL CONSIDERATIONS

As imaging technology becomes increasingly complex, it becomes essential for patients to be able to cooperate by remaining still for the longer periods of time needed to obtain images. This is especially a problem when dealing with infants and with older children who are mentally retarded. It is often helpful to explain the procedure to the child in advance. When children are particularly apprehensive about the study, parents should be encouraged to stay with the child to give reassurance. Frequently, it is necessary to sedate children under age 7 years who are undergoing MRI, and under age 5 who are undergoing x-ray CT. At UCLA, children under 18 months of age are given chloral hydrate (75 mg/kg) orally 30 minutes before imaging. Children over 18 months of age initially are given thiopental (25 mg/kg) rectally 5 minutes before imaging. If sedation is not achieved by 15 minutes, a half-dose is repeated.

Devices are now available that provide respiratory, cardiac, and temperature monitoring during the study. In sedated patients who are medically

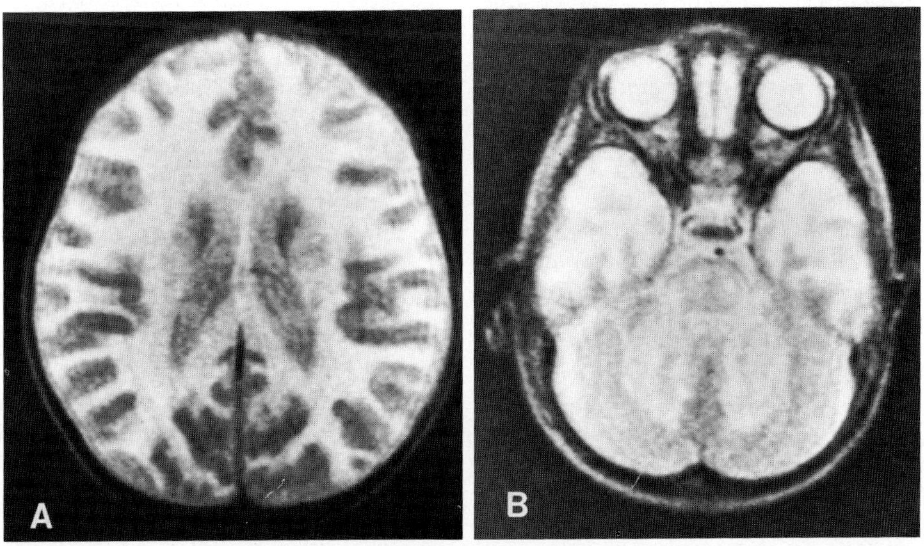

Figure 12–34. Leigh's disease, shown in axial MRI scans (SE 2000/85). (*A*) Scan through the basal ganglia reveals high signal intensity throughout the white matter and in the lentiform nuclei. (*B*) Scan through the posterior fossa shows abnormal areas of high signal intensity in the dentate nuclei.

stable, respiratory monitoring with an apnea monitor is sufficient. Alternatively, an inverted paper cup placed on the abdomen demonstrates excursion of the anterior abdominal wall with respiration and can easily be observed from outside the scanner.

It is imperative that initial scan sequences yield maximum information, since the study may have to be terminated if the child awakens or is unable to remain still. Therefore, it is important to tailor the scan in order to detect the abnormalities most suspected from the clinical history.

REFERENCES

1. Alexander, GL and Norman, RM: The Sturge-Weber syndrome. John Wright, Bristol, England, 1960.
2. Alexander, GL: Sturge-Weber syndrome. In Vinken, PJ and Bruyn, GW (eds): Handbook of Clinical Neurology, Vol 14. North-Holland, Amsterdam, 1972, pp 223–240.
3. Altman, DI, Powers, WJ, Perlman, JM, Herscovitch, P, Volpe, SL, and Volpe, JJ: Cerebral blood flow requirement for brain viability in newborn infants is lower than in adults. Ann Neurol 24:218–226, 1988.
4. Angelini, L, Broggi, G, Riva, D, and Solero, CL. A case of Lennox-Gastaut syndrome successfully treated by removal of a parietotemporal astrocytoma. Epilepsia 20:665–669, 1979.
5. Atlas, SW, Zimmerman, RA, Bilaniuk, LT, Rorke, L, Hackney, DB, Goldberg, HI, and Grossman, RI. Corpus callosum and limbic system: Neuroanatomic MR evaluation of developmental anomalies. Radiology 160:355–362, 1986.
6. Aubourg, P and Diebler, C. Adrenoleucodystrophy. Its diverse CT appearances and an evolutive or phenotypic variant: The leucodystrophy without adrenal insufficiency. Neuroradiology 24:33–42, 1982.
7. Bairamian, D, Di Chiro, G, Theodore, WH, Holmes, MD, Dorwart, RH, and Larson, SM: MR imaging and positron emission tomography of cortical heterotopia. J Comput Assist Tomogr 9:1137–1139, 1985.
8. Baram, TZ, Goldman, AM, and Percy, AK. Krabbe Disease: Specific MRI and CT findings. Neurology 36:111–115, 1986.
9. Barkovich, AJ, Kjos, BO, Jackson, DE, and Norman, D: Normal maturation of the neonatal and infant brain: MR imaging at 1.5 T. Radiology 166:173–180, 1988.
10. Barkovich, AJ, Chuang, SH, and Norman, D: MR of neuronal migration anomalies. AJNR 8:1009–1017, 1987.
11. Barkovich, AJ and Norman, D: MR imaging of schizencephaly. AJNR 9:297–302, 1988.
12. Barth, PG: Disorders of neuronal migration. Can J Neurol Sci 14: 1–16, 1987.
13. Benjamins, JA and McKhann, GM: Development, regeneration, and aging of the brain. In Siegal, GJ, Albers, RW, Agranoff, BW, and Katsman, R (eds): Basic Neurochemistry. Little, Brown & Co., Boston, 1981, pp 445–469.
14. Bentson, JR, Wilson, GH, and Newton, TH: Cerebral venous drainage pattern of the Sturge-Weber syndrome. Radiology 101:111–118, 1971.
15. Blair, E and Stanley, FJ: Intrapartum asphyxia: A rare cause of cerebral palsy. J Pediatr 112:515–519, 1988.
16. Branch, CE and Dyken, PR: Choroid plexus papilloma and infantile spasms. Ann Neurol 5:302–304, 1979.
17. Brant-Zawadski, M and Enzymann, DR: Using computed tomography of the brain to correlate low white-matter attenuation with early gestational age in neonates. Radiology 139:105–108, 1981.
18. Brody, BA, Kloman, AC, and Gilles, FH: An autopsy study of infant myelination. J Neuropathol Exp Neurol 46 (3):283–301, 1987.
19. Brown, JK, Purvis, RJ, Forfar, JO, and Cockburn, F: Neurological aspects of perinatal asphyxia. Dev Med Child Neurol 16:567–580, 1974.
20. Burton, BK: Inborn errors of metabolism: The clinical diagnosis in early infancy. Pediatrics 79:359–369, 1987.

21. Changeux JP and Danchin, A: Selective stabilization of developing synapses as a mechanism for the specification of neuronal networks. Nature 264:705–712, 1976.
22. Chugani, HT and Engel, J Jr: PET in intractable epilepsy. In Schmidt, D, Morselli, PL (eds): Intractable epilepsy: Experimental and clinical aspects. Raven Press, New York, 1986, pp 119–128.
23. Chugani, HT and Phelps, ME: Maturational changes in cerebral function in infants determined by [18]FDG positron emission tomography. Science 231: 840–843, 1986.
24. Chugani, HT, Mazziotta, JC, Engel, J Jr, and Phelps, ME: Lennox-Gastaut syndrome: Metabolic subtypes determined by 18FDG positron emission tomography. Ann Neurol 21:4–13, 1987.
25. Chugani, HT, Phelps, ME, and Mazziotta, JC: Positron emission tomography study of human brain functional development. Ann Neurol 22:487–497, 1987.
26. Chugani, HT and Phelps, ME: PET in children with seizures. Applied Radiology 17:37–49, 1988.
27. Chugani, HT, Shewmon, DA, Peacock, WJ, Shields, WB, Mazziotta, JC, and Phelps, ME: Surgical treatment of intractable neonatal onset seizures: The role of positron emission tomography. Neurology 38:1178–1188, 1988.
28. Chugani, HT, Mazziotta, JC, and Phelps, ME: Sturge-Weber syndrome: A study of cerebral glucose utilization with positron emission tomography. J Pediatr 114:244–253, 1989.
29. Cowan, WM, Fawcett, JW, O'Leary, DDM, and Stanfield, BB: Regressive events in neurogenesis. Science 225: 1258–1265, 1984.
30. Crelin, ES: Development of the nervous system. Clinical Symposia (Ciba) 26 (2), 1974.
31. Davis, PC, Hoffmann, JC Jr, Braun, IF, Ahmann, P, and Krawiecki, N. MR of Leigh's disease (subacute necrotizing encephalomyelopathy): AJNR 8:71–5, 1987.
32. Davison, AN: Myelination and diseases of the nervous system: Abnormalities of myelin composition. In: Myelination. Charles C. Thomas, Springfield, IL 1970, pp 163–183.
33. Deeb, ZL, Rothfus, WE, and Maroon, JC: Case report. MR imaging of heterotopic gray matter. J Comput Assist Tomogr 9:1140–1141, 1985.
34. De Reuck, J, Chatha, AS, and Richardson, EP: Pathogenesis and evolution of periventricular leukomalacia in infancy. Arch Neurol 27:220–236, 1972.
35. Dietrich, RB, Bradley, WG, Zaragoza, EJ, Otto, RJ, Taira, RK, Wilson, GH, Kangarloo, H: MR evaluation of early myelination patterns in normal and developmentally delayed infants. AJNR 9:69–76, 1988.
36. Dietrich, RB, Bradley, WG: Iron accumulation in the basal ganglia following severe ischemic-anoxic insults in children. Radiology 168:203–206, 1988.
37. Dietrich, RB and Bradley, WG. Normal and abnormal white matter maturation. Semin U/S, CT and MR 9:192–200, 1988.
38. Dietrich, RB, Vining, EP, Philapart, M, Hall, TR, and Kangarloo, H: Myelin disorders of childhood: Correlation of MR findings and severity of neurological impairment. Magnetic Resonance Imaging 7:21, 1989.
39. Dimauro, S, Bonilla, E, Zeviani, M, Nakaeawa, M, and Devivo, DC: Mitochondrial myopathies. Ann Neurol 17:521–538, 1985.
40. Dobbing, J and Sands, J: Quantitative growth and development of human brain. Arch Dis Child 48:757–767, 1973.
41. Doyle, LW, Nahmias, C, Firnau, G, Kenyon, DB, Garnett, ES, and Sinclair, JC: Regional cerebral glucose metabolism of newborn infants measured by positron emission tomography. Develop Med Child Neurol 25:143–151, 1983.
42. Duda, FF and Huttenlocher, PR. Computed tomography in adenoleucodystrophy: Correlation of radiological and histological findings. Radiology 120: 349–350, 1976.
43. Duffy, CJ and Rakic, P: Differentiation of granule cell dendrites in the dentrate gyrus of the rhesus monkey: A quantita-

tive Golgi study. J Comp Neurol 214:224–237, 1983.

44. Easter, SS Jr, Purves, D, Rakic, P, and Spitzer, NC: The changing view of neural specificity. Science 230:507–511, 1985.
45. Engel, J Jr, Kuhl, DE, Phelps, ME, Rausch, R, and Nuwer, M: Local cerebral metabolism during partial seizures. Neurology 33:400–413, 1983.
46. Enjolras, O, Riche, MC, and Merland, JJ: Facial port-wine stains and Sturge-Weber syndrome. Pediatrics 76:48–51, 1985.

46a. Enzman, DE, Hayward, RW, and Norman, D: Cranial computed tomographic scan appearance of Sturge-Weber disease: Unusual presentation. Radiology 122:721–723, 1977.

47. Farrell K, Chuang, S, and Becker, LE. Computed tomography in Alexander's disease. Ann Neurol 15:605–607, 1984.
48. Favata, I, Leuzzi, V, and Curatolo, P: Mental outcome in West syndrome: Prognostic value of some clinical factors. J Mental Def Res 31:9–15, 1987.
49. Finer, NN, Robertson, CM, Peters, KL, and Coward, JH: Factors affecting outcome in hypoxic-ischemic encephalopathy in term infants. Am J Dis Child 137:21–25, 1983.
50. Fischer, AQ, Anderson, JC, Shuman, RM, and Stinson, W: Pediatric Neurosonography: Clinical, Tomographic, and Neuropathologic Correlates. John Wiley & Sons, New York, 1985.
51. Fishman, MA, Agrawal, HC, Alexander, A, et al: Biochemical maturation of human central nervous system myelin. J Neurochem 24:689–694, 1975.
52. Flodmark, O, Roland, E, Hill, A, and Whitfield, M: Periventricular leukomalacia: Radiologic diagnosis. Radiology 162:119–124, 1987.
53. Freeman, JM (ed): Prenatal and Perinatal Factors Associated with Brain Disorders. NIH Publication No. 85–1149, 1985.
54. Fritz, CR, Holoprosencephaly and related entities. Neuroradiology 25:225–238, 1983.
55. Gastaut, H, Gastaut, JL, Regis, H, Bernard, R, Pinsard, N, Saint-Jean, M, Roger, J, and Dravet, C: Computerized tomography in the study of West's syndrome. Dev Med Child Neurol 20:21–27, 1978.
56. Gibbs, FA, Gibbs, EL, and Lennox, WG: The influence of blood sugar level on the wave and spike formation in petit mal epilepsy. Arch Neurol Psychiatry 41:1111–1116, 1939.
57. Gomori, J, Grossman, R, Goldberg, H, Hackney, D, Zimmerman, R, and Bilaniuk, L: High-field spin-echo MR imaging of superficial and subependymal siderosis secondary to neonatal intraventricular hemorrhage. Neuroradiology 29:339– 342, 1987.
58. Gur, RC, Sussman, NM, Alavi, A, Gur, RE, Rosen, AD, O'Connor, M, Goldberg, HI, Greenberg, JH, and Reivich, M: Positron emission tomography in two cases of childhood epileptic encephalopathy (Lennox-Gastaut syndrome). Neurology 32:1191–1195, 1982.
59. Hall, K, and Gardner-Medwin, D. CT scan appearances in Leigh's disease (subacute necrotizing encephalomyelopathy). Neuroradiology 16:48–50, 1978.
60. Han, J, Benson, J, Kaufman, B, Rekate, H, Alfidi, R, Huss, R, Sacco, D. Yoon, Y, and Morrison, S. MR imaging of pediatric cerebral abnormalities. J Comput Assist Tomogr 9: 1985.
61. Hart, ZH, Cang, CH, and Perrin, EUD. Familial poliodystrophy, mitochondrial myopathy and lactate acidemia. Arch Neurol 34:180–185, 1977.
62. Heiman-Patterson, TD, Bonilla, E, and Di Mauro, S. Cytochrome-c-oxidase in a floppy child. Neurology 32:898–900, 1982.
63. Hoffman, HJ, Hendrick, EB, Dennis, M, and Armstrong, D: Hemispherectomy for Sturge-Weber syndrome. Child's Brain 5:233–248, 1979.
64. Holland, B, Haas, D, Norman, D, Brant-Zawadski, M, and Newton, T: MRI of normal brain maturation. AJNR 7:201–208, 1986.
65. Holland, JM and Kendall, BE. Computed tomography in Alexander's disease. Neuroradiology 20:103–106, 1980.
66. Hooshmand, H: EEG and akinetic sei-

zures. Electroencephalogr Clin Neurophysiol 38:335, 1975.

67. Huttenlocher, PR: Synaptic density in human frontal cortex: Developmental changes and effects of aging. Brain Res 163:195–205, 1979.
68. Huttenlocher, PR and de Courten, C: The development of synapses in striate cortex of man. Human Neurobiol 6:1–9, 1987.
69. Hwang, PA, Gilday, DL, Ash, JM, Vimutisnthorn, J, Lambert R, Piatt, J, Hoffman, HJ, Logan, WJ, Haslam, RH: Perturbations in regional cerebral blood flow detected by SPECT scanning with 99m Tc-HmPAO correlate with EEG abnormalities in children with epilepsy. J Cereb Blood Flow Metabol (Suppl 1)7:S573, 1987.
70. Inuma, K, Yanai, K, Yanagisa, T, Fueki, N, Tada, K, Ito, M, Matsuzawa, T, and Ido, T: Cerebral glucose metabolism in five patients with Lennox-Gastaut Syndrome. Pediatr Neurol 3:12–18, 1987.
71. Jacobson, M: Developmental Neurobiology, ed 2. Plenum Press, New York, 1978, pp 302–307.
72. Jacoby, C, Yuh, W, Afifi, A, Bell, W, Schelper, R, and Sato, Y: Accelerated myelination in early Sturge-Weber syndrome demonstrated by MR imaging. J Comput Assist Tomogr 11:226–231, 1987.
73. Jeavons, PM and Bower, BD: Infantile spasms: A review of the literature and a study of 112 cases. Clin Dev Med 15:1–79, 1964.
74. Johnson, M, Pennock, J, Bydder, G, Steiner, R, Thomas, D, Hayward, R, Bryant, D, Payne, J, Levene, M, Whitelaw, A, Dubowitz, L, and Dubowitz, V: Clinical NMR imaging of the brain in children: Normal and neurologic disease. AJR 141:1005–1018, 1983.
75. Johnson, MA, Desai, S, Hugh-Jones, J, and Starer, F: MR imaging of the brain in Hurlers syndrome, AJNR 5:816–819, 1984.
76. Johnson, MA, Pennock, J, Bydder, GM, Dubowitz, L, Thomas, D, and Young, I: Serial MR imaging in neonatal cerebral injury. AJNR 8:83–92, 1987.
77. Journel, H, Roussey, M, Gandon, Y, Allaire, C, Carsin, M, and Le Marec, B: Magnetic resonance imaging in Pelizaeus-Merzbacher disease. Neuroradiology 29:403–405, 1987.
78. Kadekaro, M, Crane, AM, and Sokoloff, L: Differential effects of electrical stimulation of sciatic nerve on metabolic activity in spinal cord and dorsal root ganglion in the rat. Proc Natl Acad Sci USA 82:6010–6013, 1985.
79. Kagan, J: Emergent themes in human development. American Scientist 64:186–196, 1976.
80. Kalifa, G, Chiron, C, Sellier, N, Demange, P, Ponsot, G, Lalande, G, and Robain, O: Hemimegalencephaly: MR imaging in five children. Radiology 165:29–33, 1987.
81. Kendall, B: Dysgenesis of the corpus callosum. Neuroradiology 25:239–256, 1983.
82. Kennedy, C, Sokoloff, L: An adaptation of the nitrous oxide method to the study of the cerebral circulation in children: Normal values for cerebral blood flow and cerebral metabolic rate in childhood. J Clin Invest 36:1130–1137, 1957.
83. Kennedy, C, Sakurada, O, Shinohara, M, and Miyaoka, M: Local cerebral glucose utilization in the newborn macaque monkey. Ann Neurol 12:333–340, 1982.
84. Kerrigan, JF, Chugani, HT, Mazziotta, JC, and Phelps, ME: Patterns of cerebral glucose utilization in cerebral palsy. Neurology (Suppl 1) 30:276, 1989.
85. Kety, SS: Measurement of local blood flow by the exchange of an inert, diffusible substance. Methods Med Res 8:228–236, 1960.
86. Kortman, K and Bradley, WG: Supratentorial neoplasms. In Stark, DD and Bradley, WG (eds): Magnetic Resonance Imaging. CV Mosby, St. Louis, 1988, pp 375–413.
87. Kuhl, DE, Bevilacqua, JE, Mishkin, MM, and Sanders, TP: The brain scan in Sturge-Weber syndrome. Radiology, 103:621–626, 1972.
88. Kumar, AJ, Rosenbaum, AE, and Naidu, S: Adrenoleukodystrophy: Correlating MR imaging with CT. Radiology 165:497–504, 1987.

89. Langenstein, I, Schwendemann, G, and Kuhne, D. Neuronal lipofuscinosis: CCT findings in fourteen patients. Acta Paediatr Scand 70:857–860, 1981.
90. Larroche, JC: Developmental pathology of the neonate. Excerpta Medica (Amsterdam) :319, 1977.
91. Laster, D, Penry, J, Moody, D, Ball M, Witcofski R, and Riela A: Chronic seizure disorders: Contribution of MR imaging when CT is normal. AJNR 6:177–180, 1985.
92. Lee, B, Lipper, E, Nass, R, Ehrlich, M, Ciccio-Bloom, E, and Auld, P: MRI of the central nervous system in neonates and young children. AJNR 7:605–616, 1986.
93. Lesser, R, Modic, M, Weinstein, M, Duchesneau, P, Luders, H, Dinner, D, Morris, H, Estes, M, Chou, S, and Hahn, J: Magnetic resonance imaging (1.5 Tesla) in patients with intractable focal seizures. Arch Neurol 43:367–371, 1986.
94. Lucas-Keene, MF, and Hewer, EE: Some observations of myelination in the human central nervous system. J Anat 6:1–13, 1931.
95. Lund, JS, Boothe, RG, and Lund, RD: Development of neurons in the cerebral cortex (area 17) of the monkey (Macaca nemestrina): A Golgi study from fetal day 127 to postnatal maturity. J Comp Neurol 176:149–188, 1977.
96. MacDonald, HM, Mulligan, JC, Allen, AC, and Taylor, PM: Neonatal asphyxia. I. Relationship of obstetric and neonatal complications to neonatal mortality in 38,405 consecutive deliveries. J Pediatr 96:898–902, 1980.
97. Maiertens, P, Machen, B, Williams, J, Evans, O, Bebin, J, Bassam, B and Lum, G: Magnetic resonance imaging of mesial temporal sclerosis: Case reports. J Comput Assist Tomogr 11:136–139, 1987.
97a. Maki, Y and Semba, A: Computed tomography in Sturge-Weber disease. Child's Brain 5:51–56, 1979.
98. Martin, E, Kikinis, R, Zverrer, M, Boesch, C, Briner, J, Kewitz, G, and Kaelin, P: Developmental stages of human brain: An MR study. J Comput Assist Tomogr 12:917–922, 1988.
99. Mata, M, Fink, DJ, Gainer, H, Smith, CB, Davidsen, L, Savaki, H, Schwartz, WJ, Sokoloff, L: Activity-dependent energy metabolism in rat posterior pituitary primarily reflects sodium pump activity. N Neurochem 34:213–215, 1980.
100. Markand, ON: Slow spike-wave activity in EEG and associated clinical features: Often called "Lennox" or "Lennox-Gastaut" syndrome. Neurology 27:746–757, 1977.
101. McArdle, C, Richardson, C, Nicholas, D, Mirfakhraee, M, Hayden, C, and Amparo, E: Developmental features of the neonatal brain: MR imaging, Part I. Gray-white matter differentiation and myelination. Radiology 162:223–229, 1987.
102. McArdle, C, Richardson, C, Nicholas, D, Mirfakhraee, M, Hayden, C, and Amparo, E: Developmental features of the neonatal brain: MR imaging, Part II. Ventricular size and extracerebral space. Radiology 162:223–229, 1987.
103. McArdle, C, Richardson, C, Hayden, C, Nicholas, D, Crofford, M, and Amparo, E: Abnormalities of the neonatal brain: MR imaging, Part I. Intracranial hemorrhage. Radiology 1987.
104. McArdle, C, Richardson, C, Hayden, C, Nicholas, D, Crofford, M and Amparo, E: Abnormalities of the neonatal brain: MR imaging, Part II. Hypoxic-ischemic brain injury. Radiology May 1987.
105. Mcfaul, R, Cavanagh, N, Lake, BD. Metachromatic leukodystrophy: Review of 38 cases. Arch Dis Child 57:168–175, 1982.
105a. McMurdo Jr., S, Moore S, Brant-Zawadski M, Berg B, Koch T, Newton T, Edwards M: MR imaging of intracranial tuberous sclerosis. AJR 148:791–796, April 1987.
106. Menkes, JH: Textbook of Child Neurology, ed 3. Lea & Febiger, Philadelphia, 1985, pp 575–578.
107. Millichap, JG, Bickford, RG, Klass, DW, and Backus, RE: Infantile spasms, hypsarrhythmia, and mental retardation. A study of etiologic factors in 61 patients. Epilepsia 3:188–197, 1962.
108. Mimaki, T, Ono, J, and Yabuuchi, H: Temporal lobe astrocytoma with infan-

tile spasms. Ann Neurol 14:695–696, 1983.

109. Mintz, MC, Grossman, RI, Isaacsong, et al: MR imaging of fetal brain. J Comp Assist Tomogr 11:120–123, 1987.

110. Moore, J, Parker, C, Smith, R, and Goethe, B: Concealment of neonatal cerebral infarction of MRI by normal brain water. Pediatr Radiol 17:314–315, 1987.

111. Moser, HW, Moser, AB, Singh, I, and O'Neill, BP: Adrenoleukodystrophy: Survey of 303 cases: Biochemistry, diagnosis, and therapy. Ann Neurol 16:628–641, 1984.

112. Moser, HW: The peroxisome: Nervous system role of a previously underrated organelle. Neurology 38:1617–1627, 1988.

113. Nelson, KB and Ellenberg, JH: Antecedents of cerebral palsy: Multivariate analysis of risk. N Engl J Med 315:81–86, 1986.

114. Nowell, MA, Grossman, RI, Hackney, DB, Zimmerman, RA, Goldberg, HI, and Bilaniuk, LT: MR imaging of white matter disease in children. AJNR 9:503–509, 1988.

115. Nowell, M, Hackney, D, Zimmerman, R, Bilaniuk, L, Grossman, R, and Goldberg, H: Immature brain: Spin-echo pulse sequence parameters for high-contrast MR imaging. Radiology 162:272–273, 1987.

116. Nudo, RJ and Masterton, RB: Stimulation-induced [14C]2-deoxyglucose labeling of synaptic activity in the central auditory system. J Comp Neurol 245:553–565, 1986.

117. O'Dwyer, A, Newton, T and Hoyt, W: Radiologic features of septooptic dysplasia de Morsier syndrome. AJNR 1:443–447, 1980.

118. Olson, DM, Chugani, HT, Peacock, WJ, Shewmon, DA, Peacock, WJ, and Phelps, ME. Electrocarticographis confirmation of focal positron emission tomography abnormalities. Epilepsia 31: 731–739, 1990.

119. Oppenheim, RW: Naturally occurring cell death during neural development. Trends in Neurosciences 8:487–493, 1985.

120. Penn, R, Bernadette, T, Baldwin, L: Brain maturation followed by computed tomography. J Comput Assist Tomogr, 4(5):614–616, 1980.

121. Penner, MW, Li, KC, Gebarski, SS, and Allen, RJ: MR imaging of Pelizaeus-Merzbacher disease. J Comput Assist Tomogr 11:591–593, 1987.

122. Pennock, J, Bydder, G, Dubowitz, L, and Johnson, M: Magnetic resonance imaging of the brain in children. Magnetic Resonance Imaging 4:1–9, 1986.

123. Pennock, JM, Bydder, GM, de Vries, LS, Dubowitz, LMS, and Young, I: MRI of intracranial hemorrhage in neonates. Book of Abstracts, Socicty of Magnetic Resonance in Medicine. Sixth Annual Meeting, New York, August, 1987, p 73.

124. Peterman, S, Steiner, R, and Bydder, G: Magnetic resonance imaging of intracranial tumors in children and adolescents. AJNR 5:703–709, 1984.

125. Poser, CM and Taveras, JM: Cerebral angiography in encephalotrigeminal angiomatosis. Radiology 68:327–336, 1957.

126. Purves, D and Lichtman, JW: Elimination of synapses in the developing nervous system. Science 210:153–157, 1980.

127. Quencer, R: Maturation of normal primate white matter: Computed tomographic correlation. AJR 3:365–372, 1982.

128. Rabinowicz, T: The differentiate maturation of the human cerebral cortex. In Falkner, F and Tanner, JM (eds): Human Growth, Vol 3. Neurobiology and Nutrition. Plenum Press, New York, 1979, pp 97–103.

129. Roach, E, Williams, D, and Laster, D: Magnetic resonance imaging in tuberous sclerosis. Arch Neurol 44:, 1987.

130. Robertson, C and Finer, N: Term infants with hypoxic-ischemic encephalopathy: Outcome at 3.5 years. Dev Med Child Neurol 27:473–484, 1985.

131. Rosenberg, AA: Cerebral blood flow and oxygen metabolism after asphyxia in neonatal lambs. Pediatr Res 20:778–782, 1982.

132. Rumack, C and Johnson, ML: Perinatal and Infant Brain Imaging: Role of Ultrasound and Computed Tomography.

Year Book Medical Publishers, Chicago, 1984.

133. Sarnat, HB and Sarnat, MS: Neonatal encephalopathy following fetal distress: A clinical and electroencephalographic study. Arch Neurol 33:696–705, 1976.
134. Seay, AR, Bray, PF, and Wing, T. CT-scan in Menkes disease. Neurology 29:204–212, 1987.
135. Schellinger, D, Grant, E, and Richardson, J: Cystic periventricular leukomalacia: Sonographic and CT findings. AJNR 5:439–445, 1984.
136. Sheldon, JJ, Siddarthan, R, and Tobias, J. MR imaging of multiple sclerosis: Comparison with clinical and CT examination in 74 patients. AJNR 6:683–690, 1985.
137. Silverstein, FS, Chen, R, and Johnston, MV: The glutamate analogue quisqualic acid is neurotoxic in striatum and hippocampus of immature rat brain. Neurosci Lett 71:13–18, 1986.
138. Simon, RP, Young, RSK, Stout, S, and Cheng, J: Inhibition of excitatory neurotransmission with kynurenate reduces brain edema in neonatal anoxia. Neurosci Lett 71:361–364, 1986.
139. Schwartz, WJ, Hutchinson, HT, and Berg, BO: Computerized tomography in subacute necrotizing encephalomyelopathy (Leigh's disease). Ann Neurol 10:268–271, 1981.
140. Statz, A, Boltshauser, E, Schinzel, A, and Spiess, H: Computed tomography in Pelizeaeus-Merzbacher disease. Neuroradiology 22:103–105, 1981.
141. Szelies, B, Herholz, K, Heiss, WD, Rackl, A, Pawlik, G, Wagner, R, Ilsen, HW, and Wienhard, K: Hypometabolic cortical lesions in tuberous sclerosis with epilepsy: Demonstration by positron emission tomography. J Comput Assist Tomogr 7:946–953, 1983.
142. Townsend, JJ, Wilson, JF, Harris, T, Coulter, D, and Fife, R: Alexander's disease. Acta Neuropathol 67:163–166, 1985.
143. Theodore, WH, Rose, D, Patronas, N, et al: Cerebral glucose metabolism in the Lennox-Gastaut syndrome. Ann Neurol 21:14–21, 1987.
144. Vaghi, M, Visciani, A, Testa, D, Binelli, S, and Passerini, A: Cerebral MR findings in tuberous sclerosis. J Comput Assist Tomogr 11:403–406, 1987.
145. Volpe, JJ, Herscovitch, P, Perlman, JM, and Raichle, ME: Positron emission tomography in the newborn: Extensive impairment of regional cerebral blood flow with intraventricular hemorrhage and hemorrhagic intracerebral involvement. Pediatrics 72:589–601, 1983.
146. Volpe, JJ, Herscovitch, P, Perlman, JM, Kreusser, K, and Raichle, ME: Positron emission tomography in the asphyxiated term newborn: Parasagittal impairment of cerebral blood flow. Ann Neurol 17:287–296, 1985.
147. Volpe, JJ: Neurology of the Newborn, ed 2, WB Saunders, Philadelphia, 1987, pp 311–361.
148. Volpe, JJ: Neurology of the Newborn, ed 2, WB Saunders, Philadelphia, pp 409–453, 1987.
149. Von Hosten, C: Developmental changes in the organization of prereaching movements. Developmental Psych 20:378–388, 1984.
150. Watts, RWE, Spellacy, E, and Kendall, BE. Computed tomography studies on patients with mucopolysaccharidoses. Neuroradiology 21:9–23, 1981.
150a. Welch, J, Naheedy, MH, and Abroms, IF. Computed tomography of Sturge-Weber syndrome in infants. J Comput Assist Tomogr 4:33–36, 1980.
151. Wilson, D and Steiner, R: Periventricular leukomalacia: Evaluation with MR imaging. Radiology 160:507–511, 1986.
152. Yakovlev, P and Lecours, A: The myelogenetic cycles of regional maturation of the brain. In Minkowski, A (ed): Regional Development of the Brain in Early Life. Blackwell Scientific Publications, Oxford, pp 3–69, 1967.
153. Young, IR, Khenia, S, Thomas, D, Davis, C, Gadian, D, Cox, I, Ross, B, and Bydder, GM: Clinical magnetic susceptibility mapping of the brain. J Comput Assist Tomogr 11:2–6, 1987.
154. Young, IR, Randell, CP, Kaplan, PW, James, A, Bydder, GM, and Steiner, RE: Nuclear magnetic resonance (NMR) imaging in white matter disease of the brain using spin-echo sequences. J Comput Assist Tomogr 7:290–4, 1983.

155. Zimmerman, R, Bilaniuk, L, and Grossman, R: Computed tomography in migratory disorders of human brain development. Neuroradiology 25:257–263, 1983.

156. Zimmerman, R, Bilaniuk, L: Pediatric central nervous system. In Stark DD and Bradley, WG (eds): Magnetic Resonance Imaging. CV Mosby, St. Louis, 1988, pp 683–715.

Chapter 13

EPILOGUE: FUTURE VISIONS

John C. Mazziotta, M.D., Ph.D., and Sid Gilman, M.D.

MAGNETIC RESONANCE IMAGING
POSITRON EMISSION TOMOGRAPHY
SPECT
IMAGE INTEGRATION: MERGING STRUCTURE AND FUNCTION

In the past two decades, brain imaging with computed tomographic techniques has developed at a rapid rate. We anticipate that in the future these techniques will evolve with even greater speed. To some extent, the path of the evolutionary process can logically be predicted from research activities currently underway. Many of these activities were described in earlier chapters of this book and some will be highlighted here. It is predictable that other developments are now unforeseen. Just as the concept of making high-resolution anatomic images with magnetic fields was inconceivable 20 years ago, we will most assuredly look back from the year 2010 and take for granted the devices used in clinical practice at that time that are not conceived of today.

Whereas some advances are method-specific and will be grouped together below, others transcend methodologic categorization and are discussed later.

MAGNETIC RESONANCE IMAGING

MR Angiography

Already, striking examples exist of MR angiography of both the extracranial and intracranial vessels (Figure 13–1). Only 5 years ago, this was a mere theoretical concept, but today, such techniques are on the verge of entering routine clinical practice. MR images of flowing blood are produced through the use of gradient echo (GE) techniques with short echo times (TE)[17,18,33] (see Chapter 2). Acquired with totally noninvasive magnetic resonance techniques, these images are completely analogous to the images resulting from conventional angiography. The basic principle of MR angiography is that the protons within flowing blood constantly change orientation as they enter into or depart from the volume of tissue being imaged. This motion creates a set of phenomena that are collectively known as "time-of-flight" effects. They have the capacity of either increasing or decreasing the signal that comes from the compartment containing the flowing blood.[2,6,12] Some time-

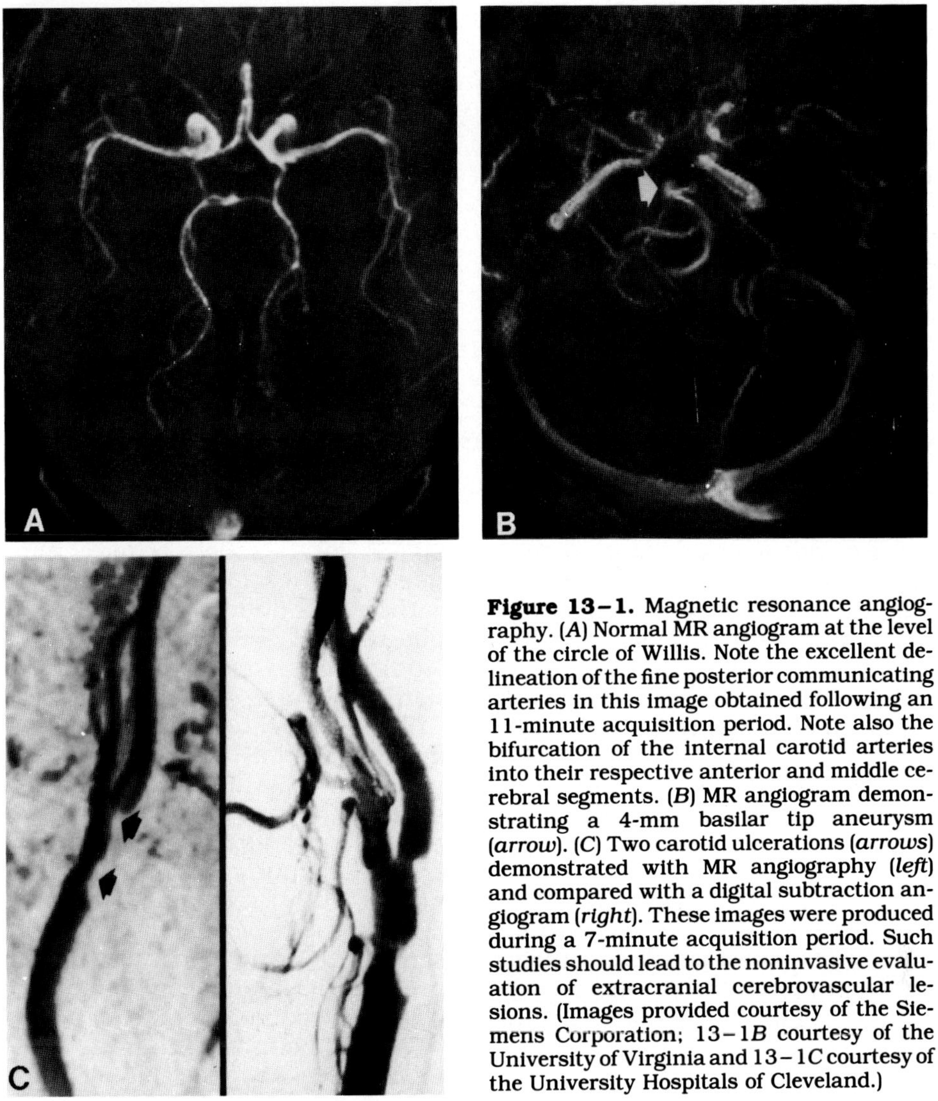

Figure 13–1. Magnetic resonance angiography. (*A*) Normal MR angiogram at the level of the circle of Willis. Note the excellent delineation of the fine posterior communicating arteries in this image obtained following an 11-minute acquisition period. Note also the bifurcation of the internal carotid arteries into their respective anterior and middle cerebral segments. (*B*) MR angiogram demonstrating a 4-mm basilar tip aneurysm (*arrow*). (*C*) Two carotid ulcerations (*arrows*) demonstrated with MR angiography (*left*) and compared with a digital subtraction angiogram (*right*). These images were produced during a 7-minute acquisition period. Such studies should lead to the noninvasive evaluation of extracranial cerebrovascular lesions. (Images provided courtesy of the Siemens Corporation; 13–1*B* courtesy of the University of Virginia and 13–1*C* courtesy of the University Hospitals of Cleveland.)

of-flight effects decrease the MR signal and are called "flow-void" effects. Others that increase the signal are called "flow-related enhancement."

The concept of focusing on a vascular signal with MR scanning dates back to 1982, when Moran[23] proposed the use of special magnetic gradients to capitalize on the unique signal resulting from flowing blood in the vascular compartment. This approach, combined with the use of three-dimensional (3-D) volume imaging (as opposed to multislice imaging), has advanced to the point where high-quality images can be obtained without even needing to gate the signal to the cardiac cycle. Currently, 3-D imaging of the extracranial or intracranial vascular system can be obtained in about 10 minutes.[33]

Ross and colleagues[33] have identified the problems with these techniques that need to be managed to make them more clinically applicable. One critical issue in imaging the neck is to optimize the positioning of cervical blood vessels to image the carotid bifurcation without overlap from the jugular vein. Other problems include limited spatial resolution, a limited volume of tissue that can be imaged in one sequence, and degradation of the image from motion.

Unlike conventional angiography, current MR angiography does not provide information about circulation time, early draining veins, or neovascularity.[33] Nevertheless, startling views of the intracranial and extracranial circulation have already been produced, and these techniques are being used in the study of cerebrovascular disease, aneurysms, arteriovenous malformations, and vascular occlusions.[33a] Aneurysms as small as 4 mm have been identified.[33]

Once MR angiography enters clinical practice, the last major vestige of invasive diagnostic neuroimaging will fall by the wayside. Already, pneumoencephalography has been supplanted by x-ray CT and MRI, myelography has been drastically reduced by the use of MRI, and angiography for diagnostic purposes will give way to MR-based techniques. This trend has resulted in the overall reduction of morbidity, mortality, and cost to the patient, since the procedures are safer than the invasive techniques and do not require hospitalization. For example, as safe as conventional angiography has become through the use of low-osmolality contrast media,[13] patients still develop allergic reactions, renal effects, and emboli from the procedures.

Three-Dimensional MRI

A logical extension of two-dimensional multislice MRI will be 3-D images produced by either volume imaging or surface rendering of multislice data (Fig. 13–2). This type of data acquisition and display provides an immediately recognizable image of the 3-D structure of the brain and the abnormalities that may affect it. Computer graphic techniques will allow the surfaces of the brain to be rendered translucent, or even stereoscopic,[24] revealing their inner structure and providing information about the complex interrelationship between cerebral structures as they exist in their normal state and in diseased states. Such a tool will be useful to the neurologist and neurosurgeon alike, for the former in understanding the site and natural history of disease, and for the latter in planning surgical procedures and observing their consequences noninvasively.

Nonproton MRI

Preliminary data already exist indicating that useful MR images can be produced with isotopes other than hydrogen. Images obtained with sodium 23[10,35] and spectroscopic information[5,14,30,34] obtained from the use of carbon-13,[7] fluorine-19,[22,36] and phosphorus-31[1,9,26,28,29] indicate that future studies may yield important information concerning physiologic processes.

The ability to produce nonproton images with MRI would provide the opportunity to evaluate natural isotopes such as sodium-23,[10,35] which are important participants in the electrophysiologic and metabolic regulation of neural tissue. In addition, if such images could be made with sufficient sensitivity and spatial resolution, tracer experiments could be performed by the introduction into the body of labeled compounds containing such isotopes.[8,22,36] An example of this approach is the use of ^{19}F-labeled drugs to evaluate neuronal function externally with nonproton MRI.[8,22,36]

At present, a major technical difficulty results from the sensitivity of current MR instruments and the amount of isotope required for imaging. While imaging with ^{23}Na has been successful with field strengths at the high end of the conventional spectrum (e.g., 1.5 T),[10,35] spectroscopic measurement of less abundant isotopes has only succeeded with magnetic field strengths that are greater than those used in conventional clinical imaging units (e.g., 1.9–4.7 T).

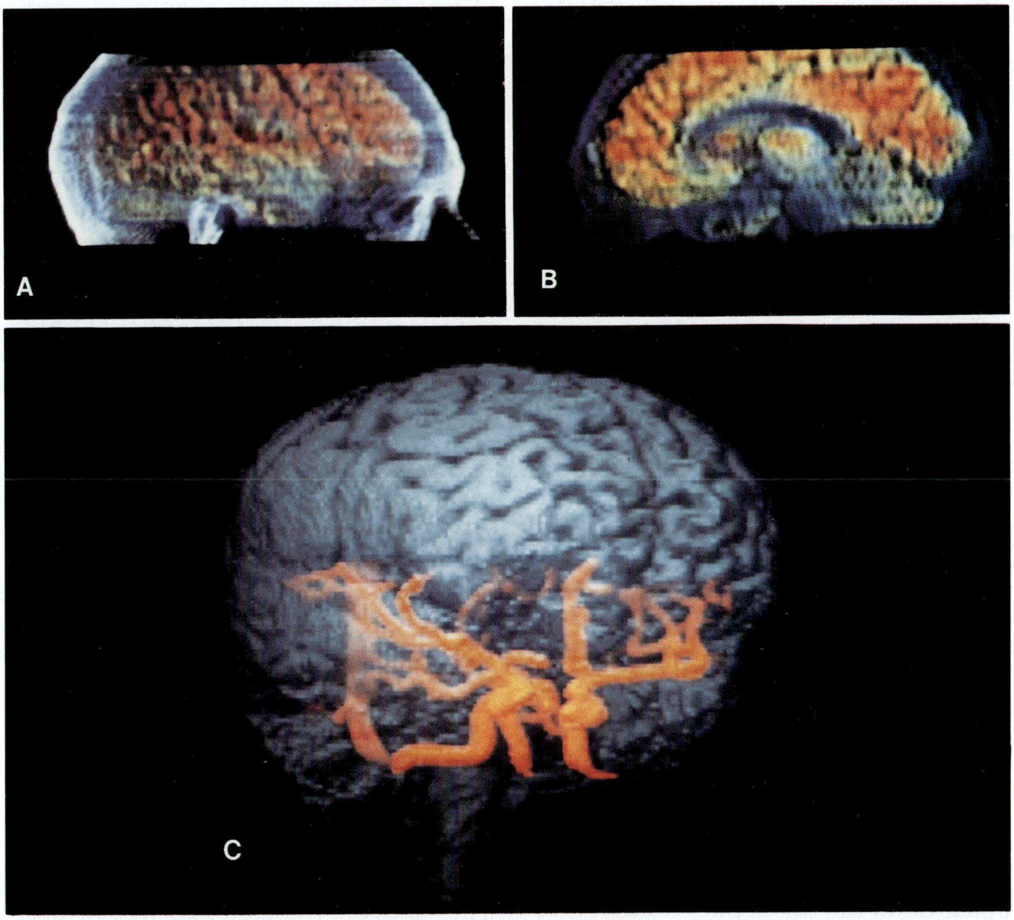

Figure 13–2. Three-dimensional image construction. Using the image integration techniques described in the text and shown schematically in Figure 13–3, these images were produced from serial MRI and PET data of a normal volunteer. A common outer boundary (i.e, the skin surface) was obtained from each image set and the resultant surfaces were fit to determine the proper translation, rotation, and scaling factors to apply in order to register and align the image sets from the two modalities.[27] Once aligned, the surface reconstruction from the MRI image set was rendered three-dimensionally using a gray-scale display. PET information was then superimposed to show cortical glucose metabolism in color. For the metabolic data, red represents high metabolic rates, whereas blue and purple represent lower rates. (*A*) Lateral surface of the head, including the skin from the MRI (gray scale). (*B*) Midsagittal surface of the brain, with skull and facial features removed. (*C*) Three-dimensional rendering of the brain obtained from MRI with three-dimensional vascular anatomy added from MR angiography. Multidimensional structure-function images of this type display vast amounts of visual information that is immediately apparent to anyone familiar with the anatomy of the region. Such approaches will be useful in studying the natural progression of disease processes, planning surgical procedures, and observing developmental processes. (Fig. 13–2*C* from D Levin, reprinted with permission from Hu et al.[11] pp 45–49.)

MR Spectroscopy

A growing literature indicates the utility of stable isotopes to produce spectra that have biologic significance for intracranial neurologic and muscular disorders.[7a] Stable ^{13}C has been used to evaluate glucose metabolism in animals through the use of specially designed surface coils and a 4.7 T magnet.[25] Similarly, brain phosphorus MR spectroscopy has been developed for the determination of intracellular pH and relative amounts of phosphate-containing metabolites in humans.[9,19,26,28,29] Ross and colleagues[32] in 1981 reported using MR spectroscopy to determine the phosphorus-containing metabolites that were altered in a subject with McArdle's muscle disease during normal aerobic and ischemic exercise.

The ultimate spatial resolution of MR spectroscopy is unclear. Based on the relatively low abundance of the isotopes that create such signals and the requirements for extremely high and very uniform magnetic fields, it appears that spatial resolution will be limited. Although MR spectroscopy has been slower in developing than other aspects of MR imaging because of these problems, there is currently sufficient interest and motivation to predict that at some level such techniques will be successful in the future.

POSITRON EMISSION TOMOGRAPHY

While PET has recently emerged as an important diagnostic tool, undoubtedly there will be an even wider range of applications for its use in the coming years. Already initial indications of promising results in psychiatric studies lead to the conservative conclusion that a biochemical imaging technique will prove extremely useful in the study of mental illness. Psychiatric disorders can be alleviated or minimized through the use of drugs, and psychiatric symptoms can be induced through the administration of drugs; hence, it seems logical that a biochemical imaging technique would have a great advantage in the study of mental illness.

New Ligands and Neurotransmitted Probes

Already a long list of positron-emitting isotope-labeled neurotransmitter and receptor ligands has been created. Many of these have been discussed in previous chapters of this text. More will achieve validation in a research environment and be transferred to clinical use. The first will undoubtedly be in the dopaminergic system, where positron-labeled analogs of L-dopa, meta-tyrosine, and other related compounds[4] are already being used in human subjects to determine their behavior and utility for the diagnosis of diseases affecting dopamine pathways. Ligands that bind to postsynaptic dopamine receptors are in a similar state of development. Compounds such as ^{18}F-labeled fluoroethylspiperone, ^{11}C-labeled methylspiperone, and ^{11}C-labeled raclopride have been employed in the study of movement disorders and psychiatric syndromes, particularly schizophrenia.

Similar ligands for the study of cholinergic, serotonergic, peptidergic, GABAergic, and opiate systems have either been developed or are under investigation. Ligands labeling NMDA receptors have been developed, but their initial use has not proved promising.

For each of these newly developed compounds labeled with positron-emitting isotopes, one will have to demonstrate its specific binding, determine the relative retention rate in neural tissue (as opposed to the off rate of its nonspecific binding), and develop appropriate models to describe its chemical behaviors, validated by quantitative data obtained in a kinetic fashion in both animal and human experiments. This process is typically a long one, taking months to a year to complete. The future availability of tomographs designed specifically to perform animal experiments (see below), however, should facilitate and expedite this process.

Concomitantly, positron-emitting, isotope-labeled drugs of the types that are currently in common use in neurology and neurosurgery will undoubtedly be developed. Already, labeled phenytoin[3] and valproate[31] have been synthesized and tested in humans. The ability to observe both the site and kinetic behavior of psychoactive drugs in vivo within the human brain will allow a more complete understanding of the in vivo pharmacokinetics of the drug-brain interaction. Our current knowledge of these interactions stems from peripheral (e.g., urine, blood, cerebrospinal fluid) analysis of metabolites or from in vitro evaluations that may or may not describe accurately the situation in cerebral tissue.

Applications to Presymptomatic Individuals

Two areas of current intense interest in the application of biochemical imaging techniques are cerebral dysfunction from genetically inherited diseases and the clinical effects of neurotoxins upon the biochemistry and physiology of neuronal tissue.

Examples of such applications with PET are already in the literature. Patients at risk for Huntington's disease have been evaluated with PET to study glucose metabolism. Data from a number of such investigations indicate that changes in glucose utilization precede structural changes in striatal anatomy as well as symptoms and signs in persons who will ultimately develop the disease. These changes may precede the onset of clinical symptoms by only a few years, so the development of probes that are more sensitive to the early manifestation of the disease may provide more useful information both for immediate clinical use and for the understanding of the natural disease process.

An example of the use of PET to detect presymptomatic toxin-induced lesions involves MPTP, a toxin that destroys dopaminergic projections and induces a clinical disorder resembling Parkinsonism. As described in Chapter 8, a series of patients were studied with PET and ^{18}F-labeled L-dopa to determine the integrity of presynaptic dopamine terminals. These studies demonstrated that the uptake and retention of labeled L-dopa in the striatum is reduced in such individuals when compared to normal controls. The resultant values in the MPTP subjects are intermediate between patients with idiopathic Parkinson's disease and control subjects[16] (see Fig. 8–13).

Functional Reorganization and Rehabilitation after Brain Injury

One of the most fundamental questions in neuroscience is how the brain functionally recovers after injury. Little information exists on a practical level about this phenomenon. The ability of PET to show functional pathways during active behavior provides the opportunity to obtain this information and from it, to develop pathophysiologically based approaches to therapy and rehabilitation.

The most striking examples of functional recovery after CNS lesions occur in childhood (see Chapter 12). Children who have had radical cerebral resections, including hemispherectomy, can maintain or reacquire the ability to move the limbs contralateral to the resected hemisphere. The imaging of functional pathways before and after such resections allows for observation of the plasticity that results in this functional maintenance or recovery of function.

Many centers are actively engaged in the development of behavioral stimulation tasks[20,21] (Fig. 3–36) to use in planning for surgical resection procedures. By developing tasks that reliably activate focal regions of the brain, we can establish functional boundaries in individual patients that can serve as limits to surgical resections so as to avoid major neurologic deficits in the patient. Such an approach may ultimately lead to the development of noninvasive Wada testing for language and memory and the visualization of motor systems and visual pathways in patients who have lesions (e.g., tumors, vascular malformations) in or around the sites of these functions.

In patients with degenerative diseases of the nervous system such as Alzheimer's, Huntington's, and Parkinson's disease, PET will allow the opportunity to observe the compensatory mechanisms used by the brain to maintain function in the face of ongoing and insidious neuronal attrition. Such data may provide clues to the compensatory capacity of the brain as well as to the natural history of the diseases themselves. This information will be useful in developing new and improved ways of providing rehabilitation to patients with acute or chronic brain injury.

PET can be used to monitor surgical interventions currently under evaluation in the treatment of degenerative brain diseases.[15] The demonstration of uptake and storage of ^{18}F-labeled L-dopa in a patient with Parkinson's disease who had received a fetal mesencephalic transplant of substantia nigra cells into his affected putamen demonstrates the principle of this approach.[15] Through the development and evaluation of new radiopharmaceuticals such as labeled nerve-growth factors and perhaps other trophic substances, PET will be able to use such approaches to evaluate the biochemical mechanisms associated with therapeutic successes and failures.

Animal Studies

The development of high-spatial-resolution (i.e., 2–3 mm) PET instruments devoted to the imaging of animal brain tissue will provide the opportunity to conduct experiments that cannot be performed in human subjects. Such techniques will allow for the validation of animal models and for the establishment of new models previously avoided because of logistic or practical problems. Once established, these animal models can provide an optimal environment for perfecting experimental therapies, understanding the natural history of disease, and testing methods of rehabilitation.[6a]

Clinical Considerations

Currently, PET is being used clinically in the presurgical evaluation of patients with intractable epilepsy (see Chapter 5), grading the malignancy of primary brain tumors, differentiating recurrent brain tumors from radiation necrosis (see Chapter 6), and in the evaluation of patients with dementia (see Chapter 9). The clinical uses of PET undoubtedly will expand into the areas of movement disorders, cerebral vascular disease, traumatic injury of the brain, and psychiatric disorders.

As commercial interest and competition in PET tomographs and cyclotrons increases in the coming years, both cost and technological complexity will be reduced. It is likely that regional cyclotrons producing relatively long-lived positron-emitting isotopes (e.g., ^{18}F, 110-minute half-life) will provide radiopharmaceuticals to PET centers in community-sized hospitals. With advancing technology, PET instruments will routinely be produced that have current state-of-the-art spatial resolution (approximately 5–6 mm in all dimensions) with substantial reductions in price. Similarly, advances in cyclotron technology have already resulted in the production of devices that are smaller in both size and weight when compared to current machines, at about half the current price. All of these advances will increase the availability and accessibility of PET. As new radiopharmaceuticals become available, commercial pressures and interests will rapidly result in the synthesis of these compounds in automated modules, making them quickly available for clinical use. Hence, it is likely that a wide range of radiopharmaceuticals will be accessible to community-based hospitals for the evaluation of patients using PET technology.

SPECT

New Choices in Ligands

Currently, SPECT imaging is limited to perfusion studies because the range of tracers and ligands is narrow. This situation is likely to change, mainly because a very large neuroscientific and neurochemical literature has accumulated on the use of iodinated tracers to study many physiologic, biochemical, and pharmacologic processes. These studies, performed either by biochemical assay or autoradiographic technique, have resulted in a wealth of information about the chemical behavior of iodinated compounds. A large number of new compounds can be made available to the SPECT imaging world by substituting ^{123}I, which emits a gamma ray and can be detected externally, for ^{125}I, which emits a beta particle and has been used in vitro. These compounds and others will require rigorous validation to determine their biochemical behavior in vivo, as well as the optimal time for imaging, and the stability of the image that results. Once this is accomplished, however, the range of biochemical measurements and the physiologic information that can be obtained with SPECT should increase dramatically.

Improved Spatial Resolution

As discussed in Chapter 4, spatial resolution has rapidly improved with SPECT technology. There is, however, a trade-off between increasing collimation, which improves spatial resolution, and diminished sensitivity, that is, a reduction in radioactive events that are detected by the system. The result is a practical limit for SPECT spatial resolution, probably in the range of about 7–8 mm. Despite this practical limitation, high-quality images that show cortical and subcortical areas should be obtainable with currently available technology. As with PET and MRI, the expansion of the consumer market for SPECT will further reduce its cost. Currently, radiopharmaceuticals used with SPECT are expensive on a unit-dose basis. It seems likely that the wider use of this technology and the greater demand for these radiopharmaceuticals will result in a reduction in such costs.

IMAGE INTEGRATION: MERGING STRUCTURE AND FUNCTION

A new phase of image integration is already underway. It involves the combination of images from multiple imaging modalities. For example, there is often a need to superimpose bony landmarks from x-ray CT with parenchymal information from MRI for purposes of radiation planning. Similarly, it is advantageous to combine structural images from MRI with functional images from PET or SPECT so that an integrated structure/function map can be constructed.[27] Already such images can be produced in both two and three dimensions (Fig. 13–2, 13–3). In the future it will be possible to produce an image combining parenchymal anatomy from MRI, vascular anatomy from MR angiography, tumor localization from a ligand-specific PET tracer, and images depicting functional activation of critical areas adjacent to the lesion from PET activation studies. This combined image would provide the optimal presurgical means of identifying a lesion, the surrounding brain anatomy, critical functional sites, and vascular territories.

Combined anatomic and functional images could be used for presurgical planning and could be displayed in the operating room as a direct guide for surgical resections. Serial images integrated over time could provide information about the natural history of disease, brain development, or recovery from injury.

Multidimensional images that compare a given patient study to a normal

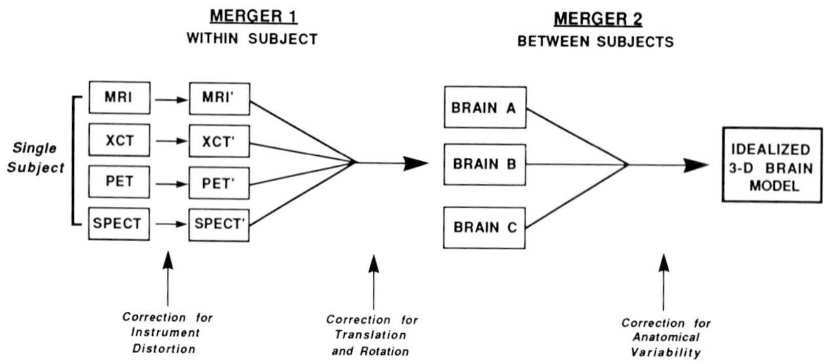

Figure 13–3. Two-step process used to merge data within a single subject from different imaging modalities (merger 1) and between different subjects from combined data sets (merger 2). Figure 13–2 illustrates the result of a merger-1 process, where MRI and PET data from the same individual are corrected for distortions, aligned, registered, scaled, and displayed as a three-dimensional rendered image. Merger 2 is a more difficult proposition that requires the distortion or warping of an individual's brain to match that of a population or an idealized model. Merger 2 permits the comparison of an individual with members of a normal control group, or of a population of patients with a specific disease.

population or to populations of patients with specific diseases would yield statistical images showing the best match for a given patient when compared to control subjects or individuals with specific diseases.

CONCLUSIONS

There is every reason to believe that the future of neuroimaging will be even richer than its past. From the events of the past two decades, it seems likely that the acceleration of knowledge of techniques and their applications will only increase with time. Technologies developed in other disciplines (e.g., radio astronomy, metallurgy, probability theory, space exploration) have already found their way into improving imaging techniques applied in medicine. This transfer of technology undoubtedly will increase in coming years.

As we noted at the outset of this epilogue, all new imaging techniques in the last two decades were initially applied to the brain. The brain has proved to be more inaccessible than other portions of the body, and the approaches that have allowed for visualizing brain structure have intrigued investigators who have sought to understand the workings of this most complicated organ. It seems likely that the development of new techniques and the integration of old techniques with the new will result in the most comprehensive understanding ever of cerebral structure and function. Imaging has played an increasingly important role, not only in the case of patients with neurologic disorders, but also in the understanding of neuronal systems and their changes with disease. The future is ripe for new opportunities for imaging to continue on this important and productive pathway.

REFERENCES

1. Arnold, D, Taylor, D, and Radda, G: Investigation of human mitochondrial myopathies by phosphorus magnetic resonance spectroscopy. Ann Neurol 18:189–196, 1985.
2. Axel, A, Shimakawa, A, and MacFall, J: A time-of-flight method of measuring flow velocity by magnetic resonance imaging. Magn Reson Imaging 4:199–205, 1986.
3. Baron, J, Roeda, D, Munari, C, Crouzel, C, Chodkiewicz, J, and Comar, D: Brain regional pharmacokinetics of ^{11}C-la-

beled diphenylhydantoin: Positron emission tomography in humans. Neurology 33:580–585, 1983.

4. Barrio, JR: Biochemical principles in radiopharmaceutical design and utilization. In Phelps, M, Mazziotta, J, and Schelbert, H (eds): Positron Emission Tomography and Autoradiography: Principles and Applications for the Brain and Heart. Raven Press, New York, 1986, pp 451–492.
5. Bottomley, PA: Human in vivo NMR spectroscopy in diagnostic medicine: Clinical tool or research probe? Radiology 170:1–15, 1989.
6. Bradley, WG and Waluch, V: Blood flow: Magnetic resonance imaging. Radiology 154:443–450, 1985.

6a. Brownell, A-L, Kano, M, McKinstry, R, Moskowitz, H, Rosen, B, Brownell, G: PET and MR studies of experimental focal stroke. J Comput Assist Tomogr 15(3):376–380, 1991.

7. Burt, CT and Koutcher, JA: Multinuclear NMR studies of naturally occurring nuclei. J Nucl Med 25:237–248, 1984.

7a. Demaerel, P, Juhanik, K, Vanetecke, P, et al: Localized ^{2}H NMR spectroscopy in fifty cases of newly diagnosed intracranial tumors. J Comput Assist Tomogr 15(1):67–76, 1991.

8. Eidelberg, D, Johnson, G, Tofts, P, Dobbin, J, Crockard, H, and Plummer, D: ^{19}F imaging of cerebral blood oxygenation in experimental middle cerebral artery occlusion: Preliminary results. J Cereb Blood Flow Metabol 8(2):276–281, 1988.
9. Gadian, D, Frackowiak, R, Crockard, H, Proctor, E, Allen, K, Williams, S, and Russell, R: Acute cerebral ischaemia: Concurrent changes in cerebral blood flow, energy metabolites, pH, and lactate measured with hydrogen clearance and ^{31}P and ^{1}H nuclear magnetic resonance spectroscopy. I. Methodology. J Cerebr Blood Flow and Metabol 7(2):199–206, 1987.
10. Hilal, S, Maudsley, A, Ra, J, Simon, H, Roschmann, P, Wittekoek, S, Cho, Z, and Mun, S: In vivo NMR imaging of sodium-23 in the human head. J Comput Assist Tomogr 9(1):1–7, 1989.
11. Hu, X, Tan, K, and Levin, D: Volumetric rendering of multi-modality, multivariable medical imaging data. In Upsan, C (ed): Proceedings of Chapel Hill Workshop on Volume Visualization. University of North Carolina, Chapel Hill, NC, 1989, pp 45–49.
12. Kaufman, L, Crooks, L, and Sheldon, PE: Evaluation of NMR imaging for detection and quantification of obstructions in vessels. Invest Radiol 77:554–560, 1982.
13. King, B, Hartman, G, Williamson, B, LeRoy, A, and Hattery, R: Low-osmolality contrast media: A current perspective. Mayo Clin Proc 64:976–985, 1989.
14. Levy, GC and Craik, DJ: Recent developments in nuclear magnetic resonance spectroscopy. Science 214:291–299, 1981.
15. Lindvall, O, Brundin, P, Widner, H, Rehncrona, S, Gustavii, B, Frackowiak, R, Leenders, K, Swale, G, Rothwell, J, Marsden, C, and Björklund, A: Grafts of fetal dopamine neurons survive and improve motor function in Parkinson's disease. Science 247:574–577, 1990.
16. Martin, W, Stoessl, A, Adam, M, Grierson, J, Ruth, T, Pate, B, Calne, D, and Langston, J: Imaging of dopamine systems in human subjects exposed to MPTP. In Markey, S, Castagnoli, N, Trevor, A, Kopin, I (eds): MPTP: A Neurotoxin Producing a Parkinsonian Syndrome. Academic Press, San Diego, Calif, 1986, pp 315–325.
17. Masaryk T, Modic M, and Ross, J: Intracranial circulation: Preliminary clinical results with three-dimensional magnetic resonance angiography. Radiology 171:793–799, 1989.
18. Masaryk, T, Modic, M, and Ruggieri, P: Three-dimensional gradient echo imaging of the carotid bifurcation: Preliminary clinical experience. Radiology 171:801–806, 1989.
19. Matthews, P, Shoubridge, E, and Arnold, D: Brain phosphorus magnetic resonance spectroscopy in acute bacterial meningitis. Arch Neurol 46:944–996, 1989.
20. Mazziotta, J, Phelps, M, and Halgren, E: Local cerebral glucose metabolic re-

sponses to audio-visual stimulation and deprivation: Studies in human subjects with positron CT. Human Neurobiol 2:11–23, 1983.

21. Mazziotta, JC and Phelps, ME: Human sensory stimulation and deprivation. PET results and strategies. Ann Neurol (Suppl 1)15:S50–S60, 1984.

22. McFarland, E, Koutcher, J, Rosen, B, Teicher, B, and Brady, T: In vivo ^{19}F NMR imaging. J Comput Assist Tomogr 9(1):8–15, 1985.

23. Moran, PR: A flow zeumatographic interface for NMR imaging in humans. Magn Reson Imaging 1:197–203, 1982.

24. Moseley, M, White, D, Wang, S, Wikström, M. Gobbel, G, and Roth, K: Stereoscopic MR imaging. J Comput Assist Tomogr 13(1):167–173, 1989.

25. Novotny, E. Rothman, D, Avison, M, Petroff, O, Lantos, G, Prichard, J, and Shulman, R: Determination of cerebral metabolic rates in vivo using stable isotopically labeled glucose (abstr). Ann Neurol 26:463, 1989.

26. Nunnally, RL and Bottomley, PA: Assessment of pharmacological treatment of myocardial infarction by phosphorus-31 NMR with surface coils. Science 211:177–180, 1981.

27. Pelizzari, C, Chen, G, Spelbring, D, Weichselbaum, R, and Chen, C: Accurate three-dimensional registration of CT, PET, and/or MR images of the brain. J Comput Assist Tomogr 13(1):20–26, 1989.

28. Petroff, O, Prichard, J, Behar, K, Alger, J, den Hollander, J, and Shulman, R: Cerebral intracellular pH by ^{31}P nuclear magnetic resonance spectroscopy. Neurology 35:781–788, 1985.

29. Petroff, O, Prichard, J, Behar, K, Rothman, D, Alger, J, and Shulman, R: Cerebral metabolism in hyper- and hypocarbia: ^{31}P and ^{1}H nuclear magnetic resonance studies. Neurology 35:1681–1685, 1985.

30. Radda, G, Rajagopalan, B, Taylor, D: Biochemistry in vivo: An appraisal of clinical magnetic resonance spectroscopy. Magnetic Resonance Quarterly 5:122–151, 1989.

31. Ramsey, RE: Valproate in brain tissue kinetically determined with PET. Neurology (Suppl 2)33:147, 1983.

32. Ross, B, Radda, G, Gadian, D, Rocker, G Esiri, M, and Falconer-Smith, J: Examination of case of suspected McArdle's syndrome by ^{31}P nuclear magnetic resonance. N Engl J Med 22:1338–1342, 1981.

33. Ross, J, Masaryk, T, Modic, M, Harik, S, Wiznitzer, M and Selman, S: Magnetic resonance angiography of the extracranial carotid arteries and intracranial vessels: A review. Neurology 39:1369–1376, 1989.

33a. Sevick, R, Tsuruda, J, Schmalbrock, P: Three-dimensional time-of-flight MR angiography in the evaluation of cerebral aneurisms. J Comput Assist Tomogr 14(6):874–881, 1990.

34. Weiner, MW: The promise of magnetic resonance spectroscopy for medical diagnosis. Invest Radiol 23:253–261, 1988.

35. Winkler, S, Thomasson, D, Sherwood, K, and Perman, W: Regional T2 and sodium concentration estimates in the normal human brain by sodium-23 MR imaging at 1.5T. J Comput Assist Tomogr 13(4):561–566, 1989.

36. Wyrwicz, A, Pszenny, M, Schofield, J, Tillman, P, Gordon, R, and Martin, P: Non-invasive observations of fluorinated anesthetics in rabbit brain by fluorine-19 nuclear magnetic resonance. Science 222:428–430, 1983.

INDEX

A page number followed by an "f" indicates a figure; a "t" following a page number indicates a table.

Abscess(es) of posterior fossa, 392, 393f
Aging, normal cerebral change, 297–300
  MRI studies, 297–298, 298f, 299f
  neurophysiologic studies of, 325
  PET and SPECT
    atrophy correction, 300
    studies, 298–300
  x-ray CT studies, 297
AIDS and dementia, 365–366
Alcoholic cerebellar degeneration, 392–394
  features, 392–393
  MRI studies, 393, 394f
  PET studies, 393–394, 395f
  x-ray CT studies, 393, 394f
Alexander's disease, 362, 366f
Aliasing artifacts
  MRI and, 55
  x-ray CT and, 9
Alzheimer's disease, 300–311, 318
  features, 300
  MRI studies, 307–310, 308–309f, 310f
  neurophysiologic studies of, 325
  PET studies, 308–309f, 310–318, 312–317t
  SPECT studies, 318
  x-ray CT studies, 300–307, 301–305t
Amipaque (metrizamide), 10, 11f, 12t, 18
Analog tracer(s) in PET, 91
Aneurysm(s) of posterior fossa, 223f, 389–390
Angiography
  conventional
    gliomas and, 172, 172f
    intracerebral metastases and, 198
    intracranial neoplasms and, 168
    meningiomas and, 192, 193f
    pituitary adenomas and, 195, 196f
  magnetic resonance, 66, 67f
    future of MRA, 458–460, 459f
    intracranial neoplasms and, 168–170
Angular coupling intervals in PET, 81
Angular momentum in MRI, 39
Annihilation coincidence detection, 74, 74f
Apical artifact in x-ray CT, 7
Arterial signature of tumors in x-ray CT, 18
Arteriovenous malformations
  cerebellar, 390–392, 391f
  structural scanning of, 225–226, 226f, 227f
Artifacts in x-ray CT, 7–9, 8f
Asymmetric multiecho in MRI, 56
Ataxia, cerebellar, imaging in differential diagnosis of, 405f
Atrophic perivascular demyelinization, 352
Atrophy correction in cerebral studies, 300

Bandwidth in MRI, 50
Beam hardening in x-ray CT, 4, 7
Behavioral activation states, 96, 96f
Binswanger's disease
  background, 326
  MRI studies, 332f
  PET studies, 332f
  x-ray CT studies, 328–329
Blood flow versus perfusion, 94
Blood-brain barrier (BBB)
  imaging of defects, 178–179, 180f
  intracerebral metastases and, 199
  meningiomas and, 194
  MRI studies, 64–65
Blurring tomography in PET, 81
Brain death documentation by
  dynamic x-ray CT, 18
  xenon x-ray CT, 22
Brain, malformations of
  cerebellar anomalies, 380–385
    Chiari malformations, 380–383, 381f
      MRI studies, 381f, 382–382
      types of, 380–382
      x-ray CT studies, 382
    Dandy-Walker syndrome
      features, 383

Brain, malformations of—*Continued*
MRI studies, 383, 384–385f
x-ray CT studies, 383, 384–385f
von Hippel-Lindau disease
features, 383
imaging studies, 383, 385, 386f
cerebral
background, 424, 425f
functional imaging, 428f, 429–432, 434–435
structural imaging, 425–429, 426f, 427f, 428f, 429f, 430ff, 431f, 435f
hamartomas and arachnoid cysts, 432, 432f
phakomatoses, 432–438
Sturge-Weber syndrome, 434–438
background, 434
correlations, 436–438
MRI studies, 434–436, 436f
PET studies, 436, 437ff
x-ray CT studies, 432–434, 433f
tuberous sclerosis, 432–434, 433f
structural imaging by MRI, 424
Brain, normal development of, 411–424
background, 411–412
functional imaging, 416–424
ethical considerations, 417–419
PET studies, 419–424, 421f, 422–423f
MRI structural imaging, 412–416
gray-white differentiation, 413f, 414, 415f, 416f, 417f, 418f, 419t
myelination, 414–416, 415f, 416f, 417f, 418f, 419f, 419t, 420f

Camera-based systems in SPECT, 114, 115f
Carotid artery disease
asymptomatic occlusion, 236–237
symptomatic occlusion, 237–238
Center-point artifact in x-ray CT, 8f, 9
Central volume principle in PET, 95
Cerebellum, disorders of, 370–405, 405f
abcesses, features and imaging, 392, 393f
alcoholic degeneration
features, 392–393
PET studies, 393–394, 395f
x-ray CT studies, 393, 394f
anomalies, 380–385
Chiari malformations, 380–383, 381f
MRI studies, 381f, 382–383
types of, 380–382
x-ray CT studies, 382
Dandy-Walker syndrome features, 383
MRI studies, 383, 384–385f
x-ray CT studies, 383, 384–385f
von Hippel-Lindau disease
features, 383
imaging studies, 383, 385, 386f
degenerative disorders, 371–378
Friedreich's ataxia, 374–377
background, 374–375
MRI studies, 375
PET studies, 375–376, 376f, 377f
x-ray CT studies, 375, 376
olivopontocerebellar atrophy, 323, 371–374,
background, 371–372
MRI studies, 372, 373ff
PET studies, 372, 374, 374f
x-ray CT studies, 372
paraneoplastic cerebellar degeneration, 377–378
background, 377–378
imaging of, 378, 378f, 379f
demyelinative disease, 378–380, 380f
neoplasms, 394–403, 398–399t
cerebellopontine-angle schwannoma
features, 402
MRI studies, 403, 404f
x-ray CT, 29f, 400–401f, 402–403, 403f, 404f
extraparenchymal tumors, 397, 400–402
features, 397, 401
MRI studies, 402
x-ray CT studies, 400–401f, 402
intra-axial tumors
MRI studies, 396–397, 397f, 398–399t
x-ray CT studies, 396–397, 397f, 398–399t
metastatic disease, 397
signs and symptoms of, 394–396
vascular disease, 385–392
aneurysms, 223f, 389–390
arteriovenous malformations, 390–392, 391f
cerebellar infarction, 387, 388f
cerebellar hemorrhage
features, 387–389
x-ray CT studies, 389, 389f
transient ischemic attacks, 385–387
features, 385
x-ray CT studies, 24f, 385–387
Cerebral blood flow (CBF), 94–97, 95f, 96f
general seizures and, 153–154, 154f
gliomas and, 181–184f, 185t, 186, 187–190f
normal values, 119–120, 120f 125, 126f, 127f
Parkinson's disease and, 260–267, 262f, 264f, 266–267f, 320f
partial seizures and, 144–145
PET approaches to, 94–97, 95f, 96f
SPECT and, 119–129
technetium 99m-HMPAO and, 123–129, 126f, 127f, 128–129f, 130f
xenon 133 and, 119–123, 120f, 122–123f, 124f
Cerebral blood volume (CBV), PET measurement, 97, 98f
Cerebral metabolism. *See* Metabolism studies in
Cerebrospinal fluid (CSF)
flow studies, 19–20
leaks and intrathecal contrast, 20
Cerebrovascular disease, 217–243
cerebral infarcts, nonhemorrhagic, 223–225, 224f, 225f
dementia and, 324–333
MRI studies, 329–331, 330f, 332f
neurophysiologic studies, 324–325
PET studies, 330f, 331–332, 332f
SPECT studies, 332–333
x-ray CT studies, 328–329
functional imaging applications
infarction, local and distant effects, 235–236, 237f
ischemic state assessment, 232–235, 233f, 234f, 235f

preischemic CVD, 218ff, 229–232, 230f, 231f
functional imaging methods
BBB integrity, 229
cerebral blood flow, 227–228
cerebral blood volume, 228
cerebral metabolism, 228–229
ischemia
luxury perfusion and, 232, 234f, 235f
pathophysiology of, 217–219, 218ff
neuroimaging in management of
carotid artery disease, 236–239
asymptomatic occlusion, 236–237
symptomatic occlusion, 237–238
cerebral infarction, 238–239
structural scanning in diagnosis, 219–227
hemorrhages and hematomas, 219–223, 220f, 221f, 222f, 223t
vascular malformations, 225–226, 226f, 227f
Cerebrum
malformations of, 425–432
background and structural imaging, 425–429, 425t, 426f, 427f, 428f, 429f, 430f
functional imaging, 428f, 429–432
normal development. *See* Brain, normal development of
Chemotoxic reactions to contrast agents, 12–13
Chiari malformations
types of, 380–382
x-ray CT studies, 382
Cisternography gas, 20–21, 22f
isotope, 19
Clearance technique in PET, 84t, 95–97, 96f
Cocaine, isotope-labeled, 100f, 104, 104f
Collimation in
PET, 83f
SPECT, 110, 113f
x-ray CT, 4
Compartment in PET, 91–92, 92f
Competitive substrate kinetics, principle of, 97–98, 98f
Compton scatter, 3, 4
SPECT and, 111, 111f, 112–113, 112f
Computed tomography, principle of, 71–73, 72f, 79–81, 80f, 81f. *See* also x-ray computed tomography.
Contrast agents
MRI and, 64–66
x-ray CT and, 10–22
inhalation (xenon), 21–22
intrathecal, 18–22, 19f
clinical applications, 20, 21f
intrathecal air, 20–21, 22f
pharmacology, 19–20, 19f
intravenous, 10–18, 11f, 12t
enhancement, 14–15
ionic versus nonionic, 14
therapy for reactions, 13–14
specific agents, 10, 11f, 12t, 18, 19
toxicity, 10, 12–14
wash-in and wash-out of, 16, 17f
Contrast in
SPECT, 100–111
x-ray CT, 6, 9
Cryogen(s) in MRI, 62
CT. See x-ray computed tomography"
CT number in x-ray CT, 5
Cupping artifact in x-ray CT, 7
Cutoff frequency in PET, 81, 81f, 82f
Cyclotron, 74, 76, 76f, 77f

Dandy-Walker syndrome
MRI studies, 383
x-ray CT studies, 383, 384–385f
Dead time
MRI and, 56, 57
PET and, 89
Dedicated systems in SPECT, 114–115, 116t, 117f
Dees, of cyclotron, 74, 76f
Dementia, 294–338
AIDS and, 365–366
characteristics of, 294–296
cortical/subcortical dementias, 294
etiology, 295–296, 296t
pathophysiology, 295
pseudodementias, 294
signs and symptoms, 294–295
degenerative disorders, 300–325
Alzheimer's disease, 300–318
background, 300
MRI studies, 307–310, 308–309f, 310f
neurophysiologic studies, 325
PET studies, 308–309f, 310–318, 312–317t
SPECT studies, 318
x-ray CT studies, 300–307, 301–305t
neurophysiologic studies of, 324–325
Parkinson's disease, 318–319
background, 318
MRI studies, 319
neurophysiologic studies, 325
PET studies, 262f, 319, 320f
SPECT studies, 319
x-ray CT studies, 318–319
Pick's disease, 319–322
background, 319–320
MRI studies, 321, 322f
PET studies, 321, 322f
SPECT studies, 321–322
progressive supranuclear palsy
background, 322–324
MRI studies, 323, 324f
neurophysiologic studies, 325
PET studies, 323–324, 324f
SPECT studies, 324
x-ray CT studies, 323
HIV encephalitis and, 365–366
neuroimaging in differential diagnosis, 336–338, 338f
normal aging and cerebral change, 297–300
MRI studies, 297–298, 298f, 299f
neurophysiologic studies of, 325
PET and SPECT
atrophy correction, 300
studies, 298–300
normal-pressure hydrocephalus, 328, 333–336

Dementia—*Continued*
characteristics of, 333–334
MRI studies, 22f, 334–336, 335f
PET and SPECT studies, 335f, 336
x-ray CT studies, 334
vascular disorders, 325–333
Binswanger's disease background, 326
MRI studies, 332f
PET studies, 332f
x-ray CT studies, 328–329
MRI studies, 329–331, 330f, 332f
multi-infarct dementia, 325–333
Hachinski Ischemic Score and, 327
x-ray CT studies, 327–328
PET studies, 330f, 331–332, 332f
SPECT studies, 332–333
subcortical arteriosclerotic encephalopathy, 328
Detector materials in PET, 83–85, 84t
Dewar (vacuum cryostat) in MRI, 62
Diatrizoate meglumine, 11f, 12t
Dilution principle in PET, 92
Dosimetry in x-ray CT, 9–10
Duty cycle in MRI, 55
Dynamic scanning with x-ray CT, 17–18
Dystonia
features, 275–276
MRI studies, 276, 277f
PET studies, 276–277
x-ray CT studies, 276

Echo in MRI, 52, 54, 63
Echo planar technique in MRI, 69
Echo time in MRI, 44–47, 45f, 49–50, 49f, 49t
Emission computerized tomography, defined, 108–109
Encephalitis subcorticalis chronica progressiva, 352
Enhancement, x-ray CT intravenous, 14–15
Epilepsy, 137–165
false localization of, 143–145, 143f
general seizures, 153–155
cerebral blood flow in, 153–154, 154f
cerebral metabolism in, 153–154, 154f
infantile spasms, 154, 444–446, 445f, 446f
Lennox-Gastaut syndrome, 154–155, 442–444, 444f
imaging evaluation strategy, 156–159, 157f, 158t
MRS studies of, 155
partial seizures, 138–153
cerebral blood flow in, 144–145
cerebral metabolism in, 144–145, 144t
localization by imaging, 151–152
MRI studies, 138–144, 139f, 140f, 141f, 142f
PET ictal studies, 148–149, 151
PET interictal studies, 145–148, 145f, 146f, 147f, 148f, 149f, 150ff
presurgical studies, 152–153, 152t
SPECT studies, 151
x-ray CT studies, 138–144, 139f, 140f, 141f, 142f
patient with, approach to, 137–138
PET neuopharmacology studies, 155–156
temporal lobe, 127, 129, 130f
Equilibrium models in PET, 94, 97
État criblé, 352
État lacunaire, 352
Ethical considerations of pediatric functional imaging, 417–419
Excited state of protons, 41
Exponential decay (T2*) in MRI, 43–46, 44f, 45f

False localization of epilepsy, 143–145, 143f
FDG (fluorine-18-labeled 2-deoxy-D-glucose)
basics of, 97–98, 98f
selected major uses
brain development, 419–424, 421f, 422–423f
glioma studies, 179–191, 181–184f, 185t, 186t, 187–191f
Huntington's at-risk studies, 252–255, 253f, 254f, 255f
Parkinson's, 261–267, 262f, 264f, 266–267f
seizure states, 144t, 145–156
Ferromagnetic substances, 41
Field of view in MRI, 54–55, 55f
First-order processes in PET, 93
Flip angle in MRI, 41
Fluorine-18-labeled 2-deoxy-D-glucose. *See* FDG
Fluorine-18-labeled levodopa (fluorodopa) studies, 262f, 263–265, 264f, 266–267f
Flux in PET, 92f, 93
Fourier transformation in MRI, 54
Free induction decay in MRI, 63
Frequency encoding in MRI, 52–53, 53f
Friedreich's ataxia
background, 374–375
MRI studies, 375
PET studies, 375–376, 376f, 377f
x-ray CT studies, 375, 376
Full width at half maximum in
PET, 82f, 85, 85f, 86f
SPECT, 110
Future visions for imaging, 458–466
Huntington's disease and, 255–256
image integration, 461f, 465–466, 466f
magnetic resonance imaging
MR angiography, 458–460, 459f
MR spectroscopy, 461–462
nonproton MRI, 460
three-dimensional MRI, 460, 461f
movement disorders and, 251t, 279–281, 280t
Parkinson's disease and, 267
positron emission tomography, 462–464
animal studies, 464
clinical considerations, 464–465
new ligands and probes, 462–463
rehabilitation after brain injury, 463–464
uses in presymptomatic individuals, 463
SPECT
improved spatial resolution, 465
new choices in ligands, 465
x-ray CT, 32

Gadolinium, pharmacokinetics of, 64–66
Gamma camera systems in SPECT, 109–110, 109f

Gas cisternography, 20–21, 22f
Gaseous xenon detectors in x-ray CT, 9
Gas-filled ionization chamber in x-ray CT, 5
Gauss, 41
Gliomas, intracerebral, 171–192
angiography and, 172, 172f
MRI studies, 176–177, 176f
PET studies of
amino acid uptake, 187, 191
CBF, 181–184f, 185t, 186, 186t, 187–190f
metabolism, 179–186, 181–184f, 185t
pH, 186–187
SPECT studies, 177–179, 178f
x-ray CT studies, 172–176, 173f, 174f, 175f
Gradient echo in MRI, 45, 69
Grays (the units), 79
Ground state of protons, 41
Gyromagnetic ratio in MRI, 42

Hachinski Ischemic Score, 327
Hamartomas and arachnoid cysts, 432, 432f
Hemorrhage(s) and hematoma(s)
cerebellar
features, 387–389
x-ray CT studies, 389, 389f
cerebral, structural scanning of, 219–223, 220f, 221f, 222f, 223t
Hepatolenticular degeneration, 272–275
background, 272–273
MRI studies, 274
x-ray CT studies, 273–274
Hexabrix (ioxaglate), 10, 11f, 12t
Hounsfield unit(s), 5, 5t
Hourglass convention in MRI, 41, 42f
Human immune deficiency virus encephalitis and dementia, 365–366
Huntington's disease
background, 246–247
future prospects for imaging, 255–256
MRI studies, 248–249, 249f
PET studies, 250–256, 250f, 251t, 252f, 253f, 254f, 255f
pneumoencephalographic studies, 247–248, 247f
x-ray CT studies, 247–248, 248f
Hypoxic-ischemic encephalopathy of newborn
MRI studies, 438–441, 439ff
x-ray CT studies, 438–440, 441f

Idiosyncratic reactions to contrast agents, 10, 12
Image formation in
MRI, 50–58
x-ray CT, 4–7, 5t, 6–7f
Image integration, future visions for, 461f, 465–466, 466f
Image reconstruction in x-ray CT, 5, 6–7f
Imaging systems
gamma camera systems, 109–110, 109f
SPECT and, 109–115, 109f
Infantile spasms, 154, 444–446, 445f, 446f
Infarction(s), cerebral
lacune (small infarctions), 352
local and distant effects of, 235–236, 237f
nonhemorrhagic, 223–225, 223f, 224f, 225f

Interpetrous lucency in x-ray CT, 7, 8f
Intra-axial cerebellar tumors, imaging of, 396–397, 397f, 398–399t
Intrathecal contrast
agents, 18–21, 19f
clinical applications, 20, 21f
intrathecal air, 20–21f, 22f
pharmacology, 19–20, 19f
x-ray CT uses, 18–21
Intravenous contrast agents, 10–18, 11f, 12t
enhancement, 14–15
ionic versus nonionic, 14
therapy for reactions, 13–14
Iodine 123, as label, 129–130
Iohexol, 11f, 12t, 18, 19
Iopamidol, 11f, 12t, 18
Iothalamate, 11f
Ioversol, 11f, 12t
Ioxaglate (Hexabrix), 10, 11f, 12t
Ischemia
assessment of, 232–235, 233f, 234f, 235f
pathophysiology of, 217–219, 218f
Ischemic (microangiopathic) leukoencephalopathy
MRI studies, 356–362, 360f, 361f, 362f
pathoanatomy of, 351–353
Iterative computations in SPECT, 113

k (magnifying constant) in x-ray CT, 5
k-edge energy, 4
k-space in MRI, 54, 54f

Labeled compounds, production of, 74–79, 75t, 76f, 77f, 77t, 78t
Lacune (small infarction), types of, 352
Larmor frequencies, 41, 51, 52f
Larmor, Sir Joseph, 41
Lattice in MRI, 46
LCMRGlc. *See* Local cerebral metabolic rate for glucose
Lennox-Gastaut syndrome, 154–155, 442–444, 444f
Lesion detection contrast in x-ray CT, 6
Leucine compartment model, 100f
Levodopa studies, 262f, 263–265, 264f, 266–267f
Line spread function in PET, 85, 85f
Linear sampling distance in PET, 81
Local cerebral metabolic rate for glucose (LCMRGlc)
basics of, 97–98, 98f
selected major uses
brain development, 419–424, 421f, 422–423f
glioma studies, 179–191, 181–184f, 185t, 186t, 187–191f
Huntington's at-risk studies, 252–255, 253f, 254f, 255f
Parkinson's, 261–267, 262f, 264f, 266–267f
seizure states, 144t, 145–156
Localization-related epilepsy, 138–153
cerebral blood flow in, 144–145
cerebral metabolism in, 144–145, 144t

MRI studies, 138–144, 139f, 140f, 141f, 142f
PET ictal studies, 148–149, 151
PET interictal studies, 145–148, 145f, 146f, 147f, 148ff, 149f, 150f
SPECT studies, 151
x-ray CT studies, 138–144, 139f, 140f, 141f, 142f
Luxury perfusion, 232, 234f, 235f

Magnetic dipole moment in MRI, 40, 40f
Magnetic resonance angiography, 66, 67f, 168
Magnetic resonance imaging (MRI), 39–70
clinical applications, 434–436, 436f
Alzheimer's, 307–310, 308–309f, 310f
carotid artery disease, 236–239
cerebral hemorrhage, 219–223
cerebral infarction, 223–225, 224f, 238–239
cerebrovascular disorders, 329–331, 330f, 332f
Chiari malformations, 381f, 382–383
Dandy-Walker syndrome, 383
dystonia, 276, 277f
epilepsy, false localization of, 143–145, 143f
extraparenchymal cerebellar tumors, 402
Friedreich's ataxia, 375
gliomas, intracerebral, 176–177, 176f
hamartomas and arachnoid cysts, 432, 432f
hypoxic-ischemic encephalopathy of newborn, 438–441, 439ff
infantile spasms, 445
intra-axial cerbellar tumors, 396–397, 397f, 398–399t
intracerebral metastases and, 198–199
ischemic leukoencephalopathy, 356–362, 360f, 361f, 362f
multiple sclerosis, 354–356, 354–355f, 357f, 358f, 379–380, 380f
neurofibromatosis, 434, 435f
normal aging and cerebral change, 297–298, 298f, 299f
normal-pressure hydrocephalus, 22f, 334–336, 335f
olivopontocerebellar atrophy, 372, 373ff
Parkinson's, 257–260, 259f, 319, 320f
partial seizures, 138–144, 139f, 140f, 141f, 142f
pediatric metabolic diseases, 447–449, 448f, 449f
phakomatoses, 432–438
Pick's disease, 321, 322f
pituitary adenomas, 197
progressive supranuclear palsy, 270, 323, 324f
vascular malformations, 225–226, 226f, 227f
von Hippel-Lindau disease, 383, 385, 386f
Wilsons's disease, 274
contraindications to use, 23
contrast agents in, 64–66
future visions of
MR angiography, 458–460, 459f
MR spectroscopy, 461–462
nonproton MRI, 460
three-dimensional MRI, 460, 461f
image formation, 50–58
2D transformation, 51–53, 52f, 53f
image formation matrix, 53–54, 54f
magnetic field gradient, 50, 50f
multiecho pulse sequence, 55–56, 56f
multislice pulse sequence, 57, 57f
orthogonal scan plane, 53f, 57–58
pulse sequence timing diagram, 53, 53f
slice select gradient, 50, 51f
spatial resolution, 54–55, 55f
varying TE, effects of, 58
varying TR, effects of, 58
instrumentation, 58–64, 59t
air core resistive magnets, 60–61, 60f
gradient magnetic field generators, 63
hybrid magnet(s), 61, 61f, 62f
iron core resistive magnet(s), 61, 61f, 62f
main magnetic field, 58–63, 59t
permanent magnet(s), 58–61, 59ff, 60f
radiofrequency subsystem, 63–64, 65f
superconductive magnet(s), 61–63, 62f, 63f
physical principles, 39–50
contrast mechanisms, 47
nuclear magnetism, 40–41, 40f
nuclear resonance, 41–42, 41f, 42f, 43f
nucleus of the atom, 39–40, 40f
proton density, 47, 48f
pulsing sequence, 46–47
spin echo, 24
T_1 relaxation, 46, 46f
T_1 and T_2 contrast mechanisms, 47, 48t
T_1 and TR effects, 47–49, 49f, 49t
T_2 relaxation, 44f, 45–46
TE and T_2 effects, 49–50, 49f, 49t
T_2^* (exponential decay), 43–46, 46f
transverse magnetization, 43–45, 44f, 45f
surface coil MRI uses, 28, 30, 64
utility in neurologic studies, 66–69
strengths, 66–68, 67f, 68f
weaknesses, 68–69
Magnetic resonance spectroscopy (MRS)
clinical uses
cerebral infarction, 238–239
epilepsy, 155
ischemic states, 232
future visions of, 461–462
Magnetic susceptibility in MRI, 41
Magnetization vector in MRI, 42, 43f, 44f
Magnet(s) in MRI, 58–63
air core resistive, 59t, 60–61
iron core (hybrid) resistive, 59t, 60f, 61, 61f, 62f
permanent, 58–61, 59ff, 59t
superconductive, 59t, 61–63, 62f, 63f
Meningiomas
angiography of, 192, 193f
BBB imaging in, 194
PET metabolic studies, 194–195
SPECT studies, 194
x-ray CT studies, 192, 193f
Metabolism studies in
Alzheimer's, 308–309f, 310–319, 310f, 312–317f
brain
malformations, 424–425, 429–432, 436, 437f

normal development, 416–424, 421f, 422–423f
cerebellar degenerative diseases, 372–374, 374f, 375f, 376f, 377f, 380, 394
cerebrovascular disease, 218f, 227–236, 230f, 234f, 235f
degenerative dementias, 324–325
dystonia, 276–277
general seizures, 144t, 153–156, 154f
gliomas, 178–192, 181–184f, 185t, 186t, 187–190f
Huntington's disease, 250–256, 250f, 252f, 253f, 254f, 255f
hypoxic-ischemic encephalopathy of newborn, 441, 442f
intracerebral metastases, 199–200
meningiomas, 194–195
normal aging, cerebral change of, 298–300, 299f
normal pressure hydrocephalus, 335f, 336
Parkinson's disease, 261–267, 262f, 264f, 266–267f, 319, 320f
Pick's disease, 321–322, 322f
pituitary adenomas, 197–198
progressive supranuclear palsy, 270–272, 271f, 323–324, 324f
tardive dyskinesia, 278–279, 278f
vascular disorders, 331–333, 332f
Wilson's disease, 274–275, 275f
Metastases, intracerebral, 198–200
angiography, 198
BBB imaging, 199
imaging modalities, 198–200
Metrizamide (Amipaque), 10, 11f, 12t, 18
Microangiopathic leukoencephalopathy, 356–362, 360f, 361f, 362f
pathoanatomy of, 351–353, 353t
Modulation transfer function
PET and, 85, 85f
SPECT and, 110–111
Movement disorders, 244–293
background, 244–246
dystonia, 275–277
MRI studies, 276, 277f
PET studies, 276–277
x-ray CT studies, 276
future of imaging in, 251t, 279–281, 280t
Huntington's disease, 246–256
background, 246–247
dopaminergic neuron studies by PET, 251–252, 252f
future prospects of imaging in, 255–256
metabolic studies of at-risk subjects, 252–255, 253f, 254f, 255f
MRI studies, 248–249, 249f
PET studies, 250–256, 250f, 251t
pneumoencephalography and, 247–248, 247f
x-ray CT studies, 247–248, 248f, 249f, 250f
Parkinson's disease, 256–267
background, 256–257
fluorine-18-labeled levodopa studies, 262f, 263–265, 264f, 266–267f
future prospects of imaging, 267
MRI studies, 257–260, 259f, 320f
PET and SPECT studies, 260–267, 262f, 264ff, 266–267f, 319, 320f
x-ray CT studies, 257, 258f
progressive supranuclear palsy, 267–272
background, 267, 269–70, 269f
MRI studies, 270, 324f
PET studies, 270–272, 271f, 324f
pneumoencephalographic studies, 269, 269f
x-ray CT studies, 270
tardive dyskinesia, 277–279, 278f
Wilson's disease, 272–275
background, 272–273
MRI studies, 274
PET and SPECT studies, 274–275, 275f
Multiecho technique in MRI, 56, 56f
Multi-infarct cognitive disorders, 325–328
Multi-infarct dementia, 325–333
Hachinski Ischemic Score and, 327
MRI studies, 329–331, 330f, 332f
PET studies, 330f, 331–332, 332f
SPECT studies, 332–333
x-ray CT studies, 327–328
Multiple sclerosis and variants, 350–351, 354–356, 378–380
MRI studies, 354–356, 354–355f, 357f, 358f, 379–380, 380f
pathoanatomy, 350–351
PET studies, 380
x-ray CT studies, 379

National Council on Radiation Protection, 79
Neoplastic disorders, intracerebral, 166–216, 167t
BBB defects, imaging of, 178–179, 180f
gliomas, 167t, 171–192
angiography and, 172, 172f
BBB defects imaging in, 178–179, 180f
MRI studies, 176–177, 176f
PET studies of amino acid uptake, 187, 191 blood flow, 181–184f, 185t, 186, 187–190f metabolism, 179–186, 181–184f, 185t other areas, 191–192 pH, 186–187
SPECT studies, 177–179, 178f
x-ray CT studies, 172–176, 173f, 174f, 175f
meningiomas, 192–195
angiography, 192, 193f
BBB imaging of, 194
PET metabolic studies, 194–195
SPECT studies, 194
x-ray CT studies, 192, 193f
metastases, 198–200
angiography, 198
BBB imaging, 199
imaging modalities, 198–200
MRA and, 168
neuroimaging evaluation of, 168–171, 169f
other CNS tumors, 200
pituitary adenomas, 195–198, 196f
angiography, 195
MRI studies, 197
PET studies, 197–198
SPECT studies, 197
x-ray CT studies, 195, 197

Neoplastic disorders, intracerebral—*Continued*
radiation necrosis versus recurrence, 203–204, 204f, 205f
remote effects of, 174f, 187–190, 190f, 200–201, 200f, 201f
treatment response, imaging of, 201–203, 202f, 203f
Net magnetic field vector in MRI, 41
Net magnetization in MRI, 42
Neurochemical systems, definitions in PET, 74f, 99–101, 100f, 101f
Neurofibromatosis, imaging of, 434, 435f
Neuroreceptor studies in Parkinson's disease, 265–267, 266f
Neurotransmitter labeling, 99–101, 100f, 129–130
Noise
in PET, 86–87, 87f
in SPECT, 113–114, 113f, 114t
Nonionic contrast agents in x-ray CT, 10
Nonorthogonal imaging in MRI, 64
Normal aging and cerebral change, 297–300
MRI studies, 297–298, 298f, 299f
neurophysiologic studies, 325
PET and SPECT
atrophy correction, 300
studies of, 298–300
x-ray CT studies, 297
Normal-pressure hydrocephalus, 328, 333–336
MRI studies, 22f, 334–336, 335f
PET and SPECT studies, 335f, 336
x-ray CT studies, 334
Nuclear magnetic resonance in MRI, 39–40
Nuclear reaction(s)
basic description, 73–76, 77t
nomenclature, 76
Nucleons in MRI, 39

Olivopontocerebellar atrophy
background, 371–372
PET studies, 372, 374, 374f
x-ray CT studies, 372
Orbit, x-ray CT examination, 26–28, 27f
Otic capsule, x-ray CT examination, 28

Paramagnetic substances, 41
Paraneoplastic cerebellar degeneration, 377–378, 378f, 379f
Parkinson's disease
features, 256–257
fluorine-18-labeled levodopa studies, 262f, 263–265, 264f, 266–267f
levodopa, effects of, 263
MRI studies, 319
PET and SPECT studies, 260–267, 262f, 264ff, 266–267f, 319, 320f
x-ray CT studies, 318–319
Partial seizures, 138–153
cerebral blood flow, 144–145
cerebral metabolism, 144–145, 144t
localization by imaging, 151–152
MRI studies, 138–144, 139f, 140f, 141f, 142f
PET studies
ictal studies, 148–149, 151
interictal studies, 145–148, 145f, 146f, 147f, 148ff, 149f, 150f
presurgical studies, 152–153, 152t
x-ray CT studies, 138–144, 139f, 140f, 141f, 142f
Partial-volume effects in x-ray CT, 7–8
Partition coefficient in PET, 92–93
Pediatric disorders, 411–450
brain, malformations of, 424–432
background, 424, 425t
cerebral, 425–432 functional imaging, 428f, 429–432 structural imaging, 425–429, 425t, 426f, 427f, 428f, 429f, 430ff, 431f
functional imaging, 424–425
hamartomas and arachnoid cysts, 432, 432f
phakomatoses
Sturge-Weber syndrome. *See* Sturge-Weber syndrome
tuberous sclerosis, 432–434, 433f
structural imaging by MRI, 424
brain, normal development of, 411–424
background, 411–412
functional imaging, 416–424
ethical considerations, 417–419
PET studies, 419–424, 421f, 422–423f
structural imaging by MRI, 412–416
gray-white differentiation, 413f, 415f, 416f, 417f, 418f
myelination, 414–416, 415f, 416f, 417f, 418f, 419f, 419t
epilepsy, childhood, 442–446
infantile spasms, 155, 444–446
background, 444–446
correlations, 446
functional imaging, 445–446, 445f, 446f
structural imaging, 445
Lennox-Gastaut syndrome, 442–444
correlations, 443
functional imaging by PET, 443, 444f
structural imaging by x-ray CT, 443
hypoxic-ischemic encephalopathy of newborn
background, 438
correlations, 441–442
functional imaging by PET, 441, 442f
structural imaging, 438–441
MRI studies, 438–441, 439ff, 440f
ultrasonographic studies, 438
x-ray CT studies, 438–440, 441f
metabolic diseases, 447–449
background, 447
structural imaging
MRI studies, 447–448, 448f, 449f
x-ray CT, 447
practical considerations, 449–450
Perfusion, cerebral
assessment by x-ray CT, 18
versus blood flow, 94
PET. See Positron emission tomography.
pH of gliomas, PET studies, 186–187
Phakomatoses, imaging of, 432–438
Photoelectric effect, 3–4
Photomultiplier tubes in SPECT, 110

Pick's disease
  MRI studies, 321, 322f
  PET studies, 321, 322f
  SPECT studies, 321–322
  x-ray CT studies, 321, 322f
Pituitary adenomas, imaging of, 195–198, 196f
Pneumoencephalography
  Huntington's disease and, 247–248, 247f
  progressive supranuclear palsy and, 269, 269f
Point spread function in SPECT, 110
Positron emission tomography (PET), 71–107
  angular coupling intervals in, 81
  basic description of, 71–73, 72f
  behavioral activation states in, 96, 96f
  blurring tomography in, 80f, 81
  central volume principle in, 95
  clearance technique in, 84t, 95–97, 96f
  clinical applications
    Alzheimer's, 308–309f, 310–318, 312–317t
    cerebellar alcoholic degeneration, 393–394, 395f
    cerebral blood flow, 84t, 94–97, 95f, 96f
    cerebral blood volume, 97, 98f
    cerebral infarction, 235–236, 238–239
    cerebrovascular disorders, 330f, 331–332, 332f
    dystonia, 276–277
    epilepsy, 144t, 155–156
    Friedreich's ataxia, 375–376, 376f, 377f
    gliomas
      blood flow studies, 181–184f, 185t, 186, 186t, 187–190f
      metabolism studies, 179–186, 181–184f, 185t
    Huntington's disease, 250–256, 250f, 251t, 252f, 253f, 254f, 255f
    hypoxic-ischemic encephalopathy of newborn, 441, 442f
    infantile spasms, 445–446, 445f, 446f
    intracerebral metastases, 199–200
    intracranial neoplasms, 170–171
    ischemic states, 232–235, 233f, 234f, 235f
    Lennox-Gastaut syndrome, 443, 444f
    meningiomas, 194–195
    multiple sclerosis, 380
    normal aging and cerebral change, 298–300
    normal-pressure hydrocephalus, 335f, 336
    olivopontocerebellar atrophy, 372, 374, 374f
    Parkinson's, 262f, 263–265, 319, 320f
    partial seizures, 152–153, 152t
    Pick's disease, 321, 322f
    pituitary adenomas, 197–198
    preischemic states, 229–232, 230ff
    progressive supranuclear palsy, 270–272, 271f, 323–324, 324f
    protein synthesis, 98–99, 99f, 100f
    Sturge-Weber syndrome, 436, 437ff
    tardive dyskinesia, 278–279, 278f
    Wilson's disease, 274–275, 275f
  collimation in, 83f
  computed tomography, principle of, 71–72, 72f, 79–81, 80f, 81f
  cutoff frequency in, 81, 81f, 82f
  dead time in, 89
  detector materials in, 83–85, 84t
  dilution principle in, 92
  epilepsy, neuropharmacology of, 144t, 155–156
  equilibrium models in, 94, 97
  first-order processes in, 93
  full width at half maximum in, 82f, 85, 85f, 86f
  future visions of, 462–464
    animal studies, 464
    clinical considerations, 464–465
    new ligands and probes, 462–463
    rehabilitation after brain injury, 463–464
    uses in presymptomatic individuals, 463
  labeled compounds in, 72, 76–78, 77t, 78f, 78t, 79f
    cyclotron and, 74, 76, 76f
    dosimetry, 78–79, 79f
    production of, 74–79
  line spread function in, 85, 85f
  linear sampling distance in, 81
  modulation transfer function in, 85, 85f
  neurochemical systems, 74f, 99–101, 100f, 101f
  neuropharmacology of epilepsy, 144t, 155–156
  neuroreceptor studies in Parkinson's, 265–267
  partition coefficient in, 92–93
  positron decay, 73–74, 73f, 74f, 75t
  primary objective of, 93
  random incidence in, 74f, 83
  recovery coefficient in, 88, 99t
  resolution in, 87, 87f
  scanners, 79–89
    annihilation coincidence detection, 74f, 82–83, 83f, 84f
    axial resolution and sampling, 89
    detectors and geometric configuration, 83–85, 84t
    efficiency and temporal resolution, 89
    partial volume effect, 87–89, 88f, 90t
    sampling requirements, 81–82, 82f
    spatial resolution, 85–86, 85f, 86f
    statistical noise, 86–87, 87ff
  signal amplification in, 82f
  single photon imaging in, 83f
  statistical resolution in, 86, 87f
  tracer kinetic modeling, 89–101
    analog tracer(s), 91
    blood flow and perfusion, 94
    cerebral blood flow, 84t, 94–97, 95f, 96f
    compartmental models, 91–92, 92f
    deoxyglucose model, 97–98, 98f
    distribution volume and partition coefficient, 92–93
    flux, 92f, 93
    neurochemical systems and, 74f, 99–101, 100f, 101f
    protein synthesis, 98–99, 99f, 100f
    rate constants, 92f, 93
    steady state, 93–94, 94f
  tracer(s) in, 78f, 91
  true coincidence in, 74f, 83, 89
Positron-emitting radioisotopes, 72–74, 75t
Positronium, 73

Positron(s), definition and description, 73–74, 73f
Precession of nucleus in MRI, 39
Precession of protons, 41–42, 41f, 42f
Precessional frequency in MRI, 42
Progressive supranuclear palsy
  background, 267, 269–70, 269f
  MRI studies, 270, 323, 324f
  PET studies, 270–272, 271f, 323–324, 324f
  pneumoencephalographic studies, 269, 269f
  SPECT studies, 324
  x-ray CT studies, 323
Protein synthesis studies, 98–99, 99f, 100f
Proton(s)
  density, 47, 48f
  excited state of, 41
  ground state of, 41
  precession of, 41–42, 41f, 42f

Quality factor in MRI, 63
Quenching in MRI, 62–63

Radiation dosage in x-ray CT, 9–10
Radiation necrosis versus recurrent tumors, 203–204, 204f, 205f
Radiofrequency coil subsystem in MRI, 42, 63–64, 65f
Radioisotopes
  PET use, 74–79, 75t, 77t, 78tt, 79t, 171
    cyclotron and, 74, 76, 76f
    dosimetry, 78–79, 79t
    production of, 74–79
  positron-emitting, 74–79, 75t, 78tt, 77t, 79t
  SPECT uses, 115–119, 118tt
Rads (the units), 79
Random incidence in PET, 74f, 83
Rate constants in PET, 92f, 93
Reactions, contrast induced, 10–14
  therapy for, 13–14
Readout gradient in MRI, 54
Receptor ligand labeling, 99–101, 100f, 129–130
Recoil electron, 3
Recovery coefficient in PET, 88, 99t
Repetition time in MRI, 46
Resolution
  PET and, 86–87, 87f
  SPECT and, 110, 113–114, 113f, 114t
  x-ray CT and, 9
Resolution volume in computed tomography, 87–88, 88f
Resonance frequency in MRI, 41
Ring artifact in x-ray CT, 9

Scanner geometry in x-ray CT, 9
Scans, single versus multiple in x-ray CT, 9–10
Scatter, 3, 4
  SPECT and, 111, 111f, 112–113, 112f
Scintillation-photomultiplier tube, x-ray CT, 5
Sensitivity in SPECT, 101, 105, 110, 113f, 114, 114t
Sequential plane in MRI, 50
Signal amplification in PET, 82f
Signal to noise ratio in MRI, 49
Single photon emission computerized tomography (SPECT), 108–130
  attenuation in, 111–112, 111f
  camera-based systems in, 114, 115f
  clinical applications
    Alzheimer's, 125–127, 126f, 128–129f, 318
    carotid occlusion, 121, 124f
    cerebral blood flow, 119–129, 126f, 127f, 128–129f, 130f
    cerebral infarction, 235–236, 237f
    cerebrovascular disorders, 125, 127f, 332–333
    gliomas, 177–179, 178f
    intracerebral metastases, 199
    intracranial neoplasms, 170–171
    meningiomas, 194
    migraine, 121, 123
    normal aging and cerebral change, 298–300
    normal-pressure hydrocephalus, 335f, 336
    Parkinson's disease, 263, 319
    partial seizures, 151, 152–153, 152t
    Pick's disease, 321–322
    pituitary adenomas, 197
    progressive supranuclear palsy, 324
    subarachnoid hemorrhage, 121
    temporal lobe epilepsy, 127, 129, 130f
    Wilson's disease, 274–275
  collimation in, 110, 113f
  contrast in, 110–111
  dedicated systems in, 114–115, 116t, 117f
  dynamic studies, 109
  emission CT defined, 108–109
  future visions of
    improved spatial resolution, 465
    new choices in ligands, 465
  imaging systems, 109–115, 109f
  iterative computations in, 113
  modular transfer function in, 110–111
  noise in, 113–114, 113f, 114t
  photomultiplier tubes in, 110
  radioisotopes used in, 115–119, 118tt
  receptor ligands labeling, 129–130
  resolution in, 110, 113–114, 113f, 114t
  scatter in, 111, 111f, 112–113, 112f
  sensitivity in, 101, 105, 110, 113f, 114, 114t
  static studies, 109
  technetium 99m-HMPAO, 123–129, 126f, 127f, 128–129f, 130f
  xenon, 119–123, 120f, 122–123f, 124f, 133
Single photon imaging in PET, 83f
Skull, x-ray CT examination, 31–32
Slice select gradient in MRI, 50, 51f, 54, 57
Soft x-rays in x-ray CT, 7
Solenoid radiofrequency coil(s), 60
Solenoidal-design magnet(s) in MRI, 60–61, 60f
Solid-state scintillation detectors in x-ray CT, 5, 9
Spatial resolution in x-ray CT, 9
SPECT. See Single photon emission computerized tomography
Spin density images in MRI, 48f, 50
Spin echo in MRI, 24, 45
Spine
  alogrithms for evaluation of, 29f
  x-ray CT examination, 28–31, 29f, 31f

Spin-spin relaxation time in MRI, 44f, 45–46
Star pattern in x-ray CT, 8–9, 8f
Static magnetic field strength in MRI, 42, 58
Statistical resolution in PET, 86–87, 87f
Steady state in PET, 92, 93–94
Sturge-Weber syndrome, 434–438
  background, 434
  correlations, 436–438
  MRI studies, 434–436, 436f
  PET studies, 436, 437ff
  x-ray CT studies, 432–434, 433f
Subcortical arteriosclerotic encephalopathy, 328
Surface coil MRI uses, 28, 30, 64

T_1, in MRI, 48
  contrast, 48
  and T_2 contrast mechanisms, 47, 48t
  and TR effects, 47–49, 49f, 49t
  -weighted image, 47–49, 49t
T_2* (exponential decay) in MRI, 43–46, 44f
Tardive dyskinesia, 277–279, 278f
TE and T2 effects, 49–50, 49f, 49t
Technetium 99m-HMPAO, 118, 188tt
  cerebral blood flow measurement, 123–129, 126f, 127f, 128–129f, 130f
    Alzheimer's disease, 125–127, 128–129f
    CVD, 127, 127f
    normal values, 125, 126f, 127f
    temporal lobe epilepsy, 127, 129, 130f
Temporal lobe epilepsy, 127, 129, 130f
Tesla in MRI, 41
Time-density curves in x-ray CT, 17–18
Tip angle in MRI, 42
Tracer kinetic assay method in PET, 71–73, 72f
Tracer(s) in PET, 78f, 91
Transient ischemic attacks, 24f, 385–387
Transverse magnetization, 43–45, 44f, 45f
True coincidence in PET, 74f, 83, 89
Tuberous sclerosis, 432–434, 433f
Tumors. *See* Cerebellum, disorders of, neoplasms; Neoplastic disorders
Tumors, recurrent, versus radiation necrosis, 203–204, 204f, 205f

Vacuum cryostat (Dewar) in MRI, 62
Vascular malformations
  cerbellar, 390–392, 391f
  structural imaging of, 225–226, 226f, 227f
View in MRI, 54
Volume imaging in MRI, 50
von Hippel-Lindau disease, 383, 385, 386f
Voxel size
  PET and, 90t
  x-ray CT and, 9

White matter disease, adult, 350–367
  differential diagnosis, 362–367, 363t, 363–364t, 365f, 366f
  MRI studies, 353–362
    ischemic leukoencephalopathy, 356–362, 360f, 361tt, 362f
    multiple sclerosis and variants, 354–356, 354–355F, 357f, 358f
    technique, 353–354
  pathoanatomy, 350–355
    microangiopathic leukoencephalopathy, 351–353, 353t
      atrophic perivascular demyelinization, 352
      encephalitis subcorticalis chronica progressiva, 352
      État criblé, 352
      État lacunaire, 352
      lacune, types of, 352
    multiple sclerosis and variants, 350–351
Wilson's disease, 272–275
  features, 272–273
  MRI and, 274
  x-ray CT and, 273–274

Xenon, stable, 21–22
Xenon 133, 119–123, 120f, 122–123f, 124f
X-ray computed tomography (x-ray CT), 3–38
  artifacts, 7–9, 8f
  clinical applications, 23–32
    Alzheimer's disease, 300–307, 301–305t
    brain examination, 23–26, 24f, 25f, 26f
    carotid artery disease, 236–239
    cerebellopontine schwannoma, 29f, 400–401f, 402–403, 403f, 404f
    cerebellum
      alcoholic degeneration of, 392–393, 394f
      extraparenchymal tumors, 400–401f, 402
      hemorrhages of, 387–389, 389f
      intra-axial tumors, 396–397, 397f, 398–399t
    cerebrovascular disorders, 328–329
    cerebrum
      hemorrhages of, 219, 221, 222–223, 222t
      infarcts of, 223–224, 223f, 225f, 238–239
    Chiari malformations, 382
    Dandy-Walker syndrome, 383, 384–385f
    dystonia, 276
    epilepsy, false localization, 143–145, 143f
    Friedreich's ataxia, 375, 376
    gliomas, intracerebral, 172–176, 173f, 174f, 175f
    hamartomas and arachnoid cysts, 432, 432f
    Huntington's disease, 247–248
    hypoxic-ischemic encephalopathy of newborn, 438–440, 441f
    infantile spasms, 445
    intracranial neoplasms, 168–169
    Lennox-Gastaut syndrome, 442–444
    metastases, intracerebral, 198, 198f
    multi-infarct dementia, 327–328
    multiple sclerosis, 379
    neurofibromatosis, 434, 435f
    normal aging and cerebral change, 297
    normal-pressure hydrocephalus, 334
    olivopontocerebellar atrophy, 372
    orbit examination, 26–28, 27f
    otic capsule examination, 28
    Parkinson's disease, 257, 258f, 318–319
    partial seizures, 138–144, 139f, 140f, 141f, 142f
    pediatric metabolic diseases, 447
    phaktomatoses, 432–434, 433f
    Pick's disease, 321, 322f

X-ray computed tomography—*Continued*
pituitary adenomas, 195, 197
progressive supranuclear palsy, 270, 323
skull examination, 31–32
spine examination, 28–31, 29f, 31f
Sturge-Weber syndrome, 434–436
transient ischemic attacks, 24f, 385–387
tuberous sclerosis, 432–434, 433f
von Hippel-Lindau disease, 383, 385
Wilson's disease, 273–274
dosimetry, 9–10
future of, 32
image formation, 4–7, 5t, 6–7f
intrathecal contrast, 18–22
clinical applications, 20, 21f
intrathecal air, 20–21, 22f
pharmacology, 19–20, 19f
intravenous contrast
delayed high-dose, 16, 17f
dynamic scanning, 17–18
enhancement of, 14–15
high-dose applications, 16
routine applications, 15–16
physical principles, 3–4, 4f
xenon in, 21–22